VOLUME SEVENTY ONE

ADVANCES IN PHARMACOLOGY

VOLUME SEVENTY ONE

ADVANCES IN PHARMACOLOGY

Pharmacology of the Blood Brain Barrier: Targeting CNS Disorders

Edited by

THOMAS P. DAVIS

Department of Pharmacology,
College of Medicine, University of Arizona,
Tucson, Arizona, USA

Serial Editor

S. J. ENNA

Department of Molecular and Integrative Physiology,
Department of Pharmacology, Toxicology and Therapeutics,
University of Kansas Medical Center, Kansas City,
Kansas, USA

Managing Editor

LYNN LECOUNT

University of Kansas Medical Center
School of Medicine, Kansas City, Kansas, USA

ELSEVIER

AMSTERDAM • BOSTON • HEIDELBERG • LONDON
NEW YORK • OXFORD • PARIS • SAN DIEGO
SAN FRANCISCO • SINGAPORE • SYDNEY • TOKYO
Academic Press is an imprint of Elsevier

Academic Press is an imprint of Elsevier
32 Jamestown Road, London NW1 7BY, UK
525 B Street, Suite 1800, San Diego, CA 92101-4495, USA
225 Wyman Street, Waltham, MA 02451, USA
The Boulevard, Langford Lane, Kidlington, Oxford OX5 1GB, UK

First edition 2014

ISBN: 978-0-12-800282-7
ISSN: 1054-3589

For information on all Academic Press publications
visit our website at http://store.elsevier.com/

CONTENTS

PREFACE

The field of blood–brain barrier (BBB) pharmacology is a relatively new area. We owe our start to the seminal work of Reese and Karnovsky in 1967, whom answered an ongoing controversy, first observed by Paul Ehrlich in 1885, that the BBB lies principally at the endothelium of cerebral capillary endothelial cells. Soon after in 1969, Brightman and Reese showed key ultrastructural evidence of protein tight junctions that function to block paracellular delivery of almost all solutes to the brain primarily due to high transendothelial cell resistance. In 2002, leaders at the National Institute of Neurological Disorders and Stroke formed a Stroke Progress Review Group (SPRG), which recognized the urgency to determine the role of the BBB in stroke. This SPRG identified the priority to "better define the molecular influences and cell-signaling mechanisms that characterize the interaction between circulating blood elements and the blood vessel wall, the extracellular matrix, glia and neurons (together, the neurovascular unit)…." (NVU). The BBB and NVU remain the most significant challenge to central nervous system (CNS) drug development from the past century. This fact drives the passion of our students and colleagues. We understand that progress in preventing, diagnosing, or treating diseases of the CNS depends upon understanding the BBB and NVU. It is often stated, "if we cannot get the drug into the brain we cannot treat a disease of the brain."

Presented in this timely volume are three sections of seminal contributions from outstanding, internationally acclaimed experts describing (1) BBB/NVU protein, ion, and receptor-mediated transporters that can be pharmacologically targeted to improve/modulate CNS drug delivery; (2) world-class experts' focus on specific targeting of CNS disorders associated with stroke, inflammation, ischemia, cancer, human African trypanosomiasis sleeping sickness, and two exciting chapters by established experts describing recent advances in engineering proteins, peptides, and antibodies to treat CNS disorders; and (3) a special innovative section on the challenges of treating complex comorbidities such as hyperglycemia/diabetes/hemorrhagic transformation/stroke; aging/metabolic syndrome/ischemic stroke; and drug abuse-induced CNS disorders.

I wish to thank each one of my valued colleagues for making this volume possible. What links each of these authors together is a strong allegiance to their chosen field that is interactive, collegial and focused on excellence. In short, we are a "tight group" of friends as well. As BBB/NVU investigators we have a unique perspective, and responsibility, to address a critical priority; that after a century of developing and testing CNS therapeutics, pharmaceutical and biotech companies remain frustrated at the enormity of problems associated with delivering drugs to the CNS. It is my hope that this volume is a source of inspiration, drug development strategy, and ideas that result in improved CNS drug development and delivery. If the chapters in this volume attain these goals and aid patient outcome, it is a success.

Thomas P. Davis
Department of Pharmacology,
College of Medicine, University of Arizona,
Tucson, Arizona, USA

CONTRIBUTORS

Thomas Abbruscato
Department of Pharmaceutical Sciences, School of Pharmacy, Texas Tech University Health Sciences Center, Amarillo, Texas, USA

Tamima Ashraf
Department of Pharmaceutical Sciences, Leslie Dan Faculty of Pharmacy, University of Toronto, Toronto, Ontario, Canada

William A. Banks
Geriatric Research Educational and Clinical Center, Veterans Affairs Puget Sound Health Care System, and Department of Medicine, Division of Gerontology and Geriatric Medicine, University of Washington, Seattle, Washington, USA

David J. Begley
King's College London, Institute of Pharmaceutical Science, London, United Kingdom

Reina Bendayan
Department of Pharmaceutical Sciences, Leslie Dan Faculty of Pharmacy, University of Toronto, Toronto, Ontario, Canada

Aliana Y. Culp
Department of Neurology, Oregon Health and Science University, Portland, Oregon, USA

Thomas P. Davis
Department of Pharmacology, College of Medicine, University of Arizona, Tucson, Arizona, USA

Nancy D. Doolittle
Department of Neurology, Oregon Health and Science University, Portland, Oregon, USA

Richard D. Egleton
Department of Pharmacology, Physiology and Toxicology, Joan C. Edwards School of Medicine, Marshall University, Huntington, West Virginia, USA

Xiang Fan
Neuroprotection Research Laboratory, Department of Neurology and Radiology, Massachusetts General Hospital, Neuroscience Program, Harvard Medical School, Boston, Massachusetts, USA

Graham K. Farrington
Biogen Idec Inc., 12 Cambridge Center, Cambridge, Massachusetts, USA

Mehmet Fidanboylu
King's College London, Institute of Pharmaceutical Sciences, London, United Kingdom

Arsalan S. Haqqani
Human Health Therapeutics Portfolio, National Research Council of Canada, Ottawa, Ontario, Canada

Ken-ichi Hosoya
Department of Pharmaceutics, Graduate School of Pharmaceutical Sciences, University of Toyama, Toyama, Japan

Jason D. Huber
The Center for Neuroscience, School of Medicine, and Department of Basic Pharmaceutical Sciences, West Virginia University, School of Pharmacy, Morgantown, West Virginia, USA

Yinghua Jiang
Neuroprotection Research Laboratory, Department of Neurology and Radiology, Massachusetts General Hospital, Neuroscience Program, Harvard Medical School, Boston, Massachusetts, USA, and Department of Neurosurgery, The First Affiliated Hospital, Chongqing Medical University, Chongqing, PR China

N. Joan Abbott
King's College London, Institute of Pharmaceutical Science, London, United Kingdom

Amy Kao
Department of Pharmaceutical Sciences, Leslie Dan Faculty of Pharmacy, University of Toronto, Toronto, Ontario, Canada

Kristin Kemmerich
Human Health Therapeutics Portfolio, National Research Council of Canada, Ottawa, Ontario, Canada

Eng H. Lo
Neuroprotection Research Laboratory, Department of Neurology and Radiology, Massachusetts General Hospital, Neuroscience Program, Harvard Medical School, Boston, Massachusetts, USA

Aric F. Logsdon
The Center for Neuroscience, School of Medicine, and Department of Basic Pharmaceutical Sciences, West Virginia University, School of Pharmacy, Morgantown, West Virginia, USA

Brandon P. Lucke-Wold
Department of Neurosurgery, and The Center for Neuroscience, West Virginia University, School of Medicine, Morgantown, West Virginia, USA

David S. Miller
Laboratory of Toxicology and Pharmacology, National Institute of Environmental Health Sciences, National Institutes of Health, Research Triangle Park, North Carolina, USA

Leslie L. Muldoon
Department of Neurology, and Department of Cell and Developmental Biology, Oregon Health and Science University, Portland, Oregon, USA

Edward A. Neuwelt
Department of Neurology; Department of Neurosurgery, Oregon Health and Science University, and Office of Research and Development, Department of Veterans Affairs Medical Center, Portland, Oregon, USA

Martha E. O'Donnell
Department of Physiology and Membrane Biology, School of Medicine, University of California, Davis, California, USA

Jane E. Preston
King's College London, Institute of Pharmaceutical Science, London, United Kingdom

Patrick T. Ronaldson
Department of Pharmacology, University of Arizona College of Medicine, Tucson, Arizona, USA

Charles L. Rosen
Department of Neurosurgery, and The Center for Neuroscience, West Virginia University, School of Medicine, Morgantown, West Virginia, USA

Therese S. Salameh
Geriatric Research Educational and Clinical Center, Veterans Affairs Puget Sound Health Care System, and Department of Medicine, Division of Gerontology and Geriatric Medicine, University of Washington, Seattle, Washington, USA

Lucy Sanchez-Covarubias
Department of Pharmacology, College of Medicine, University of Arizona, Tucson, Arizona, USA

Lisa Sanderson
King's College London, Institute of Pharmaceutical Sciences, London, United Kingdom

Karin E. Sandoval
Pharmaceutical Sciences, School of Pharmacy, Southern Illinois University, Edwardsville, Illinois, USA

Gayathri N. Sekhar
King's College London, Institute of Pharmaceutical Sciences, London, United Kingdom

Danica Stanimirovic
Human Health Therapeutics Portfolio, National Research Council of Canada, Ottawa, Ontario, Canada

Xiaochuan Sun
Neuroprotection Research Laboratory, Department of Neurology and Radiology, Massachusetts General Hospital, Neuroscience Program, Harvard Medical School, Boston, Massachusetts, USA, and Department of Neurosurgery, The First Affiliated Hospital, Chongqing Medical University, Chongqing, PR China

Masanori Tachikawa
Division of Membrane Transport and Drug Targeting, Graduate School of Pharmaceutical Sciences, Tohoku University, Sendai, Japan

Tetsuya Terasaki
Division of Membrane Transport and Drug Targeting, Graduate School of Pharmaceutical Sciences, Tohoku University, Sendai, Japan

Sarah A. Thomas
King's College London, Institute of Pharmaceutical Sciences, London, United Kingdom

Brandon J. Thompson
Department of Physiology, University of Arizona College of Medicine, Tucson, Arizona, USA

Margaret E. Tome
Department of Pharmacology, College of Medicine, University of Arizona, Tucson, Arizona, USA

Ryan C. Turner
Department of Neurosurgery, and The Center for Neuroscience, West Virginia University, School of Medicine, Morgantown, West Virginia, USA

Xiaoying Wang
Neuroprotection Research Laboratory, Department of Neurology and Radiology, Massachusetts General Hospital, Neuroscience Program, Harvard Medical School, Boston, Massachusetts, USA

Christopher P. Watson
King's College London, Institute of Pharmaceutical Sciences, London, United Kingdom

Ken A. Witt
Pharmaceutical Sciences, School of Pharmacy, Southern Illinois University, Edwardsville, Illinois, USA

Shuanglin Xiang
Neuroprotection Research Laboratory, Department of Neurology and Radiology, Massachusetts General Hospital, Neuroscience Program, Harvard Medical School, Boston, Massachusetts, USA, and Key Laboratory of Protein Chemistry and Developmental Biology of State Education Ministry of China, College of Life Sciences, Hunan Normal University, Changsha, Hunan, PR China

Zhanyang Yu
Neuroprotection Research Laboratory, Department of Neurology and Radiology, Massachusetts General Hospital, Neuroscience Program, Harvard Medical School, Boston, Massachusetts, USA

Jing Yuan
Neuroprotection Research Laboratory, Department of Neurology and Radiology, Massachusetts General Hospital, Neuroscience Program, Harvard Medical School, Boston, Massachusetts, USA, and Key Laboratory of Protein Chemistry and Developmental Biology of State Education Ministry of China, College of Life Sciences, Hunan Normal University, Changsha, Hunan, PR China

CHAPTER ONE

ABC Transporter Regulation by Signaling at the Blood–Brain Barrier: Relevance to Pharmacology

David S. Miller[1]

Laboratory of Toxicology and Pharmacology, National Institute of Environmental Health Sciences, National Institutes of Health, Research Triangle Park, North Carolina, USA

[1]Corresponding author: e-mail address: miller@niehs.nih.gov

Contents

Abstract

Brain capillary endothelial cells express multiple ATP-binding cassette transport proteins on the luminal, blood-facing, plasma membrane. There these transporters function as ATP-driven efflux pumps for xenobiotics and endogenous metabolites, providing an important element of the barrier. When the transporters limit neurotoxicant entry into the central nervous system (CNS), they are neuroprotective; when they limit therapeutic drug entry, they are obstacles to drug delivery to treat CNS diseases. Certainly, changes in the transporter expression and transport activity can have a profound effect on CNS pharmacotherapy, with increased transport activity reducing drug access to the brain and vice versa. Here, I review the signals that alter transporter expression and transport function with an emphasis on P-glycoprotein, MRP2, and breast cancer resistance protein (ABCG2) (BCRP), the efflux transporters for which we have the most detailed picture of regulation. Recent work shows that transporter protein expression can be upregulated in response to inflammatory and oxidative stress, therapeutic drugs, diet, and persistent environmental pollutants; as a consequence, drug delivery to the brain is reduced. For many of these stimuli, the transcription factor, nuclear factor kappa-light-chain-enhancer of activated B cells (NF-κB), appears to be involved. However,

Advances in Pharmacology, Volume 71
ISSN 1054-3589
http://dx.doi.org/10.1016/bs.apha.2014.06.008

NF-κB activation and nuclear translocation is often initiated by upstream signaling. In contrast, basal transport activity of P-glycoprotein and BCRP can be reduced through complex signaling pathways. Targeting such signals provides opportunities to rapidly and reversibly increase brain accumulation of drugs that are transporter substrates. The extent to which such signaling-based strategies can be utilized in the clinic remains to be seen.

ABBREVIATIONS

ABC ATP-binding cassette
AEDs antiepileptic drugs
AhR arylhydrocarbon receptor
Akt protein kinase B
BCRP breast cancer resistance protein (ABCG2)
CAR constitutive androstane receptor
CNS central nervous system
COX-2 cyclooxygenase-2
E2 17-β-estradiol
EP-1 prostaglandin E2 receptor
ER estrogen receptor
ET-1 endothelin-1
GR glucocorticoid receptor
GSK-3β glycogen synthase kinase 3 beta
iNOS inducible nitric oxide synthase
MRP multidrug resistance-associated protein (ABCC subfamily)
NF-κB nuclear factor kappa-light-chain-enhancer of activated B cells
NMDA *N*-methyl-D-aspartate
Nrf2 nuclear factor (erythroid-derived 2)-like 2
PI3-K phosphatidylinositide 3-kinase
PKCβ1 protein kinase C isoform β1
PTEN phosphatase and tensin homolog
PXR pregnane X receptor
S1P sphingosine-1-phosphate
S1PR1 sphingosine-1-phosphate receptor 1
TNF-α tumor necrosis factor-α
VDR vitamin D receptor
VEGF vascular endothelial growth factor

1. INTRODUCTION

Biological signaling refers to the transfer of information within organisms, tissues, and cells and over the dimensions of space and time. In essence, this flow of information allows the various parts of multicellular organisms and cells to communicate with each other and be aware of alterations in their extracellular and intracellular microenvironment so that they can respond appropriately and preserve homeostasis. In general, cells sense changes in their external environment as altered levels of nutrients, toxicants, stressors, and signaling molecules that might be receptor ligands or hormones. Cells then change the form of the message and respond by altered cellular function, e.g., altered pattern of gene expression, activation or inhibition of metabolism, release of additional signals. On the one hand, cell signaling is a part of a complex system of communication that governs basic cell, tissue, and organismal activities and coordinates actions and responses. On the other hand, aberrant signaling is the mechanistic basis for many diseases, including cancer and diabetes.

The traditional concept of biological signaling has invoked discrete pathways. However, we have long known that these pathways intersect, that the intersections are numerous and that the connected pathways can form complex signaling networks. It has become clear that a full understanding of cell function and regulation requires knowledge of the major signaling pathways, the underlying structure of signaling networks, the emergent features of the networks, and the ways by which changes in network structure affect the transmission and flow of information over space and time. Whether we are considering genetic or metabolic networks, the existence of complex network structures within cells has important implications. First, network structure indicates that multiple paths are available for signals to flow from point A to point B (Janes & Lauffenberger, 2013). This implies that the path taken and the integrated response can be context-dependent, i.e., determined by what else may be happening within the cell or tissue. For example, such complexity has been shown to be the basis for interaction between growth factor and proinflammatory signaling (Janes & Lauffenberger, 2013). Second, complex multicomponent signaling pathways provide opportunities for feedback, signal amplification, and interactions involving multiple signals and signaling pathways. Third, added complexity comes from the fact that signaling networks have an intrinsic spatial component, since signals often must cross multiple cellular domains, e.g., plasma membrane, cytoplasm, and nucleus.

Cellular signaling networks come in two flavors: genetic and metabolic. Genetic networks are characterized by a structure that is focused on gene expression and thus leads to alterations in the mRNA and/or protein expression of key components; these in turn affect cell function (Boucher & Jenna, 2013). Because of the time required for transcription/translation, responses mediated through genetic networks occur over timescales of tens of minutes to hours. Metabolic networks consist of proteins that function as switches turning off or on other key enzymes, channels, and transporters. They provide the capability to rapidly alter cell function, often within seconds or minutes. They also may be key elements of genetic networks, providing intermediate connections among, e.g., spatially removed elements (Janes & Lauffenberger, 2013). As shown below, it is clear that ATP-binding cassette (ABC) transporters at the blood–brain barrier respond to both genomic and nongenomic signals, resulting in changes in protein expression and activity (genomic) and in transport activity but not in protein expression (nongenomic or metabolic).

2. ABC TRANSPORTERS AT THE BLOOD–BRAIN BARRIER

This review is focused on the regulation of blood–brain barrier transporters that are members of the ABC family and that handle foreign chemicals (xenobiotics). The human genome contains 49 genes encoding ABC transporters, divided into seven different subfamilies, A–G, based on their evolutionary divergence (Moitra & Dean, 2011). The defining molecular signature of ABC family members is the presence of several consensus sequences including two ATP-binding motifs (Walker A and Walker B), as well as the ABC signature C motif (ALSGGQ) (Kuhnline Sloan et al., 2012). ABC family members include proteins that function as ATP-driven transporters on both surface and intracellular membranes, ion channels, and receptors. Mutations in some of the ABC genes result in genetic disorders such as cystic fibrosis (ABCC7, CFTR, the Cystic Fibrosis Transmembrane Regulator, a chloride channel), Dubin Johnson's syndrome (ABCC2, MRP2, a metabolite and drug transporter), progressive familial intrahepatic cholestasis (ABCB11, BSEP, a bile salt efflux pump), and retinal degeneration (ABCA4, a lipid flippase) (Moitra & Dean, 2011).

For vertebrates, three ABC subfamilies, B, C, and G, contain transporters that function as multispecific, ATP-driven efflux pumps, and largely handle foreign chemicals (xenobiotics). As a rule, these ABC transporters are expressed in all cells, but they are most highly expressed in barrier and excretory tissues. Thus, they importantly influence the peripheral and central nervous system pharmacokinetics of many signaling molecules, waste products of normal metabolism, therapeutic drugs, environmental toxicants, and drug and toxicant metabolites.

Multiple ABC transporters that handle xenobiotics are expressed in the brain capillary endothelium that makes up the blood–brain barrier (Hartz & Bauer, 2011) (Fig. 1). Certainly, for an efflux transporter to be effective in limiting blood to brain movement of drugs and neurotoxicants and driving efflux of potentially toxic metabolites, it should be localized to the luminal plasma membrane. Functional studies with wild-type and knock-out rodents as well as immunohistochemistry indicate that luminal membrane localization is certain for P-glycoprotein, MRP2, and breast cancer resistance protein (ABCG2) (BCRP) (Fig. 1). Other transporters, e.g., members of the multidrug resistance-associated protein (ABCC subfamily) (MRP) family (Dallas et al., 2006), may be expressed on both sides of the endothelium. Moreover, their distribution appears to be species-dependent (Chaves et al., 2014). They have the potential to affect both influx into and

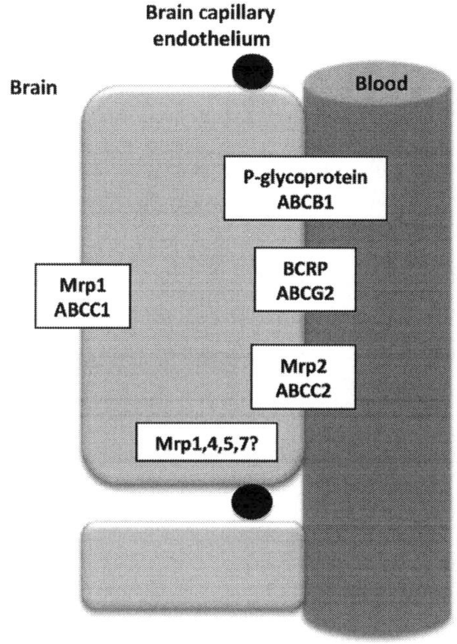

Figure 1 The distribution of ABC transporters that handle foreign chemicals, e.g., drugs and toxicants, within the brain capillary endothelium. Note that for some of the MRPs subcellular distribution is species-dependent and still unresolved (Chaves, Shawahna, Jacob, Scherrmann, & Decleves, 2014; Dallas, Miller, & Bendayan, 2006).

efflux out of the CNS. It should be noted that those ABC transporters expressed at the abluminal, CNS-facing plasma membrane of the brain capillary endothelium can facilitate transport into the brain. Indeed, the increase in expression of abluminal MRP1 (ABCC1) following experimental stroke (middle carotid artery occlusion, MCAO, followed by reperfusion) has been suggested as a way to increase brain delivery of certain therapeutics (ElAli & Hermann, 2010). Finally, for other ABC transporters, e.g., MRP5 and MRP7, there is no definitive localization in brain capillary endothelial cells, so it is not clear how they contribute to barrier function.

In addition to surface membrane localization, some studies have presented evidence for transporter localization in membranes that may be associated with internal organelles, e.g., endosomes. For example, immuno-electron microscopy and biochemical methods indicate that 30–50% of P-glycoprotein within brain capillary endothelial cells is not on the luminal membrane (Bendayan, Lee, & Bendayan, 2002; Hawkins, Rigor, & Miller, 2010). These results raise interesting possibilities with regard to regulation of transport activity through insertion and retrieval of preformed protein at surface membranes (see below). Indeed, this is one way by which transport activity can be rapidly altered while total tissue transporter protein expression remains unchanged (Hawkins, Sykes, & Miller, 2010; McCaffrey & Davis, 2012).

Finally, measurement of ABC transporter expression and activity at the blood–brain barrier pose unique challenges. For measurements of transporter expression (mRNA and protein), consider that capillaries represent <1% of brain volume. Isolation of a pure preparation of capillaries is necessary, as are specific probes and analysis methods. Selection of the appropriate antibody for Western blotting and immunostaining often presents difficulties.

Since the ABC transporters function as unidirectional, drug efflux pumps, direct measurements of substrate efflux rates are difficult to make. End points measured include: exclusion and efflux of fluorescent or radiolabeled substrates by cells, net transport of fluorescent or radiolabeled substrates across monolayers of cells, secretion of fluorescent substrates from bath into capillary lumens, and uptake into or efflux from brain *in vivo* (Kuhnline Sloan et al., 2012). Measurement of transport function, whether *in vivo* or *in vitro*, requires use of specific substrates and inhibitors. Because of overlapping substrate and inhibitor specificities, this is a problem for the MRP family of transporters, but less a problem for P-glycoprotein and BCRP.

3. ABC TRANSPORTER REGULATION

To the extent that ABC transporters expressed at the blood–brain barrier limit exposure to potentially toxic chemicals and endogenous metabolites, they are xenoprotective and neuroprotective. However, ABC transporters distinguish poorly between toxicants and therapeutic drugs. Thus, high ABC transporter expression on the luminal membrane of brain capillary endothelial cells is the major reason why it is such a challenge to deliver small molecule drugs to the brain for treatment of diseases, such as brain cancer, neuroAIDS, and epilepsy. Indeed, numerous studies have shown that increased ABC transporter expression in the tissue leads to reduced drug accumulation in the brain and that decreased expression/activity leads to increased drug accumulation. In addition, recent findings implicate the blood–brain barrier and its transporters in CNS disease progression (Zlokovic, 2008, 2011), suggesting that the barrier transporters are not just bystanders, but rather active participants and thus potential targets for therapy. Clearly, a full understanding of ABC transporter function and regulation in health and disease is needed to improve the delivery of small molecule therapeutics to the CNS and to treat CNS disease.

ABC transporter expression and transport activity at the blood–brain barrier are altered by multiple factors, including disease, stress, diet, therapy, and toxicant exposure (Miller, 2010; Miller & Cannon, 2014). Certainly, ABC transporter expression at the blood–brain barrier can be upregulated through the action of a number of ligand-activated receptors, leading to selective tightening of the barrier to both neurotoxicants and therapeutic drugs (Miller, 2010). The consequences of efflux transporter upregulation are increased neuroprotection, but reduced drug delivery. In certain situations, e.g., chemotherapy to the periphery, one might want to take advantage of these mechanisms to upregulate ABC transporter expression and augment neuroprotection. Conversely, recent studies show that targeting of blood–brain barrier signaling to manipulate transporter activity has the potential to selectively improve drug delivery to the CNS (Miller & Cannon, 2014). In spite of these recent studies, there are major gaps in our understanding of the mechanisms that establish basal transporter activity under control conditions and the mechanisms that underlie changes in ABC transporter expression in disease are not well understood.

3.1. Regulation of expression

3.1.1 Autonomous transcription factors

The top portion of the heat map in Fig. 2 shows many of the initiating signals and corresponding putative transcription factors that drive increases in the expression of three ABC transporter proteins at the blood–brain barrier. Table entries have been restricted in two ways: (1) to those signals for which we have confirmation from studies *in vivo* or *in vitro* using intact brain capillaries, and (2) to the three ABC transporters for which we have the most extensive information (P-glycoprotein, BCRP, and MRP2). Note first that several ligand-activated nuclear receptors are listed, e.g., pregnane X receptor (PXR) (Bauer et al., 2006), constitutive androstane receptor (CAR) (Wang, Sykes, & Miller, 2010), arylhydrocarbon receptor (AhR) (Wang, Hawkins, & Miller, 2011b), and GR (Narang et al., 2008). In the absence of ligand, they reside in the cytoplasm. Upon ligand binding, receptor plus ligand translocates to the nucleus where they usually find a partner

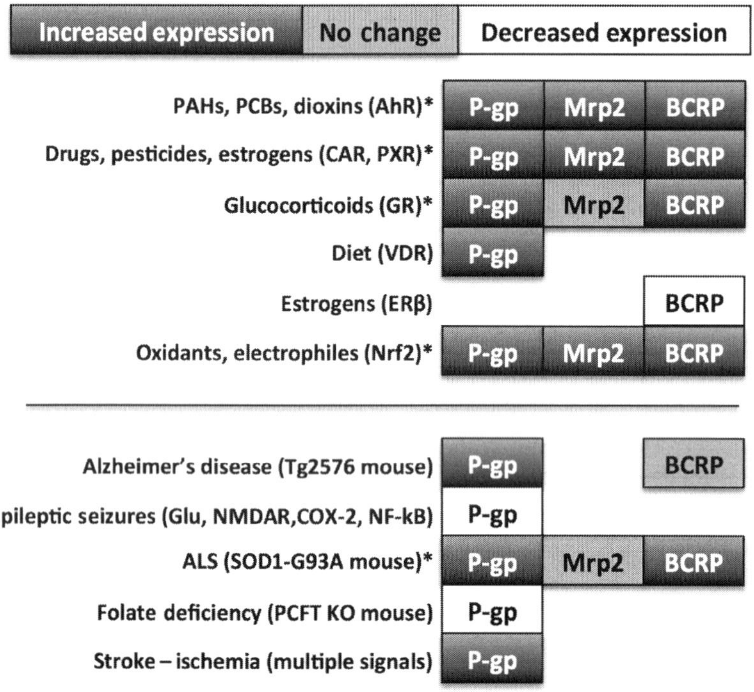

Figure 2 Heat map showing how xenobiotics and stressors alter ABC transporter protein expression at the blood–brain barrier. The figure summarizes published and unpublished data from this laboratory and others. Asterisks indicate the same mode of regulation at the blood-spinal cord barrier. See text for discussion and specific references.

protein, e.g., RXR for PXR and CAR; the heterodimer then binds to the promoter regions of target genes. Ligands for xenobiotic-activated receptors can be therapeutic drugs, toxicants, and dietary constituents. For these ligand and receptor pairs, induced transporter gene expression is part of a coordinated response to foreign chemicals that involves increased capability to metabolize xenobiotics (increased expression of Phase 1 and Phase 2 xenobiotic-metabolizing enzymes) and then excrete the metabolites or parent compounds (increased expression of efflux pumps). As one might expect, ramping up of this response profoundly affects drug absorption, distribution, metabolism, and excretion, both in the periphery and in the CNS.

3.1.2 Signaling-activated transcription factors

In contrast to the relatively simple sequence of events described above for ligand-activated nuclear receptors that appear to act autonomously, recent studies have disclosed more complicated signaling mechanisms underlying stress-induced increases in ABC transporter expression in rat and mouse brain capillaries (Fig. 3). These involve extended signaling from the plasma membrane or cytoplasm to transcription factors not directly activated by ligands. Rather, these transcription factors are maintained in a cytoplasmic complex that often facilitates polyubiquitination and directs the transcription factor to the proteasome for degradation. Upon activation, the

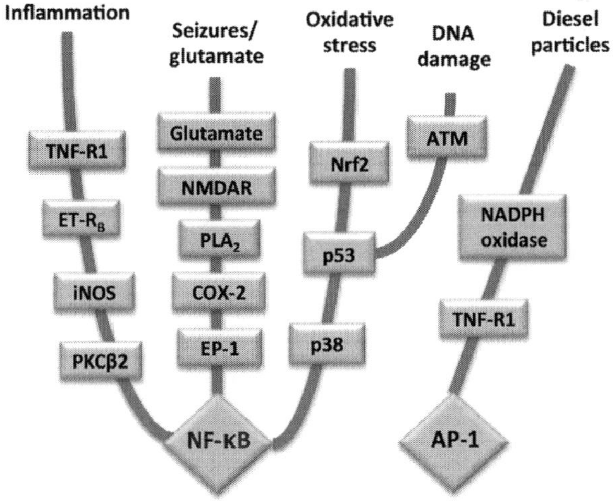

Figure 3 Signaling pathways that activate specific transcription factors that in turn induce increases in expression of ABC transporters. See text for discussion and specific references.

transcription factor translocates to the nucleus, binding to specific sequences in target gene promoters. As shown in Fig. 3, NF-κB appears to be such a transcription factor and one that targets multiple ABC transporters at the blood–brain barrier. Considering the number of stress-induced signals that converge at NF-κB (inflammation, epileptic seizures, oxidative stress), this transcription factor appears to be a stress-driven, master regulator of ABC transporter expression in brain capillaries.

Inflammation is a complex response that accompanies virtually all CNS diseases. Systemic administration of proinflammatory cytokines or bacterial endotoxin can alter P-glycoprotein expression at the blood–brain barrier and thus drug access to the CNS. Effects on transporter expression are complex, being dependent on the nature of the stimulus, the dose, and the time that transport activity/expression is assayed. Experiments with rat brain capillaries have shown complex, inside–out signaling precedes activation of NF-κB (Bauer, Hartz, & Miller, 2007). Several elements of the signaling pathway have been identified, but it is likely that additional signaling events separate them from each other (Fig. 3). Exposing vessels to TNF induces release of big-endothelin-1 (ET-1), which is converted to ET-1 by extracellular endothelin converting enzyme. ET-1 then binds to ETBR, which activates iNOS and PKCβ2 in sequence. Inhibition of NF-κB activation or nuclear translocation blocks the increase in P-glycoprotein expression and transport activity caused by TNF, sodium nitroprusside (NO generator), ET-1, or dPPA (activates PKCβ2) (Bauer et al., 2007; Rigor, Hawkins & Miller, 2010).

Consider next barrier responses to oxidative stress mediated by the molecular sensor for oxidative/electrophilic stress, nuclear factor (erythroid-derived 2)-like 2 (Nrf2) (Copple, 2012). Previous studies showed that activation of Nrf2 by sulforaphane (SFN), an electrophile and a constituent of broccoli, was neuroprotective in rodent models of ischemic stroke, traumatic brain injury (TBI), spinal cord injury (SCI), and subarachnoid hemorrhage (Alfieri et al., 2011; Chen, Fang, Zhang, Zhou, & Wang, 2011; Dash, Zhao, Orsi, Zhang, & Moore, 2009; Mao, Wang, Wang, Tian, & Xu, 2012). As a result, Nrf2 has been proposed as a therapeutic target in stroke, TBI, and SCI. However, SFN acting through Nrf2 induces expression of multiple ABC transporters in liver. We wondered whether this would also happen at the blood–brain barrier and then make it more difficult to deliver drugs to the injured brain. Indeed, SFN dosing of rats increased protein expression of P-glycoprotein, MRP2, and BCRP in brain capillaries *ex vivo* and reduced delivery to the brain of a P-glycoprotein substrate in vivo

(Wang et al., 2014). Given the large number of therapeutic drugs handled by these three efflux transporters, one would expect reduced CNS access and thus reduced drug efficacy when Nrf2 is activated for neuroprotection.

One aspect of the study is particularly interesting, showing that Nrf2 action requires elements of both metabolic and genomic signaling (Wang et al., 2014). Experiments with rat and mouse brain capillaries and mouse spinal cord capillaries show that the SFN-induced increases in transporter expression and activity are indeed mediated by Nrf2 (not seen in capillaries from Nrf2-null mice). However, Nrf2 acts indirectly, requiring functioning of p53 and NF-κB. The sequence of events is shown in Fig. 3. Although these experiments showed that Nrf2, p53, p38, and NF-κB work in concert to increase transporter expression, it is not clear how this happens. Additional support for p53 as a signaling element that activates NF-κB and increases ABC transporter expression comes from our unpublished studies in rat and mouse brain capillaries where DNA damage increases P-glycoprotein and BCRP expression through activation of ATM, p53, and NF-κB (Fig. 3)(R.E. Cannon and D.S. Miller, unpublished data).

NF-κB is not the only transcription factor that is both activated through signaling and that increases expression of ABC transporters at the blood–brain barrier. Experiments with isolated rat and mouse brain capillaries show that exposure to diesel exhaust particles *in vitro* activates a signaling pathway that involves NADPH oxidase, TNF-release, TNF-binding toTNFR1 and nuclear translocation of the transcription factor, AP-1 (Jun/Fos), resulting in increased P-glycoprotein expression (Hartz, Bauer, Block, Hong, & Miller, 2008). Note that this pathway and the proinflammatory pathway both involve signaling through TNFR1. However, the two pathways diverge at the level of the transcription factor. This is a clear example of context-dependent signaling, where in a proinflammatory context TNFR1 signals through NF-κB and in an oxidative context it signals through AP-1.

3.1.3 Altered transporter expression in disease

The bottom portion of the heat map in Fig. 2 summarizes known changes in ABC transporter expression at the blood–brain barrier associated with mouse models of disease. In most cases, underlying mechanisms are unknown, but elements of inflammatory and oxidative stress are present in the parenchyma and in the endothelium (Zlokovic, 2008). In some diseases shown, i.e., Alzheimer's disease, epilepsy, and ALS, there is good evidence for parallel changes in transporter function in the affected regions of patients' brains and spinal cords (Jablonski et al., 2012; Potschka, 2012; Vogelgesang et al., 2002).

In contrast to the other CNS diseases, substantial information is available from animal models on the signals driving increased P-glycoprotein expression following epileptic seizures. About 30% of epileptic patients exhibit resistance to antiepileptic drugs (AEDs). Several mechanisms underlie this multidrug resistance, including seizure-induced upregulation of ABC transporters at the blood–brain barrier (Loscher, Luna-Tortos, Romermann, & Fedrowitz, 2011; Potschka, 2012). Studies of the mechanism driving the increases in transporter expression focused primarily on P-glycoprotein. As with inflammation, NF-κB appears to drive the increase in expression, but following seizures, a completely different signaling sequence activates NF-κB (Fig. 3). In this case, excess glutamate, released through the increased neuronal activity, binds to an ionotropic *N*-Methyl-D-aspartate (NMDA) receptor, presumably increasing Ca^{2+} entry and activating cPLA2, which produces arachidonic acid. This metabolite is converted to PGE2 by cyclooxygenase-2 (COX-2). PGE2 efflux from the cells is mediated by an MRP, likely MRP4. Extracellular PGE2 binds to an EP-1 receptor, which then signals NF-κB activation and increased P-glycoprotein expression (Bauer et al., 2008; Pekcec et al., 2009; Zibell et al., 2009). Consistent with this sequence, inducing seizures in rats increases P-glycoprotein expression by an NMDA receptor and COX-2-dependent mechanism, and inhibiting elements of the signaling pathway improves efficacy of certain AEDs (Avemary et al., 2013).

3.2. Signals that regulate ABC transporter activity

This section is focused primarily on signals that alter P-glycoprotein and transport activity without affecting transporter protein expression. P-glycoprotein and BCRP are critical gatekeepers for many CNS-acting drugs and drug candidates (Agarwal, Hartz, Elmquist, & Bauer, 2011). Both are highly expressed at the blood–brain barrier and both are highly multispecific. In addition, studies from a number of laboratories show the two transporters work in concert to deny drugs access to the CNS. That is, the increase in brain accumulation of several drugs is much greater than additive when both transporters are knocked out or inhibited (Agarwal et al., 2011; Polli et al., 2009). Thus, for drugs that are modest substrates for both P-glycoprotein and BCRP, e.g., the tyrosine kinase inhibitor lapatinib, a large benefit for drug delivery to the CNS may be obtained by reducing transport on both transporters in concert. Given the important roles of the two transporters, singly and in combination, in limiting drug entry into the brain, a detailed understanding of the cellular signals that determine their basal transport activity could provide new options for improving small molecule drug delivery to the CNS. To date, two signals have been identified that rapidly reduce basal P-glycoprotein activity, and one signal has been identified that reduces basal BCRP activity (Miller & Cannon, 2014). In each case, transporter activity decreases but transporter protein expression level does not change. Although mechanistic studies were carried out in isolated rat and mouse brain capillaries, *in vivo* experiments demonstrate increased brain accumulation of drugs when signaling is activated. At a minimum, these findings provide a proof of principle that targeting signals that regulate basal ABC transporter activity has the potential to enhance delivery of therapeutic drugs to the brain.

3.2.1 Regulation of P-glycoprotein activity through signaling

In an initial proof-of-principle study using nude mice, Fellner et al. found that administering a P-glycoprotein inhibitor (PSC833) along with the chemotherapeutic, Taxol, twice over 5 weeks increased brain accumulation of the drug 10-fold and reduced the mass of an implanted human glioblastoma by 90% (Fellner et al., 2002). Taxol dosing alone did not alter tumor mass. Thus, inhibiting P-glycoprotein at the blood–brain barrier increased brain accumulation of Taxol sufficiently to produce a therapeutic effect in the animal model. This result suggested a simple way to circumvent this molecular barrier to drug entry into the CNS. However, the use of ABC transporter-specific inhibitors to improve drug delivery to tumors has not translated well to the clinic (Ferry, Traunecker, & Kerr, 1996; Kalvass et al., 2013; Krishna, St-Louis, & Mayer, 2000; Liang & Aszalos, 2006). As an alternative strategy, we hypothesized that basal P-glycoprotein activity (not expression) might be regulated and that identification of the signals involved in regulation could provide a means of rapidly modulating transport activity. We set out to map the signals responsible and identify "drugable" targets and suitable drugs. At the time, there was no evidence that such signals existed. Over several years, we found that basal transport activity of P-glycoprotein in rat brain capillaries is rapidly and reversibly reduced through two signaling pathways: one that is part of an extensive and complex series of events that include proinflammatory, sphingolipid, and protein kinase signaling (Hartz, Bauer, Fricker, & Miller, 2004, 2006) and a second driven by vascular endothelial growth factor (VEGF) signaling (Hawkins, Sykes, et al., 2010).

In both cases, transport activity of MRP2 and BCRP and tight junction permeability were not altered.

In searching for the first pathway, we were guided by earlier experiments in renal proximal tubule showing rapid loss of P-glycoprotein transport activity through by ET-1, ET_BR, NO, and a classical PKC isoform (Masereeuw, Terlouw, van Aubel, Russel, & Miller, 2000). Initial experiments with isolated rat brain capillaries showed similar signaling rapidly and reversibly reduced P-glycoprotein transport activity (Hartz et al., 2004). This effect occurred without a change in transporter expression nor in tight junction permeability. Signaling did not affect transport activity of BCRP nor Mrp2.

Other experiments identified TNFR1 as being upstream of ET-1 release and protein kinase C isoform β1 (PKCβ1) as the critical isoform downstream of NOS (Hartz et al., 2006; Rigor et al., 2010). Importantly, specifically activating PKCβ1 with a phorbol ester derivative (dPPA) *in vivo* increased rat brain accumulation of a P-glycoprotein substrate without affecting tight junction permeability (Rigor et al., 2010). Note that PKCβ1 signaling also reduces P-glycoprotein activity after a xenobiotic-induced increase in blood–brain barrier transporter expression. AhR activation by a dioxin increases blood–brain barrier P-glycoprotein expression *in vitro* and *in vivo* (Wang et al., 2011b). Activating PKCβ1 with dPPA reversed the effect of P-glycoprotein induction on transporter activity in rat brain capillaries exposed to dioxin *in vitro*, in brain capillaries from TCDD-dosed rats and in intact TCDD-dosed animals (Wang, Hawkins, & Miller, 2011a). Thus, by targeting signaling to P-glycoprotein (Fig. 4), access of drugs to the CNS can be increased even in a drug-resistant population, one in which blood–brain barrier transporter expression had been induced two- to three-fold.

At this point, we knew that basal transporter activity could be rapidly and reversibly modulated *in vitro* and *in vivo*. However, the signaling elements identified did not provide a way to safely target the pathway in the clinic. Exploring events downstream of PKCβ1 in rat and mouse brain capillaries, we recently identified multiple sphingolipid-based steps, involving sphingosine kinase, sphingosine-1-phosphate (S1P), and sphingosine-1-phosphate receptor 1 (S1PR1) (Fig. 4) (Cannon, Peart, Hawkins, Campos, & Miller, 2012). Immunostaining of rat brain capillaries localized S1PR1 to both the luminal and abluminal plasma membranes of the endothelial cells. In rat brain capillaries, sphingosine, S1P, and S1PR1 agonists rapidly reduced P-glycoprotein transport activity. These effects were

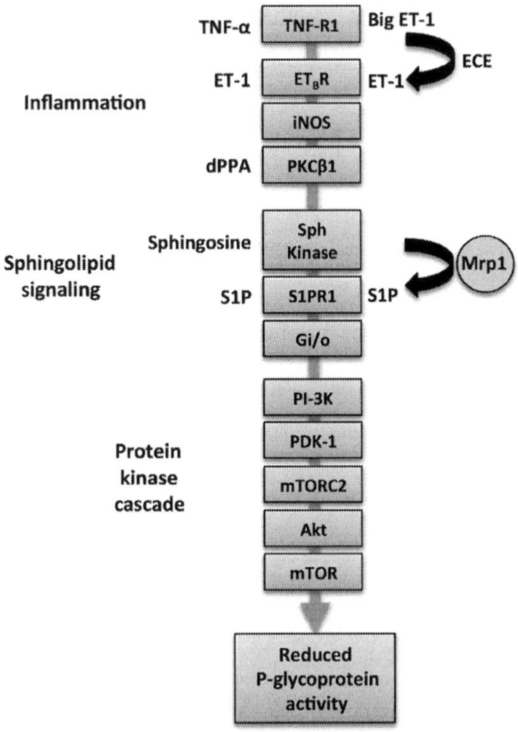

Figure 4 An extended signaling pathway that regulates basal P-glycoprotein activity at the blood–brain barrier. Activation of the pathway *in vitro* (isolated brain capillaries) causes rapid and reversible loss of transport activity. Activation of the pathway *in vivo* rapidly increases drug delivery to the brain. See text for discussion and specific references.

blocked by S1PR1 antagonists; the sphingosine effect was blocked by a sphingosine kinase inhibitor (Cannon et al., 2012). Importantly, the receptor could be targeted with Fingolimod (Gilenya, FTY720), a prodrug, prescribed for patients with relapsing–remitting multiple sclerosis. FTY720 generates a phosphorylated, S1P analog (FTY720P), that is, a S1PR agonist; both the prodrug and its phosphorylated metabolite rapidly reduced P-glycoprotein transport activity in brain capillaries (Cannon et al., 2012).

Importantly, *in situ* brain perfusion in rats showed that dosing with S1P, S1PR1 agonists, FTY720 or FTY220P, rapidly and specifically increased brain uptake of three radiolabeled drugs that are P-glycoprotein substrates (Cannon et al., 2012). For Taxol, the chemotherapeutic used in the initial mouse study with the implanted human glioblastoma (Fellner et al., 2002), brain accumulation increased fivefold. Brain uptake of ^{14}C-sucrose, a sensitive measure of changes in tight junction permeability, was not altered by S1P, S1PR1 agonists, FTY720 or FTY220P (Cannon et al., 2012).

Recent progress in extending this signaling pathway has come in two areas: identifying the transporter that pumps S1P out of the endothelial cells and identifying signaling elements downstream of S1PR1. First, following action of sphingosine kinase, S1P (and FTY720P) must exit the cells to bind S1PR1. However, S1P is sufficiently polar so that passive membrane permeability and thus access to external S1PR binding sites is limited. In other cells, ABCA1 and MRP1 have been implicated in S1P efflux from cells (Kim, Takabe, Milstien, & Spiegel, 2009; Mitra et al., 2006). In addition, a novel S1P transporter (Spns2), not a member of the ABC transporter family, was discovered in zebra fish (Hisano, Kobayashi, Kawahara, Yamaguchi, & Nishi, 2011; Kawahara et al., 2009), and an ortholog of this transporter is expressed in mammals (Fukuhara et al., 2012). Using brain capillaries from MRP1 knock-out mice, Cartwright et al. identified MRP1 as the ABC transporter that mediates S1P efflux from brain capillary endothelial cells (Cartwright, Campos, Cannon, & Miller, 2013). In those capillaries, signaling upstream of sphingosine kinase, e.g., that initiated by tumor necrosis factor-α (TNF-α), sphingosine, or FTY720, no longer reduced P-glycoprotein activity. In contrast, signaling by S1P and FTY720P was as effective as in capillaries from wild-type mice (Cartwright et al., 2013).

Second, experiments with rat brain capillaries show a protein kinase cascade downstream of S1PR1. At the blood–brain barrier, S1PR1 is coupled to $G_{i/o}$ (Cannon et al., 2012). This G-protein is capable of signaling through pathways involving phospholipase C, Ras/MAPK, PI-3kinase, or adenyl cyclase. Our experiments using specific inhibitors of the PI-3K pathway indicate that signaling to P-glycoprotein occurs through activation of a canonical PI-3kinase/PDK1/protein kinase B (Akt)/mTOR pathway (Fig. 4) (R.E. Cannon and D.S. Miller, unpublished observations).

3.2.2 Regulation of P-glycoprotein activity through VEGF signaling

Hawkins et al. found that exposing isolated rat brain capillaries to VEGF acting through flk-1 and Src kinase rapidly and reversibly decreases P-glycoprotein transport activity, without changing transporter expression or tight junction permeability (Hawkins, Sykes, et al., 2010). In intact rats, intracerebroventricular injection of VEGF increases brain accumulation of the P-glycoprotein substrates, ^{3}H-morphine, and ^{3}H-verapamil, but not the tight junction marker, ^{14}C-sucrose. These VEGF effects on

P-glycoprotein-mediated transport are blocked by systemic administration of a Src kinase inhibitor (Hawkins, Sykes, et al., 2010). Taken together, these findings imply that P-glycoprotein activity is acutely diminished in pathological conditions associated with increased brain VEGF expression. They also imply that once the more downstream elements of VEGF signaling to P-glycoprotein are identified, there could be elements additional that modulate P-glycoprotein activity acutely and thus can be targeted to improve drug delivery to the brain.

3.2.3 Regulation of BCRP activity through estrogen signaling

Estradiol reduces BCRP transport activity in mouse and rat brain capillaries by inducing transporter trafficking away from the plasma membrane, transporter protein degradation, and reduced transporter transcription (Hartz, Madole, Miller, & Bauer, 2010; Hartz, Mahringer, Miller, & Bauer, 2010; Mahringer & Fricker, 2010). Rodent brain capillaries express both ERα and ERβ, with expression of the latter dominating at both the mRNA and proteins levels (Hartz, Madole, et al., 2010; Hartz, Mahringer, et al., 2010). Exposing rat and mouse brain capillaries to subnanomolar to nanomolar concentrations of 17-β-estradiol (E2) rapidly and reversibly reduces BCRP-mediated transport activity without altering protein expression (Hartz, Madole, et al., 2010; Hartz, Mahringer, et al., 2010). The reduction in activity is not altered by inhibitors of transcription and translation, but is blocked by Brefeldin A, an inhibitor of intracellular vesicle trafficking. Both estrogen receptor (ER) subtypes, ERα and ERβ, are involved since capillaries isolated from ERα-null mice or ERβ-null mice do not show reduced BCRP transport activity in response to E2. The rapid response to E2 and the lack of effect of inhibitors of transcription and translation point to a nonclassical mechanism of E2 action (Hartz, Madole, et al., 2010; Hartz, Mahringer, et al., 2010).

Extending the time of exposure to E2 reduces BCRP mRNA and protein expression (Hartz, Madole, et al., 2010; Mahringer & Fricker, 2010). These effects are mediated by ERβ, which signals through PTEN, PI3-K, Akt, and GSK-3β (Fig. 5). ERα is not involved. Such signaling increases ubiquitination of BCRP protein, which leads to transporter protein degradation at the proteasome E2 also reduces BCRP mRNA after 90 min of exposure, although it is not clear whether this is a result of reduced transcription, increased mRNA degradation, or both (Mahringer & Fricker, 2010). Dosing mice with E2 (0.1 mg/kg by i.p. injection) recapitulates the complex time course of changes in BCRP activity and expression seen in

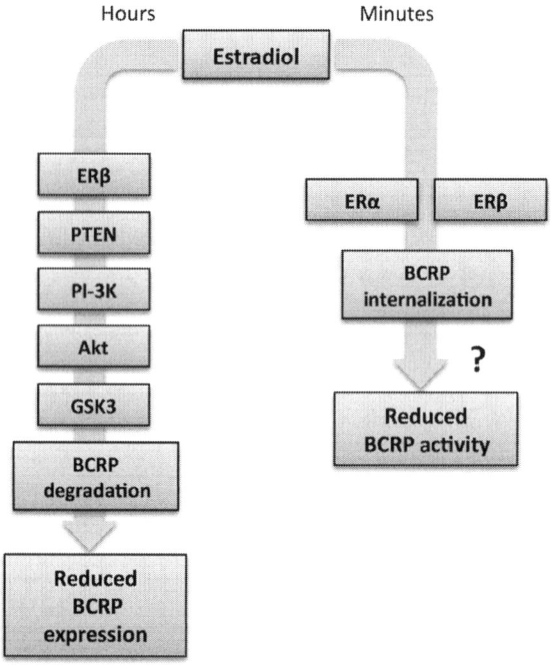

Figure 5 Signals underlying the loss of BCRP transport activity and protein expression following estradiol exposure. See text for discussion and specific references.

E2-exposed brain capillaries (Hartz, Madole, et al., 2010). These studies suggest two estrogen-based strategies for reducing basal BCRP activity at the blood–brain barrier, with ERα-specific agonists rapidly and reversibly reducing transport activity and ERβ-specific agonists initially reducing transport activity but then sending transporter protein to the proteasome for degradation.

3.2.4 Mechanisms underlying reduced ABC transporter activity

By what mechanisms do intracellular signals rapidly reduce ABC transporter activity when transporter protein expression is not altered? For many proteins that function primarily at the cell surface, a fraction of total cellular protein is stored away from the surface in intracellular vesicular compartments. In hepatocytes, P-glycoprotein and other ABC transporters move rapidly in both directions between intracellular, membrane-bound compartments and the canalicular membrane (Kipp, Pichetshote, & Arias, 2001). In brain capillary endothelial cells, both immunoelectron microscopy and our biochemical measurements indicate that a significant fraction of total P-glycoprotein protein is not present in the luminal plasma membrane (Bendayan et al., 2002; Hawkins, Rigor, et al., 2010). Experiments in rat using an *in vivo* protease K protection assay in which the protease was infused into the brain's vasculature examined this possibility for signaling initiated by VEGF and by PKCβ1 (Hawkins, Rigor, et al., 2010). In control experiments, protease K infusion reduced levels of luminal plasma membrane proteins (Western blots of P-glycoprotein, MRP2), but did not alter levels of intracellular proteins (β-actin) or levels of proteins localized to the abluminal plasma membrane (Na,K-ATPase) (Hawkins, Rigor, et al., 2010). VEGF caused reduced proteolysis of P-glycoprotein, but not of MRP2 (transport activity of MRP2 is not affected by VEGF) (Hawkins, Rigor, et al., 2010). These findings indicate that VEGF signaling drives the transporter away from the luminal surface, perhaps to a subapical or vesicular compartment where it cannot contribute to efflux transport at the luminal plasma membrane. Such trafficking is reversible.

In contrast, PKCβ1 activation by dPPA did not change protease K-induced proteolysis of P-glycoprotein, indicating no movement of the transporter away from the luminal membrane surface. How transport activity is lost as a consequence of TNF-αPKCβ1/S1PR1 signaling remains unknown. Loss of activity could be the result of covalent modification of the transport protein, perhaps through phosphorylation–dephosphorylation, acetylation, redox reactions, or cross-linking at cysteines, or through changes in membrane microenvironment that induce allosteric effects, e.g., noncovalent associations with other proteins or membrane phospholipids and altered local ion activities. In this regard, both caveoli and lipid rafts have been implicated in the regulation of P-glycoprotein in brain endothelial cells (Barakat et al., 2007, 2008; Zhong, Hennig, & Toborek, 2010) and of BCRP in tumor cells (Storch, Ehehalt, Haefeli, & Weiss, 2007). Recent experiments using an animal model of peripheral inflammatory pain (λ-carageenan model in rats) show complex changes in membrane protein biochemistry that accompanies altered P-glycoprotein activity (McCaffrey et al., 2012). These experiments showed that increased transport activity *in vivo* was driven by protein–protein interactions, i.e., a concerted redistribution of P-glycoprotein and caveolin-1, involving disassembly of high-molecular-weight P-glycoprotein-containing structures. Movement into and out of these structures could very well alter transport activity.

4. CONCLUSION

Delivery of small molecule drugs designed to access CNS targets remains a problem in the clinic. High expression of certain ABC transporters at the blood–brain barrier contributes substantially to the problem. Recent progress in understanding the regulation of these transporters provides good news and bad news. The good news is that the basal activities of P-glycoprotein and BCRP appear to be regulated and the signaling pathways responsible contain multiple elements that could be manipulated with drugs already in use in the clinic (Miller & Cannon, 2014). If that could be done, efflux transport through those transporters could be rapidly and reversibly reduced. This would provide a window in time when part of the barrier is down and drugs that are transporter substrates could enter the CNS unimpeded.

The bad news is threefold. First, studies that identified pathways that signal reduced transporter activity have not yet provided a strategy that is immediately translatable to the clinic (Kalvass et al., 2013). Second, little is known about the extent to which drug-metabolizing enzymes in the blood–brain barrier present an additional obstacle to the delivery of biologically active drugs to the CNS. It is clear that the capillary endothelium expresses a number of Phase 1 and Phase 2 enzymes and that enzyme expression (like ABC transporter expression) can be induced through xenobiotic-activated nuclear receptors, e.g., PXR, CAR, and AhR (Bauer, Hartz, Fricker, & Miller, 2004; Wang et al., 2010, 2011b). However, for the blood–brain barrier, the effect of these enzymes on drug pharmacokinetics and how well they are coupled to efflux transporters remain to be determined. Third, the list of stressors that upregulate ABC transporter expression at the blood–brain barrier is growing (Fig. 2). Given the breadth of the list, it is hard to believe that a substantial portion of the human population is not already induced and thus multidrug resistant. If that were the case, it would be interesting to know whether a modified diet could be designed that would reduce blood–brain barrier transporter expression and transport activity in patients prior to CNS pharmacotherapy.

CONFLICT OF INTEREST

I have no conflicts of interest to declare.

ACKNOWLEDGMENTS

This work was supported by the Intramural Research Program of the National Institute of Environmental Health Sciences, National Institutes of Health. I thank all past and present members of the Miller Laboratory for insightful discussions.

REFERENCES

Agarwal, S., Hartz, A. M., Elmquist, W. F., & Bauer, B. (2011). Breast cancer resistance protein and P-glycoprotein in brain cancer: Two gatekeepers team up. *Current Pharmaceutical Design, 17*, 2793–2802.

Alfieri, A., Srivastava, S., Siow, R. C., Modo, M., Fraser, P. A., & Mann, G. E. (2011). Targeting the Nrf2-Keap1 antioxidant defence pathway for neurovascular protection in stroke. *The Journal of Physiology, 589*, 4125–4136.

Avemary, J., Salvamoser, J. D., Peraud, A., Remi, J., Noachtar, S., Fricker, G., et al. (2013). Dynamic regulation of P-glycoprotein in human brain capillaries. *Molecular Pharmaceutics, 10*, 3333–3341.

Barakat, S., Demeule, M., Pilorget, A., Regina, A., Gingras, D., Baggetto, L. G., et al. (2007). Modulation of P-glycoprotein function by caveolin-1 phosphorylation. *Journal of Neurochemistry, 101*, 1–8.

Barakat, S., Turcotte, S., Demeule, M., Lachambre, M. P., Regina, A., Baggetto, L. G., et al. (2008). Regulation of brain endothelial cells migration and angiogenesis by P-glycoprotein/caveolin-1 interaction. *Biochemical and Biophysical Research Communications, 372*, 440–446.

Bauer, B., Hartz, A. M., Fricker, G., & Miller, D. S. (2004). Pregnane X receptor up-regulation of P-glycoprotein expression and transport function at the blood-brain barrier. *Molecular Pharmacology, 66*, 413–419.

Bauer, B., Hartz, A. M., & Miller, D. S. (2007). Tumor necrosis factor alpha and endothelin-1 increase P-glycoprotein expression and transport activity at the blood-brain barrier. *Molecular Pharmacology, 71*, 667–675.

Bauer, B., Hartz, A. M., Pekcec, A., Toellner, K., Miller, D. S., & Potschka, H. (2008). Seizure-induced up-regulation of P-glycoprotein at the blood-brain barrier through glutamate and cyclooxygenase-2 signaling. *Molecular Pharmacology, 73*, 1444–1453.

Bauer, B., Yang, X., Hartz, A. M., Olson, E. R., Zhao, R., Kalvass, J. C., et al. (2006). In vivo activation of human pregnane X receptor tightens the blood-brain barrier to methadone through P-glycoprotein up-regulation. *Molecular Pharmacology, 70*, 1212–1219.

Bendayan, R., Lee, G., & Bendayan, M. (2002). Functional expression and localization of P-glycoprotein at the blood brain barrier. *Microscopy Research and Technique, 57*, 365–380.

Boucher, B., & Jenna, S. (2013). Genetic interaction networks: better understanding to better predict. *Frontiers in genetics, 4*, 290.

Cannon, R. E., Peart, J. C., Hawkins, B. T., Campos, C. R., & Miller, D. S. (2012). Targeting blood-brain barrier sphingolipid signaling reduces basal P-glycoprotein activity and improves drug delivery to the brain. *Proceedings of the National Academy of Sciences of the United States of America, 109*, 15930–15935.

Cartwright, T. A., Campos, C. R., Cannon, R. E., & Miller, D. S. (2013). Mrp1 is essential for sphingolipid signaling to p-glycoprotein in mouse blood-brain and blood-spinal cord barriers. *Journal of Cerebral Blood Flow and Metabolism, 33*, 381–388.

Chaves, C., Shawahna, R., Jacob, A., Scherrmann, J. M., & Decleves, X. (2014). Human ABC transporters at blood-CNS interfaces as determinants of CNS drug penetration. *Current Pharmaceutical Design, 20*, 1450–1462.

Chen, G., Fang, Q., Zhang, J., Zhou, D., & Wang, Z. (2011). Role of the Nrf2-ARE pathway in early brain injury after experimental subarachnoid hemorrhage. *Journal of Neuroscience Research, 89*, 515–523.

Copple, I. M. (2012). The Keap1-Nrf2 cell defense pathway—a promising therapeutic target? *Advances in Pharmacology, 63*, 43–79.

Dallas, S., Miller, D. S., & Bendayan, R. (2006). Multidrug resistance-associated proteins: Expression and function in the central nervous system. *Pharmacological Reviews, 58*, 140–161.

Dash, P. K., Zhao, J., Orsi, S. A., Zhang, M., & Moore, A. N. (2009). Sulforaphane improves cognitive function administered following traumatic brain injury. *Neuroscience Letters, 460*, 103–107.

ElAli, A., & Hermann, D. M. (2010). Apolipoprotein E controls ATP-binding cassette transporters in the ischemic brain. *Science Signaling, 3*, ra72.
Fellner, S., Bauer, B., Miller, D. S., Schaffrik, M., Fankhanel, M., Spruss, T., et al. (2002). Transport of paclitaxel (Taxol) across the blood-brain barrier in vitro and in vivo. *The Journal of Clinical Investigation, 110*, 1309–1318.
Ferry, D. R., Traunecker, H., & Kerr, D. J. (1996). Clinical trials of P-glycoprotein reversal in solid tumours. *European Journal of Cancer, 32A*, 1070–1081.
Fukuhara, S., Simmons, S., Kawamura, S., Inoue, A., Orba, Y., Tokudome, T., et al. (2012). The sphingosine-1-phosphate transporter Spns2 expressed on endothelial cells regulates lymphocyte trafficking in mice. *The Journal of Clinical Investigation, 122*, 1416–1426.
Hartz, A. M., & Bauer, B. (2011). ABC transporters in the CNS—An inventory. *Current Pharmaceutical Biotechnology, 12*, 656–673.
Hartz, A. M., Bauer, B., Block, M. L., Hong, J. S., & Miller, D. S. (2008). Diesel exhaust particles induce oxidative stress, proinflammatory signaling, and P-glycoprotein up-regulation at the blood-brain barrier. *The FASEB Journal, 22*, 2723–2733.
Hartz, A. M., Bauer, B., Fricker, G., & Miller, D. S. (2004). Rapid regulation of P-glycoprotein at the blood-brain barrier by endothelin-1. *Molecular Pharmacology, 66*, 387–394.
Hartz, A. M., Bauer, B., Fricker, G., & Miller, D. S. (2006). Rapid modulation of P-glycoprotein-mediated transport at the blood-brain barrier by tumor necrosis factor-alpha and lipopolysaccharide. *Molecular Pharmacology, 69*, 462–470.
Hartz, A. M., Madole, E. K., Miller, D. S., & Bauer, B. (2010). Estrogen receptor beta signaling through phosphatase and tensin homolog/phosphoinositide 3-kinase/Akt/glycogen synthase kinase 3 down-regulates blood-brain barrier breast cancer resistance protein. *The Journal of Pharmacology and Experimental Therapeutics, 334*, 467–476.
Hartz, A. M., Mahringer, A., Miller, D. S., & Bauer, B. (2010). 17-Beta-estradiol: A powerful modulator of blood-brain barrier BCRP activity. *Journal of Cerebral Blood Flow and Metabolism, 30*, 1742–1755.
Hawkins, B. T., Rigor, R. R., & Miller, D. S. (2010). Rapid loss of blood-brain barrier P-glycoprotein activity through transporter internalization demonstrated using a novel in situ proteolysis protection assay. *Journal of Cerebral Blood Flow and Metabolism, 30*, 1593–1597.
Hawkins, B. T., Sykes, D. B., & Miller, D. S. (2010). Rapid, reversible modulation of blood-brain barrier P-glycoprotein transport activity by vascular endothelial growth factor. *Journal of Neuroscience, 30*, 1417–1425.
Hisano, Y., Kobayashi, N., Kawahara, A., Yamaguchi, A., & Nishi, T. (2011). The sphingosine 1-phosphate transporter, SPNS2, functions as a transporter of the phosphorylated form of the immunomodulating agent FTY720. *The Journal of Biological Chemistry, 286*, 1758–1766.
Jablonski, M. R., Jacob, D. A., Campos, C., Miller, D. S., Maragakis, N. J., Pasinelli, P., et al. (2012). Selective increase of two ABC drug efflux transporters at the blood-spinal cord barrier suggests induced pharmacoresistance in ALS. *Neurobiology of Disease, 47*, 194–200.
Janes, K. A., & Lauffenberger, D. A. (2013). Models of cell signaling networks – what biologists can gain from them. *Journal of Cell Science, 126*, 849–855.
Kalvass, J. C., Polli, J. W., Bourdet, D. L., Feng, B., Huang, S. M., Liu, X., et al. (2013). Why clinical modulation of efflux transport at the human blood-brain barrier is unlikely: The ITC evidence-based position. *Clinical Pharmacology and Therapeutics, 94*, 80–94.
Kawahara, A., Nishi, T., Hisano, Y., Fukui, H., Yamaguchi, A., & Mochizuki, N. (2009). The sphingolipid transporter spns2 functions in migration of zebrafish myocardial precursors. *Science, 323*, 524–527.
Kim, R. H., Takabe, K., Milstien, S., & Spiegel, S. (2009). Export and functions of sphingosine-1-phosphate. *Biochimica et Biophysica Acta, 1791*, 692–696.

Kipp, H., Pichetshote, N., & Arias, I. M. (2001). Transporters on demand: Intrahepatic pools of canalicular ATP binding cassette transporters in rat liver. *The Journal of Biological Chemistry, 276*, 7218–7224.

Krishna, R., St-Louis, M., & Mayer, L. D. (2000). Increased intracellular drug accumulation and complete chemosensitization achieved in multidrug-resistant solid tumors by co-administering valspodar (PSC 833) with sterically stabilized liposomal doxorubicin. *International Journal of Cancer, 85*, 131–141.

Kuhnline Sloan, C. D., Nandi, P., Linz, T. H., Aldrich, J. V., Audus, K. L., & Lunte, S. M. (2012). Analytical and biological methods for probing the blood-brain barrier. *Annual Review of Analytical Chemistry (Palo Alto, California), 5*, 505–531.

Liang, X. J., & Aszalos, A. (2006). Multidrug transporters as drug targets. *Current Drug Targets*, 7, 911–921.

Loscher, W., Luna-Tortos, C., Romermann, K., & Fedrowitz, M. (2011). Do ATP-binding cassette transporters cause pharmacoresistance in epilepsy? Problems and approaches in determining which antiepileptic drugs are affected. *Current Pharmaceutical Design, 17*, 2808–2828.

Mahringer, A., & Fricker, G. (2010). BCRP at the blood-brain barrier: Genomic regulation by 17beta-estradiol. *Molecular Pharmaceutics*, 7, 1835–1847.

Mao, L., Wang, H. D., Wang, X. L., Tian, L., & Xu, J. Y. (2012). Disruption of Nrf2 exacerbated the damage after spinal cord injury in mice. *Journal of Trauma and Acute Care Surgery, 72*, 189–198.

Masereeuw, R., Terlouw, S. A., van Aubel, R. A., Russel, F. G., & Miller, D. S. (2000). Endothelin B receptor-mediated regulation of ATP-driven drug secretion in renal proximal tubule. *Molecular Pharmacology, 57*, 59–67.

McCaffrey, G., & Davis, T. P. (2012). Physiology and pathophysiology of the blood-brain barrier: P-glycoprotein and occludin trafficking as therapeutic targets to optimize central nervous system drug delivery. *Journal of Investigative Medicine, 60*, 1131–1140.

McCaffrey, G., Staatz, W. D., Sanchez-Covarrubias, L., Finch, J. D., Demarco, K., Laracuente, M. L., et al. (2012). P-glycoprotein trafficking at the blood-brain barrier altered by peripheral inflammatory hyperalgesia. *Journal of Neurochemistry, 122*, 962–975.

Miller, D. S. (2010). Regulation of P-glycoprotein and other ABC drug transporters at the blood-brain barrier. *Trends in Pharmacological Sciences, 31*, 246–254.

Miller, D. S., & Cannon, R. E. (2014). Signaling pathways that regulate basal ABC transporter activity at the blood-brain barrier. *Current Pharmaceutical Design, 20*, 1463–1471.

Mitra, P., Oskeritzian, C. A., Payne, S. G., Beaven, M. A., Milstien, S., & Spiegel, S. (2006). Role of ABCC1 in export of sphingosine-1-phosphate from mast cells. *Proceedings of the National Academy of Sciences of the United States of America, 103*, 16394–16399.

Moitra, K., & Dean, M. (2011). Evolution of ABC transporters by gene duplication and their role in human disease. *Biological Chemistry, 392*, 29–37.

Narang, V. S., Fraga, C., Kumar, N., Shen, J., Throm, S., Stewart, C. F., et al. (2008). Dexamethasone increases expression and activity of multidrug resistance transporters at the rat blood-brain barrier. *American Journal of Physiology Cell Physiology. 295*, C440–C450.

Pekcec, A., Unkruer, B., Schlichtiger, J., Soerensen, J., Hartz, A. M., Bauer, B., et al. (2009). Targeting prostaglandin E2 EP1 receptors prevents seizure-associated P-glycoprotein up-regulation. *The Journal of Pharmacology and Experimental Therapeutics, 330*, 939–947.

Polli, J. W., Olson, K. L., Chism, J. P., John-Williams, L. S., Yeager, R. L., Woodard, S. M., et al. (2009). An unexpected synergist role of P-glycoprotein and breast cancer resistance protein on the central nervous system penetration of the tyrosine kinase inhibitor lapatinib (N-{3-chloro-4-[(3-fluorobenzyl)oxy]phenyl}-6-[5-({[2-(methylsulfonyl)ethy l]amino}methyl)-2-furyl]-4-quinazolinamine; GW572016). *Drug Metabolism and Disposition, 37*, 439–442.

Potschka, H. (2012). Role of CNS efflux drug transporters in antiepileptic drug delivery: Overcoming CNS efflux drug transport. *Advanced Drug Delivery Reviews*, *64*, 943–952.

Rigor, R. R., Hawkins, B. T., & Miller, D. S. (2010). Activation of PKC isoform beta(I) at the blood-brain barrier rapidly decreases P-glycoprotein activity and enhances drug delivery to the brain. *Journal of Cerebral Blood Flow and Metabolism*, *30*, 1373–1383.

Storch, C. H., Ehehalt, R., Haefeli, W. E., & Weiss, J. (2007). Localization of the human breast cancer resistance protein (BCRP/ABCG2) in lipid rafts/caveolae and modulation of its activity by cholesterol in vitro. *The Journal of Pharmacology and Experimental Therapeutics*, *323*, 257–264.

Vogelgesang, S., Cascorbi, I., Schroeder, E., Pahnke, J., Kroemer, H. K., Siegmund, W., et al. (2002). Deposition of Alzheimer's beta-amyloid is inversely correlated with P-glycoprotein expression in the brains of elderly non-demented humans. *Pharmacogenetics*, *12*, 535–541.

Wang, X., Campos, C. R., Peart, J., Smith, L. K., Boni, J. L., Cannon, R. E., et al. (2014). Nrf2 upregulates ABC transporter expression and activity at the blood-brain and blood-spinal cord barriers. *Journal of Neuroscience*, *34*, 8585–8593.

Wang, X., Hawkins, B. T., & Miller, D. S. (2011a). Activating PKC-beta1 at the blood-brain barrier reverses induction of P-glycoprotein activity by dioxin and restores drug delivery to the CNS. *Journal of Cerebral Blood Flow and Metabolism*, *31*, 1371–1375.

Wang, X., Hawkins, B. T., & Miller, D. S. (2011b). Aryl hydrocarbon receptor-mediated up-regulation of ATP-driven xenobiotic efflux transporters at the blood-brain barrier. *The FASEB Journal*, *25*, 644–652.

Wang, X., Sykes, D. B., & Miller, D. S. (2010). Constitutive androstane receptor-mediated up-regulation of ATP-driven xenobiotic efflux transporters at the blood-brain barrier. *Molecular Pharmacology*, *78*, 376–383.

Zhong, Y., Hennig, B., & Toborek, M. (2010). Intact lipid rafts regulate HIV-1 Tat protein-induced activation of the Rho signaling and upregulation of P-glycoprotein in brain endothelial cells. *Journal of Cerebral Blood Flow and Metabolism*, *30*, 522–533.

Zibell, G., Unkruer, B., Pekcec, A., Hartz, A. M., Bauer, B., Miller, D. S., et al. (2009). Prevention of seizure-induced up-regulation of endothelial P-glycoprotein by COX-2 inhibition. *Neuropharmacology*, *56*, 849–855.

Zlokovic, B. V. (2008). The blood-brain barrier in health and chronic neurodegenerative disorders. *Neuron*, *57*, 178–201.

Zlokovic, B. V. (2011). Neurovascular pathways to neurodegeneration in Alzheimer's disease and other disorders. *Nature Reviews. Neuroscience*, *12*, 723–738.

CHAPTER TWO

P-glycoprotein Trafficking as a Therapeutic Target to Optimize CNS Drug Delivery

Thomas P. Davis[1], Lucy Sanchez-Covarubias, Margaret E. Tome
Department of Pharmacology, College of Medicine, University of Arizona, Tucson, Arizona, USA
[1]Corresponding author: e-mail address: davistp@email.arizona.edu

Contents

Abstract

The primary function of the blood–brain barrier (BBB)/neurovascular unit is to protect the central nervous system (CNS) from potentially harmful xenobiotic substances and maintain CNS homeostasis. Restricted access to the CNS is maintained via a combination of tight junction proteins as well as a variety of efflux and influx transporters that limits the transcellular and paracellular movement of solutes. Of the transporters identified at the BBB, P-glycoprotein (P-gp) has emerged as the transporter that is the greatest obstacle to effective CNS drug delivery. In this chapter, we provide data to support intracellular protein trafficking of P-gp within cerebral capillary microvessels as a potential target for improved drug delivery. We show that pain-induced changes in P-gp trafficking are associated with changes in P-gp's association with caveolin-1, a key scaffolding/trafficking protein that colocalizes with P-gp at the luminal membrane of brain microvessels. Changes in colocalization with the phosphorylated and nonphosphorylated forms of caveolin-1, by pain, are accompanied by dynamic changes in the distribution, relocalization, and activation of P-gp "pools" between microvascular endothelial cell subcellular compartments. Since redox-sensitive processes may be involved in signaling disassembly of higher-order structures of P-gp, we feel that

Advances in Pharmacology, Volume 71
ISSN 1054-3589
http://dx.doi.org/10.1016/bs.apha.2014.06.009

manipulating redox signaling, via specific protein targeting at the BBB, may protect disulfide bond integrity of P-gp reservoirs and control trafficking to the membrane surface, providing improved CNS drug delivery. The advantage of therapeutic drug "relocalization" of a protein is that the physiological impact can be modified, temporarily or long term, despite pathology-induced changes in gene transcription.

ABBREVIATIONS

ALK1 activin-like receptor kinase-1
ALK5 activin-like receptor kinase-5
BBB blood–brain barrier
BCRP/Bcrp breast cancer resistance protein
BCSF brain cerebral spinal fluid
CNS central nervous system
MBE4 mouse brain endothelial cells
MCTs/Mcts monocarboxylate transporters
MRPs/Mrps multidrug resistance proteins
NSAID nonsteroidal anti-inflammatory drug
NVU neurovascular unit
OATP/Oatp organic anion-transporting peptides
OATs/Oats organic anion transporters
OCTs/Octs organic cation transporters
P-gp P-glycoprotein
S1P sphingosine-1-phosphate
S1PR sphingosine-1-phosphate receptor
TEER transendothelial electrical resistance
TGF-β transforming growth factor β
VEGF vascular endothelial growth factor

1. INTRODUCTION

The blood–brain barrier (BBB) is a formidable physical and biochemical barrier to effective drug delivery to the brain, thus limiting the ability to effectively treat central nervous system (CNS) disorders. Within the past decade, intense research efforts have focused on directly targeting the BBB for optimization of drug delivery (Ronaldson & Davis, 2013). Such BBB targets include influx organic anion-transporting peptides (Oatp1a4) and efflux P-glycoprotein (P-gp) transporters that are expressed at the level of the brain microvascular endothelium. Instead of physically circumventing the BBB by using various tissue disruption/damaging, mechanical techniques such as osmotic shock, microdialysis, or intracerebroventricular injection, targeting transporters enables the development of novel chemical approaches to utilize endogenous barrier components to deliver drugs to the brain, thereby providing a unique opportunity to improve efficacy of existing therapies while promoting development of new ones (Ronaldson & Davis, 2013). This chapter provides an overview of BBB biology and focuses on the "800 pound gorilla," known as the P-gp transporter, which is responsible for many failures of CNS developmental therapeutics. Furthermore, we highlight various techniques that have been developed to circumvent the BBB for CNS drug delivery, with a particular emphasis on opportunities provided by targeting endogenous BBB transporter systems, such as P-gp and Oatp1a4.

2. THE BBB/NEUROVASCULAR UNIT

The neurovascular unit (NVU) comprises cellular constituents (i.e., endothelial cells, astrocytes, microglia, pericytes, neurons) and the extracellular matrix (Ronaldson & Davis, 2013) (Fig. 1). The concept of the NVU emphasizes that brain function and dysfunction requires coordinated interaction between the various NVU components. Disruption of any NVU component, as a result of a physiological, pathological, or pharmacological stressor, can alter BBB integrity, subsequently modifying brain microvascular permeability and drug delivery (Hawkins & Davis, 2005; Rolfe & Brown, 1997; Ronaldson & Davis, 2013).

3. ENDOTHELIAL CELLS AND THE BBB

The CNS is the most sensitive and critical organ system in the human body. Therefore, proper function requires precise regulation of the brain extracellular milieu. Additionally, CNS metabolic demands are considerable, with the CNS accounting for approximately 20% of overall oxygen consumption in humans (Oldendorf, Cornford, & Brown, 1977). The interface between the brain and the systemic circulation must possess highly selective and efficient mechanisms that are capable of facilitating nutrient transport, regulating ion balance, and providing a barrier to potentially toxic substances. Specifically, brain entry of some substances must be permitted while permeation of others must be limited. This homeostatic function of the cerebral microvasculature occurs primarily at the level of brain microvascular endothelial cells, the principal cell type of the BBB/NVU.

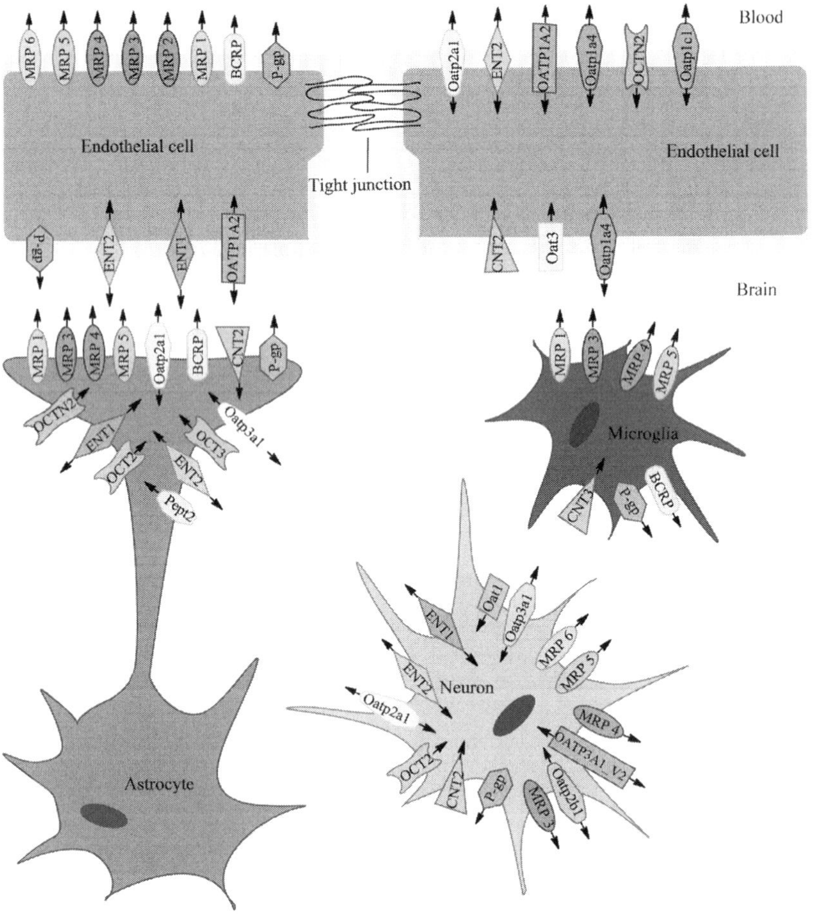

Figure 1 Transporters expressed in cells comprising the neurovascular unit (NVU). A large number of transporters are expressed on capillary endothelial cells, astrocytes, microglia, and neurons. Transporter systems aid in transport of nutrients, peptides, drugs, and ions into the brain parenchyma and as well as efflux of waste and potentially neurotoxic substance out of the brain. Arrows indicate the proposed direction of substrate transport. *Adapted from Sanchez-Covarrubias, Slosky, Thompson, Davis, and Ronaldson (2014).*

Compared to peripheral vasculature, BBB endothelial cells are characterized by increased mitochondrial content, high transendothelial electrical resistance (TEER), minimal pinocytosis activity, and lack of fenestrations (Hawkins & Davis, 2005; Oldendorf et al., 1977). Increased mitochondrial content is essential for these cells to maintain various active transport mechanisms such as those utilized to transport ions, nutrients, and waste products into and out of the brain parenchyma, thus contributing to the precise regulation of the CNS microenvironment and ensures proper neuronal function. Cell polarity of endothelial cells is ascribed to differing functional expression of transporter proteins and metabolic enzymes that are differentially expressed on the luminal and abluminal membranes. Such different biochemical characteristics of the luminal and abluminal plasma membranes further contribute to the high selectivity of the BBB (Betz, Firth, & Goldstein, 1980; Sanchez del Pino, Peterson, & Hawkins, 1995; Vorbrodt & Dobrogowska, 2003).

Of the many transporters expressed at the BBB endothelium, several have been implicated in influx and/or efflux of drugs into the CNS. Examples of efflux transporters include P-gp (Bendayan, Lee, & Bendayan, 2002), breast cancer resistance protein (BCRP in humans; Bcrp in rodents), and multidrug resistance proteins (MRPs in humans; Mrps in rodents). Additionally, transporters that facilitate drug entry into the brain are also expressed at the BBB. For example, OATPs (humans)/Oatps (rodents), whose transporters are bidirectional and have been shown to mediate drug transport into the brain, are also expressed on capillary endothelial cells. Other examples of uptake transporters that are endogenously expressed at the BBB include organic anion transporters (OATs in humans; Oats in rodents), organic cation transporters (OCTs in humans; Octs in rodents), nucleoside transporters, monocarboxylate transporters (MCTs in humans; Mcts in rodents), and mechanisms for peptide transport. Figure 1 is a representation of the location of several of these transporters on NVU cell types.

4. TRANSPORT ACROSS THE BRAIN BARRIERS

Several disorders of the CNS remain difficult to treat pharmacologically due to an inability of many drugs to attain efficacious concentrations in the brain. In part, this is due to active efflux transport processes that restrict blood-to-brain drug uptake. However, drugs may still cross brain barriers (i.e., BBB, brain cerebral spinal fluid (BCSF) barrier) and accumulate in the CNS by various mechanisms that favor uptake including passive diffusion, transcytosis, carrier-mediated transport, and endocytosis. A brief description of each process is provided in Fig. 2.

5. P-GLYCOPROTEIN

P-gp is a 170-kDa efflux transporter encoded by the MDR gene (Gottesman, Hrycyna, Schoenlein, Germann, & Pastan, 1995). Two MDR isoforms have been identified in human tissues, MDR-1 and

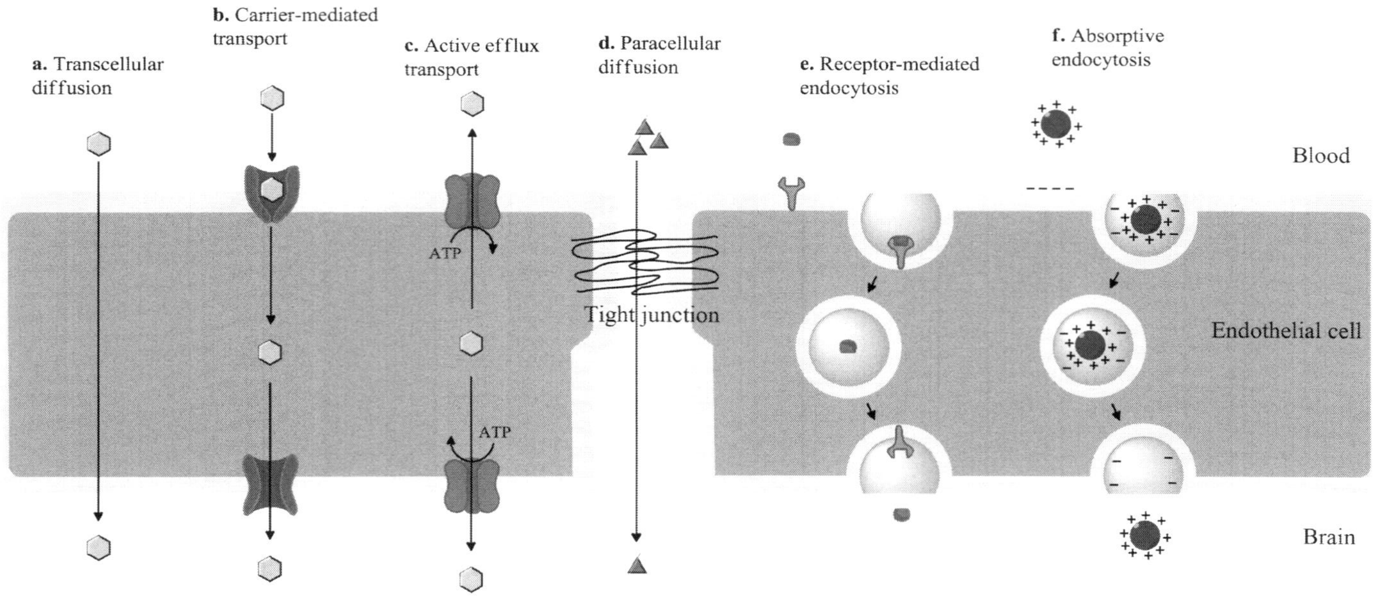

Figure 2 Methods of drug transport across the blood–brain barrier. This figure describes the various routes of delivery of xenobiotics across the BBB from transcytosis to paracellular delivery to various types of transporter-based delivery. *Adapted from Sanchez-Covarrubias et al. (2014).*

MDR-2 (Chen et al., 1986; Roninson et al., 1986); however, P-gp expression in rodent tissues is encoded by three distinct mdr isoforms (mdr-1a, mdr-1b, and mdr-2 in rats and mdr-1, mdr-2, and mdr-3 in mice). While over expression of MDR-1/mdr-1a/mdr-1b confers the MDR phenotype (Gottesman et al., 1995; Ueda, Cardarelli, Gottesman, & Pastan, 1987), MDR-2/mdr-2 is primarily expressed in the liver and is involved in transport of phosphatidylcholine into bile (Gottesman et al., 1995; Smit et al., 1993). In humans, the MDR-1 gene product is 1280 amino acids in length and consists of two homologous halves, each containing six transmembrane domains. Each homologous half also contains one ATP-binding site. Two to four glycosylation sites have been located on the first extracellular loop. Although glycosylation is necessary for localization to the plasma membrane, it is not necessary for transport function. Studies using glycosylation-deficient P-gp found lower levels of this transporter at the cell surface but transport function remained unaffected (Gribar, Ramachandra, Hrycyna, Dey, & Ambudkar, 2000). Mature P-gp is phosphorylated on the linker region between the two homologous halves (TM6–TM7) (Gottesman et al., 1995). Phosphorylation may protect nonglycosylated P-gp from being degraded by endoplasmic reticulum proteases or from undergoing proteasomal degradation prior to glycosylation and trafficking to the plasma membrane. For example, *in vitro* studies have demonstrated that activation of Pim-1 kinase, a serine/threonine kinase, decreased P-gp degradation and increased cell surface expression (Xie, Burcu, Linn, Qiu, & Baer, 2010), which suggests that phosphorylation may be a critical step in processing of a mature and functional P-gp transporter and a potential point to target for improved CNS drug delivery (Ronaldson & Davis, 2013). Studies using rat brain endothelial cells *in vitro* have also demonstrated that the physical interaction between P-gp with caveolin-1 is enhanced by tyrosine-14-phosphorylation of caveolin-1 (Barakat et al., 2007).

Since its initial discovery in Chinese hamster ovary cells (Ling & Thompson, 1974), P-gp expression has been observed in multiple barrier and nonbarrier cell types, including kidney, liver, gastrointestinal tract, placenta, and testes (Juliano & Ling, 1976). In the brain, P-gp is localized to both the luminal and abluminal membranes of the BBB endothelium (Bendayan, Ronaldson, Gingras, & Bendayan, 2006) and to the apical plasma membrane of choroid plexus epithelial cells (Rao et al., 1999). Expression of P-gp at the BBB likely evolved to protect the CNS from exposure to potentially neurotoxic xenobiotics and to maintain the precise homeostatic environment required for proper neuronal function (Sharom,

2007). Evolution favors adaptation and the maintenance of homeostasis and this is why P-gp has evolved as central to brain function during times of stress. The importance of P-gp's role in CNS protection is highlighted by studies using mdr-1a/mdr-1b knockout mice. Mdr-1a/mdr-1b null mice showed a 100-fold increase in brain uptake of ivermectin, a neurotoxic pesticide, when compared to their wild-type counterparts. Furthermore, mdr-1a/mdr-1b null mice displayed multiple symptoms of ivermectin toxicity (i.e., tremors, paralysis, coma, and death) that are directly attributed to increased brain penetration (Schinkel et al., 1994). Similar observations were reported in collies where increased sensitivity to ivermectin was directly correlated to a complete absence of the mdr-1 gene (Doran et al., 2005). Additionally, P-gp expression has been detected in brain parenchyma cellular compartments such as astrocytes, microglia, and neurons (Golden & Pardridge, 1999; Lee, Dallas, Hong, & Bendayan, 2001; Ronaldson, Bendayan, Gingras, Piquette-Miller, & Bendayan, 2004; Schlachetzki & Pardridge, 2003; Volk et al., 2004). Each of these observations points to the real possibility that P-gp has developed and evolved as the primary "gate keeper" that is critical in maintaining a safe, nontoxic environment in the brain and CNS that limits entry of many potentially toxic drugs such as morphine and other opioids (Fig. 3).

P-gp also has an immense substrate and drug profile that renders it a formidable obstacle to any/all CNS drug delivery. In fact, the number of compounds known to be P-gp substrates is continuously expanding as more and more research is done. P-gp substrates are generally nonpolar, weakly amphipathic compounds that vary considerably in molecular size. For example, P-gp is known to transport small molecule drugs such as daunorubicin (563.99 Da) as well as larger molecules such as actinomycin D (1255.42 Da) (Sharom, 2007). The list of known substrate categories includes, but is not limited to, antibiotics, calcium channel blockers, cardiac glycosides, chemotherapeutics, immunosuppressants, antiepileptics, antidepressants, and HIV-1 protease inhibitors (Demeule et al., 2002; Sun et al., 2004) (Fig. 4). Additionally, recent studies have demonstrated that many HMG CoA reductase inhibitors (i.e., pitavastatin, pravastatin) are transported across biological membranes by P-gp (Shirasaka, Suzuki, Nakanishi, & Tamai, 2011; Shirasaka, Suzuki, Shichiri, Nakanishi, & Tamai, 2011). Studies have also shown that opioid analgesic drugs such as morphine and the opioid peptide DPDPE are directly extruded from brain tissue by P-gp (Fig. 3) (Chen & Pollack, 1997, 1998; Ronaldson, Finch, Demarco, Quigley, & Davis, 2011; Seelbach, Brooks, Egleton, & Davis, 2007).

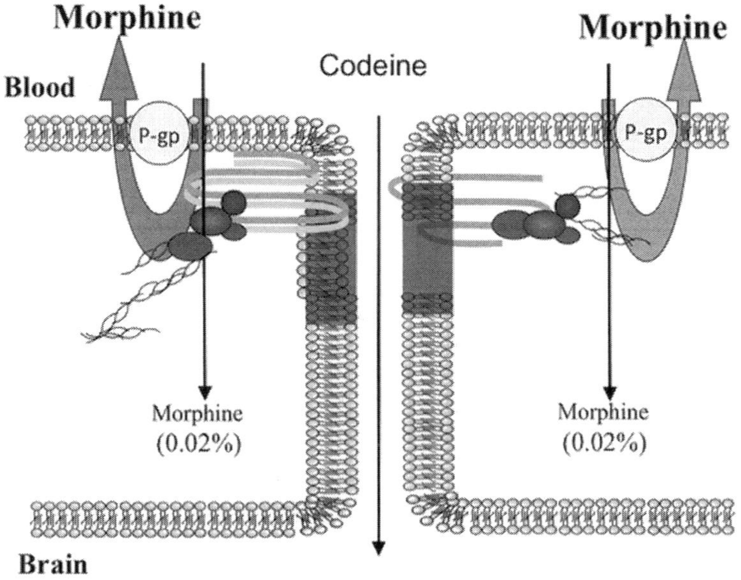

Figure 3 P-glycoprotein transporter—can it be targeted? Although preclinical evidence suggests that P-glycoprotein transport activity can be modulated with small molecule inhibitors, clinical evidence indicates that this approach cannot work. Use of small molecule inhibitors to block P-glycoprotein in clinical settings has resulted in significant toxicity associated with increased deposition of drug in peripheral tissues or due to high concentrations of the inhibitor itself. Morphine is a good example of the perils of blocking P-glycoprotein to increase drug delivery to the brain. In the setting of functional P-glycoprotein, only 0.02% of systemic morphine is able to permeate the blood–brain barrier. Blockade of P-glycoprotein at the blood–brain barrier would significantly increase this amount and lead to clinically significant adverse drug reactions (i.e., seizures).

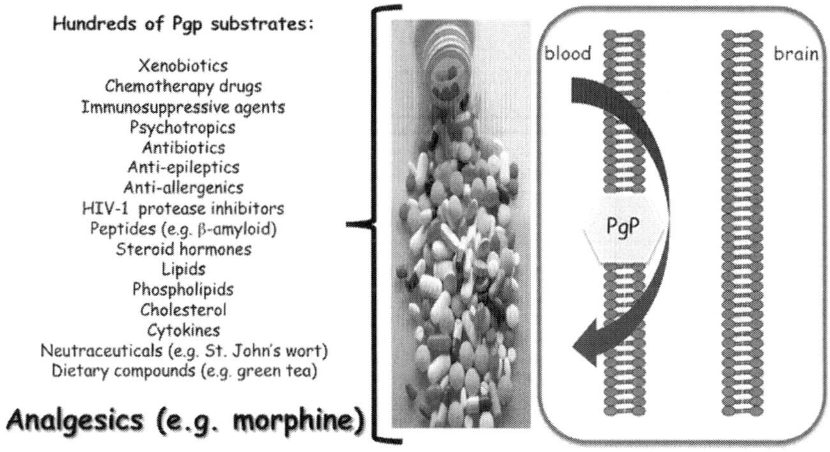

Figure 4 P-glycoprotein (P-gp) at the blood–brain barrier: the greatest molecular challenge to CNS drug delivery. Note the significant cross section of drugs and xenobiotics that are all substrates for P-gp.

Endogenous substrates of P-gp may include cytokines, lipids, steroid hormones, and peptides (Sharom, 2007).

Additionally, several substrates of P-gp have been found to be competitive transport inhibitors. Examples of such drugs include calcium channel blockers (i.e., verapamil), antipsychotics (i.e., chlorpromazine), immunosuppressive agents (i.e., cyclosporine A), and the cyclosporine A analog PSC 833 (i.e., valspodar) (Sharom, 2007). HMG CoA reductase inhibitors have also been found to block P-gp transport function, and several studies are exploring the possibility of using these drugs to reverse P-gp-induced drug resistance in tumor cells (Goard et al., 2010).

6. DRUG DELIVERY TO THE CNS: STRATEGIES DEVELOPED TO CIRCUMVENT BRAIN BARRIER SITES

The BBB is a formidable obstacle to drug delivery. Transcellular permeability of compounds across the BBB is complex and regulated by expression of various transporter proteins (Fig. 2). In fact, the overall balance of these transporters is a critical determinant in CNS permeation of multiple therapeutic drugs. Restricted entry of therapeutic compounds into the CNS results in ineffectual treatment of CNS disorders such as epilepsy, brain cancer, HIV-associated neurocognitive disease, cerebral hypoxia, ischemic stroke, and peripheral inflammatory pain. Therefore, several therapeutic strategies have been developed to circumvent the BBB and improve CNS drug delivery. Among those developed, some efforts have involved invasive procedures such as forced, mechanical opening of the BBB that can cause undesirable side effects and extensive tissue pathology. Other efforts have focused on circumventing those efflux transporters (i.e., P-gp, MRPs/Mrps, BCRP/Bcrp) that severely limit entry of therapeutic compounds into the brain. While efflux transporter inhibition has achieved modest success in improving CNS drug permeability, their utility is greatly limited by adverse drug reactions that may occur due to increased drug concentrations in the brain and other peripheral tissues. Recently, there is a growing interest in exploiting other transport systems to improve drug delivery, including targeting endogenous influx transporters expressed at brain barrier sites such as Oatp1a4. The following section will provide a brief overview of several methods for drug delivery to the CNS that have been developed to date as well as suggest novel approaches based on recent findings.

7. INHIBITION OF BRAIN BARRIER EFFLUX TRANSPORTERS

In order to circumvent efflux transporters at brain barrier sites, particularly P-gp, pharmacological inhibitors have been developed with the intent of enabling greater penetration of drugs into the CNS. Such studies have shown mixed results with regard to efficacy and safety of these inhibitory compounds. The first generation of P-gp inhibitors was identified in the early 1980s. Despite their ability to inhibit P-gp transport activity and increase delivery cellular drug permeation, the doses required to be effective inhibitors were extremely high and resulted in both toxicity and unwanted pharmacokinetic interactions (Thomas & Coley, 2003). Second-generation inhibitors, such as PSC833 (i.e., valspodar), are much more potent than their predecessors and do exhibit less toxicity. However, PSC833 demonstrated disappointing results in clinical studies, with only modest increases in CNS drug delivery (Thomas & Coley, 2003). Additionally, this generation of inhibitors significantly inhibited metabolism and excretion of cytotoxic agents. These unexpected effects necessitated reduction in chemotherapy doses to levels that were no longer efficacious (Thomas & Coley, 2003).

An ability to selectively modulate P-gp activity has the potential to impact treatment of numerous CNS pathologies and alter disease progression. Accumulated research suggests that P-gp affects CNS drug uptake in a plethora of diseases including inflammation, pain, epilepsy, HIV, brain cancer (McCaffrey et al., 2012; Miller, Bauer, & Hartz, 2008; Seelbach et al., 2007; Zhang, Kwan, Zuo, & Baum, 2012), and cerebral ischemia (Miller et al., 2008; Spudich et al., 2006; Thompson & Ronaldson, this volume). These data support a role for P-gp in treatment response. Although there is consensus that P-gp plays a role in the ability to treat disease at the level of the CNS, there are inconsistencies in the data particularly when P-gp inhibitors are used. Further, the failure of available P-gp inhibitors to improve clinical outcome has been discouraging. There is also some evidence that P-gp is involved in Alzheimer disease (Cirrito et al., 2005; Hartz, Miller, & Bauer, 2010); decreased P-gp function has been observed in Alzheimer patients compared to healthy control subjects (van Assema et al., 2012). These data suggest that P-gp can impact disease progression. However, there is a study showing that β-amyloid clearance in a rat Alzheimer disease model did not decrease after treatment with P-gp inhibitors (Ito, Ohtsuki, & Terasaki, 2006). Each of the pathologies in which P-gp potentially plays a role is complex and the contribution of P-gp to treatment response or pathogenesis is still being defined. The complexity of this issue indicates that an understanding of signaling and trafficking pathways that lead to increased (or decreased) P-gp activity in each pathological condition is necessary to identify novel drug targets and regulate P-gp in a context-dependent way. A more nuanced approach to P-gp regulation may succeed where direct inhibition of P-gp has failed.

Recent work elucidating mechanisms that regulate changes in P-gp functional expression has suggested discrete signaling pathways that can be targeted to impair P-gp function and improve CNS drug delivery. Targeting such pathways is an attractive alternative to global inhibition of P-gp as it can lead more precise control of P-gp in specific target tissues and/or preservation of basal P-gp activity, which is critical for neuroprotection (Ronaldson & Davis, 2013). Recently, the role of sphingolipid signaling in regulating basal levels of P-gp activity was investigated. Using a confocal-based activity assay that used rat brain capillaries, investigators determined that basal activity levels were regulated via signaling through the sphingosine-1-phosphate receptor (S1PR) (Cannon, Peart, Hawkins, Campos, & Miller, 2012). Exposure of brain capillaries to sphingosine-1-phosphate (S1P), a bioactive lipid metabolite and endogenous ligand for S1PR1, resulted in a reduction in P-gp-mediated drug efflux (Cannon et al., 2012). Removal of S1P from the capillary media restored P-gp efflux activity to levels seen in the control group, demonstrating that signaling via S1PR can allow for transient modulation of P-gp-mediated efflux activity. Changes in P-gp function observed in isolated brain capillaries were validated *in vivo* using the *in situ* perfusion technique. Animals treated with S1P or the S1P analog, fingolimod (FTY720), exhibited increased brain uptake of radiolabeled verapamil, loperamide, and paclitaxel, demonstrating reduced P-gp activity *in vivo* (Cannon et al., 2012). The use of an S1PR1-specific antagonist or inhibition of G-protein-coupled receptor signaling blocked this effect (Cannon et al., 2012). While targeting S1PR1 directly may prove to be a useful method for controlling efflux transport at the BBB, data from this study also suggest that additional targets for therapeutic development lie downstream in the S1PR signaling pathway. Characterization of the signaling events that result in S1P production (Cannon et al., 2012 and references therein) and the recent finding that Mrp1 is critical for the sphingolipid signaling events that alter P-gp activity at the mouse BBB (Cartwright, Campos, Cannon, & Miller, 2013) indicate that there is also potential for therapeutic intervention upstream of S1PR signaling.

Our studies measuring the effects of peripheral inflammatory pain, induced by λ-carrageenan injection into the rat footpad, on CNS drug delivery indicate that the protein–protein interactions that govern P-gp trafficking and complex formation are also potential drug targets. Protein transport from one subcellular location to another results directly from specific protein–protein interactions that are governed by unique motifs encoded within a protein's primary sequence. P-gp has a binding motif in its N-terminus for caveolin-1, a key scaffolding protein. Studies using rat brain endothelial cells *in vitro* have demonstrated that the physical interaction between P-gp with caveolin-1 is enhanced by tyrosine-14-phosphorylation of caveolin-1, and that the binding of P-gp to caveolin-1 negatively regulates P-gp function (Barakat et al., 2007). Our *in vivo* work showed that peripheral inflammatory pain causes a redistribution of P-gp, total caveolin-1, and tyrosine-14-phosphorylated caveolin-1 in rat brain microvessels, suggesting movement of these proteins to different subcellular locations (McCaffrey et al., 2012) (Fig. 5). Trafficking of these proteins is accompanied by increased P-gp activity (McCaffrey et al., 2012) and decreased accumulation of morphine in the brain (Seelbach et al., 2007). These data suggest that a further characterization of peripheral inflammatory pain-induced trafficking events will identify potential therapeutic targets. Additionally, demonstration of a vascular endothelial growth factor (VEGF)-induced rapid reduction of P-gp efflux function at the BBB through endocytosis further highlights the potential that therapeutic manipulation of a trafficking pathway may have in temporarily reducing P-gp efflux activity at the luminal membrane (Hawkins, Rigor, & Miller, 2010).

Peripheral inflammatory pain causes disassembly of high molecular weight complexes containing P-gp (McCaffrey et al., 2012). The disassembly process includes a loss or rearrangement of disulfide bonds that are accessible to aqueous reducing agents (McCaffrey et al., 2012). These data suggest that redox processes are involved in the activation/trafficking of P-gp. Recent data indicate that drug-mediated ATPase activity in P-gp depends on formation of specific disulfide bonds after the binding of the ATP molecule (Loo, Bartlett, & Clarke, 2013). The redox-dependent changes we see could be direct, i.e., rearrangements of disulfide bonds within P-gp complexes catalyzed by enzymatic processes, or occur via redox-dependent signaling pathways. An ability to block disassembly of higher-order P-gp complexes and maintain a major portion of the P-gp in an inactive form in reservoirs would provide a unique opportunity to titrate P-gp activity as described in Fig. 6. This would allow maintenance of basal P-gp activity

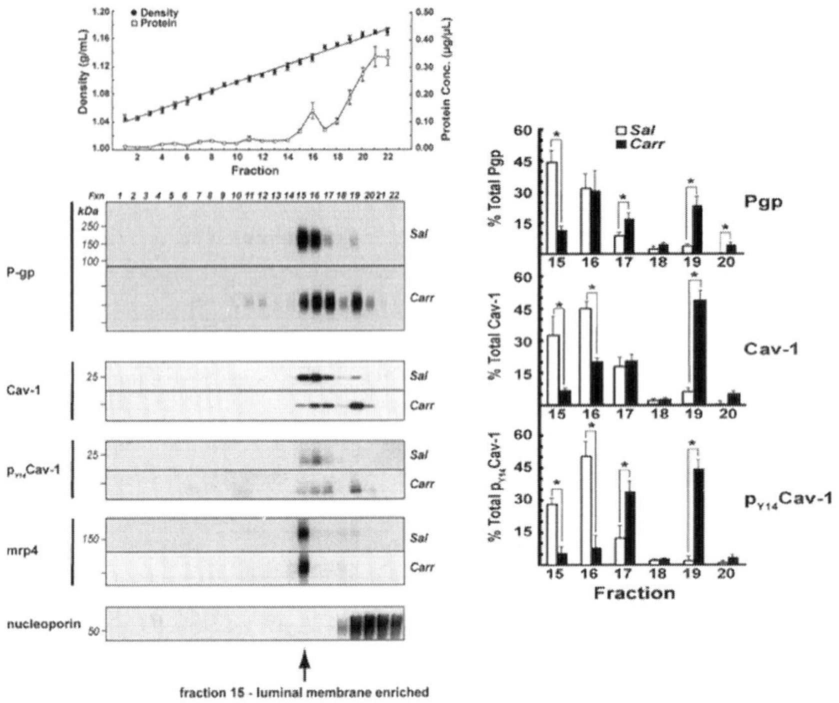

Figure 5 P-glycoprotein (P-gp) trafficking within caveolin-enriched domains modulated by peripheral inflammatory pain. These data show that the previously characterized increase, *in vivo*, of P-glycoprotein functional activity, at 3 h postinflammatory pain, was associated with a dynamic redistribution of P-glycoprotein between microvascular endothelial cell subcellular compartments. The top panel shows the typical OptiPrep density gradient profile of fractions from previously intact rat microvessels. P-gp and the key scaffolding protein caveolin were both shown to be associated with luminal membrane-enriched fractions 15 and 16 (bottom panel) and dynamically trafficked to higher-density fractions after the pain stimulus. No trafficking change was noted for the brain efflux transporter Mrp4 after a peripheral pain stimulus to the rats. *Adapted from McCaffrey et al. (2012).*

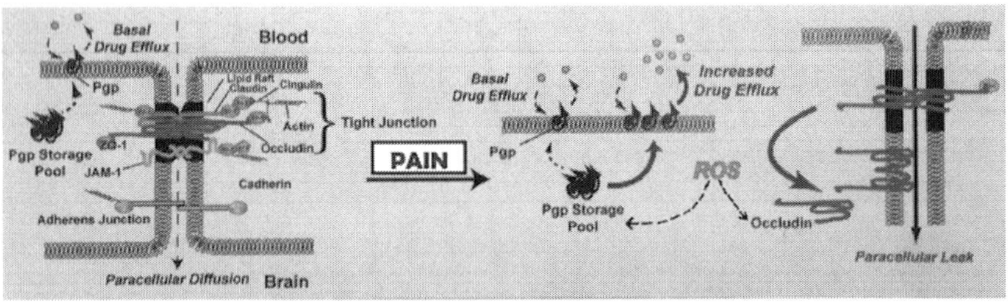

Figure 6 Model indicating proposed molecular targets of peripheral inflammatory pain-induced reactive oxygen species (ROS) that account for the compromised blood–brain barrier observed during peripheral inflammatory pain.

to protect against xenobiotic toxicity while preventing the increased P-gp activity that inhibits effective CNS drug delivery. With the increasing availability of redox-based therapeutics, characterizing the redox reactions and signaling that occur during P-gp trafficking/activation after a peripheral inflammatory pain stimulus could suggest new applications of redox-based drugs to improve CNS drug delivery (Fig. 6).

Our studies measuring the effects of peripheral inflammatory pain on CNS drug delivery indicate that transforming growth factor-β1 (TGF-β1) signaling could also be manipulated to improve drug uptake into the brain. TGF-β1 is a critical regulator of brain microvascular homeostasis (Lebrin, Deckers, Bertolino, & ten Dijke, 2005). During peripheral inflammatory pain, serum TGF-β1 decreased concomitant with activin receptor-like kinase-1 (ALK1)/activin receptor-like kinase-5 (ALK5) signaling (Ronaldson, Demarco, Sanchez-Covarrubias, Solinsky, & Davis, 2009). Administration of diclofenac, a commonly prescribed nonsteroidal anti-inflammatory drug (NSAID), prevented decreases in serum TGF-β as well as reduced microvascular expression of ALK1/ALK5, suggesting that inflammatory pain in the periphery is directly involved in overall regulation of the TGF-β signaling pathway (Ronaldson et al., 2011). Furthermore, pharmacological inhibition of TGF-β/ALK5 signaling using SB431542 increased the Oatp1a4 drug uptake transporter functional expression both in animals subjected to peripheral inflammatory pain and in corresponding saline controls (Ronaldson et al., 2011). Although studies in immortalized mouse brain endothelial cells (MBE4) have shown involvement of ALK5-mediated signaling in P-gp transporter regulation (Dohgu et al., 2004), we are the first to report TGF-β/ALK5 signaling regulation of any endogenous BBB drug uptake transporter. Our work on TGF-β/ALK5 signaling demonstrated that this pathway could regulate permeability at the BBB both by altering the structure of tight junction protein complexes and by increasing functional expression of an influx transporter. Furthermore, these studies highlight the potential of the TGF-β/ALK5 pathway as a pharmacological target that can be utilized to precisely control functional expression of a BBB influx transporter for optimization of CNS drug delivery.

8. CONCLUSION

The field of BBB biology and particularly the study of endogenous xenobiotic transport systems have rapidly advanced over the past two decades. For example, it is now well established that tight junctions between the capillary endothelial cells effectively limit paracellular drug diffusion while expression of various efflux transporters (i.e., P-gp, OATPs/Oatps, MRPs/Mrps, BCRP/Bcrp) interacts with a multitude of therapeutic compounds, further restricting their influx or efflux at the brain parenchyma. Additionally, many previous studies reported on the controversial ability of drug transporters (i.e., Oatp1a4 and P-gp) to act as facilitators of brain drug uptake. Now, it is beginning to be appreciated that endogenous BBB transporters can facilitate uptake of xenobiotics from blood to the brain, thereby rendering these transport proteins potential targets for optimizing CNS drug delivery. Furthermore, molecular machinery involved in regulating endogenous BBB transport systems (i.e., TGF-β/ALK5 signaling, nuclear receptor systems, protein–protein signaling) and mechanisms governing intracellular trafficking of BBB transporters are just now being identified and characterized. These critical discoveries have identified multiple molecular targets that can be exploited for optimization of CNS delivery of therapeutic agents. Such studies are particularly critical for newly developed therapeutics such as opioid analgesic peptides. In fact, many novel opioid peptides have been recently produced and have shown analgesic efficacy (Largent Milnes et al., 2010; Yamamoto et al., 2009); however, molecular and trafficking mechanisms involved in their CNS delivery have yet to be identified. Discovery of mechanisms that determine brain permeation of these peptides will undoubtedly enable more efficient analgesia and an improved utility of these compounds as potential therapeutics. Perhaps targeting of novel opioid peptides to influx transporters such as Oatp1a4, or efflux transporters such as P-gp, which are already known to be involved in opioid peptide transport at the BBB (Ronaldson et al., 2011), will lead to significant advancements in the field of opioid pharmacology and pain management. Additionally, identification and characterization of intracellular signaling pathways, such as reactive oxygen species-sensitive pathways (Lochhead et al., 2010, 2012), and protein trafficking mechanisms (Hawkins & Davis, 2005; Lochhead et al., 2010; McCaffrey et al., 2012; Ronaldson & Davis, 2013) that can regulate functional expression/activity of uptake or efflux transporters provides an additional approach for pharmacological modulation/control of drug transporter systems in an effort to deliver therapeutics to the CNS. Future work will continue to provide more insight on the interplay of tight junction protein complexes, transporters, and intracellular protein–protein signaling pathways at the BBB and how these systems can be effectively targeted. Therapeutic manipulation of protein trafficking is only recently emerging as a novel means of modulating protein function. The advantage of therapeutic drug development focused on "relocalization" of a protein, such as P-gp or Oatp1a4, is that its physiological impact can be modified, temporarily or long term, despite pathology-induced changes in gene transcription. By targeting the trafficking of P-gp or Oatp1a4 as a novel, reversible means of optimizing CNS drug delivery, data derived from studies described in this chapter and ongoing work in several laboratories to understand the composition of the storage pools of transporters and how they are released in response to stress will enable achievement of more precise drug concentrations within the CNS and improved treatment for pathological conditions.

CONFLICT OF INTEREST

The authors have no conflicts of interest to report.

ACKNOWLEDGMENTS

The authors acknowledge the financial support by the NINDS and NIDA of the NIH. RO1 Grants NS 42652-15 and DA 11271-16 to T. P. D. funded this work.

REFERENCES

Barakat, S., Demeule, M., Pilorget, A., Regina, A., Gingras, D., Baggetto, L. G., et al. (2007). Modulation of p-glycoprotein function by caveolin-1 phosphorylation. *Journal of Neurochemistry*, *101*, 1–8.

Bendayan, R., Lee, G., & Bendayan, M. (2002). Functional expression and localization of P-glycoprotein at the blood brain barrier. *Microscopy Research and Technique*, *57*, 365–380.

Bendayan, R., Ronaldson, P. T., Gingras, D., & Bendayan, M. (2006). In situ localization of P-glycoprotein (ABCB1) in human and rat brain. *The Journal of Histochemistry and Cytochemistry*, *54*, 1159–1167.

Betz, A. L., Firth, J. A., & Goldstein, G. W. (1980). Polarity of the blood-brain barrier: Distribution of enzymes between the luminal and antiluminal membranes of brain capillary endothelial cells. *Brain Research*, *192*, 17–28.

Cannon, R. E., Peart, J. C., Hawkins, B. T., Campos, C. R., & Miller, D. S. (2012). Targeting blood-brain barrier sphingolipid signaling reduces basal P-glycoprotein activity and improves drug delivery to the brain. *Proceedings of the National Academy of Sciences of the United States of America*, *109*, 15930–15935.

Cartwright, T. A., Campos, C. R., Cannon, R. E., & Miller, D. S. (2013). Mrp1 is essential for sphingolipid signaling to p-glycoprotein in mouse blood-brain and blood-spinal cord barriers. *Journal of Cerebral Blood Flow and Metabolism*, *33*, 381–388.

Chen, C. J., Chin, J. E., Ueda, K., Clark, D. P., Pastan, I., Gottesman, M. M., et al. (1986). Internal duplication and homology with bacterial transport proteins in the mdr1 (P-glycoprotein) gene from multidrug-resistant human cells. *Cell*, *47*, 381–389.

Chen, C., & Pollack, G. M. (1997). Extensive biliary excretion of the model opioid peptide [D-PEN2,5] enkephalin in rats. *Pharmaceutical Research*, *14*, 345–350.

Chen, C., & Pollack, G. M. (1998). Altered disposition and antinociception of [D-penicillamine(2,5)] enkephalin in mdr1a-gene-deficient mice. *The Journal of Pharmacology and Experimental Therapeutics*, *287*, 545–552.

Cirrito, J. R., Deane, R., Fagan, A. M., Spinner, M. L., Parsadanian, M., Finn, M. B., et al. (2005). P-glycoprotein deficiency at the blood-brain barrier increases amyloid-beta deposition in an Alzheimer disease mouse model. *Journal of Clinical Investigation, 115*, 3285–3290.

Demeule, M., Regina, A., Jodoin, J., Laplante, A., Dagenais, C., Berthelet, F., et al. (2002). Drug transport to the brain: Key roles for the efflux pump P-glycoprotein in the blood-brain barrier. *Vascular Pharmacology, 38*, 339–348.

Dohgu, S., Yamauchi, A., Takata, F., Naito, M., Tsuruo, T., Higuchi, S., et al. (2004). Transforming growth factor-beta1 upregulates the tight junction and P-glycoprotein of brain microvascular endothelial cells. *Cellular and Molecular Neurobiology, 24*, 491–497.

Doran, A., Obach, R. S., Smith, B. J., Hosea, N. A., Becker, S., Callegari, E., et al. (2005). The impact of P-glycoprotein on the disposition of drugs targeted for indications of the central nervous system: Evaluation using the MDR1A/1B knockout mouse model. *Drug Metabolism and Disposition, 33*, 165–174.

Goard, C. A., Mather, R. G., Vinepal, B., Clendening, J. W., Martirosyan, A., Boutros, P. C., et al. (2010). Differential interactions between statins and P-glycoprotein: Implications for exploiting statins as anticancer agents. *International Journal of Cancer, 127*, 2936–2948.

Golden, P. L., & Pardridge, W. M. (1999). P-Glycoprotein on astrocyte foot processes of unfixed isolated human brain capillaries. *Brain Research, 819*, 143–146.

Gottesman, M. M., Hrycyna, C. A., Schoenlein, P. V., Germann, U. A., & Pastan, I. (1995). Genetic analysis of the multidrug transporter. *Annual Review of Genetics, 29*, 607–649.

Gribar, J. J., Ramachandra, M., Hrycyna, C. A., Dey, S., & Ambudkar, S. V. (2000). Functional characterization of glycosylation-deficient human P-glycoprotein using a vaccinia virus expression system. *The Journal of Membrane Biology, 173*, 203–214.

Hartz, A. M., Miller, D. S., & Bauer, B. (2010). Restoring blood-brain barrier P-glycoprotein reduces brain amyloid-beta in a mouse model of Alzheimer's disease. *Molecular Pharmacology, 77*, 715–723.

Hawkins, B. T., & Davis, T. P. (2005). The blood-brain barrier/neurovascular unit in health and disease. *Pharmacological Reviews, 57*, 173–185.

Hawkins, B. T., Rigor, R. R., & Miller, D. S. (2010). Rapid loss of blood-brain barrier P-glycoprotein activity through transporter internalization demonstrated using a novel in situ proteolysis protection assay. *Journal of Cerebral Blood Flow and Metabolism, 30*, 1593–1597.

Ito, S., Ohtsuki, S., & Terasaki, T. (2006). Functional characterization of the brain-to-blood efflux clearance of human amyloid-beta peptide (1–40) across the rat blood-brain barrier. *Neuroscience Research, 56*, 246–252.

Juliano, R. L., & Ling, V. (1976). A surface glycoprotein modulating drug permeability in Chinese hamster ovary cell mutants. *Biochimica et Biophysica Acta, 455*, 152–162.

Largent-Milnes, T. M., Yamamoto, T., Nair, P., Moulton, J. W., Hruby, V. J., Lai, J., et al. (2010). Spinal or systemic TY005, a peptidic opioid agonist/neurokinin 1 antagonist, attenuates pain with reduced tolerance. *British Journal of Pharmacology, 161*, 986–1001.

Lebrin, F., Deckers, M., Bertolino, P., & ten Dijke, P. (2005). TGF-beta receptor function in the endothelium. *Cardiovascular Research, 65*, 599–608.

Lee, G., Dallas, S., Hong, M., & Bendayan, R. (2001). Drug transporters in the central nervous system: Brain barriers and brain parenchyma considerations. *Pharmacological Reviews, 53*, 569–596.

Ling, V., & Thompson, L. H. (1974). Reduced permeability in CHO cells as a mechanism of resistance to colchicine. *Journal of Cellular Physiology, 83*, 103–116.

Lochhead, J. J., McCaffrey, G., Quigley, C. E., Finch, J., Demarco, K. M., Nametz, N., et al. (2010). Oxidative stress increases blood-brain barrier permeability and induces alterations in occludin during hypoxia-reoxygenation. *Journal of Cerebral Blood Flow and Metabolism, 30*, 1625–1636.

Lochhead, J. J., McCaffrey, G., Sanchez-Covarrubias, L., Finch, J. D., Demarco, K. M., Quigley, C. E., et al. (2012). Tempol modulates changes in xenobiotic permeability and occludin oligomeric assemblies at the blood-brain barrier during inflammatory pain. *American Journal of Physiology Heart and Circulatory Physiology, 302*, H582–H593.

Loo, T. W., Bartlett, M. C., & Clarke, D. M. (2013). Human P-glycoprotein contains a greasy ball-and-socket joint at the second transmission interface. *The Journal of Biological Chemistry, 288*, 20326–20333.

McCaffrey, G., Staatz, W. D., Sanchez-Covarrubias, L., Finch, J. D., Demarco, K., Laracuente, M. L., et al. (2012). P-glycoprotein trafficking at the blood-brain barrier altered by peripheral inflammatory hyperalgesia. *Journal of Neurochemistry, 122*, 962–975.

Miller, D. S., Bauer, B., & Hartz, A. M. (2008). Modulation of P-glycoprotein at the blood-brain barrier: Opportunities to improve central nervous system pharmacotherapy. *Pharmacological Reviews, 60*, 196–209.

Oldendorf, W. H., Cornford, M. E., & Brown, W. J. (1977). The large apparent work capability of the blood-brain barrier: A study of the mitochondrial content of capillary endothelial cells in brain and other tissues of the rat. *Annals of Neurology, 1*, 409–417.

Rao, V. V., Dahlheimer, J. L., Bardgett, M. E., Snyder, A. Z., Finch, R. A., Sartorelli, A. C., et al. (1999). Choroid plexus epithelial expression of MDR1 P glycoprotein and multidrug resistance-associated protein contribute to the blood-cerebrospinal-fluid drug-permeability barrier. *Proceedings of the National Academy of Sciences of the United States of America, 96*, 3900–3905.

Rolfe, D. F., & Brown, G. C. (1997). Cellular energy utilization and molecular origin of standard metabolic rate in mammals. *Physiological Reviews*, 77, 731–758.

Ronaldson, P. T., Bendayan, M., Gingras, D., Piquette-Miller, M., & Bendayan, R. (2004). Cellular localization and functional expression of P-glycoprotein in rat astrocyte cultures. *Journal of Neurochemistry, 89*, 788–800.

Ronaldson, P. T., & Davis, T. P. (2013). Targeted drug delivery to treat pain and cerebral hypoxia. *Pharmacological Reviews, 65*, 291–314.

Ronaldson, P. T., Demarco, K. M., Sanchez-Covarrubias, L., Solinsky, C. M., & Davis, T. P. (2009). Transforming growth factor-beta signaling alters substrate permeability and tight junction protein expression at the blood-brain barrier during inflammatory pain. *Journal of Cerebral Blood Flow and Metabolism, 29*, 1084–1098.

Ronaldson, P. T., Finch, J. D., Demarco, K. M., Quigley, C. E., & Davis, T. P. (2011). Inflammatory pain signals an increase in functional expression of organic anion transporting polypeptide 1a4 at the blood-brain barrier. *The Journal of Pharmacology and Experimental Therapeutics, 336*, 827–839.

Roninson, I. B., Chin, J. E., Choi, K. G., Gros, P., Housman, D. E., Fojo, A., et al. (1986). Isolation of human mdr DNA sequences amplified in multidrug-resistant KB carcinoma cells. *Proceedings of the National Academy of Sciences of the United States of America, 83*, 4538–4542.

Sanchez del Pino, M. M., Peterson, D. R., & Hawkins, R. A. (1995). Neutral amino acid transport characterization of isolated luminal and abluminal membranes of the blood-brain barrier. *The Journal of Biological Chemistry, 270*, 14913–14918.

Sanchez-Covarrubias, L., Slosky, L. M., Thompson, B. J., Davis, T. P., & Ronaldson, P. T. (2014). Transporters at CNS barrier sites: Obstacles or opportunities for drug delivery? *Current Pharmaceutical Design, 20*, 1422–1449.

Schinkel, A. H., Smit, J. J., van Tellingen, O., Beijnen, J. H., Wagenaar, E., van Deemter, L., et al. (1994). Disruption of the mouse mdr1a P-glycoprotein gene leads to a deficiency in the blood-brain barrier and to increased sensitivity to drugs. *Cell*, 77, 491–502.

Schlachetzki, F., & Pardridge, W. M. (2003). P-glycoprotein and caveolin-1alpha in endothelium and astrocytes of primate brain. *Neuroreport, 14*, 2041–2046.
Seelbach, M. J., Brooks, T. A., Egleton, R. D., & Davis, T. P. (2007). Peripheral inflammatory hyperalgesia modulates morphine delivery to the brain: A role for P-glycoprotein. *Journal of Neurochemistry, 102*, 1677–1690.
Sharom, F. J. (2007). Multidrug resistance protein: P-glycoprotein. In G. You, & M. E. Morris (Eds.), *Drug transporters: Molecular characterization and role in drug disposition* (pp. 263–318). Hoboken, NJ: John Wiley & Sons.
Shirasaka, Y., Suzuki, K., Nakanishi, T., & Tamai, I. (2011). Differential effect of grapefruit juice on intestinal absorption of statins due to inhibition of organic anion transporting polypeptide and/or P-glycoprotein. *Journal of Pharmaceutical Sciences, 100*, 3843–3853.
Shirasaka, Y., Suzuki, K., Shichiri, M., Nakanishi, T., & Tamai, I. (2011). Intestinal absorption of HMG-CoA reductase inhibitor pitavastatin mediated by organic anion transporting polypeptide and P-glycoprotein/multidrug resistance 1. *Drug Metabolism and Pharmacokinetics, 26*, 171–179.
Smit, J. J., Schinkel, A. H., Oude Elferink, R. P., Groen, A. K., Wagenaar, E., van Deemter, L., et al. (1993). Homozygous disruption of the murine mdr2 P-glycoprotein gene leads to a complete absence of phospholipid from bile and to liver disease. *Cell, 75*, 451–462.
Spudich, A., Kilic, E., Xing, H., Kilic, U., Rentsch, K. M., Wunderli-Allenspach, H., et al. (2006). Inhibition of multidrug resistance transporter-1 facilitates neuroprotective therapies after focal cerebral ischemia. *Nature Neuroscience, 9*, 487–488.
Sun, J., He, Z. G., Cheng, G., Wang, S. J., Hao, X. H., & Zou, M. J. (2004). Multidrug resistance P-glycoprotein: Crucial significance in drug disposition and interaction. *Medical Science Monitor, 10*, RA5–RA14.
Thomas, H., & Coley, H. M. (2003). Overcoming multidrug resistance in cancer: An update on the clinical strategy of inhibiting p-glycoprotein. *Cancer Control, 10*, 159–165.
Ueda, K., Cardarelli, C., Gottesman, M. M., & Pastan, I. (1987). Expression of a full-length cDNA for the human "MDR1" gene confers resistance to colchicine, doxorubicin, and vinblastine. *Proceedings of the National Academy of Sciences of the United States of America, 84*, 3004–3008.
van Assema, D. M., Lubberink, M., Bauer, M., van der Flier, W. M., Schuit, R. C., Windhorst, A. D., et al. (2012). Blood-brain barrier P-glycoprotein function in Alzheimer's disease. *Brain, 135*, 181–189.
Volk, H. A., Burkhardt, K., Potschka, H., Chen, J., Becker, A., & Loscher, W. (2004). Neuronal expression of the drug efflux transporter P-glycoprotein in the rat hippocampus after limbic seizures. *Neuroscience, 123*, 751–759.
Vorbrodt, A. W., & Dobrogowska, D. H. (2003). Molecular anatomy of intercellular junctions in brain endothelial and epithelial barriers: Electron microscopist's view. *Brain Research. Brain Research Reviews, 42*, 221–242.
Xie, Y., Burcu, M., Linn, D. E., Qiu, Y., & Baer, M. R. (2010). Pim-1 kinase protects P-glycoprotein from degradation and enables its glycosylation and cell surface expression. *Molecular Pharmacology, 78*, 310–318.
Yamamoto, T., Nair, P., Jacobsen, N. E., Vagner, J., Kulkarni, V., Davis, P., et al. (2009). Improving metabolic stability by glycosylation: Bifunctional peptide derivatives that are opioid receptor agonists and neurokinin 1 receptor antagonists. *Journal of Medicinal Chemistry, 52*, 5164–5175.
Zhang, C., Kwan, P., Zuo, Z., & Baum, L. (2012). The transport of antiepileptic drugs by P-glycoprotein. *Advanced Drug Delivery Reviews, 64*, 930–942.

CHAPTER THREE

Functional Expression of Drug Transporters in Glial Cells: Potential Role on Drug Delivery to the CNS

Tamima Ashraf, Amy Kao, Reina Bendayan[1]
Department of Pharmaceutical Sciences, Leslie Dan Faculty of Pharmacy, University of Toronto, Toronto, Ontario, Canada
[1]Corresponding author: e-mail address: r.bendayan@utoronto.ca

Contents

Abstract

Drug permeability in the central nervous system (CNS) across blood–brain and blood–cerebrospinal fluid barriers is an important determinant of neurological disorders therapeutic efficacy and is highly regulated by the expression of membrane-associated transporters belonging to the ATP-binding cassette (ABC) and solute carrier (SLC) superfamilies. Functional expression of ABC efflux transporters exists not only at the brain barriers (primary biochemical barrier) but also in astrocytes, microglia, neurons, and oligodendrocytes can significantly restrict drug penetration into these cells, thus creating a secondary biochemical barrier to permeability in brain parenchyma. In contrast, SLC

Advances in Pharmacology, Volume 71
ISSN 1054-3589
http://dx.doi.org/10.1016/bs.apha.2014.06.010

members primarily contribute to the uptake of endogenous substrates (i.e., hormones, neurotransmitters) and pharmacological agents and can play a critical role in maintaining CNS homeostasis and drug response. In this chapter, we review the functional expression and localization of drug transporters in the brain, their role in CNS drug delivery, and their regulation in neuropathological conditions.

ABBREVIATIONS

Aβ amyloid-β
ABC ATP-binding cassette
AD Alzheimer's disease
AEDs antiepileptic drugs
BBB blood–brain barrier
BCRP breast cancer resistance protein
BCSFB blood-cerebrospinal fluid barrier
BMECs brain microvessel endothelial cells
CNS central nervous system
CNTs concentrative nucleoside transporters
CSF Cerebrospinal fluid
ENTs equilibrative nucleoside transporters
GFAP Glial fibrillary acidic protein
GSH glutathione
GSSG glutathione disulfide
HIV-1 human immunodeficiency virus type-1
LPS Lipopolysaccharide
LTC_4 Leukotrienes C_4
LTD_4 Leukotrienes D_4
LTE_4 Leukotrienes E_4
MAPK mitogen-activated protein kinase pathway
MCTs monocarboxylate transporters
MDR multidrug resistance
MRP multidrug resistance-associated protein
NF-κB nuclear factor-κB
OAT Organic anion transporter
OATP Organic anion transporting polypeptide
OCT Organic cation transporter
OCTN Organic carnitine transporter
PD Parkinson's disease
P-gp P-glycoprotein
PMEA 9-(2-phosphonomethoxyethyl)-adenine
SLC solute carrier
TEA tetraethyl ammonium
TMD Transmembrane domain

1. INTRODUCTION

Effective pharmacotherapy of central nervous system (CNS) diseases and/or infections is dependent on the permeability of drugs across the blood–brain barrier (BBB) and blood–cerebrospinal fluid barrier (BCSFB) as well as into brain parenchymal cellular compartments. Permeability of a number of drugs across the BBB can be significantly restricted due to the expression of drug efflux transporters belonging to ATP-binding cassette (ABC) superfamily. Cellular membranes of parenchymal cells are also known to express functional drug efflux transporters. Studies have demonstrated expression of ABC transporters in astrocytes, microglia, oligodendrocytes, and neurons. Over a decade ago, our laboratory has proposed that cellular membranes of parenchymal cells can serve as a secondary barrier to drug permeability within the CNS (Lee, Dallas, Hong, & Bendayan, 2001). In addition to ABC transporters, many members of the solute carrier (SLC) transporter family are also expressed at the level of the BBB, BCSFB, and in brain parenchymal cellular compartments that allow uptake of endogenously secreted compounds (i.e., nutrients, hormones, neurotransmitters) as well as pharmacological agents. Functional expression of both ABC and SLC transporters in the brain plays a major role in regulating CNS drug disposition. The objective of this chapter are (i) to review the localization, function, and substrate specificity of both ABC and SLC family members in brain parenchymal cellular compartments; (ii) to discuss the regulation of these transporters in brain parenchyma in the context of neurological disorders; and (iii) to address the potential role that these transporters may play in drug delivery and disposition in the brain.

2. PHYSIOLOGICAL ROLE OF THE BBB AND BRAIN PARENCHYMAL CELLULAR COMPARTMENTS

The BBB is a highly dynamic physical as well as biochemical barrier (Reese & Karnovsky, 1967). Tight junctions formed between brain microvessel endothelial cells (BMECs) lining the capillary wall restrict paracellular entry, whereas efflux/influx transporters, ion channels, and receptors expressed by BMECs regulate the transcellular traffic of solutes, nutrients, and numerous xenobiotics (Abbott, Patabendige, Dolman, Yusof, &

Begley, 2010). These endothelial cells are surrounded by basal lamina, pericytes, astrocyte end-feet, and neurons. This multilayer unit is collectively referred to as neurovascular unit (Neuwelt et al., 2011). Each of the cellular units in the brain parenchyma plays a critical role in maintaining a functional BBB and brain homeostasis. Astrocytes maintain the integrity of the BBB by providing cytoskeletal support and protect the CNS from neurotoxicity by controlling the extracellular K^+ and glutamate concentration. Astrocytes also secrete various neurotrophic factors that are essential for the growth of neurons, maintenance of endothelial tight junctions, and differentiation of microglia (Abbott, Ronnback, & Hansson, 2006). Neurons transmit nerve signals through axonal processes and form the basic structural and functional component of the CNS. Besides astrocytes and neurons, the other two cell types present within the brain parenchyma are microglia and oligodendrocytes. Microglia are the brain resident immunocompetent cells that become activated during injury or pathological stimuli. Oligodendrocytes mainly form insulating myelin sheath around neuronal axons to protect them from injury. Numerous uptake transporters are expressed in brain parenchymal cells and play an important role in the traffic of many endogenous (i.e., neurotransmitters) as well as exogenous compounds. Functional expression of multiple drug efflux transporters has also been detected in brain parenchymal cellular units, particularly in astrocytes, microglia, and neurons. Therefore, cellular membranes of parenchymal cells can act as a secondary biochemical barrier to drug permeability in the brain (Lee, Dallas, et al., 2001). In addition to BBB and brain parenchyma compartments, epithelial cells lining the fenestrated capillary surrounding choroid plexus also express many influx/efflux transporters which can contribute to the regulation of drug permeability into/out of the CNS (Pardridge, 2012).

3. FUNCTIONAL EXPRESSION OF DRUG TRANSPORTERS IN GLIAL CELLS

3.1. ABC drug efflux transporters

The ABC superfamily is one of the largest and best characterized families of eukaryotic efflux transporters. These transporters are typically membrane-bound proteins that use ATP to actively expel potentially harmful exogenous or endogenous molecules and their conjugates. Within the ABC superfamily (50 known members), there are seven subfamilies (A–G). ABC family members are classified based on two consensus sequences: the two ATP-binding motifs (Walker A and Walker B) and the ABC signature C motif

(ALSGGQ). Three most extensively studied ABC proteins are the P-glycoprotein (P-gp), multidrug resistance proteins (MRPs), and breast cancer resistance protein (BCRP). These transporters were discovered in cancer cell lines that displayed resistance to a number of structurally diverse anticancer agents—a phenotype known as multidrug resistance (MDR) (Juliano & Ling, 1976). Upon completion of the human genome sequencing project, several other human MRP homologues have been found and characterized. Currently, there are 13 known isoforms of MRP (MRP1–13). In addition to conferring MDR, ABC transporters have also been identified to regulate the absorption, distribution, excretion, and clearance of several xenobiotics including pharmacological agents as well as metabolites. Polymorphisms or mutations of several of these transporters can result in interindividual differences in drug disposition as well as a number of disorders such as cystic fibrosis, Grönblad–Strandberg syndrome, Tangier disease, and Stargardt disease (Sissung et al., 2010). Localization of different ABC transporters in brain cellular compartments has been summarized in Figs. 1 and 2 and Table 1.

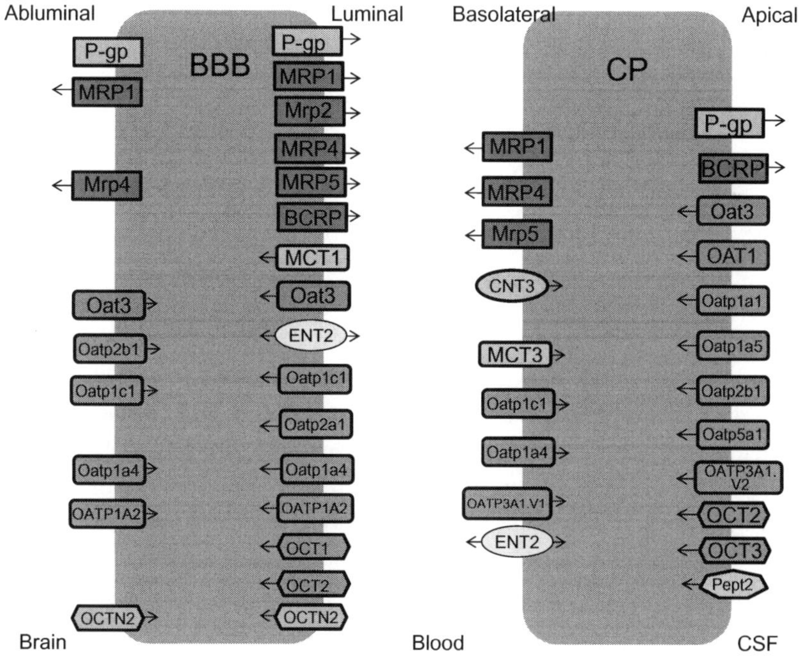

Figure 1 Localization of ABC and SLC transporters at the BBB and BCSFB. The arrows indicate the direction of substrate transport.

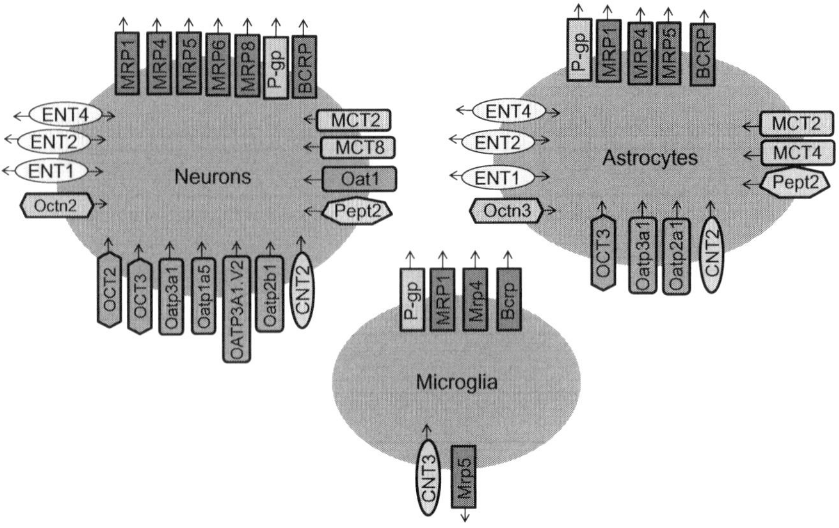

Figure 2 Localization of ABC and SLC transporters in astrocytes, microglia, and neurons. The arrows indicate the direction of substrate transport.

3.1.1 P-glycoprotein

The most extensively studied ABC transporter is the protein product encoded by the *ABCB1 (MDR1)* gene called P-gp. It was discovered in 1970 in Toronto by Victor Ling in a colchicine-resistant Chinese hamster ovary cell line (Juliano & Ling, 1976). Two isoforms of the *MDR* gene in humans (*MDR1, MDR2*) and three in rodents (*Mdr1a, Mdr1b,* and *Mdr2*) have been cloned and sequenced to date. P-gp is a 170-kDa membrane-associated glycoprotein. Topology studies reported P-gp as a transmembrane protein composed of 1276–1280 amino acids with amino- and carboxy-termini located intracellularly (Loscher & Potschka, 2005; Sharom, 2011). Structurally, P-gp has two homologous halves connected by a linker sequence. Each half contains six α-helical transmembrane domains and a nucleotide-binding domain. The nucleotide-binding domains are critical for transporter function since ATP is required to bind and hydrolyze at both nucleotide-binding domains to actively transport P-gp substrates out of the cell. The linker sequence contains several post-translational modification sites (i.e., phosphorylation, glycosylation sites) that are assumed to be necessary for correct protein folding and trafficking. Crystal structure of human P-gp is constructed based on homology models from various organisms (e.g., *Caenorhabditis elegans*, mouse, bacterial

Table 1 CNS expression/localization and substrate specificity of ABC transporters

Name	Gene	CNS expression/localization	Substrates
P-gp (ABCB1)[a]	*MDR1*	Luminal and abluminal membranes of BMECs, apical membrane of choroid plexus epithelium, astrocytes, pericytes, neurons	Anticancer, antiretroviral drugs, psychotropic drugs, antiepileptic drugs, antimicrobials, antihistamines, steroids, immunosuppressants, β-blockers, calcium channel blockers, cardiac glycosides, analgesics
P-gp (Abcb1)[b]	*mdr1a* and *mdr1b*	Luminal and abluminal membranes of BMECs, apical membrane of choroid plexus epithelium, astrocytes, microglia, pericytes, neurons	
BCRP (ABCG2)	*ABCG2*	Luminal membrane of BMECs, apical membrane of choroid plexus epithelium, astrocytes, neurons	Folic acid, vitamin K3, riboflavin, porphyrins, pheophorbide, estrone-3-sulfate, β-estradiol-17-β-D-glucuronide, dehydroepiandrosterone sulfate, uric acid, anticancer agents, antiretroviral drugs, antibiotics, calcium channel blockers, HMG-CoA reductase inhibitors, fluorescent dyes, carcinogens, tyrosine kinase inhibitors, phototoxins
Bcrp (Abcg2)	*Abcg2*	Luminal membrane of BMECs, apical membrane of choroid plexus epithelium, astrocytes, neurons, microglia, pericytes	
MRP1 (ABCC1)	*ABCC1*	Luminal membrane of BMECs, basolateral membrane of choroid plexus epithelium, astrocytes, microglia, neurons	LTC_4, LTE_4, LTD_4, GSH, GSSG and glucuronate, sulfate conjugates, folate, antiretroviral drugs, anticancer agents, antibiotics, metalloids, fluorescent dyes, toxins
Mrp1 (Abcc1)	*Abcc1*	Luminal membrane of BMECs, basolateral membrane of choroid plexus epithelium, astrocytes, microglia, neurons, oligodendrocytes	
MRP2 (ABCC2)	*ABCC2*	Not detected	Substrates are similar to the ones listed for MRP1

Continued

Table 1 CNS expression/localization and substrate specificity of ABC transporters—cont'd

Name	Gene	CNS expression/localization	Substrates
Mrp2 (Abcc2)	*Abcc2*	Luminal membrane of BMECs	
MRP3 (ABCC3)	*ABCC3*	Not detected	LTC_4, β-estradiol-17-β-D-glucuronide, glucuronide conjugates, cholylglycine, dehydroepiandrosterone sulfate, anticancer agents
Mrp3 (Abcc3)	*Abcc3*	BMECs, choroid plexus epithelium	
MRP4 (ABCC4)	*ABCC4*	Luminal membrane of BMECs, basolateral membrane of choroid plexus epithelium, astrocytes, neurons	Cyclic GMP/AMP, LTC_4, GSH conjugates, prostaglandins E_1, E_2, and $F_{2\alpha}$, thromboxane B_2, dehydroepiandrosterone sulfate, β-estradiol-17-β-D-glucuronide, folate, urate, ADP, cholate, cholylglycine, cholytaurine, eicosanoids, conjugated steroid and bile salts, nucleotide and purine analogs, 9-(2-phosphonomethoxyethyl)-adenine, 6-thioguanine, 6-mercaptopurine, antiretroviral drugs, anticancer drugs
Mrp4 (Abcc4)	*Abcc4*	Luminal and abluminal membrane of BMECs, basolateral membranes of choroid plexus epithelium, astrocytes, microglia	
MRP5 (ABCC5)	*ABCC5*	Luminal membrane of BMECs, astrocytes, neurons	Cyclic GMP/AMP, folate, cyclic nucleotides, nucleoside analogs, glutathione, methotrexate, 9-(2-phosphonomethoxyethyl)-adenine, 6-thioguanine, 6-mercaptopurine, heavy metals, antiretrovirals drugs
Mrp5 (Abcc5)	*Abcc5*	Luminal membrane of BMECs, basolateral membrane of choroid plexus epithelium, astrocytes, microglia	
MRP6 (ABCC6)	*ABCC6*	Neurons	LTC_4, *N*-ethylmaleimide, anticancer drugs
Mrp6 (Abcc6)	*Abcc6*	Unknown	

Table 1 CNS expression/localization and substrate specificity of ABC transporters—cont'd

Name	Gene	CNS expression/localization	Substrates
MRP8 (ABCC11)	*ABCC11*	Neurons	Cyclic GMP/AMP, cholylglycine, glycocholate, taurocholate, folate, GSH conjugates LTC_4, β-estradiol-17-β-D-glucuronide, estrone-3-sulfate, dehydroepiandrosterone sulfate, glycocholate, taurocholate, estrone 3-sulfate, folic acid, 9-(2-phosphonomethoxyethyl)-adenine, 5-fluorouracil, purine and pyrimidine nucleotide derivatives, anticancer drugs, methotrexate

[a]Gene nomenclature follows conventional use of uppercase letters for human protein expression.
[b]Gene nomenclature follows conventional use of only the first letter uppercase and remaining letters are lowercase for non human protein expression.
Abbreviations follow those used in the text.
Adapted from Ashraf, Kis, Banerjee, and Bendayan (2012).

Sav1866). Based on these models, it has recently been reported that intermolecular attractions (e.g., salt bridges, hydrogen bonds, van der Waals forces) between transmembrane domains and nucleotide-binding domains can promote human P-gp maturation as well as protein biosynthesis and folding (Loo & Clarke, 2013). X-ray crystal structures of mouse P-gp show a pretransport state of P-gp that consists of an internal cavity with a nucleotide-free inward facing structure. Upon ATP binding and hydrolysis at the nucleotide-binding domains, a conformational change into an outward facing structure releases the substrate (Aller et al., 2009). This model has recently been refined to identify drug-binding amino acids that were previously unrecognized (Li, Jaimes, & Aller, 2014).

Since its discovery, a large number of P-gp substrates and inhibitors have been identified. Pharmacologically relevant agents include anticancer (e.g., dasatinib, menadione, methotrexate, vincristine, vinblastine, doxorubicin), antiretroviral drugs (e.g., darunavir, atazanavir, saquinavir, indinavir, ritonavir, abacavir, raltegravir, maraviroc), psychotropic drugs (e.g., olanzapine, chlorpromazine, respiridone, haloperidol, quetiapine, fluphenazine, amitryptiline, paroxetine, venlafaxine), antiepileptic drugs (AEDs) (e.g., phenytoin, phenobarbital, acetazolamide), antimicrobials (e.g., erythromycin, salinomycin), antihistamines (e.g., fexofenadine), steroids (e.g., dexamethasone), immunosuppressants (e.g., cyclosporine, sirolimus, tacrolimus), β-blockers (e.g., bunitrolol), calcium channel blockers (e.g., azidopine, diltiazem, nifedipine), cardiac glycosides (e.g., digoxin), and analgesics (e.g., morphine, methadone, fentanyl) (Darby, Callaghan, & McMahon, 2011; Loscher & Potschka, 2005; Sharom, 2011).

In the periphery, P-gp is expressed in tissues directly involved in the absorption or elimination of pharmacological agents. In the CNS, P-gp has been localized at the BBB, both the luminal and abluminal membranes of BMECs, at the apical side of choroid plexus epithelium as well as in brain parenchymal cells: astrocytes, microglia, pericytes, and neurons (Bendayan, Ronaldson, Gingras, & Bendayan, 2006; Berezowski, Landry, Dehouck, Cecchelli, & Fenart, 2004; Virgintino et al., 2002). At the BBB, functional activity of P-gp has been extensively evaluated *in vitro*, in several mammalian BMECs cell culture systems, *in situ*, in isolated brain capillaries (Miller et al., 2000), and *in vivo*, in transgenic knockout animal models lacking P-gp (Kim et al., 1998; Robillard et al., 2014).

In astrocytes, membrane localization and distribution of P-gp were first documented in human and primate brain tissues immunostained with MRK16 monoclonal murine antibody (Pardridge, Golden, Kang, & Bickel, 1997). Confocal immunofluorescent microscopy later confirmed P-gp localization in astrocyte foot processes proximal to the brain microvasculature (Golden & Pardridge, 1999; Pardridge et al., 1997). Using immunogold cytochemistry, our laboratory also confirmed P-gp localization at the luminal and abluminal surface of BMECs as well as in pericytes and astrocyte foot processes (Bendayan et al., 2006). Expression of P-gp has also been reported in primary cultures of fetal rat astrocytes, human glioma cell lines, rhesus monkey astrocytes, and an immortalized rat astrocyte cell line CTX-TNA2 (Ballerini et al., 2002; Ronaldson & Bendayan, 2006; Ronaldson, Bendayan, Gingras, Piquette-Miller, & Bendayan, 2004; Spiegl-Kreinecker et al., 2002). In an immortalized rat brain endothelial cell line system (RBE4) cultured individually or cocultured with pericytes and astrocytes, a significant increase in the luminal efflux of P-gp substrates was observed in the coculture system, suggesting that pericytes and astrocytes can effectively improve BBB integrity and in turn induce P-gp transporter activity (Al, Taboada, Gassmann, & Ogunshola, 2011).

A recent investigation on the spatial distribution of P-gp in immortalized human cerebral microvascular endothelial cells (hCMEC/D3) showed that P-gp is randomly distributed in clusters over the plasma membrane (Huber et al., 2012). In addition to P-gp expression at the plasma membrane, subcellular localization of P-gp has also been reported. Work from our laboratory detected P-gp expression in caveolae, Golgi apparatus, nuclear envelope, cytoplasmic vesicles of BMECs, and primary cultures of rat astrocytes (Bendayan et al., 2006; Ronaldson, Lee, Dallas, & Bendayan, 2004). In addition, we also demonstrated expression and localization of the transporter at the nuclear membrane of RBE4 cells and microglia cells in culture (Babakhanian, Bendayan, & Bendayan, 2007). Such localization is also observed in several cancer cell lines and it is proposed that the transporter may play a role in MDR by preventing anticancer drugs from gaining access to the DNA (Babakhanian et al., 2007; Szaflarski et al., 2013).

Localization of P-gp in microglia was first observed by our group using immunocytochemical techniques that displayed P-gp localization along the plasma membrane and nuclear envelope of the continuous rat microglia cell line, MLS-9 (Lee, Schlichter, Bendayan, & Bendayan, 2001). In addition, we investigated functional expression of P-gp in microglia in the context of human immunodeficiency virus (HIV)-1 pharmacotherapy (Lee, Schlichter, et al., 2001; Ronaldson, Lee, et al., 2004). Regulation of P-gp along with other ABC transporters has also been demonstrated in the mouse BV-2 microglia cell line where exposure to lipopolysaccharide (LPS) significantly reduced functional expression of ABC transporters (e.g., Mdr1, Bcrp, Mrp4), presumably, through interactions with the nuclear factor-κB (NF-κB) pathway (Gibson, Hossain, Richardson, & Aleksunes, 2012).

Although the expression of P-gp in oligodendrocytes is not known, studies in human neural stem cells which can differentiate into oligodendrocytes have demonstrated expression of *MDR1* transcript and functional protein (Islam et al., 2005; Yamamoto et al., 2009). At this level of cellular differentiation, functional significance of P-gp may serve to protect stem cells from exposure to xenobiotics or other potentially toxic substances. In the developing human CNS, selected neuronal cells have demonstrated positive P-gp immunostaining, particularly in the large pyramidal neurons of the brainstem and thalamus as well as in the Purkinje cells of the cerebellum (Daood, Tsai, Ahdab-Barmada, & Watchko, 2008). In rats, P-gp does not appear to colocalize with neuronal markers in the hippocampal hilus (Unkruer et al., 2009). However, in a rat model of tuberous sclerosis and refractory epilepsy, high expression of the transporter in dysplastic neurons, as well as astrocytes and microglia, was observed in the hippocampus, striatum, and cerebral cortex (Lazarowski, Ramos, Garcia-Rivello, Brusco, & Girardi, 2004).

At the BBB, it is well established that P-gp significantly restricts the permeability of several drugs which results in subtherapeutic CNS drug concentrations. To enhance brain accumulation, coadministration of small-molecule P-gp inhibitors (e.g., cyclosporine A, biricodar, laniquidar) with anticancer drugs has been clinically investigated, however, with unsuccessful results (Darby et al., 2011; Saneja, Khare, Alam, Dubey, & Gupta, 2014). This is largely due to nonspecificity to P-gp activity and/or nonselective distribution to nontarget organs leading to systemic toxicity. Furthermore, toxicity can be amplified by the high doses necessary for effective transporter inhibition and the reduced elimination of drugs causing systemic accumulation (Binkhathlan & Lavasanifar, 2013). In order to overcome these obstacles, current research has focused on drug delivery systems including nanoparticles (Punfa, Yodkeeree, Pitchakarn, Ampasavate, & Limtrakul, 2012), microparticles (Gong et al., 2012), micelles (Jin, Mo, Ding, Zheng, & Zhang, 2014), as well as the development of novel P-gp inhibitors with improved specificity (Kaddoumi et al., 2007).

It has been reported that P-gp expression at the BBB and parenchymal compartments can be regulated by physiological or pathological stimuli. These stimuli include proinflammatory cytokines, polypeptide hormone endothelin-1, viral proteins, bacterial LPS, amyloid-β (Aβ), as well as pharmacological agents (e.g., antiretrovirals) (Ashraf, Ronaldson, Persidsky, & Bendayan, 2011; Chan, Patel, Cummins, & Bendayan, 2013; Miller, 2010; Ronaldson & Bendayan, 2006; Zastre et al., 2009). At the cellular and molecular level, several signaling cascades have been investigated in the context of the aforementioned stimuli and P-gp expression. These pathways include the mitogen-activated protein kinase (MAPK) pathway, NF-κB, nuclear receptors (i.e., pregnane-X-receptor, constitutive androstane receptor), protein kinase C, protein kinase Akt, and Rho pathways (Ashraf et al., 2011; Gibson et al., 2012; Katayama, Yoshioka, Tsukahara, Mitsuhashi, & Sugimoto, 2007; Lemmen, Tozakidis, Bele, & Galla, 2013; Miller, 2010). P-gp regulatory pathways may present an attractive approach to reduce or prevent P-gp-mediated drug efflux in the CNS.

3.1.2 MDR-associated proteins

Another drug transport subfamily of the ABC superfamily is constituted by 13 multidrug resistance-associated proteins (MRP1–13) encoded by the

ABCC1–13 genes. Of the 13 isoforms, 9 (*ABCC1–6* and *ABCC10–12*) genes encode transporter proteins. ABCC7–9 and ABCC13 do not participate in drug transport activity but, instead, function as an ion channel (cystic fibrosis transmembrane regulator gene), sulfonylurea surface receptors 1 and 2, and a truncated protein. The nine MRP isoforms involved in drug transport can be further divided into two groups (MRP1-3, MRP6-7 and MRP4-5, MRP8-9) according to their membrane topology. MRP1–3 and MRP6–7 contain three transmembrane domains (TMD_0, TMD_1, TMD_2) with a 5+6+6 transmembrane α-helix configuration. The nucleotide-binding domains (NBD_1, NBD_2) are sandwiched between TMD_1 and TMD_2, and TMD_2 and the C-terminus, respectively. The cytoplasmic linker sequence that connects TMD_0 and TMD_1 is essential for a functional and active transporter. MRP4, MRP5, MRP8, and possibly MRP9 are considered to be "short" MRPs, as they do not contain TMD_0, and do not retain the cytoplasmic linker; they are arranged in a 6 +6 transmembrane helix (Dallas, Miller, & Bendayan, 2006; He, Li, Kanwar, & Zhou, 2011).

MRP1 is a 190-kDa protein encoded by the *ABCC1* gene. It was first isolated in the H69AR human lung carcinoma cell line that displayed MDR phenotype in the absence of P-gp overexpression (Cole et al., 1992). The substrate profile of MRP1 includes lipophilic anions as well as neutral or mildly positive lipophilic compounds (Kruh & Belinsky, 2003). MRP1 substrates include leukotrienes C_4, E_4, and D_4 (LTC_4, LTE4, and LTD_4), glutathione (GSH), glutathione disulfide (GSSG) and glucuronate conjugates (e.g., S-glutathionyl prostaglandin A_2, glucuronosylbilirubin), sulfate conjugates (e.g., estrone-3-sulfate), folate, antiretroviral drugs (e.g., atazanavir, saquinavir, ritonavir,indinavir, emtricitabine), anticancer agents (e.g., methotrexate, vinca alkaloids, doxorubicin, daunorubicin, epipodophyllotoxin, vincristine, vinblastine, irinotecan, paclitaxel), antibiotics (e.g., difloxacin, anthracyclines), metalloids (e.g., sodium arsenite, sodium arsenate, potassium antimonite), dyes (e.g., carboxydichlorofluorescein, calcein), toxins (e.g., methoxychlor), and others (Kruh & Belinsky, 2003; Zhou et al., 2008).

In the periphery, MRP1 is reported to be ubiquitously expressed in peripheral tissues (i.e., lung, testes, kidney, and placenta). In the CNS, MRP1 localizes at the basolateral membrane of choroid plexus epithelial cells as well as at the luminal and abluminal membranes of BMECs (Gazzin et al., 2011; Rao et al., 1999). Expression of *Mrp1* mRNA was observed in bovine BMECs cocultured with pericytes as well as in pericyte monolayer cell cultures (Berezowski et al., 2004). In brain parenchyma, *Mrp1* mRNA expression has been identified in rat astrocytes, microglia, oligodendrocytes, and neurons (Hirrlinger, Konig, & Dringen, 2002). Expression of *MRP1/Mrp1* has also been detected at the mRNA level in primary cultures of rat astrocytes, human astrocytoma, and glioblastoma cells of epileptic brains (Decleves et al., 2002; Hirrlinger et al., 2002). At the protein level, studies have revealed expression of MRP1 at the plasma membrane of astroglial foot processes, rodent reactive and nonreactive astrocytes but not in human nonreactive astrocytes (Aronica et al., 2003; Lazarowski et al., 2004; Mercier, Masseguin, Roux, Gabrion, & Scherrmann, 2004; Nies et al., 2004). Subcellular expression of Mrp1 has also been documented at the perinuclear regions of the Golgi apparatus in cultured mouse astroglial cells (Gennuso et al., 2004). This group also evaluated the functional expression of Mrp1 and reported a regulatory effect of unconjugated bilirubin on the trafficking of the transporter to the plasma membrane. Functional expression of Mrp1 has also been reported in primary cultures of rat astrocytes (Ronaldson & Bendayan, 2008). A depletion of cellular GSH and increase in extracellular GSH content were observed when cultured astrocytes were exposed to protease inhibitors (e.g., indinavir or nelfinavir); this effect was found to be attenuated in the presence of an MRP-specific inhibitor (MK571), suggesting involvement of Mrp-mediated transport activity (Brandmann, Tulpule, Schmidt, & Dringen, 2012). Furthermore, our group and others have documented that Mrp1 is involved in GSH and GSSG export in cultured astrocytes, suggesting a protective role of this transporter in the context of brain cellular inflammation and oxidative stress (Hirrlinger et al., 2001; Minich et al., 2006; Ronaldson & Bendayan, 2008).

Mrp1/Mrp1 expression and function have been demonstrated by our group in a continuous rat microglial cell line (MLS-9) and in primary cultures of rat microglia (Dallas, Zhu, Baruchel, Schlichter, & Bendayan, 2003). Another group identified weak but detectable levels of MRP1 at the protein level in human brain tumor tissues using immunohistochemical analysis (Lazarowski et al., 2006). MRP1 expression and localization studies in oligodendrocytes are limited. Oligodendrocyte-enriched primary cultures from rats revealed low levels of *Mrp1* mRNA expression (Hirrlinger et al., 2002). In the rat oligodendrocyte cell line, OLN-93, functional expression of Mrp1 appears to mediate GSH-conjugate export upon formaldehyde treatment (Tulpule et al., 2012). Further studies are needed to confirm MRP1 involvement in formaldehyde-mediated GSH export since other MRP isoforms (MRP2, MRP4) are known to transport GSH and

GSSG as well. Neuronal expression of MRP1 remains unclear. Using immunofluorescence techniques, MRP1 was not detected in neurons or glial cells in human cerebral cortex and subcortical white matter (Nies et al., 2004). However, immunocytochemistry detected MRP1 expression in hypertrophic hilar neurons and hippocampal CA1 region residual neurons (Aronica et al., 2004). The functional expression of MRP1 has been investigated in a drosophila genetic seizure model; overexpression of human MRP1 in drosophila neurons was able to confer resistance to commonly used AEDs such as phenytoin and valproic acid (Bao et al., 2011).

MRP2 exhibits approximately 49% sequence homology with MRP1 and is encoded by the *ABCC2* gene. Similar substrate profiles have been documented for MRP1 and MRP2 but are distinguishable based on the degree of substrate affinity and transport kinetics. MRP2 has lower affinity for GSH and glucuronate conjugates and can be allosterically regulated by bile acids and other amphipathic anions (Kruh & Belinsky, 2003). In the CNS, Mrp2 has been localized at the luminal membrane of BMECs and brain capillaries but negligible amounts could be detected at the BCSFB (Choudhuri, Cherrington, Li, & Klaassen, 2003; Miller et al., 2000). MRP2/Mrp2 localization, functional expression, and regulation within brain parenchyma cells have not been extensively investigated. At the mRNA level, but not protein, *Mrp2* expression was observed in embryonic rat astrocytes and MLS-9 microglia cell cultures (Dallas et al., 2003; Hirrlinger et al., 2002) as well as pericyte cultures (Yousif, Marie-Claire, Roux, Scherrmann, & Decleves, 2007). MRP2 protein expression functional data within the brain parenchyma is currently lacking.

MRP3, encoded by the *ABCC3* gene, was identified in the human expressed sequence tag library and shares 83% sequence homology with MRP1 (Kool et al., 1997). Despite the structural resemblance, MRP3 affinity for GSH and glucuronate conjugates is significantly lower than MRP1 (Sodani, Patel, Kathawala, & Chen, 2012). Within the CNS, MRP3/Mrp3 expression has not been detected in human and bovine BMECs (Berezowski et al., 2004; Kool et al., 1997; Zhang, Han, Elmquist, & Miller, 2000). *Mrp3* mRNA quantification revealed abundant expression in rat astrocytes and microglia and to a lesser extent in oligodendrocytes and neurons (Hirrlinger et al., 2002). Our laboratory also detected *Mrp3* transcript expression in rat MLS-9 microglia cell line (unpublished data). Evidence also suggests *Mrp3* gene expression in pericytes as well as in rat olfactory neurons (Thiebaud et al., 2011; Yousif et al., 2007). However, in human brain tissues, immunofluorescence localization was unable to detect MRP3 neuronal or glial cell staining (Nies et al., 2004). Overall, it appears that this transporter may not play a significant role in human brain.

MRP4 and MRP5 are encoded by the *ABCC4* and *ABCC5* genes, respectively, and were identified in a human expressed sequence tag library following the discovery of MRP1 and MRP2 (Kool et al., 1997). Initial investigation of MRP4 revealed very low expression in several human cancer cell lines of various origins (e.g., lung, bladder, ovarian, testicular, epidermal). Tissue-specific pattern of MRP4 has mainly localized this transporter to the apical membrane of renal proximal tubules and basolateral plasma membranes of tubuloacinar cells (Hoque, Conseil, & Cole, 2009; Lee, Klein-Szanto, & Kruh, 2000). Since MRP5 resembles MRP4 in structure, their substrate profiles overlap and include transport of endogenous compounds such as cyclic nucleotides (cAMP, cGMP), eicosanoids, urate, conjugated steroid and bile salts, folate, nucleotide, and purine analogs as well as pharmacological agents such as antiretroviral drugs (e.g., abacavir, zidovudine monophosphate, tenofovir, and ganciclovir) and anticancer drugs (e.g., 6-mercaptopurine, 6-thioguanine, methotrexate) (Zelcer et al., 2003). Localization and cellular distribution in the CNS of MRP4 and MRP5 have been primarily reported at the luminal membrane of brain capillary endothelial cells and at the basolateral membrane of the choroid plexus epithelium (Nies et al., 2004; Roberts et al., 2008; Zhang, Schuetz, Elmquist, & Miller, 2004). Pertinent to brain parenchymal compartments, our laboratory detected Mrp4 expression in primary cultures of rat astrocytes (Ronaldson & Bendayan, 2008) and characterized the functional expression of Mrp4/Mrp5 in a rat microglia cell line (MLS-9) (Dallas, Schlichter, & Bendayan, 2004). We have shown that Mrp4/Mrp5-mediated transport of 9-(2-phosphonomethoxyethyl)-adenine (PMEA) was GSH independent and could be significantly inhibited by several MRP inhibitors. In addition, rodent *Mrp4* mRNA levels were reported in rat astrocytes and microglia cultures with weak expression in oligodendrocytes and neurons; whereas *Mrp5* gene expression was ubiquitously expressed at low levels in brain parenchymal cells (Berezowski et al., 2004; Hirrlinger et al., 2002). In humans, both MRP4 and MRP5 expression and localization have been reported in astrocytes and MRP5 has been detected in neurons proximal to dysembryoplastic neuroepithelial tumors and pyramidal neurons (Bronger et al., 2005; Nies et al., 2004; Vogelgesang, Kunert-Keil, et al., 2004; Vogelgesang, Warzok, et al., 2004). In addition, another group identified Mrp5 expression in rat neurons within cytosolic vesicles as well as an upregulation of protein in peri-infarcted areas (Dazert et al., 2006). Furthermore, regulatory mechanisms of Mrp4/Mrp5 were investigated in a mouse BV-2 microglia cell model exposed to LPS; upon treatment, Mrp4 was downregulated, whereas Mrp5 was upregulated at both mRNA and protein level. This effect appeared to be mediated, in part, by NF-KB signaling pathway (Gibson et al., 2012).

MRP6, encoded by the *ABCC6* gene, was discovered during the human genome sequencing project (Kool, van der Linden, De, Baas, & Borst, 1999). Substrates of MRP6 include chemotherapeutic drugs (e.g., etoposide, doxorubicin, and daunorubicin) and GSH conjugates (i.e., LTC4, *N*-ethymaleimide *S*-glutathione) (Belinsky, Chen, Shchaveleva, Zeng, & Kruh, 2002; Zhou et al., 2008). Tissue distribution of *MRP6/Mrp6* transcripts had predominantly been identified in the liver and kidney with trace amounts in other tissues. Localization and cellular distribution of MRP6/Mrp6 in the CNS reveal *Mrp6* mRNA expression in primary cultures of bovine BMECs and in capillary-enriched fractions of bovine brain homogenate (Zhang et al., 2000). However, in human brain parenchyma, *MRP6*/MRP6 expression remains controversial. No detectable levels of mRNA or protein were observed in human brain tissues (Nies et al., 2004). However, in another study, expression of *MRP6*/MRP6 mRNA and protein was observed in neurons (Beck, Hayashi, Dang, Hayashi, & Boyd, 2005). Further studies are needed to elucidate the expression and function of this transporter in the mammalian brain.

MRP7 is encoded by the *ABCC10* gene and is characterized as a lipophilic anion transporter that confers resistance to anticancer drugs, i.e., docetaxel, vincristine, daunorubicin, epothilone B, taxanes (e.g., paclitaxel), antivirals (e.g., 2′,3′-dideoxycytidine, PMEA), nucleoside analogs, and other lipophilic anions (Malofeeva, Domanitskaya, Gudima, & Hopper-Borge, 2012). Notably, the transport of docetaxel, a chemotherapeutic agent, is primarily MRP7-mediated and can be used to distinguish from other MRPs. *MRP7* transcripts have been found in several peripheral tissues of various species including human, murine, and rat (Kao, Huang, & Chang, 2002; Takayanagi et al., 2004). In addition, various peripheral tumor specimens have shown detectable levels of *MRP7* transcripts (Mohelnikova-Duchonova et al., 2013). Expression in the CNS remains unclear; in one study, brain endothelial and glial cells in culture did not show detectable levels of *Mrp7* transcripts (Berezowski et al., 2004). However, another recent study reported high mRNA levels in BMECs isolated from human, rat, mouse, pig, and cow brain (Warren et al., 2009). MRP7 function has been shown using inhibitors such as tariquidar and tandutinib in an MRP7-transfected human kidney cell line, HEK293 (Deng et al., 2013; Sun, Chen, et al., 2013; Sun, Li, et al., 2013); however, functional expression and regulation in brain cellular compartments are yet to be characterized.

MRP8 is encoded by the *ABCC11* gene and has been characterized to confer resistance to several purine and pyrimidine nucleotide derivatives, anticancer drugs (e.g., 5-fluoro-2′-deoxyuridine-5′-monophosphate), steroid hormones (dexamethasone, progesterone), and several lipophilic anions (e.g., glycocholate, taurocholate, dehydroepiandrosterone, estrone-3-sulfate, folic acid, methotrexate) (Bera, Lee, Salvatore, Lee, & Pastan, 2001; Bortfeld et al., 2006; Honorat et al., 2011, 2013). In peripheral tissues, immunofluorescence microscopy detected MRP8 protein localization at the apical membrane of canine renal epithelial cells (MDCKII) and human hepatocyte cell line system (HepG2) (Bortfeld et al., 2006). In breast cancer tissues, a downregulation of MRP8 protein expression was detected when compared to normal breast tissue (Sosonkina, Nakashima, Ohta, Niikawa, & Starenki, 2011). However, MRP8 localization and expression within the CNS have been largely understudied. Within the human brain parenchymal compartments, neurons are the only cells known to date which express MRP8; the transporter was found at the axonal membrane of neurons and was predicted to mediate steroid efflux (Bortfeld et al., 2006).

MRP9 is encoded by the *ABCC12* gene and appears to be the product of a gene duplication event (Bera et al., 2002). Substrate profile of MRP9 has not been well characterized. In the brain, mRNA transcripts have been detected but cellular localization has not been examined (Bera et al., 2002). Although MRP9-overexpressing HEK293 cells have been reported to show resistance to antiretroviral drugs (i.e., atazanavir, lopinavir, ritonavir), the functional activity of this transporter in cellular brain compartments has yet to be examined (Bierman et al., 2010).

3.1.3 Breast cancer resistance protein

The BCRP belongs to the ABCG subfamily of the ABC efflux transporters and is encoded by the *ABCG2* gene. It was discovered in the multidrug-resistant human breast cancer cell line MCF-7/AdrVp; in the absence of overexpressed transporters (i.e., P-gp and MRPs), these breast cancer cells continued to displayed MDR phenotype against various anticancer drugs (e.g., mitoxantrone, methotrexate, and doxorubicin) (Doyle et al., 1998). Each BCRP monomer is approximately 70-kDa membrane-associated "half-transporter" that is composed of 663 amino acids and requires homodimerization to become an active transporter. Structural topology studies and protein sequence analysis report BCRP in two homologous halves each containing a single nucleotide-binding domain and a six α-helical transmembrane domain region. Furthermore, posttranslational modifications (i.e., glycosylation) do not appear to contribute to function or plasma membrane localization of BCRP (Diop & Hrycyna, 2005).

BCRP substrate specificity profile significantly overlaps with P-gp. These two efflux proteins are thought to act in concert to exert a synergistic effect in limiting drug tissue penetration, especially at the BBB (Agarwal, Hartz, Elmquist, & Bauer, 2011). Substrates include tyrosine kinase inhibitors (e.g., imatinib, gefitinib), sulfoconjugated organic anions, and hydrophobic and amphiphilic compounds including anticancer drugs (e.g., daunorubicin, bisantrene, irinotecan, methotrexate, mitoxantrone, topotecan), phototoxins (e.g., pheophorbide-A), antiretrovirals (e.g., zidovudine), fluorescent compounds (e.g., BODIPY prazosin), and physiological substrates (e.g., GSH, steroid hormones, folic acid) (Cygalova, Hofman, Ceckova, & Staud, 2009).

Localization of BCRP/Bcrp at the BBB has been detected in several cell systems including human BMECs, mouse brain capillaries, and an immortalized rat brain microvessel endothelial cell line (Lee et al., 2007; Zhang et al., 2003). A porcine Bcrp homologous protein, known as brain MDR protein, was discovered and characterized by Eisenblätter and colleagues in endothelial cells of porcine brain capillaries (Eisenblatter & Galla, 2002). This homologous protein showed 86% amino acid sequence homology to BCRP and conferred drug resistance to several anticancer agents (e.g., mitoxantrone, doxorubicin, daunorubicin, topotecan, and camptothecin derivatives) (Eisenblatter, Huwel, & Galla, 2003). The Bcrp porcine homologue displayed weak expression in pericytes (Eisenblatter et al., 2003). In addition, studies have shown increased BCRP protein expression at the luminal cell surface of blood vessels isolated from refractory epileptic brains and newly formed primary glial tumor capillaries but not in astrocytes or neuronal cells (Aronica et al., 2005). In contrast, another group demonstrated *BCRP*/BCRP expression (mRNA and protein) in primary cultures of fetal human astrocytes. Our laboratory also confirmed protein expression of BCRP in primary cultures of human BMECs, immortalized rat brain microvessel endothelial cell line RBE4, primary cultures of rat astrocytes, and rat brain microglial cell line (MLS-9) (Lee et al., 2007). *Bcrp*/Bcrp expression has also been detected at both mRNA and protein level in mouse microglia BV-2 cell system (Gibson et al., 2012). Although BCRP is predominantly localized at the plasma membrane, subcellular localization has also been reported. In human-derived glioblastoma (LN229, T98, A172, U87, U118, U138) and astrocytoma (1321N1) cell lines, BCRP localization was observed at the nuclear envelope and cell surface, by confocal immunofluorescence microscopy (Bhatia et al., 2012). This finding is in agreement with subcellular localization of BCRP in the mitochondria of renal epithelial LLC-PK1 cells and perinuclear regions from various human cancer cells (i.e., nasopharyngeal, ovarian, breast, human head and neck squamous cell carcinoma) (Lemos et al., 2009; Takada, Suzuki, Gotoh, & Sugiyama, 2005).

BCRP localization in neurons is controversial. There was no evidence of BCRP immunostaining in perivascular astrocytes or neurons during CNS maturation (Daood et al., 2008). However, in a stroke study, Bcrp was found to localize within surviving neurons from peri-infarcted area and along the wall of the lateral and third ventricles (Dazert et al., 2006). In addition, refractory epileptic brains revealed high expression of BCRP in dysplastic neurons from transmantle cortical dysplasia and bilateral cortical dysplasia (Lazarowski et al., 2007).

Although expression of BCRP in brain cellular compartments has been demonstrated, functional activity of BCRP in these cells remains inconclusive. Functionally active BCRP has been reported in isolated rodent (rat and mice) brain capillaries, cultured human and rodent BMECs, and immortalized rat astrocyte cell line (Cantrill, Skinner, Rothwell, & Penny, 2012; Hartz, Mahringer, Miller, & Bauer, 2010). However, several studies have suggested lack of BCRP-mediated transport in cultured cell systems and primary cultures of human brain microvessel endothelial cells and the RBE4 cell line (Hori et al., 2004; Zhang et al., 2003). In primary cultures of rat astrocytes and in a rat brain microglia cell line (MLS-9), lack of BCRP-mediated transport of mitoxantrone, an established BCRP substrate was observed (Lee et al., 2007).

Altered BCRP expression has also been reported at the level of the BBB and brain parenchyma. LPS-induced inflammation in porcine BMECs and mouse BV-2 microglial cells appears to downregulate Bcrp and other ABC transporter function by 40–70% (Gibson et al., 2012). A recent investigation on the effect of chronic renal failure on transporters at the BBB showed significantly downregulated mRNA and protein expression of several transporters (e.g., Bcrp, Mrp2–4, Oat3, Oatp2–3, and P-gp) in rat brain biopsies as well as in cultured rat astrocytes and brain endothelial cells incubated with chronic renal failure serum (Naud et al., 2012). *In vivo*, expression of Bcrp, along with P-gp, at the BBB can limit therapeutic agents from exerting therapeutic actions in the brain. A recent study investigating CNS penetration of the anticancer drug, sorafenib, in Bcrp1 and Mdr1 knockout mice demonstrated that Bcrp, together with P-gp, at the BBB directly restricted sorafenib distribution into the brain (Agarwal, Sane, Ohlfest, & Elmquist, 2011).

3.2. SLC drug transporters

The SLC membrane transporters constitute the largest and highly conserved superfamily of transporters. To date, 48 SLC families have been identified. Members of the SLC family are highly expressed in the BBB, BCSFB, and brain parenchyma. In this section, we discuss brain region and/or cell-specific localization as well as known functions of organic anion-transporting polypeptides (OATPs), organic anion transporters (OATs), organic cation transporting systems, nucleoside transporters, peptide transporters, and monocarboxylate transporters (MCTs). Localization of different SLC transporters in brain cellular compartments has been summarized in Figs. 1 and 2 and Table 2.

3.2.1 Organic anion-transporting polypeptides

OATPs (OATP in humans; Oatp in rodents) belong to the SLCO/Slco family (formerly termed as SLC21 family). To date, more than 40 members of OATP/Oatp family have been identified from human, rat, and mouse (Hagenbuch & Meier, 2003). OATPs mediate the uptake of several endogenously synthesized compounds (i.e., bile salt, hormone steroid conjugate) as well as a number of drugs including HMG-CoA-reductase inhibitors, anticancer agents, antibiotics, and cardiac glycosides (Hagenbuch & Gui, 2008; Konig, Seithel, Gradhand, & Fromm, 2006; Kullak-Ublick et al., 2001). Structurally, the OATP/Oatp family members share a similar membrane topology of 12 transmembrane domains, with a large extracellular loop between transmembrane domains 9 and 10 and a conserved amino acid sequence (i.e., D-X-RW-(I,V)-GAWW-X-G-(F,L)-L) between extracellular loop 3 and transmembrane domain 6 (Hagenbuch & Meier, 2003; Ronaldson & Davis, 2013). A number of OATP/Oatp isoforms have been identified at the BBB as well as in brain parenchyma. Due to the wide substrate preference of OATPs and their brain cellular localization, members of this family can be potentially targeted for improving CNS drug delivery for treatment of various diseases. For example, opioid analgesics are substrates

Table 2 CNS expression, localization, and substrate specificity of SLC transporters

Name	Gene	CNS expression/ localization	Substrates
Organic anion-transporting polypeptides (OATPs)			
OATP1A2	*SLCO1A2*	Luminal and abluminal membranes of BMECs	Bile acids (cholate, taurocholate, glycocholate, taurochenodeoxycholate, tauroursodeoxycholate), estrone-3-sulfate, estradiol-17β-glucuronide, dehydroepiandrosterone sulfate, T3, T4, ciprofloxacin, erythromycin, fexofenadine, β-blockers, darunavir, lopinavir, saquinavir, pitavastatin, rosuvastatin, *N*-methyl-quinidine
OATP3A1_V1	*SLCO3A1*	Basolateral membrane of choroid plexus epithelial cells, glial cells	Prostaglandin E_1, E_2, T_4, cyclic oligopeptides, vasopressin
OATP3A1_V2	*SLCO3A1*	Apical membrane of choroid plexus epithelial cells, neurons	
Oatp1a4	*Slco1a4*	Luminal and abluminal membrane of BMECs	Bile acids (cholate, glycocholate, taurocholate), estrone-3-sulfate, estradiol-17β-glucuronide, dehydroepiandrosterone sulfate, T3, T4, prostaglandins E_2,folate, methotrexate, digoxin, rosuvastatin, fexofenadine, ouabain, β-lactam antibiotics, zidovidine, ochratoxin A, *N*-methyl-quinidine, *N*-methyl-quinine
Oatp1c1	*Slco1c1*	Luminal and abluminal membranes of BMECs, basolateral membrane of choroid plexus epithelial cells	T3, T4, β-estradiol-17-β-D-glucuronide, cerivastatin, troglitazone sulfate

Oatp2a1	*Slco2a1*	Luminal membrane of BMECs, astrocytes, pericytes, choroid plexus epithelial cells	Prostaglandins E_1, E_2, and $F_{2\alpha}$, thromboxane B_2
Oatp2b1	*Slco2b1*	Abluminal membrane of BMECs, apical membrane of choroid plexus epithelial cells, neurons	Taurocholate, LTC_4, prostaglandins E_1, E_2, and D_2, thromboxane B_2, estrone-3-sulfate, iloprost
Organic anion transporters (OATs)			
OAT1	*SLC22A6*	Apical membrane of choroid plexus epithelium	Cyclic AMP/GMP, medium chain fatty acids, α-ketoglutarate, citrulline, prostaglandins E_2 and $F_{2\alpha}$, urate, vanilmandelic acid, hydroxycinnamic acids, indoxyl sulfate, acetylsalicylate, salicylate, stavudine, lamivudine, didanosine, zidovudine, zalcitabine, acyclovir, adefovir, cidofovir, cephaloridine, cimetidine, edaravone sulfate, furosemide, ganciclovir, ibuprofen, indomethacin, ketoprofen, methotrexate, penicillin G, tetracycline, trifluridine, *p*-aminohippurate, ochratoxin A
OAT3	*SLC22A8*	BMECs, choroid plexus	Cyclic AMP/GMP, dehydroepiandrosterone sulfate, prostaglandins E_2 and $F_{2\alpha}$, cortisol, estrone-3-sulfate, estradiol-17β-glucuronide, choline, taurocholate, glycocholate, glutarate, GSH, urate, vanilmandelic acid, hydroxycinnamic acid conjugates, indoxyl sulfate, pravastatin, tetracycline, antiretroviral drugs, activated oseltamivir, allopurinol, benzylpenicillin, cefazolin, cephaloridine, cimetidine, famotidine, fexofenadine, indomethacin, salicylate, ketoprofen, ibuprofen, edaravone sulfate, methotrexate, topotecan, 6-mercaptopurine, 5-fluorouracil, *p*-aminohippurate, ochratoxin A, perfluorooctanoic acid, aflatoxin B1

Continued

Table 2 CNS expression, localization, and substrate specificity of SLC transporters—cont'd

Name	Gene	CNS expression/ localization	Substrates
Oat1	*Slc22a6*	Apical membrane of choroid plexus epithelium, neurons	Cyclic AMP/GMP, urate, indoxyl sulfate, antibiotics, diuretics, nonsteroidal anti-inflammatory drugs, uricosuric drugs, valproic acid, zidovudine, zalcitabine, *p*-aminohippurate
Oat3	*Slc22a8*	Abluminal and luminal membrane of BMECs, apical membrane of choroid plexus epithelium	Estrone-3-sulfate, cyclic AMP/GMP, urate, indoxyl sulfate, antibiotics, diuretics, nonsteroidal anti-inflammatory drug, benzylpenicillin, indoxylsulfate, homovanillic acid, uricosuric drugs, *p*-aminohippurate
Organic cation transporters (OCTs)			
OCT1	*SLC22A1*	Luminal membrane of BMECs	Choline, acetylcholine, dopamine, serotonin, putrescin, cyclo(His-Pro), salsolinol, agmatine, spermine, spermidine, quinidine, quinine, acyclovir, ganciclovir, lamivudine, zalcitabine, cimetidine, metformin, oxaliplatin, picoplatin, diphenylhydramine, ranitidine, famotidine, atropine, desipramine, 1-methyl-4-phenylpyridinium, tetraethylammonium, tetrapropylammonium, tetrabutylammonium, *N*-methylnicotinamide, *N*-methyl-quinine, tetrabutylammonium, aflatoxin B1, ethidiumbromide
OCT2	*SLC22A2*	Luminal membrane of BMECs, neurons, apical membrane of choroid plexus epithelial cells	Choline, acetylcholine, dopamine, norepinephrine, epinephrine, serotonin, histamine, agmatine, cyclo (His-pro), salsolinol, putrescine, quinine, famotidine, ranitidine, amantadine, metformin, lamivudine, zalcitabine, cimetidine, oxaliplatin, picoplatin, cisplatin, memantine, etilefrine, amiloride, paraquat, 1-methyl-4-phenylpyridinium, tetraethylammonium, *N*-methylnicotinamide, aflatoxin B1
OCT3	*SLC22A3*	Astrocytes, neurons, apical membrane of choroid plexus epithelial cells	Dopamine, norepinephrine, epinephrine, serotonin, histamine, agmatine, lidocaine, quinidine, metformin, atropine, guanidine, etilefrine, oxaliplatin, lamivudine, 1-methyl-4-phenylpyridinium, tetraethylammonium

Organic cation/carnitine transporter (OCTN)			
OCTN2	*SLC22A5*	Luminal and abluminal membranes of BMECs	L-Carnitine,choline, quinidine, verapamil, oxaliplatin, ipratropium, tiotropium, cephaloridine, mildronate, pyrilamine, spironolactone, tetraethylammonium, valproic acid
Octn2	*Slc22a5*	Neurons	
Octn3	*Slc22a9*	Astrocytes	L-Carnitine
Concentrative nucleoside transporters			
Rat/mouse CNT2	*Slc28a2*	BMECs, choroid plexus epithelium, neurons, astrocytes	Adenosine, cladribine, clofarabine, cytidine, didanosine, fialuridine, 5-fluorouridine, formycin B, inosine, guanosine, ribavirin, tiazofurin, uridine
Rat/mouse CNT3	*Slc28a3*	Basolateral membrane of choroid plexus, microglia	Adenosine, benzamide riboside, cladribine, clofarabine, cytarabine, cytidine, didanosine, fludarabine, 5-fluorouridine, gemcitabine, guanosine, inosine, 6-mercaptopurine, ribavirin, uridine, 6-thioguanine, tiazofurin, thymidine, zalcitabine, zebularine, zidovudine
Equilibrative nucleoside transporters			
Rat/mouse ENT1	*Slc29a1*	BMECs, choroid plexus epithelium, neurons, astrocytes	Adenine, adenosine, clofarabine, cytidine, fialuridine, gemcitabine, guanine, guanosine, hypoxanthine, inosine, thymidine, tiazofurin, uridine
Rat/mouse ENT2	*Slc29a2*	Luminal membrane of BMECs, basolateral side of choroid plexus epithelium, astrocytes, neurons	Adenine, adenosine, clofarabine, cytidine, fialuridine, gemcitabine, guanine, guanosine, hypoxanthine, inosine, thymidine, tiazofurin, uridine

Continued

Table 2 CNS expression, localization, and substrate specificity of SLC transporters—cont'd

Name	Gene	CNS expression/ localization	Substrates
ENT4	*SLC29A4*	Astrocytes, epithelial cells of choroid plexus	Serotonin, norepinephrine, epinephrine
Rat/mouse ENT4	*SSlc29a4*	Neurons	
Peptide transporter			
Pept2	*Slc15a2*	Astrocytes, neurons, apical membrane of choroid plexus	5-Aminolevulinic acid, bestatin, cefadroxil, glycylsarcosine, L-kyotorphin
Monocarboxylate transporters (MCTs)			
MCT1	*SLC16A1*	BMECs	Lactate, pyruvate, ketone bodies, β-hydroxybutyrate, acetoacetate, γ-aminobutyric acid, β-lactam antibiotics, statins
Rat MCT1	*Slc16a1*	Luminal membrane of BMECs, oligodendrocytes	
MCT2	*SLC16A7*	Astrocytes, neurons	Lactate, pyruvate, ketone bodies, β-hydroxybutyrate
Mouse MCT3	*Slc16a8*	Basolateral membrane of choroid plexus epithelial cells	Lactate
MCT4	*SLC16A3*	Astrocytes	Lactate, ketone bodies, butyrate, statins
MCT8	*SLC16A2*	Brain microvessels, neurons, choroid plexus epithelial cells	Thyroid hormones (T_2, T_3, T_4)

Abbreviations follow those used in the text.
Adapted from Ashraf, Kis, Banerjee, and Bendayan (2012).

for OATP/Oatps and these transporters can be targeted for effective delivery of drugs for the treatment of pain and/or cerebral hypoxia (Ronaldson & Davis, 2013).

3.2.1.1 Human OATP isoforms

The human OATP family consists of 11 members (Hagenbuch & Meier, 2003). Multiple OATP isoforms have been identified in the brain. In particular, OATP1A2 is highly expressed in the brain and testes (Kullak-Ublick, Hagenbuch, Stieger, Wolkoff, & Meier, 1994). Immunofluorescence staining of human brain frontal cortex tissue showed OATP1A2 localization at both the apical and basolateral side of brain microvascular endothelium, whereas astrocytes and neurons remained immunonegative (Gao et al., 2000). OATP1A2-mediated transport of bile acids, cholate, taurocholate, glycocholate, taurochenodeoxycholate, and tauroursodeoxycholate has been shown in *Xenopus* oocytes (Kullak-Ublick et al., 1995). Other substrates of OATP1A2 include steroid hormones and conjugates, thyroid hormones, antibiotics (i.e., ciprofloxacin, erythromycin), fexofenadine, β-blockers (i.e., atenolol, labetalol, talinolol), HIV-1 protease inhibitors (i.e., darunavir, lopinavir, saquinavir), HMG-CoA reductase inhibitors (i.e., pitavastatin, rosuvastatin), as well as organic cations like *N*-methyl-quinidine (Kullak-Ublick et al., 1995, 1994; Ronaldson & Davis, 2013).

Two different splice variants of *OATP3A1* have been detected in human brains that are designated as *OATP3A1_v1* and *OATP3A1_v2*, respectively (Huber et al., 2007). At the cellular level, OATP3A1_v1 is expressed at the basolateral membrane of choroid plexus epithelial cells as well as in glial cells in the gray matter of frontal cortex (Huber et al., 2007). In contrast, OATP3A1_v2 was found to be expressed at the apical membrane of choroid plexus epithelial cells and in neurons of both gray and white matter of frontal cortex (Huber et al., 2007). Using *Xenopus laevis* oocytes and stably transfected cell lines, these OATP isoforms were found to be involved in the transport of prostaglandin (PGE1 and PGE2), thyroxine and the cyclic oligopeptides BQ-123 (endothelin receptor antagonist), and vasopressin (Huber et al., 2007). Gene expression of *OATP2B1* and *OATP4A1* has been reported in brain tissue (Fujiwara et al., 2001; Kullak-Ublick et al., 2001). Transcripts of *OATP1C1* have also been detected in different brain regions. At the BBB, low expression of OATP1C1 has been detected in brain microvessels (Roberts et al., 2008). In contrast to other OATPs, OATP1C1 showed a more selective substrate preference and has been characterized as a high-affinity thyroid hormone transporter (Pizzagalli et al., 2002).

OATP2A1 has been cloned and characterized as a prostaglandin transporter (Lu, Kanai, Bao, & Schuster, 1996). Transcripts of *OATP2A1* have been found in adult as well as fetal human brain tissue (Lu et al., 1996). Protein expression of OATP2A1 has only been detected in choroid/retinal pigment epithelium (Kraft et al., 2010). Although expression of a number of OATP isoforms has been reported in brain cellular compartments, a comprehensive understanding of the localization and function of these transporters in brain cellular compartments is lacking.

3.2.1.2 Rodent OATP isoforms

Rat Oatp1a1 was the first cloned and characterized member of the OATP/Oatp family, and transcripts of this rodent *Oatp* isoform have been detected in the brain (Jacquemin, Hagenbuch, Stieger, Wolkoff, & Meier, 1994). Several other Oatp isoforms have also been identified in rodent brain. Oatp1a4 expression has been observed in rat brain capillaries as well as ependymal cells (Roberts et al., 2008). Using immunohistochemical analysis, Oatp1a4 has been localized at both the luminal and abluminal membrane of mouse brain endothelial cells. However, Oatp1a4 immunoreactivity did not colocalize with glial fibrillary acidic protein (GFAP), indicating that Oatp1a4 is not expressed in astrocytes (Ose et al., 2010). Functional expression of Oatp1a4 was observed in rat brain microvessels where transport of atorvastatin and taurocholate (established Oatp1a4 substrate) was inhibited in the presence of Oatp inhibitors. This study suggests that Oatps are involved in drug permeability to CNS (Thompson et al., 2014). Another recent study demonstrated by *in situ* brain perfusion that uptake of Aβ in mouse brain is partly mediated by Oatp1a4, suggesting the significance of this transporter as a potential target for inhibiting Aβ accumulation in the brain of Alzheimer's patients (Do et al., 2013).

Another Oatp isoform that has been identified at the BBB is Oatp1c1. In rodents, this isoform was found to be strongly expressed in BMECs and in choroid plexus (Sugiyama, Kusuhara, Lee, & Sugiyama, 2003). Oatp1c1 has been characterized as a high-affinity, Na^+-independent thyroid transporter. Furthermore, Oatp1c1 knockout animals showed a decrease in thyroid levels in the brain, suggesting an important role of this transport protein in mediating thyroid uptake across the BBB (Mayerl, Visser, Darras, Horn, & Heuer, 2012). Oatp2a1 expression has been shown in primary cultures of BMECs, astrocytes, pericytes, and choroid plexus epithelial cells, and a role of this transporter in prostaglandin transport and maintaining prostaglandin homeostasis in the brain have been implicated (Kis et al., 2006). At the choroid plexus epithelium, other isoforms of Oatps have also been identified including Oatp1a1, Oatp1a5, Oatp1a6, Oatp1c1, and Oatp4a1.

In brain parenchyma, rat Oatp3a1 was found to be widely distributed in the brain with a specific localization in somatoneurons and astroglial cells (Huber et al., 2007). Expression of Oatp2a1 has also been reported in primary cultures of rat astrocytes (Kis et al., 2006). Neuronal expression of Oatp1a5 and Oatp2b1 has been observed in mouse and rat neurons (Feurstein, Kleinteich, Heussner, Stemmer, & Dietrich, 2010; Nishio et al., 2000). Gene expression of several other rodent *Oatps* has also been detected in the brain, including *Oatp3a1, Oatp4a1*, and *Oatp5a1*, although their cellular distribution and localization are still unknown.

3.2.2 Organic anion transporter family

OATs/Oats belong to the SLC22 family and the members include OAT1, OAT2, OAT3, OAT4, OAT5, OAT6, and OAT10. OATs/Oats can be Na^+-independent or Na^+-dependent exchangers or ATP-dependent active transporters. OATs have 12 membrane spanning domains with intracellular carboxy- and amino-terminus. Substrates of OATs include neurotransmitter metabolites, antimetabolites, xanthine-related compounds, HMG-CoA reductase inhibitors, nonsteroidal anti-inflammatory drugs, antiretrovirals, toxins, steroid hormones, and their metabolites. OAT/Oat isoforms have been identified in different brain cellular compartments including brain capillaries, choroid plexus epithelial cells, and neurons (Bahn et al., 2005; Kikuchi, Kusuhara, Sugiyama, & Sugiyama, 2003). The expression of OAT/Oat isoforms in glial cells has not been characterized yet. In the brain, OATs/Oats are involved in maintaining the uptake and/or clearance of organic anionic drugs, steroid hormones, toxins, neurotransmitters, and their metabolites.

OAT1 was the first identified member of the SLC22 family (Sekine, Watanabe, Hosoyamada, Kanai, & Endou, 1997; Sweet, Wolff, & Pritchard, 1997). Human OAT1 is highly expressed in kidney and weaker expression has been detected in brain, choroid plexus, spinal cord, and iris-cilliary bodies (Alebouyeh et al., 2003; Hilgendorf et al., 2007). Murine *Oat1* mRNA expression was found in fetal brain in choroid plexus, dura mater, root ganglions, spinal cord, and highest gene expression was observed during embryogenesis which dramatically decreased toward adulthood

(Pavlova et al., 2000). This temporal Oat1 expression in the developing brain suggests a role for Oat1 during formation of CNS structures. At the protein level, murine Oat1 was found to be expressed in cortical and hippocampal neurons as well as in choroid plexus ependymal cells (Bahn et al., 2005). Gene expression of *Oat1* and *Oat3* has also been reported in mouse choroid plexus. In choroid plexus derived from mice lacking either Oat1 or Oat3, probenecid-inhibitable transport of Oat substrate, 6-carboxyfluorescein was observed suggesting functional role of Oat1 and Oat3 in choroid plexus (Nagle, Wu, Eraly, & Nigam, 2013). This study also demonstrated interaction of several antiretroviral drugs, i.e., zidovudine, tenofovir, and lamivudine with both Oat1 and Oat3 in choroid plexus (Nagle et al., 2013). Expression of OAT1/Oat1 at the apical side of choroid plexus epithelial cells suggests a role of this transporter in CSF-to-blood transport of anionic drugs and neurotransmitter metabolites.

OAT2/Oat2 has been originally cloned in rat liver. In the brain, only *Oat2* mRNA has been detected in rat choroid plexus (Choudhuri et al., 2003). Unlike Oat2/Oat2, OAT3/Oat3 has been detected at both the gene and protein level in the brain. *OAT3* transcripts have been reported in a human BMEC line (BB19) (Kusch-Poddar, Drewe, Fux, & Gutmann, 2005). Immunohistochemical analysis confirmed abluminal as well as luminal localization of rat Oat3 in brain capillary endothelial cells (Kikuchi et al., 2003). A study by Ohtsuki et al. demonstrated that Oat3 is involved in the transport of indoxyl sulfate, a uremic toxin, from the brain to the circulating blood (Ohtsuki et al., 2002). In addition, homovanillic acid and 5-hydroxyindole acetic acid, metabolites of neurotransmitter dopamine and serotonin, strongly inhibited Oat3-mediated uptake of indoxyl sulfate in *X. laevis* oocytes, suggesting that Oat3 may play an important role in the removal of toxins as well as neurotransmitter metabolites from the brain (Ohtsuki et al., 2002). Oat3 functional expression at the BBB is also an important determinant of brain permeation of several drugs. For example, Oat3-mediated transport of anti-influenza drug oseltamivir was observed in the murine BBB (Ose et al., 2009). In addition, functional expression of rat Oat3 has been demonstrated in brain capillary endothelial cells where Oat3-mediated transport of the organic anions, *para*-aminohippurate and benzylpenicillin, was observed (Kikuchi et al., 2003). Nagata et al. reported localization of rat Oat3, but not Oat1, in the choroid plexus. Immunohistochemical analysis revealed brush border localization of Oat3 in rat choroid plexus epithelial cells (Nagata, Kusuhara, Endou, & Sugiyama, 2002). Rat Oat3-mediated uptake of *para*-aminohippurate and benzylpenicillin was also observed in isolated rat choroid plexus, suggesting that this transporter may play a role in removing organic anions from the CSF (Nagata et al., 2002). In humans, plasma membrane and cytoplasmic localization of OAT3 have been demonstrated in choroid plexus (Alebouyeh et al., 2003).

Studies have shown *OAT4* gene expression in BB19, a human BMEC line as well as in choroid plexus epithelial cells (Kusch-Poddar et al., 2005). *OAT5* has been identified at the gene level in human liver; however, the protein and functional expression of this transporter in other tissues including the brain is still unknown. OAT6 has not been detected in human tissue. However, mouse Oat6 has been found in olfactory mucosa (Monte, Nagle, Eraly, & Nigam, 2004). Among the OAT isoforms, OAT7 is the only liver-specific OAT and has not been detected in other tissues. OAT10, previously known as the orphan transporter hORCTLC3 (human organic cation transporter-like 3), is a high-affinity urate and nicotinate exchanger and is strongly expressed in the kidney; however, weaker expression has been detected in brain, heart, and intestine (Bahn et al., 2008; Nishiwaki, Daigo, Tamari, Fujii, & Nakamura, 1998).

3.2.3 Organic cation transporter systems

Membrane transport of organic cations is mediated by members of the organic cation transporters (OCTs) and organic carnitine transporters (OCTNs). In the CNS, these transport systems regulate the uptake or excretion of endogenous and exogenous organic cations at the BBB, glial cells, neurons, and BCSFB. In particular, OCTs play an important role in the transport of several neurotransmitters (i.e., dopamine, norepinephrine) in the brain, whereas OCTNs mediate the transport of carnitine. L-Carnitine (β-hydroxy-γ-trimethylaminobutyric acid) is a small, highly polar zwitterion that plays an essential role in cotransport of long-chain fatty acids across the inner mitochondrial membrane for β-oxidation and ATP generation. Carnitine and its metabolite (i.e., acetyl-L-carnitine) are present in the CNS and are known to have different physiological roles including control of acetylcholine synthesis in brain parenchyma.

3.2.3.1 Organic cation transporters

Members of the OCT/Oct family (SLC22A1) include OCT1/Oct1, OCT2/Oct2, and OCT3/Oct3. OCTs mediate transport of organic cations by facilitated diffusion. The direction of the transport is dependent upon the ion gradient. OCTs mediate transport of a number of endogenous compounds including tetraethyl ammonium, 1-methyl-4-phenylpyridinium, choline, acetylcholine, prostaglandins, and monoamine neurotransmitters (i.e., dopamine, epinephrine, norepinephrine, histamine). In addition, a larger number of drugs have also been recognized as OCT substrates including antidiabetics (i.e., metformin), antivirals (e.g., acyclovir, lamivudine, zalcitabine), acid-lowering agents (e.g., cimetidine, famotidine, ranitidine), antineoplastic agents (e.g., cisplatin), quinidine, and quinine. OCTs share similar predicted membrane topology of 12 α-helical transmembrane domains, a large extracellular loop between domains 1 and 2 and a large intracellular loop between domains 6 and 7 (Koepsell, 2013).

OCTs are expressed at the BBB, glial cells, neurons, and BCSFB. OCT1 expression has been detected in BMECs (Lin et al., 2010). OCT2 is primarily expressed in the kidney, but protein expression of this transporter has also been detected in other organs including the brain. In the CNS, human OCT2 has been detected at the luminal side of BMECs, in neurons and in choroid plexus (Bacq et al., 2012; Koepsell, Schmitt, & Gorboulev, 2003; Lin et al., 2010). Recently, OCT2 protein expression has been reported in cholinergic neurons and motor neurons in the anterior horn of the spinal cord (Nakata, Matsui, Kobayashi, Kobayashi, & Anzai, 2013). Bacq et al. demonstrated that Oct2 plays an important functional role in the clearance of serotonin and norepinephrine in the brain (Bacq et al., 2012).

OCT3 is considered to be the most abundant OCT isoform in the brain. OCT3 is a high-capacity transporter of dopamine and other amines and has been implicated in the regulation of aminergic neurotransmission in the brain. *OCT3*/OCT3 gene and protein expression has been detected in neurons, astrocytes, and epithelial cells of the choroid plexus (Wang et al., 2007). Using immunohistochemical analysis, Hill and Gasser have also demonstrated OCT3 expression in intercalated cells (a group of GABAergic neurons) in the amygdala (Hill & Gasser, 2013). Oct3 is abundantly expressed in dopaminergic neurons of the substantia nigra, nonaminergic neurons of the ventral tegmental area, substantia nigra reticulata, locus coeruleus, hippocampus, and cortex (Vialou et al., 2008). In rodents, Oct3 expression has been detected in astrocytes in the hippocampus, substantia nigra reticulata, and several hypothalamic nuclei. Oct3-deficient mice show altered behavioral response to changes in osmolarity, altered monoamine neurotransmission in the brain, increased sensitivity to psychostimulants, and increased levels of stress and anxiety (Vialou, Amphoux, Zwart, Giros, & Gautron, 2004; Vialou et al., 2008). These studies indicate the potential for Oct3 as a target for the treatment of anxiety disorders that involve aminergic neurotransmission (i.e., panic disorder).

3.2.3.2 Carnitine/cation transporters

Mammalian members of the OCTN family include human OCTN1 (*SLC22A4*), OCTN2 (*SLC22A5*), and OCTN3 (*SLC22A21*) and rodent Octn1, Octn2, and Octn3. OCTN2 and OCTN3 have been characterized as high-affinity carnitine transporters. OCTN2-mediated carnitine transport is Na^+ dependent, whereas OCTN3 has been shown to transport carnitine independent of sodium. Substrates of OCTNs include carnitine, tetraethyl ammonium, quinidine, choline, nicotine, cimetidine, and clonidine. Similar to other SLC22 family members, topological predictions of OCTNs suggest 12 α-helical transmembrane domains, an intracellular amino- and carboxy-terminus (Koepsell, Lips, & Volk, 2007).

Expression of Octn1 and Octn2 has been identified in mouse brain hippocampus, hypothalamus, cerebellum, and motor cortex (Lamhonwah et al., 2008). Both gene and protein expression of rat *Octn1*/Octn1 have been found in spinal cord, choroid plexus, hippocampus, cortex, cerebellum, nuclei of cranial nerves V and VII, and Purkinje cell dendrites (Lamhonwah et al., 2008). OCTN2/Octn2 has been detected at the BBB and in brain parenchyma. OCTN2/Octn2 expression has been reported in primary cultures of BMECs isolated from humans and rodents. A recent study has reported *OCTN2* mRNA expression in a human BMEC line, hCMEC/D3 cells (Okura, Kato, & Deguchi, 2014). [^{3}H]L-Carnitine uptake was found to be significantly decreased in hCMEC/D3 cells treated with silencing RNA designed against OCTN2. This study suggests that OCTN2 is involved in the transport of L-carnitine at the human BBB (Okura et al., 2014). Colocalization of Octn2 with neuronal cell marker, microtubule-associated protein-2, was observed in mouse brain as well as in primary cultures of cortical neurons (Nakamichi et al., 2012). In parenchymal cells, *OCTN2* mRNA expression was detected in neurons from hippocampus, cerebellum, spinal cord, and superior cervical ganglion. Functional expression of Octn1 and Octn2 has also been demonstrated in neurons. Octn1- and Octn2-mediated transport of the chemotherapeutic agent, oxaliplatin, has been shown in primary cultures of rat dorsal root ganglion neurons where neuronal accumulation and neurotoxicity associated with oxaliplatin were observed (Jong, Nakanishi, Liu, Tamai, & McKeage, 2011). Based on these findings, the authors anticipated that oxaliplatin-associated neuronal loss could be prevented by transient inhibition of Octn1. However, it is not known if Octn1 is also involved in the excretion of this agent and further studies are required to determine if inhibition of Octn1 has the potential to prevent oxaliplatin-induced neuropathy.

Octn3/Octn3 mRNA and protein expression has been detected in rat astrocytes where Octn3 expression was found to be upregulated when cells were exposed to the peroxisome proliferator–activator agonist (WY-14,643), suggesting that OCTN3 may play a role in peroxisome fatty acid metabolism in astrocytes (Januszewicz et al., 2009).

3.2.4 Nucleoside membrane transport systems

Nucleosides are essential precursors of DNA and RNA synthesis. Nucleoside transporters play a critical role in the brain in the transport of nucleosides for the biosynthesis of nucleic acids as well as in the regulation of endogenous adenosine concentrations. By regulating the levels of adenosine to interact with cell surface adenosine receptors, nucleoside transporters can modulate neurotransmission. In addition, a number of nucleoside-derived anticancer and antiviral drugs depend on nucleoside transport systems for uptake into the cells.

3.2.4.1 Concentrative nucleoside transporters

Concentrative nucleoside transporters (CNTs) belong to the SLC28 family and are comprised of three members. CNT1–3 are encoded by *SLC28A1, SLC28A2*, and *SLC28A3* genes, respectively. CNTs are active transporters of nucleosides and nucleoside-derived drugs and mediate transport of their substrates against their concentration gradient. CNT1 exhibits selectivity for pyrimidine nucleosides, CNT2 for purine nucleosides, and CNT3 is broadly selective for both purine and pyrimidine nucleosides. In human tissues, CNT1 and CNT2 translocate nucleosides using a Na^+-dependent mechanism, whereas CNT3 can use both proton and Na^+-dependent mechanisms as mode of transport. CNTs are widely distributed in prokaryotes and eukaryotes; however, equilibrative nucleoside transporters (ENTs) have been detected only in eukaryotes. CNTs transport a number of pyrimidine (i.e., gemcitabine, 5-flurouridine, zidovudine) and purine (i.e., ribavirin, fludarabine, cladribine) nucleoside derivatives as well as nucleobase derivatives (i.e., 6-mercaptopurine, 6- thioguanine). A crystal structure of a Na^+-dependent CNT from *Vibrio cholerae* bound to uridine has recently been identified (Johnson, Cheong, & Lee, 2012). The structure reveals eight transmembrane helices, two helix-turn-helix hairpins with opposite orientation, and three interfacial helices that are parallel to the membrane (Johnson et al., 2012). Human CNTs are predicted to have three more transmembrane helices than prokaryotic CNTs.

In human brain tissues, gene expression of *CNT1* and *CNT2* has been detected at low levels (Lu, Chen, & Klaassen, 2004). At the cellular level, *CNT1* expression was found to be absent at the gene level in primary cultures of mouse astrocytes and neurons, but *CNT2* and *CNT3* were found to be present (Li, Gu, Hertz, & Peng, 2013; Peng et al., 2005). Compared to *CNT1*, *CNT2* gene expression was found abundant in the brain, in particular, in neurons expressed in amygdala, hippocampus, neocortical regions, and the cerebellum (Guillen-Gomez et al., 2004). CNT2 protein expression has also been detected at the BBB in rats. Redzic et al. have reported gene and protein expression of CNT2 in primary cultures of rat BMECs as well as in rat choroid plexus epithelial cells (Redzic et al., 2005). CNT3 has been localized at the basolateral membranes of choroid plexus epithelial cells in rat and rabbit. Human *CNT3* transcripts have also been detected in choroid plexus (Redzic, Malatiali, Grujicic, & Isakovic, 2010). Human CNT3-mediated transport of several antiretroviral agents (i.e., zidovudine, zalcitabine, didanosine) has been demonstrated in *Xenopus* oocytes. Our laboratory characterized Na^+-dependent uptake of the pyrimidine nucleoside probe thymidine in a rat microglia cell line (MLS-9), suggesting CNT3-like transport properties in microglia (Hong, Schlichter, & Bendayan, 2000).

3.2.4.2 Equilibrative nucleoside transporters

ENTs transport nucleosides and/or nucleobases down their concentration gradient. The direction of the transport is dictated by the extracellular/intracellular gradient. Four nucleoside transporters have been identified. They are encoded by four SLC29 family genes: *SLC29A1, SLC29A2, SLC29A3* and *SLC29A4*. ENT1, ENT2, and ENT4 are membrane proteins, whereas ENT3 is primarily located intracellularly (Young, Yao, Sun, Cass, & Baldwin, 2008). The proposed membrane topology of human ENT1 includes 11 transmembrane helices, a cytoplasmic N-terminus, an extracellular C-terminus, and a large cytoplasmic loop linking two transmembrane domains, TMD_6 and TMD_7. A conserved PWN motif near the N-terminus contributes to the ENT1 function and membrane processing (Nivillac et al., 2009).

In human brain, protein expression of ENT1 was found to be predominant in the frontal and parietal lobes of the cerebral cortex, thalamus, midbrain, and basal ganglia (Jennings et al., 2001). In these regions, colocalization of ENT1 and adenosine receptor (A1) was also observed, suggesting ENT1-mediated regulation of adenosine signaling (Jennings et al., 2001). ENT1 and ENT2 expression has also been confirmed in BMECs, choroid plexus epithelium, astrocytes, and neurons. Transcripts of mouse *ENT1* and *ENT2* have been reported in primary cultures of mouse astrocytes (Peng et al., 2005). Redzic et al. have detected gene and protein expression of *ENT1*/ENT1 and *ENT2*/ENT2 in primary culture of rat BMECs as well as in rat choroid plexus epithelial cells (Redzic et al., 2005). Rat *ENT1* has been detected in pyrimidal neurons of the hippocampus, granule neurons of the dentate gyrus, Purkinji and granule neurons of the cerebellum, and cortical and strial neurons (Anderson, Xiong, et al., 1999). Similar to *ENT1*, *ENT2* transcripts have also been detected in neuronal and glial cells of human and rat brain, including cortex, striatum, hippocampus, and cerebellum (Anderson, Baldwin, Young, Cass, & Parkinson, 1999). In adult cynomolgus monkey brain microvessels, ENT1 membrane protein expression has been detected (Ito et al., 2011). Human ENT2 protein is highly expressed in the cerebellum, thalamus, medulla, midbrain, and brainstem regions, particularly the pons, and is expressed weakly in cerebral cortex and basal ganglia. ENT2 was found to be localized to the luminal side in endothelial cells, whereas at choroid plexus epithelium basolateral localization of this transporter was observed. Human *ENT1–3* have been detected at the gene level in choroid plexus with *ENT3* transcripts being the most abundant(Redzic et al., 2010).

ENT4 mediates Na^+-independent, low-affinity, and high-capacity transport of monoamine neurotransmitters (Engel, Zhou, & Wang, 2004). *ENT4* gene expression has been detected in human brain tissue in cerebral cortex, cerebellum, medulla, occipital pole, frontal and temporal lobes, and putamen (Engel et al., 2004). *ENT4*/ENT4 expression has been previously detected in mouse brain using RT-PCR, *in situ* hybridization, and immunohistochemistry. Both gene and protein expression of mouse *ENT4*/ENT4 were found to be abundant in forebrain cortex, olfactory tubercle, ventral striatum, hippocampal CA 1–3 regions, dentate gyrus, cerebellum, and epithelial cells of the choroid plexus. Using dual-fluorescence immunohistochemistry against markers for microtubule-associated protein-2 and GFAP, mouse ENT4 was found to be localized in neurons, but not in astrocytes (Dahlin, Xia, Kong, Hevner, & Wang, 2007). This group also confirmed protein expression of ENT4 in primary cultures of rat neurons (Dahlin et al., 2007). Li et al. have compared expression of *ENTs* in freshly isolated astrocytes and neurons from mouse brain (Li et al., 2013). Transcripts of all four *ENT* isoforms were detected in primary cultures of mouse astrocytes and neurons. However, *ENT2* and *ENT4* transcripts were found to be equally present in mouse astrocyte and neurons, whereas *ENT3* gene expression was more profound in astrocytes than in neurons.

Human ENT4 and OCT3 share similar substrate preference toward monoamines. ENT4 prefers 5-hydroxytryptamine and dopamine, whereas OCT prefers norepinephrine and epinephrine (Engel et al., 2004). The affinity of ENT4 toward monoamines and its wide distribution in the brain and in particular in neurons suggest a role of this transporter in maintaining the baseline levels of monoamines within the brain. A recent study demonstrated that ENT4 along with OCT3 and histamine-*N*-methyl-transferase in primary cultures of human astrocytes plays a role in the clearance of histamine from extracellular space to regulate extraneuronal histamine concentration (Yoshikawa et al., 2013).

3.2.5 Peptide transporters

Peptide transporters belong to SLC15 family and consist of four members: PEPT1, PEPT2, PhT1, and PhT2. Peptide transporters mediate proton-coupled transport of a broad range of peptides as well as peptidomimetics across the cellular membranes. Topological predictions of human PEPT1 suggest a structure of 12 transmembrane helices with a long intracellular loop between transmembrane domains 9 and 10. Crystal structures of prokaryotic homologues of mammalian peptide transporters have been solved (Newstead et al., 2011; Solcan et al., 2012). PEPT1 and PEPT2 transport a number of dipeptides, tripeptides, and peptide-like drugs. Substrates of these transporters include amino β-lactam antibiotics (i.e., cefadroxil), angiotensin-converting enzyme inhibitors (i.e., captopril), selected renin inhibitors, antiviral (acyclovir), photosensitizing agent (5-aminolevulinic acid), dopamine receptor antagonists, and antitumor agents (Rubio-Aliaga & Daniel, 2008). Peptide transporters expressed at the BBB and brain parenchymal cells regulate the uptake of peptides or peptidomimetics into the cell, whereas these transporters at the choroid plexus play a role in the removal of peptides or peptidomimetics from CSF to limit their exposure in the brain.

Pept1 is a low-affinity, high-capacity transporter that is predominantly expressed in the intestine. Pept1 has not been detected at the level of the BBB or in parenchyma. In contrast to Pept1, Pept2 is a high-affinity, low-capacity transporter that has a broader tissue distribution with highest expression in kidney. In the brain, *Pept2* mRNA transcripts have been detected in rat astrocytes, subependymal cells, ependymal cells, and epithelial cells of the choroid plexus (Berger & Hediger, 1999). Protein expression of Pept2 has been reported in cortex, olfactory bulb, basal ganglia, cerebellum, hindbrain, epithelial cells of the choroid plexus, and ependymal cells

(Shen, Smith, Keep, & Brosius, 2004). At the cellular level, Pept2 protein expression has been found in neurons, astrocytes, and apical membranes of choroid plexus epithelial cells.

Localization of Pept2 in brain parenchymal cellular compartments as well as in choroid plexus epithelial cells suggests a functional role of this transporter in the uptake or clearance of neuropeptides in the brain. For example, using primary cultures of neonatal astrocytes isolated from wild-type and Pept2 knockout mice, Xiang et al. demonstrate Pept2-mediated uptake of 5-aminolevulinic acid and carnosine in astrocytes, suggesting an important role of PEPT2 in the uptake of peptides into glial cells (Xiang, Hu, Smith, & Keep, 2006). Studies performed in *Pept2−/−* mice suggest a role of PEPT2 in the clearance of peptidomimetics from the CSF (Ocheltree et al., 2004a, 2004b). A decrease in Pept2-mediated clearance of peptides Gly-Sar and peptide-like drugs (i.e., cefadroxil) was also observed in choroid plexus epithelial cells isolated from Pept2-knockout mice (Smith et al., 2011).

PhT1 and PhT2, the other two members of the peptide transporter family, are peptide/histidine transporters (Sakata et al., 2001; Yamashita et al., 1997). Using *in situ* hybridization, Yamashita et al. detected mRNA transcripts of *PhT1* throughout whole brain, with higher expression in hippocampus, choroid plexus, cerebellum, and pontine nucleus (Yamashita et al., 1997). At the cellular level, gene expression was identified in neurons and other nonneuronal cells (Yamashita et al., 1997). *PhT2* transcripts has also been detected in the brain, although the expression was weaker compared to lung, spleen, and thymus (Sakata et al., 2001). Although gene expression of *PhT1* and *PhT2* has been reported in the brain, their functional role in brain parenchymal cells remains unknown.

3.2.6 Monocarboxylate transporters

Glucose is the major source of metabolic fuel in the CNS. However, monocarboxylic acids (i.e., lactate, pyruvate) can be utilized by the brain cells as alternative energy source. MCTs mediate the transport of monocarboxylic acids into brain cellular compartments. MCTs belong to the SLC16A family, and to date, 14 members of this family have been identified. Among these 14 members, only 7 members of the MCT family are known to be functionally active. Predicted membrane topology of MCT transporters suggests 12 transmembrane helices, intracellular N- and C-terminus, and a large cytosolic loop between transmembrane domains 6 and 7. MCTs 1–4 have been characterized as H^+-dependent transporters, whereas MCT6,

8, and 10 have been characterized as H^+- and Na^+-independent transporters of diuretics, aromatic amino acids, and thyroid hormone. Other substrates of MCTs include γ-hydroxy butyrate, salicylic acid, 3-hydroxy-3-methyl-glutaryl-coenzyme A reductase inhibitors, and bumetanide (Halestrap & Wilson, 2012).

MCTs are ubiquitously expressed in different tissues including brain, liver, kidney, and intestine. At the BBB, MCT1 expression has been detected in the luminal membrane of BMECs (Gerhart, Enerson, Zhdankina, Leino, & Drewes, 1997). MCT1 protein expression has also been detected in rat brain endothelial cell line, RBE4, as well as in brain microvessels isolated from adult cynomolgus monkey (Ito et al., 2011; Smith, Uhernik, Li, Liu, & Drewes, 2012). MCT1-mediated uptake of benzoate has also been characterized in both immortalized and primary cultures of BMECs (Kido, Tamai, Okamoto, Suzuki, & Tsuji, 2000). In brain parenchyma, MCT1 is strongly expressed in oligodendrocytes (Morrison, Lee, & Rothstein, 2013). Recent data suggest that oligodendrocytes may transfer energy metabolites to axons using MCT1 and downregulation of MCT1 can result in axonal and/or neuronal loss *in vitro* or *in vivo* (Lee et al., 2012). Using confocal microscopy, MCT2 protein expression has been localized in neurons. Functional expression of MTC2 has been demonstrated in the hypothalamic neuronal cell line, GT1–7 (Cortes-Campos et al., 2013). Studies suggest that MCT2 plays an important role in providing neurons with lactate as an energy sources (Wilson et al., 2013). Altered distribution of MCT2 has been observed in astrocytes in human epileptogenic hippocampus. Loss of MCT2 on astrocyte end-feet was associated with an upregulation of MCT2 protein on astrocyte membranes facing synapses, suggesting a compensatory mechanism to maintain the exchange of monocarboxylates within the parenchyma and the flux across the BBB (Lauritzen et al., 2012).

MCT3 has been localized at the basolateral membrane of retinal pigment epithelium and choroid plexus. Expression of MCT4 has been observed in cells with high glycolytic rates such as white skeletal muscle fibers, astrocytes, white blood cells, and chondrocytes. Recently, overexpression of MCT1 and MCT4 has been detected in human glioblastoma. Using the MCT inhibitor, α-cyano-4-hydroxycinnamic acid, in an animal model for glioblastoma, a decrease in tumor size and blood vessel formation was observed, suggesting MCT1 as a potential therapeutic target for glioblastoma treatment (Miranda-Goncalves et al., 2013). MCT8 is a highly specific thyroid hormone transporter and has been implicated in neurodevelopment.

Mutations within the MCT8 gene have been associated with various X-linked mental retardation syndromes where subjects may develop psychomotor and cognitive impairments (Holden et al., 2005; Schwartz et al., 2005). Patients also demonstrate abnormalities in the serum profile of thyroid hormone concentrations (Schwartz et al., 2005). Immunohistochemical staining of human fetal brain tissue revealed MCT8 expression in neurons of the cortex, epithelial cells of the choroid plexus, and ependymal cells as well as in brain microvessels (Chan, Hancox, et al., 2013; Ito et al., 2011). Transport studies in Mct8-deficient mice revealed a strongly diminished uptake of T_3 at the BBB or BCSF barrier, whereas the transport of T_4 into the brain was not impeded (Ceballos et al., 2009).

4. REGULATION OF DRUG TRANSPORTERS IN GLIAL CELLS IN THE CONTEXT OF NEUROPATHOLOGIES

Drug transporters expressed in brain parenchyma can play a significant role in the efficacy of therapeutic agents once they have crossed the BBB. For a number of pathological conditions (i.e., tumor, viral infection), it is critical for the drug to permeate into the parenchymal cells. In this section, we discuss different classes of drugs, their permeability into the brain, and their interaction with transporters.

4.1. Gliomas

Gliomas are the most common tumors in the brain. The expression of ABC transporters in brain tumors can limit the permeability of chemotherapeutic agents into the cells. Upregulation of P-gp, BCRP, and MRP1 has been reported in a number of neuroblastomas, astrocytomas, and glioblastomas, suggesting their contribution in generating resistance toward a number of therapeutic substrates. For example, enhanced P-gp expression has been reported in both gliomas and glioblastomas (Regina et al., 2001). Increased expression of MRP1 in neuroblastoma has been found to be associated with poor pharmacological treatment outcome (Haber et al., 2006). Similarly, others have demonstrated inadequate penetration of other chemotherapeutic agents (i.e., gefitinib, sorafenib) due to active efflux transport processes by P-gp and BCRP (Agarwal & Elmquist, 2012; Agarwal, Hartz, et al., 2011; Agarwal, Sane, Gallardo, Ohlfest, & Elmquist, 2010; Agarwal, Sane, et al., 2011). For example, gefitinib, a specific epidermal growth factor receptor-associated tyrosine kinase inhibitor, has been shown to be actively effluxed at the BBB by P-gp and Bcrp, limiting its distribution in the CNS. Using *Mdr1a/b* (−/−) *Bcrp1* (−/−) triple knockout mouse model, the authors have further demonstrated enhanced CNS distribution of gefitinib due to the absence of P-gp and Bcrp (Agarwal et al., 2010). Erlotinib was also found to be effluxed by both P-gp and Bcrp in mice (de Vries et al., 2012).

Many studies have attempted to reverse MDR *in vitro* or *in vivo*. Coadministration of the dual P-gp/BCRP inhibitor elacridar was able to significantly enhance brain distribution of gefitinib (Agarwal et al., 2010). Another study has reported inhibition of ABC transporter-mediated drug efflux by gefitinib *in vivo*, suggesting that gefitinib can increase the apparent bioavailability of coadministered drugs that are substrates for the transporters (Leggas et al., 2006). In a neuroblastoma cell line, increased expression of P-gp and MRP1 was detected, and after administration of low-intensity pulsed ultrasound, the expression of P-gp was significantly decreased (Sun, Chen, et al., 2013; Sun, Li, et al., 2013). Enhanced BCRP expression has also been found in nuclear fractions of several glioblastoma and astrocytoma cell lines as well as human glioblastoma tumor cell lines (Bhatia et al., 2012). Inhibition of BCRP using fumitremorgin C or downregulation of BCRP using small interfering RNA resulted in increased mitoxantrone cytotoxicity in glioblastoma Ln229 cell line (Bhatia et al., 2012). Increased MRP1 expression has been detected in glioblastoma multiforme biopsies. *In vitro*, concurrent administration of anticancer drugs along with an MRP1inhibitor in human glioblastoma T98G and G44 cells resulted in decreased cell viability (Peignan et al., 2011). Another study demonstrated that targeting hypoxia-inducible factor-1α using siRNA resulted in reduced MRP1 expression and increased cellular susceptibility to chemotherapeutic agents (Chen et al., 2009). Although many potential mechanisms have been explored to reverse MDR, further studies are needed to determine the permeability and efficacy of different chemotherapeutic agents against brain tumors.

4.2. Brain HIV-1 infection

HIV-1-associated neurological disorder is another neuropathological condition where drug transporters play an important role in determining the availability of antiretroviral drugs (Ronaldson, Persidsky, & Bendayan, 2008). About 50% of patients with HIV-1 infection develop neurocognitive deficits. In the brain, microglia hosts the productive infection of the HIV-1 virus and astrocytes host the latent virus. These cells are known to secrete many neurotoxic factors, chemokines, proinflammatory cytokines, nitric oxide, and glutamate during brain HIV-1 infection (Genis et al., 1992; Sacktor et al., 2004; Wang et al., 2003). In addition, shed viral proteins (i.e., tat, gp120, vpr) are also known to induce inflammatory and oxidative stress response in glial cells (Guha et al., 2012; Ronaldson & Bendayan, 2006, 2008). Chronic HIV-1 infection may result in elevated monocyte/macrophage infiltration into the brain, myelin pallor, multinucleated giant cells, activated microglia, reactive astrocytosis (proliferation and activation of astrocytes), and presence of microglial nodules. These neuropathological conditions are collectively termed as HIV-encephalitis (HIVE). Prolonged brain inflammation, oxidative stress, and neuronal loss associated with HIV-1 infection can ultimately lead to development of neurocognitive disorders in infected individuals (Heaton et al., 2011; Warriner et al., 2010).

Treatment of brain HIV-1 infection remains challenging. Poor permeability of antiretroviral drugs is one of the major obstacles to therapy. A number of HIV- protease inhibitors and nucleoside reverse transcriptase inhibitors exhibit low penetration into the brain due to the expression of drug efflux transporters both at the level of BBB and in brain parenchyma. Furthermore, studies suggest that functional expression of these transporters in the brain may get altered during HIV-1 infection. Increased P-gp staining has been observed in postmortem brain tissue from HIV-1-infected patients who were on antiretroviral therapy (Langford et al., 2004). Since antiretroviral drugs can modulate the expression of transporters *in vitro* and *in vivo*, it remains unclear if this increased P-gp immunoreactivity is due to therapy itself or due to HIV-associated pathogenesis. In contrast, decreased protein expression has been reported in brain autopsy samples from patients with HIVE not receiving therapy and in brain tissue from severe combined immunodeficiency mice model of HIVE (Persidsky, Zheng, Miller, & Gendelman, 2000). Using cell culture systems, many groups have demonstrated altered P-gp expression in human or rodent brain cellular compartments. Persidsky et al. reported decreased functional expression of P-gp in primary cultures of human BMECs exposed to TNF-α, IL-1β, IFN-γ, and supernatants from HIV-1-infected macrophages (Persidsky et al., 2000). In both murine BMECs and astrocytes, HIV-1 viral transactivator protein tat exposure resulted in an upregulation of P-gp expression (Hayashi et al., 2005). In our hands, we observed that HIV-1 gp120 can induce secretion of proinflammatory cytokines (IL-6, IL1-β, and TNF-α) by interacting with CCR5 chemokine receptors in primary cultures of rat astrocytes and significantly decrease functional expression of P-gp (Ronaldson & Bendayan,

2006). Our group also examined the effect of different cytokines on P-gp expression and demonstrated that IL-6 could profoundly decrease P-gp expression, whereas TNF-α or IL-1β exposure resulted in a modest enhancement in P-gp expression (Ronaldson & Bendayan, 2006). We have further confirmed similar findings in human astrocytes. Primary cultures of human fetal astrocytes exposed to R5-tropic and dual-tropic HIV-1 isolates led to a significant downregulation of P-gp expression (Ashraf et al., 2011). We also observed gp120 and IL-6-mediated downregulation of P-gp in human fetal astrocytes. This P-gp downregulation was attenuated by NF-κB inhibitory peptide SN50, suggesting an involvement of the NF-κB pathway in P-gp regulation (Ashraf et al., 2011).

In regard to Mrp1 regulation, in primary cultures of rat astrocytes, we have observed an increase in functional expression of this transporter in response to gp120 treatment which correlated with an enhanced efflux of GSH and GSSG, implying a potential role of MRP1 in regulating oxidative stress in glial cells (Ronaldson & Bendayan, 2008). In addition, *Mrp1*/Mrp1 expression was found to be upregulated at both the gene and protein level when cells were exposed to TNF-α in primary cultures of rat astrocytes (Ronaldson, Ashraf, & Bendayan, 2010). Inhibition of NF-κB using inhibitory peptide (SN50) or a pharmacological inhibitor (BAY-11-7082) attenuated gp120-mediated TNF-α release and Mrp1 upregulation, suggesting a role of the NF-κB pathway in Mrp1 regulation. Using inhibitor of NF-κB or JNK pathway in cultured astrocytes treated with TNF-α, we have further demonstrated that NF-κB is not directly involved in the regulation of Mrp1, but mediates its effect by activating JNK pathway which in turn results in the release of TNF-α (Ronaldson et al., 2010). Others have also investigated the involvement of signaling pathways in the regulation of transporters in the context of HIV-1 infection. For example, Hayashi et al. demonstrated Tat-induced upregulation of Mrp1 at the mRNA and protein level in cultured astrocytes with an involvement of the MAPK pathway (Hayashi et al., 2006). Zhong et al. have reported the involvement of intact lipid rafts and Rho signaling pathways in Tat-mediated P-gp upregulation (Zhong, Hennig, & Toborek, 2010). These observations provide evidence that ABC transporters are regulated during HIV-associated neuroinflammation which may result in altered brain permeability of antiretroviral drugs. Several SLC transporters (i.e., nucleoside transporter) have also been implicated in the uptake of antiretrovirals into the brain. However, the regulation of these transporters in the context of brain HIV-1 infection is not yet characterized.

4.3. Epilepsy

Epilepsy is another neurological disorder that is known to alter the expression of drug transporters (Tishler et al., 1995). Tishler and colleagues detected increased P-gp expression in brain capillary endothelial cells isolated from pharmacoresistant epileptic patients (Tishler et al., 1995). Upregulated P-gp expression has also been reported in reactive astrocytes in brain tissue of epileptic patients (Tishler et al., 1995; Volk, Potschka, & Loscher, 2004). Among other ABC transporters, ABCG2, MRP1, MRP2, and MRP5 were found to be upregulated during epilepsy. Abcg2 expression was increased in a rat model of epilepsy (van Vliet, Redeker, Aronica, Edelbroek, & Gorter, 2005). Increased MRP1 expression has been detected in several brain abnormalities characteristic of refractory epilepsy including dysplastic neurons and reactive astrocytes (Sisodiya et al., 2006). MRP2 and MRP5 expression has been found to be upregulated in brain tissue of pharmacoresistant epileptic patients.

Several studies have demonstrated that anti-epileptic drugs (AEDs) are substrates of ABC transporters and upregulation of these transporters are associated with reduced brain penetration of these drugs (Luna-Tortos, Fedrowitz, & Loscher, 2008). In a rat brain model of medically intractable epilepsy, mRNA and protein expression of P-gp was found to be upregulated in cerebral tissue compared to normal rat brain tissue (Ma, Wang, Chen, & Yuan, 2013). Concentrations of phenytoin and carbamazepine were also found to be very low in the extracellular fluid in these epileptic rats. However, after administration of verapamil, concentrations of phenytoin and carbamazepine increased in the extracellular fluid. These results suggest P-gp involvement in developing resistance to AEDs during epilepsy (Ma et al., 2013). In contrast, others have suggested that AEDs may not be substrates of ABC transporters and it is still inconclusive which AEDs are substrates of ABC transporters (Luna-Tortos, Fedrowitz, & Loscher, 2010). In Mdr1 knockout mice, brain permeation of phenytoin and carbamazepine were no different than wild-type animals, whereas significant penetration of topiramate, lamotrigine, and gabapentin was observed (Sills et al., 2002). Since increased expression of ABC transporters has been observed at the level of BBB and the parenchyma during pharmacoresistant epilepsy, further investigation is necessary to determine the role of transporters at the level of brain parenchyma and their interaction with AEDs.

It is also inconclusive if AEDs can modulate the expression of transporters. Lombardo et al. demonstrated that three-day exposure of AEDs (phenobarbital, phenytoin, carbamazepine, topiramate, tiagabine, and levetiracetam) induced the expression of P-gp in the rat BMEC cell line, GPNT (Lombardo, Pellitteri, Balazy, & Cardile, 2008). In contrast, phenobarbital, phenytoin, and carbamazepine did not have any effect on the functional expression of P-gp in this cell line. Another group also tested the effect of different AEDs on functional expression of P-gp in rat and human endothelial cells lines and reported that only carbamazepine resulted in a significant increase in P-gp function in hCMEC/D3 cells (Alms, Fedrowitz, Romermann, Noack, & Loscher, 2014). Yang et al. reported AED-mediated induction of P-gp expression in both endothelial and astroglial cells. In contrast, phenobarbital, phenytoin, and carbamazepine did not alter P-gp functional expression in brain capillary endothelial cells (Ambroziak et al., 2010). Another study has demonstrated that glutamate released during an epileptic seizure induces P-gp expression in mouse as well as in human brain capillaries via N-methyl-D-aspartate receptor (Avemary et al., 2013). Using antagonist against this receptor, functional activity of P-gp was inhibited, suggesting that P-gp is upregulated during disease state and NMDA receptor antagonist may serve as therapeutic intervention to reverse transporter-associated drug resistance (Avemary et al., 2013).

4.4. Parkinson's disease

ABC transporters are also known to be regulated during neurodegenerative diseases such as Parkinson's and Alzheimer's. Parkinson's disease (PD) is characterized by loss of neurons in the substantia nigra and formation of Lewy bodies. Clinically, PD is characterized by bradykinesia, akinesia, muscle rigidity, and tremor. Accumulation of endogenous or exogenous toxins can lead to the pathology of PD (Bartels & Leenders, 2009; Westerlund, Hoffer, & Olson, 2010). Several P-gp substrates have been implicated in the pathophysiology of PD. For example, several pesticides are known to induce oxidative stress and subsequent neuronal death that can contribute to the development of PD (Lai, Marion, Teschke, & Tsui, 2002). On the other hand, some toxins have been found to not be P-gp substrates. Using knockout animals, Lacher et al. demonstrated that paraquat, a Parkinson's associated neurotoxicant, is not a P-gp substrate (Lacher et al., 2014).

Reduced *MDR1* gene expression has been reported in brain capillary endothelial cells isolated from autopsy samples of PD patients (Westerlund, Belin, Olson, & Galter, 2008). Permeation of a radiolabeled P-gp substrate, verapamil, was also found to be elevated in patients with advanced PD (Bartels et al., 2008; Kortekaas et al., 2005). Although it was speculated that

MRP1- and MRP2-mediated transport of GSH conjugates of toxic substances may have beneficial effects in PD, inhibiting different MRP isoforms in mice did not affect 1-methyl-4-phenyl-1,2,3,6-tetrahydropyridine-induced neurotoxicity (Plangar, Zadori, Szalardy, Vecsei, & Klivenyi, 2013). A recent study has demonstrated that Mrp7 expression in dopaminergic neurons inhibits methylmercury, an environmental pollutant, induced neuronal toxicity (VanDuyn & Nass, 2014). Genetic knockdown of Mrp7 resulted in a twofold increase in stress response in the endoplasmic reticulum and led to animal death indicating a neuroprotective role of Mrp7 (VanDuyn & Nass, 2014).

Although antiparkinsonian drugs, i.e., bromocriptine, are known to interact with P-gp *in vitro*, it is still inconclusive if these drugs are substrates or inhibitors of P-gp *in vivo*. P-gp-mediated efflux of rhodamine123 and calcein AM efflux was inhibited by bromocriptine in P-gp-overexpressing cells (Shiraki et al., 2002). However, studies performed in mdr1a knockout animal suggest that bromocriptine is not a P-gp inhibitor (Vautier et al., 2006). Since accumulation of xenobiotics due to impaired function of drug transporters may increase the risk of PD, it is important to understand transporter-mediated clearance of neurotoxins in brain cellular compartments.

4.5. Alzheimer's disease

Alzheimer's disease (AD) is characterized by deposition of amyloid plaques within the brain parenchyma. It is clinically characterized by the decline of cognitive performance including memory and mental processing. In cases with several capillary cerebral amyloid angiopathy, Aβ accumulates in the capillary wall (Attems, Jellinger, & Lintner, 2005; Thal, Griffin, & Braak, 2008). It has been hypothesized that impaired clearance of Aβ due to functional changes in Aβ transporters at the BBB may contribute to the pathogenesis of AD (Vogelgesang, Kunert-Keil, et al., 2004; Vogelgesang, Warzok, et al., 2004).

Studies have indicated that P-gp may play a role in Aβ transport. After injecting [^{125}I] Aβ40 and [^{125}I] Aβ42 in mdr1a/1b knockout mice and wild-type mice, clearance of these peptides was found to be slower compared to wild-type controls (Cirrito et al., 2005). Silverberg et al. reported reduction of P-gp expression in brain capillaries and increased accumulation of Aβ in aging rats (Silverberg et al., 2010). Reduced P-gp expression was also observed in brain capillaries isolated from transgenic mouse model of AD, suggesting a role of P-gp in Aβ transport across the BBB (Hartz,

Miller, & Bauer, 2010). Using radiolabeled-verapamil and positron emission tomography, increased [^{11}C]verapamil was detected in brains of AD patients compared to age-matched healthy individuals, suggesting decreased P-gp functional activity at the BBB (van Assema et al., 2012). A recent study has detected a dramatic decrease in P-gp and BCRP expression in capillaries isolated from cerebral amyloid angiopathy cases.

Alteration of other ABC transporters has also been reported in the context of AD. Increased ABCG2 expression has been detected in microvessels isolated from brain tissue obtained from transgenic Alzheimer's mouse model as well as from patients with cerebral amyloid angiopathy (Xiong et al., 2009). In Abcg2 knockout mice, Aβ accumulation was found to be higher compared to wild-type mice. Similarly, Krohn et al. reported that Mrp1 deficiency resulted in increased Aβ brain accumulation in genetically modified AD mice (Krohn et al., 2011). Increased MRP1 expression has also been found in hippocampal tissue of AD patients, suggesting a protective role of this transporter in the pathogenesis of AD (Sultana & Butterfield, 2004). In a mouse model of AD, 1α,25-dihydroxy vitamin D3 induced P-gp expression, reduced cerebral Aβ accumulation, and resulted in improved cognition in the animals (Durk et al., 2012, 2014). Overall, ABC transporters may play a critical role in the pathogenesis of AD and could be a potential target to modulate disease progression and/or treatment of AD. However, further studies are required to fully characterize the role of these drug transporters in Aβ trafficking in parenchymal cells in the context of AD.

4.6. Drugs of abuse, analgesics, and anesthetics

The ABC efflux transporters are neuroprotective as they synergistically expel potentially harmful substances out of the brain. However, substances such as drugs of abuse (e.g., cocaine, LSD, cannabinoids), narcotics (morphine), and anesthetics are still able to successfully penetrate across the BBB and into the CNS.

Marijuana is a commonly used illegal drug and its frequent use can lead to addiction and dependence (Fratta & Fattore, 2013). The active chemical agents in marijuana can interact with cannabinoid receptors in neurons in order to induce psychotropic effects, analgesia, and memory impairment. Studies have also shown that these active ingredients can also interact with cannabinoid receptors in glial cells and affect the pathogenesis of diseases associated with neuroinflammation (i.e., multiple sclerosis) (Stella, 2004). Marijuana can also alter transporter expression or function. For example, cannabinol, one of the four major active ingredients of marijuana, has been shown to significantly inhibit P-gp-mediated drug transport in rat BMECs, suggesting potential drug–drug interactions when taken with other P-gp substrates (Zhu et al., 2006). In another study, decreased P-gp expression was observed in CEM/VLB(100) cells after 72 h of exposure to cannabinoids which correlated with an increase in intracellular accumulation of Rhodamine123, a fluorescent P-gp substrate, suggesting the efficacy of plant-derived cannabinoids in reversing MDR phenotype (Holland et al., 2006). A number of studies suggest that plant-derived cannabinoid may exhibit potential for therapeutic applications. Further studies are required to understand the cellular mechanisms of plant-derived cannabinoids as well as their effect on transporters in glial cells.

Cocaine is another well-known drug of abuse. It has been well established that cocaine has a profound effect on the integrity of BBB through downregulation of tight junction proteins and upregulation of cellular adhesion molecules (Dietrich, 2009). Within the brain parenchymal cells, cocaine is highly toxic. Recent studies of chronic cocaine exposure in glial cells (astrocytes and microglial) indicate toxicity leading to dysfunction and cell death (Badisa & Goodman, 2012; Costa, Yao, Yang, & Buch, 2013). Cocaine-induced cytotoxicity may involve mechanisms associated with endoplasmic reticulum stress, namely, the unfolded protein response. Multiple endoplasmic reticulum stress signaling mediators (i.e., PERK, Elf2α, CHOP) have been reported to exhibit increased levels upon cocaine administration in striatal neurons and BV-2 microglial cell line (Choe, Ahn, Yang, Go, & Wang, 2011; Costa et al., 2013). Cocaine is known to exert its effect by interacting with dopamine transporters. However, it is yet to be elucidated if cocaine has any effect on ABC or SLC transporters.

Opioids are the most effective analgesics used in pharmacological pain management. Opioids exert their analgesic effect by binding to specific receptors (i.e., mu-, kappa-, and delta-opioid receptors) that are localized to neural tissue within the CNS. Glial cells have also been the focus of opioid addiction research and are anticipated to play a fundamental role in eliciting positive reinforcements through inflammatory effects. For example, upon acute and chronic morphine administration, astrocyte activation was observed in several regions of the brain in humans and rodents (Cooper, Jones, & Comer, 2012). Astrocyte activation leads to inflammation, generation of reactive oxygen species, and proinflammatory markers, ultimately resulting in opioid and morphine tolerance (Shah, Kumar, Simon, Singh, & Kumar, 2013; Shen, Tsai, & Wong, 2012). The signaling cascades responsible for opioid addiction and tolerance remain unidentified. However, a recent study suggested involvement of cytokine IL-1β and ERK 1/2 in mice astrocytes. Microglia cells treated with morphine show increased secretion of cytokines and chemokines that are able to modulate neuronal behavior (e.g., IL-10, CCL25, CCL4, CCL17) (Horvath & DeLeo, 2009; Schwarz, Smith, & Bilbo, 2013). Furthermore, permanent reductions in oligodendrocytes and neurons have been observed in morphine treated rats (Rafati, Noorafshan, & Torabi, 2013). In one study, morphine has been shown to decrease P-gp and Bcrp expression at the rat BBB following increasing doses of morphine (Yousif et al., 2012). However, this has not been observed at the astrocyte and neuronal level using immunofluorescence and *in situ* hybridization in rats or human tissue (Yousif et al., 2008). Furthermore, it appears that astrocytes and microglial cells lack the μ-opioid receptor that is believed to be necessary for glial activation undermining theories of direct activation by morphine (Kao et al., 2012). Additional research is necessary to delineate the significance of ABC transporters in the pharmacokinetics and pharmacodynamics of morphine within the brain parenchyma.

General anesthetics such as isoflurane, pentobarbital, midazolam, ketamine, and propofol have been known to have a suppressive effect on cytokine secretion in microglia (Tanaka et al., 2013). In a recent investigation in primary cultures of mice glial cells and BV-2 microglia cell line, LPS-induced IL-1β expression was inhibited upon anesthetic administration but mRNA levels of NF-κB and AP-1 activation was unaffected (Tanaka et al., 2013). Since inflammatory mediators are known to regulate transporter expression, changes in inflammatory conditions due to anesthetic administration may alter expression of ABC transporters at the BBB (von Wedel-Parlow, Wolte, & Galla, 2009). The effect of general anesthesia on ABC efflux transporter expression in brain parenchymal cells is yet to be investigated.

5. CONCLUSION

It is clear that drug transporters at the level of brain parenchyma play a major role in maintaining the homeostasis of the CNS during normal physiological conditions and constitute important determinants of drug disposition across the BBB, BCSFB, and into brain parenchymal cells during neuropathological conditions. Brain expression of these transporters with a wide variety of substrate specificity has important implications in the pharmacotherapy of neurological disorders. However, functional relevance of several SLC and ABC transporters in brain parenchyma cells is yet to be discovered. In addition, overlapping substrate specificity of these drug transporters may result in unexpected drug–drug interactions leading to pharmacotherapy failure in the brain. Further investigation is required to elucidate the functional role of each transporter in each of the brain cellular compartments. Understanding the substrate specificity and physiological role of these transporters may allow to identify and/or develop novel therapeutic agents that can readily penetrate across the BBB as well as brain parenchymal cellular membranes.

CONFLICTS OF INTEREST

None to declare.

ACKNOWLEDGMENTS

This work is supported by the Canadian Institutes of Health Research (CIHR) and the Ontario, HIV Treatment Network (OHTN), Ministry of Health of Ontario. Dr. R. Bendayan is a career scientist of the OHTN.

REFERENCES

Abbott, N. J., Patabendige, A. A., Dolman, D. E., Yusof, S. R., & Begley, D. J. (2010). Structure and function of the blood-brain barrier. *Neurobiology of Disease*, *37*, 13–25.

Abbott, N. J., Ronnback, L., & Hansson, E. (2006). Astrocyte-endothelial interactions at the blood-brain barrier. *Nature Reviews. Neuroscience*, *7*, 41–53.

Agarwal, S., & Elmquist, W. F. (2012). Insight into the cooperation of P-glycoprotein (ABCB1) and breast cancer resistance protein (ABCG2) at the blood-brain barrier: A case study examining sorafenib efflux clearance. *Molecular Pharmaceutics*, *9*(3), 678–684.

Agarwal, S., Hartz, A. M., Elmquist, W. F., & Bauer, B. (2011). Breast cancer resistance protein and P-glycoprotein in brain cancer: Two gatekeepers team up. *Current Pharmaceutical Design*, *17*(26), 2793–2802.

Agarwal, S., Sane, R., Gallardo, J. L., Ohlfest, J. R., & Elmquist, W. F. (2010). Distribution of gefitinib to the brain is limited by P-glycoprotein (ABCB1) and breast cancer resistance protein (ABCG2)-mediated active efflux. *The Journal of Pharmacology and Experimental Therapeutics*, *334*, 147–155.

Agarwal, S., Sane, R., Ohlfest, J. R., & Elmquist, W. F. (2011). The role of the breast cancer resistance protein (ABCG2) in the distribution of sorafenib to the brain. *The Journal of Pharmacology and Experimental Therapeutics*, *336*, 223–233.

Al, A. A., Taboada, C. B., Gassmann, M., & Ogunshola, O. O. (2011). Astrocytes and pericytes differentially modulate blood-brain barrier characteristics during development and hypoxic insult. *Journal of Cerebral Blood Flow and Metabolism*, *31*(2), 693–705.

Alebouyeh, M., Takeda, M., Onozato, M. L., Tojo, A., Noshiro, R., Hasannejad, H., et al. (2003). Expression of human organic anion transporters in the choroid plexus and their interactions with neurotransmitter metabolites. *Journal of Pharmacological Sciences*, *93*(4), 430–436.

Aller, S. G., Yu, J., Ward, A., Weng, Y., Chittaboina, S., Zhuo, R., et al. (2009). Structure of P-glycoprotein reveals a molecular basis for poly-specific drug binding. *Science*, *323*, 1718–1722.

Alms, D., Fedrowitz, M., Romermann, K., Noack, A., & Loscher, W. (2014). Marked differences in the effect of antiepileptic and cytostatic drugs on the functionality of p-glycoprotein in human and rat brain capillary endothelial cell lines. *Pharmaceutical Research*, *31*(6), 1588–1604.

Ambroziak, K., Kuteykin-Teplyakov, K., Luna-Tortos, C., Al-Falah, M., Fedrowitz, M., & Loscher, W. (2010). Exposure to antiepileptic drugs does not alter the functionality of P-glycoprotein in brain capillary endothelial and kidney cell lines. *European Journal of Pharmacology*, *628*, 57–66.

Anderson, C. M., Baldwin, S. A., Young, J. D., Cass, C. E., & Parkinson, F. E. (1999). Distribution of mRNA encoding a nitrobenzylthioinosine-insensitive nucleoside transporter (ENT2) in rat brain. *Brain Research. Molecular Brain Research*, *70*(2), 293–297.

Anderson, C. M., Xiong, W., Geiger, J. D., Young, J. D., Cass, C. E., Baldwin, S. A., et al. (1999). Distribution of equilibrative, nitrobenzylthioinosine-sensitive nucleoside transporters (ENT1) in brain. *Journal of Neurochemistry*, *73*(2), 867–873.

Aronica, E., Gorter, J. A., Jansen, G. H., van Veelen, C. W., van Rijen, P. C., Leenstra, S., et al. (2003). Expression and cellular distribution of multidrug transporter proteins in two major causes of medically intractable epilepsy: Focal cortical dysplasia and glioneuronal tumors. *Neuroscience*, *118*, 417–429.

Aronica, E., Gorter, J. A., Ramkema, M., Redeker, S., Ozbas-Gerceker, F., van Vliet, E. A., et al. (2004). Expression and cellular distribution of multidrug resistance-related proteins in the hippocampus of patients with mesial temporal lobe epilepsy. *Epilepsia*, *45*(5), 441–451.

Aronica, E., Gorter, J. A., Redeker, S., van Vliet, E. A., Ramkema, M., Scheffer, G. L., et al. (2005). Localization of breast cancer resistance protein (BCRP) in microvessel endothelium of human control and epileptic brain. *Epilepsia*, *46*, 849–857.

Ashraf, T., Kis, O., Banerjee, N., & Bendayan, R. (2012). Drug transporters at the brain barriers: Expression and regulation by neurological disorders. *Advances in Experimental Medicine and Biology*, *763*, 20–69.

Ashraf, T., Ronaldson, P. T., Persidsky, Y., & Bendayan, R. (2011). Regulation of P-glycoprotein by human immunodeficiency virus-1 in primary cultures of human fetal astrocytes. *Journal of Neuroscience Research*, *89*, 1773–1782.

Attems, J., Jellinger, K. A., & Lintner, F. (2005). Alzheimer's disease pathology influences severity and topographical distribution of cerebral amyloid angiopathy. *Acta Neuropathologica*, *110*(3), 222–231.

Avemary, J., Salvamoser, J. D., Peraud, A., Remi, J., Noachtar, S., Fricker, G., et al. (2013). Dynamic regulation of P-glycoprotein in human brain capillaries. *Molecular Pharmaceutics*, *10*(9), 3333–3341.

Babakhanian, K., Bendayan, M., & Bendayan, R. (2007). Localization of P-glycoprotein at the nuclear envelope of rat brain cells. *Biochemical and Biophysical Research Communications*, *361*, 301–306.

Bacq, A., Balasse, L., Biala, G., Guiard, B., Gardier, A. M., Schinkel, A., et al. (2012). Organic cation transporter 2 controls brain norepinephrine and serotonin clearance and antidepressant response. *Molecular Psychiatry*, *17*(9), 926–939.

Badisa, R. B., & Goodman, C. B. (2012). Effects of chronic cocaine in rat C6 astroglial cells. *International Journal of Molecular Medicine*, *30*(3), 687–692.

Bahn, A., Hagos, Y., Reuter, S., Balen, D., Brzica, H., Krick, W., et al. (2008). Identification of a new urate and high affinity nicotinate transporter, hOAT10 (SLC22A13). *The Journal of Biological Chemistry*, *283*(24), 16332–16341.

Bahn, A., Ljubojevic, M., Lorenz, H., Schultz, C., Ghebremedhin, E., Ugele, B., et al. (2005). Murine renal organic anion transporters mOAT1 and mOAT3 facilitate the transport of neuroactive tryptophan metabolites. *American Journal of Physiology. Cell Physiology, 289*(5), C1075–C1084.

Ballerini, P., Di, I. P., Ciccarelli, R., Nargi, E., D'Alimonte, I., Traversa, U., et al. (2002). Glial cells express multiple ATP binding cassette proteins which are involved in ATP release. *Neuroreport, 13*, 1789–1792.

Bao, G. S., Wang, W. A., Wang, T. Z., Huang, J. K., He, H., Liu, Z., et al. (2011). Overexpression of human MRP1 in neurons causes resistance to antiepileptic drugs in Drosophila seizure mutants. *Journal of Neurogenetics, 25*(4), 201–206.

Bartels, A. L., & Leenders, K. L. (2009). Parkinson's disease: The syndrome, the pathogenesis and pathophysiology. *Cortex, 45*, 915–921.

Bartels, A. L., Willemsen, A. T., Kortekaas, R., de Jong, B. M., de Vries, R., de Klerk, O., et al. (2008). Decreased blood-brain barrier P-glycoprotein function in the progression of Parkinson's disease, PSP and MSA. *Journal of Neural Transmission, 115*, 1001–1009.

Beck, K., Hayashi, K., Dang, K., Hayashi, M., & Boyd, C. D. (2005). Analysis of ABCC6 (MRP6) in normal human tissues. *Histochemistry and Cell Biology, 123*, 517–528.

Belinsky, M. G., Chen, Z. S., Shchaveleva, I., Zeng, H., & Kruh, G. D. (2002). Characterization of the drug resistance and transport properties of multidrug resistance protein 6 (MRP6, ABCC6). *Cancer Research, 62*(21), 6172–6177.

Bendayan, R., Ronaldson, P. T., Gingras, D., & Bendayan, M. (2006). In situ localization of P-glycoprotein (ABCB1) in human and rat brain. *Journal of Histochemistry and Cytochemistry, 54*, 1159–1167.

Bera, T. K., Iavarone, C., Kumar, V., Lee, S., Lee, B., & Pastan, I. (2002). MRP9, an unusual truncated member of the ABC transporter superfamily, is highly expressed in breast cancer. *Proceedings of the National Academy of Sciences of the United States of America, 99*, 6997–7002.

Bera, T. K., Lee, S., Salvatore, G., Lee, B., & Pastan, I. (2001). MRP8, a new member of ABC transporter superfamily, identified by EST database mining and gene prediction program, is highly expressed in breast cancer. *Molecular Medicine, 7*, 509–516.

Berezowski, V., Landry, C., Dehouck, M. P., Cecchelli, R., & Fenart, L. (2004). Contribution of glial cells and pericytes to the mRNA profiles of P-glycoprotein and multidrug resistance-associated proteins in an in vitro model of the blood-brain barrier. *Brain Research, 1018*, 1–9.

Berger, U. V., & Hediger, M. A. (1999). Distribution of peptide transporter PEPT2 mRNA in the rat nervous system. *Anatomy and Embryology, 199*, 439–449.

Bhatia, P., Bernier, M., Sanghvi, M., Moaddel, R., Schwarting, R., Ramamoorthy, A., et al. (2012). Breast cancer resistance protein (BCRP/ABCG2) localises to the nucleus in glioblastoma multiforme cells. *Xenobiotica, 42*(8), 748–755.

Bierman, W. F., Scheffer, G. L., Schoonderwoerd, A., Jansen, G., van Agtmael, M. A., Danner, S. A., et al. (2010). Protease inhibitors atazanavir, lopinavir and ritonavir are potent blockers, but poor substrates, of ABC transporters in a broad panel of ABC transporter-overexpressing cell lines. *Journal of Antimicrobial Chemotherapy, 65*, 1672–1680.

Binkhathlan, Z., & Lavasanifar, A. (2013). P-glycoprotein inhibition as a therapeutic approach for overcoming multidrug resistance in cancer: Current status and future perspectives. *Current Cancer Drug Targets, 13*(3), 326–346.

Bortfeld, M., Rius, M., Konig, J., Herold-Mende, C., Nies, A. T., & Keppler, D. (2006). Human multidrug resistance protein 8 (MRP8/ABCC11), an apical efflux pump for steroid sulfates, is an axonal protein of the CNS and peripheral nervous system. *Neuroscience, 137*, 1247–1257.

Brandmann, M., Tulpule, K., Schmidt, M. M., & Dringen, R. (2012). The antiretroviral protease inhibitors indinavir and nelfinavir stimulate Mrp1-mediated GSH export from cultured brain astrocytes. *Journal of Neurochemistry, 120*, 78–92.

Bronger, H., Konig, J., Kopplow, K., Steiner, H. H., Ahmadi, R., Herold-Mende, C., et al. (2005). ABCC drug efflux pumps and organic anion uptake transporters in human gliomas and the blood-tumor barrier. *Cancer Research, 65,* 11419–11428.

Cantrill, C. A., Skinner, R. A., Rothwell, N. J., & Penny, J. I. (2012). An immortalised astrocyte cell line maintains the in vivo phenotype of a primary porcine in vitro blood-brain barrier model. *Brain Research, 1479,* 17–30.

Ceballos, A., Belinchon, M. M., Sanchez-Mendoza, E., Grijota-Martinez, C., Dumitrescu, A. M., Refetoff, S., et al. (2009). Importance of monocarboxylate transporter 8 for the blood-brain barrier-dependent availability of 3,5,3'-triiodo-L-thyronine. *Endocrinology, 150*(5), 2491–2496.

Chan, S. Y., Hancox, L. A., Martin-Santos, A., Loubiere, L. S., Walter, M. N., Gonzalez, A. M., et al. (2013). MCT8 expression in human fetal cerebral cortex is reduced in severe intrauterine growth restriction. *Journal of Endocrinology, 220*(2), 85–95.

Chan, G. N., Patel, R., Cummins, C. L., & Bendayan, R. (2013). Induction of p-glycoprotein by antiretroviral drugs in human brain microvessel endothelial cells. *Antimicrobial Agents and Chemotherapy, 57*(9), 4481–4488.

Chen, L., Feng, P., Li, S., Long, D., Cheng, J., Lu, Y., et al. (2009). Effect of hypoxia-inducible factor-1alpha silencing on the sensitivity of human brain glioma cells to doxorubicin and etoposide. *Neurochemical Research, 34,* 984–990.

Choe, E. S., Ahn, S. M., Yang, J. H., Go, B. S., & Wang, J. Q. (2011). Linking cocaine to endoplasmic reticulum in striatal neurons: Role of glutamate receptors. *Basal Ganglia, 1*(2), 59–63.

Choudhuri, S., Cherrington, N. J., Li, N., & Klaassen, C. D. (2003). Constitutive expression of various xenobiotic and endobiotic transporter mRNAs in the choroid plexus of rats. *Drug Metabolism and Disposition, 31,* 1337–1345.

Cirrito, J. R., Deane, R., Fagan, A. M., Spinner, M. L., Parsadanian, M., Finn, M. B., et al. (2005). P-glycoprotein deficiency at the blood-brain barrier increases amyloid-beta deposition in an Alzheimer disease mouse model. *The Journal of Clinical Investigation, 115,* 3285–3290.

Cole, S. P., Bhardwaj, G., Gerlach, J. H., Mackie, J. E., Grant, C. E., Almquist, K. C., et al. (1992). Overexpression of a transporter gene in a multidrug-resistant human lung cancer cell line. *Science, 258,* 1650–1654.

Cooper, Z. D., Jones, J. D., & Comer, S. D. (2012). Glial modulators: A novel pharmacological approach to altering the behavioral effects of abused substances. *Expert Opinion on Investigational Drugs, 21*(2), 169–178.

Cortes-Campos, C., Elizondo, R., Carril, C., Martinez, F., Boric, K., Nualart, F., et al. (2013). MCT2 expression and lactate influx in anorexigenic and orexigenic neurons of the arcuate nucleus. *PLoS One, 8*((4), e62532.

Costa, B. M., Yao, H., Yang, L., & Buch, S. (2013). Role of endoplasmic reticulum (ER) stress in cocaine-induced microglial cell death. *Journal of Neuroimmune Pharmacology, 8*(3), 705–714.

Cygalova, L. H., Hofman, J., Ceckova, M., & Staud, F. (2009). Transplacental pharmacokinetics of glyburide, rhodamine 123, and BODIPY FL prazosin: Effect of drug efflux transporters and lipid solubility. *The Journal of Pharmacology and Experimental Therapeutics, 331,* 1118–1125.

Dahlin, A., Xia, L., Kong, W., Hevner, R., & Wang, J. (2007). Expression and immunolocalization of the plasma membrane monoamine transporter in the brain. *Neuroscience, 146*(3), 1193–1211.

Dallas, S., Miller, D. S., & Bendayan, R. (2006). Multidrug resistance-associated proteins: Expression and function in the central nervous system. *Pharmacological Reviews, 58*(2), 140–161.

Dallas, S., Schlichter, L., & Bendayan, R. (2004). Multidrug resistance protein (MRP) 4- and MRP 5-mediated efflux of 9-(2-phosphonylmethoxyethyl)adenine by microglia. *The Journal of Pharmacology and Experimental Therapeutics*, *309*, 1221–1229.

Dallas, S., Zhu, X., Baruchel, S., Schlichter, L., & Bendayan, R. (2003). Functional expression of the multidrug resistance protein 1 in microglia. *The Journal of Pharmacology and Experimental Therapeutics*, *307*, 282–290.

Daood, M., Tsai, C., Ahdab-Barmada, M., & Watchko, J. F. (2008). ABC transporter (P-gp/ABCB1, MRP1/ABCC1, BCRP/ABCG2) expression in the developing human CNS. *Neuropediatrics*, *39*, 211–218.

Darby, R. A., Callaghan, R., & McMahon, R. M. (2011). P-glycoprotein inhibition: The past, the present and the future. *Current Drug Metabolism*, *12*(8), 722–731.

Dazert, P., Suofu, Y., Grube, M., Popa-Wagner, A., Kroemer, H. K., Jedlitschky, G., et al. (2006). Differential regulation of transport proteins in the periinfarct region following reversible middle cerebral artery occlusion in rats. *Neuroscience*, *142*, 1071–1079.

Decleves, X., Fajac, A., Lehmann-Che, J., Tardy, M., Mercier, C., Hurbain, I., et al. (2002). Molecular and functional MDR1-Pgp and MRPs expression in human glioblastoma multiforme cell lines. *International Journal of Cancer*, *98*, 173–180.

Deng, W., Dai, C. L., Chen, J. J., Kathawala, R. J., Sun, Y. L., Chen, H. F., et al. (2013). Tandutinib (MLN518) reverses multidrug resistance by inhibiting the efflux activity of the multidrug resistance protein 7 (ABCC10). *Oncology Reports*, *29*(6), 2479–2485.

de Vries, N. A., Buckle, T., Zhao, J., Beijnen, J. H., Schellens, J. H., & van Tellingen, O. (2012). Restricted brain penetration of the tyrosine kinase inhibitor erlotinib due to the drug transporters P-gp and BCRP. *Investigational New Drugs*, *30*(2), 443–449.

Dietrich, J. B. (2009). Alteration of blood-brain barrier function by methamphetamine and cocaine. *Cell and Tissue Research*, *336*(3), 385–392.

Diop, N. K., & Hrycyna, C. A. (2005). N-Linked glycosylation of the human ABC transporter ABCG2 on asparagine 596 is not essential for expression, transport activity, or trafficking to the plasma membrane. *Biochemistry*, *44*(14), 5420–5429.

Do, T. M., Bedussi, B., Chasseigneaux, S., Dodacki, A., Yapo, C., Chacun, H., et al. (2013). Oatp1a4 and an L-thyroxine-sensitive transporter mediate the mouse blood-brain barrier transport of amyloid-beta peptide. *Journal of Alzheimer's Disease*, *36*(3), 555–561.

Doyle, L. A., Yang, W., Abruzzo, L. V., Krogmann, T., Gao, Y., Rishi, A. K., et al. (1998). A multidrug resistance transporter from human MCF-7 breast cancer cells. *Proceedings of the National Academy of Sciences of the United States of America*, *95*, 15665–15670.

Durk, M. R., Chan, G. N., Campos, C. R., Peart, J. C., Chow, E. C., Lee, E., et al. (2012). 1alpha,25-Dihydroxyvitamin D3-liganded vitamin D receptor increases expression and transport activity of P-glycoprotein in isolated rat brain capillaries and human and rat brain microvessel endothelial cells. *Journal of Neurochemistry*, *123*(6), 944–953.

Durk, M. R., Han, K., Chow, E. C., Ahrens, R., Henderson, J. T., Fraser, P. E., et al. (2014). 1alpha,25-Dihydroxyvitamin D3 reduces cerebral amyloid-beta accumulation and improves cognition in mouse models of Alzheimer's disease. *Journal of Neuroscience*, *34*(21), 7091–7101.

Eisenblatter, T., & Galla, H. J. (2002). A new multidrug resistance protein at the blood-brain barrier. *Biochemical and Biophysical Research Communications*, *293*, 1273–1278.

Eisenblatter, T., Huwel, S., & Galla, H. J. (2003). Characterisation of the brain multidrug resistance protein (BMDP/ABCG2/BCRP) expressed at the blood-brain barrier. *Brain Research*, *971*, 221–231.

Engel, K., Zhou, M., & Wang, J. (2004). Identification and characterization of a novel monoamine transporter in the human brain. *The Journal of Biological Chemistry*, *279*, 50042–50049.

Feurstein, D., Kleinteich, J., Heussner, A. H., Stemmer, K., & Dietrich, D. R. (2010). Investigation of microcystin congener-dependent uptake into primary murine neurons. *Environmental Health Perspectives*, *118*(10), 1370–1375.

Fratta, W., & Fattore, L. (2013). Molecular mechanisms of cannabinoid addiction. *Current Opinion in Neurobiology*, *23*(4), 487–492.

Fujiwara, K., Adachi, H., Nishio, T., Unno, M., Tokui, T., Okabe, M., et al. (2001). Identification of thyroid hormone transporters in humans: Different molecules are involved in a tissue-specific manner. *Endocrinology*, *142*(5), 2005–2012.

Gao, B., Hagenbuch, B., Kullak-Ublick, G. A., Benke, D., Aguzzi, A., & Meier, P. J. (2000). Organic anion-transporting polypeptides mediate transport of opioid peptides across blood-brain barrier. *The Journal of Pharmacology and Experimental Therapeutics*, *294*, 73–79.

Gazzin, S., Berengeno, A. L., Strazielle, N., Fazzari, F., Raseni, A., Ostrow, J. D., et al. (2011). Modulation of Mrp1 (ABCc1) and Pgp (ABCb1) by bilirubin at the blood-CSF and blood-brain barriers in the Gunn rat. *PLoS One*, *6*, e16165.

Genis, P., Jett, M., Bernton, E. W., Boyle, T., Gelbard, H. A., Dzenko, K., et al. (1992). Cytokines and arachidonic metabolites produced during human immunodeficiency virus (HIV)-infected macrophage-astroglia interactions: Implications for the neuropathogenesis of HIV disease. *Journal of Experimental Medicine*, *176*, 1703–1718.

Gennuso, F., Fernetti, C., Tirolo, C., Testa, N., L'Episcopo, F., Caniglia, S., et al. (2004). Bilirubin protects astrocytes from its own toxicity by inducing up-regulation and translocation of multidrug resistance-associated protein 1 (Mrp1). *Proceedings of the National Academy of Sciences of the United States of America*, *101*, 2470–2475.

Gerhart, D. Z., Enerson, B. E., Zhdankina, O. Y., Leino, R. L., & Drewes, L. R. (1997). Expression of monocarboxylate transporter MCT1 by brain endothelium and glia in adult and suckling rats. *The American Journal of Physiology*, *273*(1 Pt 1), E207–E213.

Gibson, C. J., Hossain, M. M., Richardson, J. R., & Aleksunes, L. M. (2012). Inflammatory regulation of ATP binding cassette efflux transporter expression and function in microglia. *The Journal of Pharmacology and Experimental Therapeutics*, *343*(3), 650–660.

Golden, P. L., & Pardridge, W. M. (1999). P-Glycoprotein on astrocyte foot processes of unfixed isolated human brain capillaries. *Brain Research*, *819*, 143–146.

Gong, J., Jaiswal, R., Mathys, J. M., Combes, V., Grau, G. E., & Bebawy, M. (2012). Microparticles and their emerging role in cancer multidrug resistance. *Cancer Treatment Reviews*, *38*, 226–234.

Guha, D., Nagilla, P., Redinger, C., Srinivasan, A., Schatten, G. P., & Ayyavoo, V. (2012). Neuronal apoptosis by HIV-1 Vpr: Contribution of proinflammatory molecular networks from infected target cells. *Journal of Neuroinflammation*, *9*, 138.

Guillen-Gomez, E., Calbet, M., Casado, J., de Lecea, L., Soriano, E., Pastor-Anglada, M., et al. (2004). Distribution of CNT2 and ENT1 transcripts in rat brain: Selective decrease of CNT2 mRNA in the cerebral cortex of sleep-deprived rats. *Journal of Neurochemistry*, *90*(4), 883–893.

Haber, M., Smith, J., Bordow, S. B., Flemming, C., Cohn, S. L., London, W. B., et al. (2006). Association of high-level MRP1 expression with poor clinical outcome in a large prospective study of primary neuroblastoma. *Journal of Clinical Oncology*, *24*, 1546–1553.

Hagenbuch, B., & Gui, C. (2008). Xenobiotic transporters of the human organic anion transporting polypeptides (OATP) family. *Xenobiotica*, *38*, 778–801.

Hagenbuch, B., & Meier, P. J. (2003). The superfamily of organic anion transporting polypeptides. *Biochimica et Biophysica Acta*, *1609*(1), 1–18.

Halestrap, A. P., & Wilson, M. C. (2012). The monocarboxylate transporter family—Role and regulation. *IUBMB Life*, *64*(2), 109–119.

Hartz, A. M., Mahringer, A., Miller, D. S., & Bauer, B. (2010). 17-beta-Estradiol: A powerful modulator of blood-brain barrier BCRP activity. *Journal of Cerebral Blood Flow and Metabolism*, *30*, 1742–1755.

Hartz, A. M., Miller, D. S., & Bauer, B. (2010). Restoring blood-brain barrier P-glycoprotein reduces brain amyloid-beta in a mouse model of Alzheimer's disease. *Molecular Pharmacology*, 77, 715–723.

Hayashi, K., Pu, H., Andras, I. E., Eum, S. Y., Yamauchi, A., Hennig, B., et al. (2006). HIV-TAT protein upregulates expression of multidrug resistance protein 1 in the blood-brain barrier. *Journal of Cerebral Blood Flow and Metabolism*, *26*, 1052–1065.

Hayashi, K., Pu, H., Tian, J., Andras, I. E., Lee, Y. W., Hennig, B., et al. (2005). HIV-Tat protein induces P-glycoprotein expression in brain microvascular endothelial cells. *Journal of Neurochemistry*, *93*, 1231–1241.

He, S. M., Li, R., Kanwar, J. R., & Zhou, S. F. (2011). Structural and functional properties of human multidrug resistance protein 1 (MRP1/ABCC1). *Current Medicinal Chemistry*, *18*, 439–481.

Heaton, R. K., Franklin, D. R., Ellis, R. J., McCutchan, J. A., Letendre, S. L., Leblanc, S., et al. (2011). HIV-associated neurocognitive disorders before and during the era of combination antiretroviral therapy: Differences in rates, nature, and predictors. *Journal of Neurovirology*, *17*, 3–16.

Hilgendorf, C., Ahlin, G., Seithel, A., Artursson, P., Ungell, A. L., & Karlsson, J. (2007). Expression of thirty-six drug transporter genes in human intestine, liver, kidney, and organotypic cell lines. *Drug Metabolism and Disposition*, *35*(8), 1333–1340.

Hill, J. E., & Gasser, P. J. (2013). Organic cation transporter 3 is densely expressed in the intercalated cell groups of the amygdala: Anatomical evidence for a stress hormone-sensitive dopamine clearance system. *Journal of Chemical Neuroanatomy*, *52*, 36–43.

Hirrlinger, J., Konig, J., & Dringen, R. (2002). Expression of mRNAs of multidrug resistance proteins (Mrps) in cultured rat astrocytes, oligodendrocytes, microglial cells and neurones. *Journal of Neurochemistry*, *82*, 716–719.

Hirrlinger, J., Konig, J., Keppler, D., Lindenau, J., Schulz, J. B., & Dringen, R. (2001). The multidrug resistance protein MRP1 mediates the release of glutathione disulfide from rat astrocytes during oxidative stress. *Journal of Neurochemistry*, *76*, 627–636.

Holden, K. R., Zuniga, O. F., May, M. M., Su, H., Molinero, M. R., Rogers, R. C., et al. (2005). X-linked MCT8 gene mutations: Characterization of the pediatric neurologic phenotype. *Journal of Child Neurology*, *20*(10), 852–857.

Holland, M. L., Panetta, J. A., Hoskins, J. M., Bebawy, M., Roufogalis, B. D., Allen, J. D., et al. (2006). The effects of cannabinoids on P-glycoprotein transport and expression in multidrug resistant cells. *Biochemical Pharmacology*, *71*(8), 1146–1154.

Hong, M., Schlichter, L., & Bendayan, R. (2000). A Na(+)-dependent nucleoside transporter in microglia. *The Journal of Pharmacology and Experimental Therapeutics*, *292*, 366–374.

Honorat, M., Mesnier, A., Vendrell, J., Di, P. A., Lin, V., Dumontet, C., et al. (2011). MRP8/ABCC11 expression is regulated by dexamethasone in breast cancer cells and is associated to progesterone receptor status in breast tumors. *International Journal of Breast Cancer*, *2011*, 807380.

Honorat, M., Terreux, R., Falson, P., Di, P. A., Dumontet, C., & Payen, L. (2013). Localization of putative binding sites for cyclic guanosine monophosphate and the anti-cancer drug 5-fluoro-2′-deoxyuridine-5′-monophosphate on ABCC11 in silico models. *BMC Structural Biology*, *13*, 7–13.

Hoque, M. T., Conseil, G., & Cole, S. P. (2009). Involvement of NHERF1 in apical membrane localization of MRP4 in polarized kidney cells. *Biochemical and Biophysical Research Communications*, *379*(1), 60–64.

Hori, S., Ohtsuki, S., Tachikawa, M., Kimura, N., Kondo, T., Watanabe, M., et al. (2004). Functional expression of rat ABCG2 on the luminal side of brain capillaries and its enhancement by astrocyte-derived soluble factor(s). *Journal of Neurochemistry*, *90*, 526–536.

Horvath, R. J., & DeLeo, J. A. (2009). Morphine enhances microglial migration through modulation of P2X4 receptor signaling. *Journal of Neuroscience*, *29*(4), 998–1005.

Huber, O., Brunner, A., Maier, P., Kaufmann, R., Couraud, P. O., Cremer, C., et al. (2012). Localization microscopy (SPDM) reveals clustered formations of P-glycoprotein in a human blood-brain barrier model. *PLoS One*, 7(9), e44776.

Huber, R. D., Gao, B., Sidler Pfandler, M. A., Zhang-Fu, W., Leuthold, S., Hagenbuch, B., et al. (2007). Characterization of two splice variants of human organic anion transporting polypeptide 3A1 isolated from human brain. *American Journal of Physiology. Cell Physiology*, *292*, C795–C806.

Islam, M. O., Kanemura, Y., Tajria, J., Mori, H., Kobayashi, S., Shofuda, T., et al. (2005). Characterization of ABC transporter ABCB1 expressed in human neural stem/progenitor cells. *FEBS Letters*, *579*(17), 3473–3480.

Ito, K., Uchida, Y., Ohtsuki, S., Aizawa, S., Kawakami, H., Katsukura, Y., et al. (2011). Quantitative membrane protein expression at the blood-brain barrier of adult and younger cynomolgus monkeys. *Journal of Pharmaceutical Sciences*, *100*(9), 3939–3950.

Jacquemin, E., Hagenbuch, B., Stieger, B., Wolkoff, A. W., & Meier, P. J. (1994). Expression cloning of a rat liver Na(+)-independent organic anion transporter. *Proceedings of the National Academy of Sciences of the United States of America*, *91*(1), 133–137.

Januszewicz, E., Pajak, B., Gajkowska, B., Samluk, L., Djavadian, R. L., Hinton, B. T., et al. (2009). Organic cation/carnitine transporter OCTN3 is present in astrocytes and is up-regulated by peroxisome proliferators-activator receptor agonist. *The International Journal of Biochemistry & Cell Biology*, *41*(12), 2599–2609.

Jennings, L. L., Hao, C., Cabrita, M. A., Vickers, M. F., Baldwin, S. A., Young, J. D., et al. (2001). Distinct regional distribution of human equilibrative nucleoside transporter proteins 1 and 2 (hENT1 and hENT2) in the central nervous system. *Neuropharmacology*, *40*(5), 722–731.

Jin, X., Mo, R., Ding, Y., Zheng, W., & Zhang, C. (2014). Paclitaxel-loaded N-octyl-O-sulfate chitosan micelles for superior cancer therapeutic efficacy and overcoming drug resistance. *Molecular Pharmaceutics*, *11*, 145–157.

Johnson, Z. L., Cheong, C. G., & Lee, S. Y. (2012). Crystal structure of a concentrative nucleoside transporter from Vibrio cholerae at 2.4 A. *Nature*, *483*(7390), 489–493.

Jong, N. N., Nakanishi, T., Liu, J. J., Tamai, I., & McKeage, M. J. (2011). Oxaliplatin transport mediated by organic cation/carnitine transporters OCTN1 and OCTN2 in overexpressing human embryonic kidney 293 cells and rat dorsal root ganglion neurons. *The Journal of Pharmacology and Experimental Therapeutics*, *338*(2), 537–547.

Juliano, R. L., & Ling, V. (1976). A surface glycoprotein modulating drug permeability in Chinese hamster ovary cell mutants. *Biochimica et Biophysica Acta*, *455*, 152–162.

Kaddoumi, A., Choi, S. U., Kinman, L., Whittington, D., Tsai, C. C., Ho, R. J., et al. (2007). Inhibition of P-glycoprotein activity at the primate blood-brain barrier increases the distribution of nelfinavir into the brain but not into the cerebrospinal fluid. *Drug Metabolism and Disposition*, *35*, 1459–1462.

Kao, H. H., Huang, J. D., & Chang, M. S. (2002). cDNA cloning and genomic organization of the murine MRP7, a new ATP-binding cassette transporter. *Gene*, *286*, 299–306.

Kao, S. C., Zhao, X., Lee, C. Y., Atianjoh, F. E., Gauda, E. B., Yaster, M., et al. (2012). Absence of mu opioid receptor mRNA expression in astrocytes and microglia of rat spinal cord. *Neuroreport*, *23*(6), 378–384.

Katayama, K., Yoshioka, S., Tsukahara, S., Mitsuhashi, J., & Sugimoto, Y. (2007). Inhibition of the mitogen-activated protein kinase pathway results in the down-regulation of P-glycoprotein. *Molecular Cancer Therapeutics*, *6*, 2092–2102.

Kido, Y., Tamai, I., Okamoto, M., Suzuki, F., & Tsuji, A. (2000). Functional clarification of MCT1-mediated transport of monocarboxylic acids at the blood-brain barrier using in vitro cultured cells and in vivo BUI studies. *Pharmaceutical Research*, *17*(1), 55–62.

Kikuchi, R., Kusuhara, H., Sugiyama, D., & Sugiyama, Y. (2003). Contribution of organic anion transporter 3 (Slc22a8) to the elimination of p-aminohippuric acid and benzylpenicillin across the blood-brain barrier. *The Journal of Pharmacology and Experimental Therapeutics*, *306*(1), 51–58.

Kim, R. B., Fromm, M. F., Wandel, C., Leake, B., Wood, A. J., Roden, D. M., et al. (1998). The drug transporter P-glycoprotein limits oral absorption and brain entry of HIV-1 protease inhibitors. *Journal of Clinical Investigation, 101*, 289–294.

Kis, B., Isse, T., Snipes, J. A., Chen, L., Yamashita, H., Ueta, Y., et al. (2006). Effects of LPS stimulation on the expression of prostaglandin carriers in the cells of the blood-brain and blood-cerebrospinal fluid barriers. *Journal of Applied Physiology, 100*(4), 1392–1399.

Koepsell, H. (2013). The SLC22 family with transporters of organic cations, anions and zwitterions. *Molecular Aspects of Medicine, 34*(2–3), 413–435.

Koepsell, H., Lips, K., & Volk, C. (2007). Polyspecific organic cation transporters: Structure, function, physiological roles, and biopharmaceutical implications. *Pharmaceutical Research, 24*, 1227–1251.

Koepsell, H., Schmitt, B. M., & Gorboulev, V. (2003). Organic cation transporters. *Reviews of Physiology, Biochemistry and Pharmacology, 150*, 36–90.

Konig, J., Seithel, A., Gradhand, U., & Fromm, M. F. (2006). Pharmacogenomics of human OATP transporters. *Naunyn-Schmiedeberg's Archives of Pharmacology, 372*(6), 432–443.

Kool, M., De, H. M., Scheffer, G. L., Scheper, R. J., van Eijk, M. J., Juijn, J. A., et al. (1997). Analysis of expression of cMOAT (MRP2), MRP3, MRP4, and MRP5, homologues of the multidrug resistance-associated protein gene (MRP1), in human cancer cell lines. *Cancer Research, 57*(16), 3537–3547.

Kool, M., van der Linden, M., De, H. M., Baas, F., & Borst, P. (1999). Expression of human MRP6, a homologue of the multidrug resistance protein gene MRP1, in tissues and cancer cells. *Cancer Research, 59*(1), 175–182.

Kortekaas, R., Leenders, K. L., van Oostrom, J. C., Vaalburg, W., Bart, J., Willemsen, A. T., et al. (2005). Blood-brain barrier dysfunction in parkinsonian midbrain in vivo. *Annals of Neurology, 57*, 176–179.

Kraft, M. E., Glaeser, H., Mandery, K., Konig, J., Auge, D., Fromm, M. F., et al. (2010). The prostaglandin transporter OATP2A1 is expressed in human ocular tissues and transports the antiglaucoma prostanoid latanoprost. *Investigative Ophthalmology & Visual Science, 51*(5), 2504–2511.

Krohn, M., Lange, C., Hofrichter, J., Scheffler, K., Stenzel, J., Steffen, J., et al. (2011). Cerebral amyloid-beta proteostasis is regulated by the membrane transport protein ABCC1 in mice. *The Journal of Clinical Investigation, 121*(10), 3924–3931.

Kruh, G. D., & Belinsky, M. G. (2003). The MRP family of drug efflux pumps. *Oncogene, 22*, 7537–7552.

Kullak-Ublick, G. A., Hagenbuch, B., Stieger, B., Schteingart, C. D., Hofmann, A. F., Wolkoff, A. W., et al. (1995). Molecular and functional characterization of an organic anion transporting polypeptide cloned from human liver. *Gastroenterology, 109*(4), 1274–1282.

Kullak-Ublick, G. A., Hagenbuch, B., Stieger, B., Wolkoff, A. W., & Meier, P. J. (1994). Functional characterization of the basolateral rat liver organic anion transporting polypeptide. *Hepatology, 20*(2), 411–416.

Kullak-Ublick, G. A., Ismair, M. G., Stieger, B., Landmann, L., Huber, R., Pizzagalli, F., et al. (2001). Organic anion-transporting polypeptide B (OATP-B) and its functional comparison with three other OATPs of human liver. *Gastroenterology, 120*, 525–533.

Kusch-Poddar, M., Drewe, J., Fux, I., & Gutmann, H. (2005). Evaluation of the immortalized human brain capillary endothelial cell line BB19 as a human cell culture model for the blood-brain barrier. *Brain Research, 1064*, 21–31.

Lacher, S. E., Gremaud, J. N., Skagen, K., Steed, E., Dalton, R., Sugden, K. D., et al. (2014). Absence of P-glycoprotein transport in the pharmacokinetics and toxicity of the herbicide paraquat. *The Journal of Pharmacology and Experimental Therapeutics, 348*(2), 336–345.

Lai, B. C., Marion, S. A., Teschke, K., & Tsui, J. K. (2002). Occupational and environmental risk factors for Parkinson's disease. *Parkinsonism & Related Disorders, 8*(5), 297–309.

Lamhonwah, A. M., Hawkins, C. E., Tam, C., Wong, J., Mai, L., & Tein, I. (2008). Expression patterns of the organic cation/carnitine transporter family in adult murine brain. *Brain Development*, *30*, 31–42.

Langford, D., Grigorian, A., Hurford, R., Adame, A., Ellis, R. J., Hansen, L., et al. (2004). Altered P-glycoprotein expression in AIDS patients with HIV encephalitis. *Journal of Neuropathology and Experimental Neurology*, *63*, 1038–1047.

Lauritzen, F., Heuser, K., de Lanerolle, N. C., Lee, T. S., Spencer, D. D., Kim, J. H., et al. (2012). Redistribution of monocarboxylate transporter 2 on the surface of astrocytes in the human epileptogenic hippocampus. *Glia*, *60*(7), 1172–1181.

Lazarowski, A., Czornyj, L., Lubienieki, F., Girardi, E., Vazquez, S., & D'Giano, C. (2007). ABC transporters during epilepsy and mechanisms underlying multidrug resistance in refractory epilepsy. *Epilepsia*, *48*(Suppl. 5), 140–149.

Lazarowski, A. J., Lubieniecki, F. J., Camarero, S. A., Pomata, H. H., Bartuluchi, M. A., Sevlever, G., et al. (2006). New proteins configure a brain drug resistance map in tuberous sclerosis. *Pediatric Neurology*, *34*(1), 20–24.

Lazarowski, A., Ramos, A. J., Garcia-Rivello, H., Brusco, A., & Girardi, E. (2004). Neuronal and glial expression of the multidrug resistance gene product in an experimental epilepsy model. *Cellular and Molecular Neurobiology*, *24*(1), 77–85.

Lee, G., Babakhanian, K., Ramaswamy, M., Prat, A., Wosik, K., & Bendayan, R. (2007). Expression of the ATP-binding cassette membrane transporter, ABCG2, in human and rodent brain microvessel endothelial and glial cell culture systems. *Pharmaceutical Research*, *24*, 1262–1274.

Lee, G., Dallas, S., Hong, M., & Bendayan, R. (2001). Drug transporters in the central nervous system: Brain barriers and brain parenchyma considerations. *Pharmacological Reviews*, *53*, 569–596.

Lee, K., Klein-Szanto, A. J., & Kruh, G. D. (2000). Analysis of the MRP4 drug resistance profile in transfected NIH3T3 cells. *Journal of the National Cancer Institute*, *92*(23), 1934–1940.

Lee, Y., Morrison, B. M., Li, Y., Lengacher, S., Farah, M. H., Hoffman, P. N., et al. (2012). Oligodendroglia metabolically support axons and contribute to neurodegeneration. *Nature*, *487*(7408), 443–448.

Lee, G., Schlichter, L., Bendayan, M., & Bendayan, R. (2001). Functional expression of P-glycoprotein in rat brain microglia. *The Journal of Pharmacology and Experimental Therapeutics*, *299*, 204–212.

Leggas, M., Panetta, J. C., Zhuang, Y., Schuetz, J. D., Johnston, B., Bai, F., et al. (2006). Gefitinib modulates the function of multiple ATP-binding cassette transporters in vivo. *Cancer Research*, *66*(9), 4802–4807.

Lemmen, J., Tozakidis, I. E., Bele, P., & Galla, H. J. (2013). Constitutive androstane receptor upregulates Abcb1 and Abcg2 at the blood-brain barrier after CITCO activation. *Brain Research*, *1501*, 68–80.

Lemos, C., Kathmann, I., Giovannetti, E., Belien, J. A., Scheffer, G. L., Calhau, C., et al. (2009). Cellular folate status modulates the expression of BCRP and MRP multidrug transporters in cancer cell lines from different origins. *Molecular Cancer Therapeutics*, *8*(3), 655–664.

Li, B., Gu, L., Hertz, L., & Peng, L. (2013). Expression of nucleoside transporter in freshly isolated neurons and astrocytes from mouse brain. *Neurochemical Research*, *38*(11), 2351–2358.

Li, J., Jaimes, K. F., & Aller, S. G. (2014). Refined structures of mouse P-glycoprotein. *Protein Sciences*, *23*(1), 34–46.

Lin, C. J., Tai, Y., Huang, M. T., Tsai, Y. F., Hsu, H. J., Tzen, K. Y., et al. (2010). Cellular localization of the organic cation transporters, OCT1 and OCT2, in brain microvessel endothelial cells and its implication for MPTP transport across the blood-brain barrier and MPTP-induced dopaminergic toxicity in rodents. *Journal of Neurochemistry*, *114*(3), 717–727.

Lombardo, L., Pellitteri, R., Balazy, M., & Cardile, V. (2008). Induction of nuclear receptors and drug resistance in the brain microvascular endothelial cells treated with antiepileptic drugs. *Current Neurovascular Research*, *5*(2), 82–92.

Loo, T. W., & Clarke, D. M. (2013). A salt bridge in intracellular loop 2 is essential for folding of human p-glycoprotein. *Biochemistry*, *52*(19), 3194–3196.

Loscher, W., & Potschka, H. (2005). Drug resistance in brain diseases and the role of drug efflux transporters. *Nature Reviews Neuroscience*, *6*, 591–602.

Lu, H., Chen, C., & Klaassen, C. (2004). Tissue distribution of concentrative and equilibrative nucleoside transporters in male and female rats and mice. *Drug Metabolism and Disposition*, *32*, 1455–1461.

Lu, R., Kanai, N., Bao, Y., & Schuster, V. L. (1996). Cloning, in vitro expression, and tissue distribution of a human prostaglandin transporter cDNA(hPGT). *The Journal of Clinical Investigation*, *98*(5), 1142–1149.

Luna-Tortos, C., Fedrowitz, M., & Loscher, W. (2008). Several major antiepileptic drugs are substrates for human P-glycoprotein. *Neuropharmacology*, *55*, 1364–1375.

Luna-Tortos, C., Fedrowitz, M., & Loscher, W. (2010). Evaluation of transport of common antiepileptic drugs by human multidrug resistance-associated proteins (MRP1, 2 and 5) that are overexpressed in pharmacoresistant epilepsy. *Neuropharmacology*, *58*, 1019–1032.

Ma, A., Wang, C., Chen, Y., & Yuan, W. (2013). P-glycoprotein alters blood-brain barrier penetration of antiepileptic drugs in rats with medically intractable epilepsy. *Drug Design, Development and Therapy*, *7*, 1447–1454.

Malofeeva, E. V., Domanitskaya, N., Gudima, M., & Hopper-Borge, E. A. (2012). Modulation of the ATPase and transport activities of broad-acting multidrug resistance factor ABCC10 (MRP7). *Cancer Research*, *72*(24), 6457–6467.

Mayerl, S., Visser, T. J., Darras, V. M., Horn, S., & Heuer, H. (2012). Impact of Oatp1c1 deficiency on thyroid hormone metabolism and action in the mouse brain. *Endocrinology*, *153*(3), 1528–1537.

Mercier, C., Masseguin, C., Roux, F., Gabrion, J., & Scherrmann, J. M. (2004). Expression of P-glycoprotein (ABCB1) and Mrp1 (ABCC1) in adult rat brain: Focus on astrocytes. *Brain Research*, *1021*, 32–40.

Miller, D. S. (2010). Regulation of P-glycoprotein and other ABC drug transporters at the blood-brain barrier. *Trends in Pharmacological Sciences*, *31*, 246–254.

Miller, D. S., Nobmann, S. N., Gutmann, H., Toeroek, M., Drewe, J., & Fricker, G. (2000). Xenobiotic transport across isolated brain microvessels studied by confocal microscopy. *Molecular Pharmacology*, *58*, 1357–1367.

Minich, T., Riemer, J., Schulz, J. B., Wielinga, P., Wijnholds, J., & Dringen, R. (2006). The multidrug resistance protein 1 (Mrp1), but not Mrp5, mediates export of glutathione and glutathione disulfide from brain astrocytes. *Journal of Neurochemistry*, *97*, 373–384.

Miranda-Goncalves, V., Honavar, M., Pinheiro, C., Martinho, O., Pires, M. M., Pinheiro, C., et al. (2013). Monocarboxylate transporters (MCTs) in gliomas: Expression and exploitation as therapeutic targets. *Neuro-Oncology*, *15*(2), 172–188.

Mohelnikova-Duchonova, B., Brynychova, V., Oliverius, M., Honsova, E., Kala, Z., Muckova, K., et al. (2013). Differences in transcript levels of ABC transporters between pancreatic adenocarcinoma and nonneoplastic tissues. *Pancreas*, *42*(4), 707–716.

Monte, J. C., Nagle, M. A., Eraly, S. A., & Nigam, S. K. (2004). Identification of a novel murine organic anion transporter family member, OAT6, expressed in olfactory mucosa. *Biochemical and Biophysical Research Communications*, *323*(2), 429–436.

Morrison, B. M., Lee, Y., & Rothstein, J. D. (2013). Oligodendroglia: Metabolic supporters of axons. *Trends in Cell Biology*, *23*(12), 644–651.

Nagata, Y., Kusuhara, H., Endou, H., & Sugiyama, Y. (2002). Expression and functional characterization of rat organic anion transporter 3 (rOat3) in the choroid plexus. *Molecular Pharmacology*, *61*(5), 982–988.

Nagle, M. A., Wu, W., Eraly, S. A., & Nigam, S. K. (2013). Organic anion transport pathways in antiviral handling in choroid plexus in Oat1 (Slc22a6) and Oat3 (Slc22a8) deficient tissue. *Neuroscience Letters*, *534*, 133–138.

Nakamichi, N., Taguchi, T., Hosotani, H., Wakayama, T., Shimizu, T., Sugiura, T., et al. (2012). Functional expression of carnitine/organic cation transporter OCTN1 in mouse brain neurons: Possible involvement in neuronal differentiation. *Neurochemistry International*, *61*(7), 1121–1132.

Nakata, T., Matsui, T., Kobayashi, K., Kobayashi, Y., & Anzai, N. (2013). Organic cation transporter 2 (SLC22A2), a low-affinity and high-capacity choline transporter, is preferentially enriched on synaptic vesicles in cholinergic neurons. *Neuroscience*, *252*, 212–221.

Naud, J., Laurin, L. P., Michaud, J., Beauchemin, S., Leblond, F. A., & Pichette, V. (2012). Effects of chronic renal failure on brain drug transporters in rats. *Drug Metabolism and Disposition*, *40*(1), 39–46.

Neuwelt, E. A., Bauer, B., Fahlke, C., Fricker, G., Iadecola, C., Janigro, D., et al. (2011). Engaging neuroscience to advance translational research in brain barrier biology. *Nature Reviews. Neuroscience*, *12*, 169–182.

Newstead, S., Drew, D., Cameron, A. D., Postis, V. L., Xia, X., Fowler, P. W., et al. (2011). Crystal structure of a prokaryotic homologue of the mammalian oligopeptide-proton symporters, PepT1 and PepT2. *The EMBO Journal*, *30*(2), 417–426.

Nies, A. T., Jedlitschky, G., Konig, J., Herold-Mende, C., Steiner, H. H., Schmitt, H. P., et al. (2004). Expression and immunolocalization of the multidrug resistance proteins, MRP1-MRP6 (ABCC1-ABCC6), in human brain. *Neuroscience*, *129*, 349–360.

Nishio, T., Adachi, H., Nakagomi, R., Tokui, T., Sato, E., Tanemoto, M., et al. (2000). Molecular identification of a rat novel organic anion transporter moat1, which transports prostaglandin D(2), leukotriene C(4), and taurocholate. *Biochemical and Biophysical Research Communications*, *275*(3), 831–838.

Nishiwaki, T., Daigo, Y., Tamari, M., Fujii, Y., & Nakamura, Y. (1998). Molecular cloning, mapping, and characterization of two novel human genes, ORCTL3 and ORCTL4, bearing homology to organic-cation transporters. *Cytogenetics and Cell Genetics*, *83*(3–4), 251–255.

Nivillac, N. M., Wasal, K., Villani, D. F., Naydenova, Z., Hanna, W. J., & Coe, I. R. (2009). Disrupted plasma membrane localization and loss of function reveal regions of human equilibrative nucleoside transporter 1 involved in structural integrity and activity. *Biochimica et Biophysica Acta*, *1788*(10), 2326–2334.

Ocheltree, S. M., Shen, H., Hu, Y., Xiang, J., Keep, R. F., & Smith, D. E. (2004a). Mechanisms of cefadroxil uptake in the choroid plexus: Studies in wild-type and PEPT2 knockout mice. *The Journal of Pharmacology and Experimental Therapeutics*, *308*(2), 462–467.

Ocheltree, S. M., Shen, H., Hu, Y., Xiang, J., Keep, R. F., & Smith, D. E. (2004b). Role of PEPT2 in the choroid plexus uptake of glycylsarcosine and 5-aminolevulinic acid: Studies in wild-type and null mice. *Pharmaceutical Research*, *21*(9), 1680–1685.

Ohtsuki, S., Asaba, H., Takanaga, H., Deguchi, T., Hosoya, K., Otagiri, M., et al. (2002). Role of blood-brain barrier organic anion transporter 3 (OAT3) in the efflux of indoxyl sulfate, a uremic toxin: Its involvement in neurotransmitter metabolite clearance from the brain. *Journal of Neurochemistry*, *83*(1), 57–66.

Okura, T., Kato, S., & Deguchi, Y. (2014). Functional expression of organic cation/carnitine transporter 2 (OCTN2/SLC22A5) in human brain capillary endothelial cell line hCMEC/D3, a human blood-brain barrier model. *Drug Metabolism and Pharmacokinetics*, *29*(1), 69–74.

Ose, A., Ito, M., Kusuhara, H., Yamatsugu, K., Kanai, M., Shibasaki, M., et al. (2009). Limited brain distribution of [3R,4R,5S]-4-acetamido-5-amino-3-(1-ethylpropoxy)-1-cyclohexene-1-carboxylate phosphate (Ro 64-0802), a pharmacologically active form of oseltamivir, by active efflux across the blood-brain barrier mediated by organic anion transporter 3 (Oat3/Slc22a8) and multidrug resistance-associated protein 4 (Mrp4/Abcc4). *Drug Metabolism and Disposition, 37*(2), 315–321.

Ose, A., Kusuhara, H., Endo, C., Tohyama, K., Miyajima, M., Kitamura, S., et al. (2010). Functional characterization of mouse organic anion transporting peptide 1a4 in the uptake and efflux of drugs across the blood-brain barrier. *Drug Metabolism and Disposition, 38*, 168–176.

Pardridge, W. M. (2012). Drug transport across the blood-brain barrier. *Journal of Cerebral Blood Flow and Metabolism, 32*(11), 1959–1972.

Pardridge, W. M., Golden, P. L., Kang, Y. S., & Bickel, U. (1997). Brain microvascular and astrocyte localization of P-glycoprotein. *Journal of Neurochemistry, 68*, 1278–1285.

Pavlova, A., Sakurai, H., Leclercq, B., Beier, D. R., Yu, A. S., & Nigam, S. K. (2000). Developmentally regulated expression of organic ion transporters NKT (OAT1), OCT1, NLT (OAT2), and Roct. *American Journal of Physiology. Renal Physiology, 278*(4), F635–F643.

Peignan, L., Garrido, W., Segura, R., Melo, R., Rojas, D., Carcamo, J. G., et al. (2011). Combined use of anticancer drugs and an inhibitor of multiple drug resistance-associated protein-1 increases sensitivity and decreases survival of glioblastoma multiforme cells in vitro. *Neurochemical Research, 36*(8), 1397–1406.

Peng, L., Huang, R., Yu, A. C., Fung, K. Y., Rathbone, M. P., & Hertz, L. (2005). Nucleoside transporter expression and function in cultured mouse astrocytes. *Glia, 52*(1), 25–35.

Persidsky, Y., Zheng, J., Miller, D., & Gendelman, H. E. (2000). Mononuclear phagocytes mediate blood-brain barrier compromise and neuronal injury during HIV-1-associated dementia. *Journal of Leukocyte Biology, 68*(3), 413–422.

Pizzagalli, F., Hagenbuch, B., Stieger, B., Klenk, U., Folkers, G., & Meier, P. J. (2002). Identification of a novel human organic anion transporting polypeptide as a high affinity thyroxine transporter. *Molecular Endocrinology, 16*(10), 2283–2296.

Plangar, I., Zadori, D., Szalardy, L., Vecsei, L., & Klivenyi, P. (2013). Assessment of the role of multidrug resistance-associated proteins in MPTP neurotoxicity in mice. *Ideggyogyaszati Szemle, 66*(11-12), 407–414.

Punfa, W., Yodkeeree, S., Pitchakarn, P., Ampasavate, C., & Limtrakul, P. (2012). Enhancement of cellular uptake and cytotoxicity of curcumin-loaded PLGA nanoparticles by conjugation with anti-P-glycoprotein in drug resistance cancer cells. *Acta Pharmacologica Sinica, 33*, 823–831.

Rafati, A., Noorafshan, A., & Torabi, N. (2013). Stereological study of the effects of morphine consumption and abstinence on the number of the neurons and oligodendrocytes in medial prefrontal cortex of rats. *Anatomy and Cell Biology, 46*(3), 191–197.

Rao, V. V., Dahlheimer, J. L., Bardgett, M. E., Snyder, A. Z., Finch, R. A., Sartorelli, A. C., et al. (1999). Choroid plexus epithelial expression of MDR1 P glycoprotein and multidrug resistance-associated protein contribute to the blood-cerebrospinal-fluid drug-permeability barrier. *Proceedings of the National Academy of Sciences of the United States of America, 96*, 3900–3905.

Redzic, Z. B., Biringer, J., Barnes, K., Baldwin, S. A., Al-Sarraf, H., Nicola, P. A., et al. (2005). Polarized distribution of nucleoside transporters in rat brain endothelial and choroid plexus epithelial cells. *Journal of Neurochemistry, 94*, 1420–1426.

Redzic, Z. B., Malatiali, S. A., Grujicic, D., & Isakovic, A. J. (2010). Expression and functional activity of nucleoside transporters in human choroid plexus. *Cerebrospinal Fluid Research, 7*, 2.

Reese, T. S., & Karnovsky, M. J. (1967). Fine structural localization of a blood-brain barrier to exogenous peroxidase. *Journal of Cell Biology, 34*, 207–217.

Regina, A., Demeule, M., Laplante, A., Jodoin, J., Dagenais, C., Berthelet, F., et al. (2001). Multidrug resistance in brain tumors: Roles of the blood-brain barrier. *Cancer Metastasis Reviews, 20*, 13–25.

Roberts, L. M., Black, D. S., Raman, C., Woodford, K., Zhou, M., Haggerty, J. E., et al. (2008). Subcellular localization of transporters along the rat blood-brain barrier and blood-cerebral-spinal fluid barrier by in vivo biotinylation. *Neuroscience, 155*, 423–438.

Robillard, K. R., Chan, G. N., Zhang, G., la Porte, C., Cameron, W., & Bendayan, R. (2014). Role of P-glycoprotein in the distribution of the HIV protease inhibitor atazanavir in the brain and male genital tract. *Antimicrobial Agents and Chemotherapy, 58*, 1713–1722.

Ronaldson, P. T., Ashraf, T., & Bendayan, R. (2010). Regulation of multidrug resistance protein 1 by tumor necrosis factor alpha in cultured glial cells: Involvement of nuclear factor-kappaB and c-Jun N-terminal kinase signaling pathways. *Molecular Pharmacology*, 77, 644–659.

Ronaldson, P. T., & Bendayan, R. (2006). HIV-1 viral envelope glycoprotein gp120 triggers an inflammatory response in cultured rat astrocytes and regulates the functional expression of P-glycoprotein. *Molecular Pharmacology, 70*, 1087–1098.

Ronaldson, P. T., & Bendayan, R. (2008). HIV-1 viral envelope glycoprotein gp120 produces oxidative stress and regulates the functional expression of multidrug resistance protein-1 (Mrp1) in glial cells. *Journal of Neurochemistry, 106*, 1298–1313.

Ronaldson, P. T., Bendayan, M., Gingras, D., Piquette-Miller, M., & Bendayan, R. (2004). Cellular localization and functional expression of P-glycoprotein in rat astrocyte cultures. *Journal of Neurochemistry, 89*, 788–800.

Ronaldson, P. T., & Davis, T. P. (2013). Targeted drug delivery to treat pain and cerebral hypoxia. *Pharmacological Reviews, 65*(1), 291–314.

Ronaldson, P. T., Lee, G., Dallas, S., & Bendayan, R. (2004). Involvement of P-glycoprotein in the transport of saquinavir and indinavir in rat brain microvessel endothelial and microglia cell lines. *Pharmaceutical Research, 21*, 811–818.

Ronaldson, P. T., Persidsky, Y., & Bendayan, R. (2008). Regulation of ABC membrane transporters in glial cells: Relevance to the pharmacotherapy of brain HIV-1 infection. *Glia, 56*, 1711–1735.

Rubio-Aliaga, I., & Daniel, H. (2008). Peptide transporters and their roles in physiological processes and drug disposition. *Xenobiotica, 38*, 1022–1042.

Sacktor, N., Haughey, N., Cutler, R., Tamara, A., Turchan, J., Pardo, C., et al. (2004). Novel markers of oxidative stress in actively progressive HIV dementia. *Journal of Neuroimmunology, 157*(1–2), 176–184.

Sakata, K., Yamashita, T., Maeda, M., Moriyama, Y., Shimada, S., & Tohyama, M. (2001). Cloning of a lymphatic peptide/histidine transporter. *Biochemical Journal, 356*(Pt 1), 53–60.

Saneja, A., Khare, V., Alam, N., Dubey, R. D., & Gupta, P. N. (2014). Advances in P-glycoprotein-based approaches for delivering anticancer drugs: Pharmacokinetic perspective and clinical relevance. *Expert Opinion on Drug Delivery, 11*(1), 121–138.

Schwartz, C. E., May, M. M., Carpenter, N. J., Rogers, R. C., Martin, J., Bialer, M. G., et al. (2005). Allan-Herndon-Dudley syndrome and the monocarboxylate transporter 8 (MCT8) gene. *American Journal of Human Genetics*, 77(1), 41–53.

Schwarz, J. M., Smith, S. H., & Bilbo, S. D. (2013). FACS analysis of neuronal-glial interactions in the nucleus accumbens following morphine administration. *Psychopharmacology, 230*(4), 525–535.

Sekine, T., Watanabe, N., Hosoyamada, M., Kanai, Y., & Endou, H. (1997). Expression cloning and characterization of a novel multispecific organic anion transporter. *The Journal of Biological Chemistry, 272*(30), 18526–18529.

Shah, A., Kumar, S., Simon, S. D., Singh, D. P., & Kumar, A. (2013). HIV gp120- and methamphetamine-mediated oxidative stress induces astrocyte apoptosis via cytochrome P450 2E1. *Cell Death and Disease, 4*, e850.

Sharom, F. J. (2011). The P-glycoprotein multidrug transporter. *Essays in Biochemistry*, *50*, 161–178.

Shen, H., Smith, D. E., Keep, R. F., & Brosius, F. C., III (2004). Immunolocalization of the proton-coupled oligopeptide transporter PEPT2 in developing rat brain. *Molecular Pharmaceutics*, *1*(4), 248–256.

Shen, C. H., Tsai, R. Y., & Wong, C. S. (2012). Role of neuroinflammation in morphine tolerance: Effect of tumor necrosis factor-alpha. *Acta Anaesthesiologica Taiwanica*, *50*(4), 178–182.

Shiraki, N., Okamura, K., Tokunaga, J., Ohmura, T., Yasuda, K., Kawaguchi, T., et al. (2002). Bromocriptine reverses P-glycoprotein-mediated multidrug resistance in tumor cells. *Japanese Journal of Cancer Research*, *93*, 209–215.

Sills, G. J., Kwan, P., Butler, E., de Lange, E. C., van den Berg, D. J., & Brodie, M. J. (2002). P-glycoprotein-mediated efflux of antiepileptic drugs: Preliminary studies in mdr1a knockout mice. *Epilepsy and Behavior*, *3*(5), 427–432.

Silverberg, G. D., Messier, A. A., Miller, M. C., Machan, J. T., Majmudar, S. S., Stopa, E. G., et al. (2010). Amyloid efflux transporter expression at the blood-brain barrier declines in normal aging. *Journal of Neuropathology and Experimental Neurology*, *69*, 1034–1043.

Sisodiya, S. M., Martinian, L., Scheffer, G. L., van der Valk, P., Scheper, R. J., Harding, B. N., et al. (2006). Vascular colocalization of P-glycoprotein, multidrug-resistance associated protein 1, breast cancer resistance protein and major vault protein in human epileptogenic pathologies. *Neuropathology and Applied Neurobiology*, *32*, 51–63.

Sissung, T. M., Baum, C. E., Kirkland, C. T., Gao, R., Gardner, E. R., & Figg, W. D. (2010). Pharmacogenetics of membrane transporters: An update on current approaches. *Molecular Biotechnology*, *44*, 152–167.

Smith, D. E., Hu, Y., Shen, H., Nagaraja, T. N., Fenstermacher, J. D., & Keep, R. F. (2011). Distribution of glycylsarcosine and cefadroxil among cerebrospinal fluid, choroid plexus, and brain parenchyma after intracerebroventricular injection is markedly different between wild-type and Pept2 null mice. *Journal of Cerebral Blood Flow and Metabolism*, *31*(1), 250–261.

Smith, J. P., Uhernik, A. L., Li, L., Liu, Z., & Drewes, L. R. (2012). Regulation of Mct1 by cAMP-dependent internalization in rat brain endothelial cells. *Brain Research*, *1480*, 1–11.

Sodani, K., Patel, A., Kathawala, R. J., & Chen, Z. S. (2012). Multidrug resistance associated proteins in multidrug resistance. *Chinese Journal of Cancer*, *31*, 58–72.

Solcan, N., Kwok, J., Fowler, P. W., Cameron, A. D., Drew, D., Iwata, S., et al. (2012). Alternating access mechanism in the POT family of oligopeptide transporters. *The EMBO Journal*, *31*(16), 3411–3421.

Sosonkina, N., Nakashima, M., Ohta, T., Niikawa, N., & Starenki, D. (2011). Down-regulation of ABCC11 protein (MRP8) in human breast cancer. *Experimental Oncology*, *33*(1), 42–46.

Spiegl-Kreinecker, S., Buchroithner, J., Elbling, L., Steiner, E., Wurm, G., Bodenteich, A., et al. (2002). Expression and functional activity of the ABC-transporter proteins P-glycoprotein and multidrug-resistance protein 1 in human brain tumor cells and astrocytes. *Journal of Neuro-Oncology*, *57*, 27–36.

Stella, N. (2004). Cannabinoid signaling in glial cells. *Glia*, *48*(4), 267–277.

Sugiyama, D., Kusuhara, H., Lee, Y. J., & Sugiyama, Y. (2003). Involvement of multidrug resistance associated protein 1 (Mrp1) in the efflux transport of 17beta estradiol-D-17beta-glucuronide (E217betaG) across the blood-brain barrier. *Pharmaceutical Research*, *20*, 1394–1400.

Sultana, R., & Butterfield, D. A. (2004). Oxidatively modified GST and MRP1 in Alzheimer's disease brain: Implications for accumulation of reactive lipid peroxidation products. *Neurochemical Research*, *29*, 2215–2220.

Sun, Y. L., Chen, J. J., Kumar, P., Chen, K., Sodani, K., Patel, A., et al. (2013). Reversal of MRP7 (ABCC10)-mediated multidrug resistance by tariquidar. *PLoS One*, *8*(2), e55576.

Sun, Y., Li, Q., Xu, Y., Pu, C., Zhao, L., Guo, Z., et al. (2013). Study of the mechanisms underlying the reversal of multidrug resistance of human neuroblastoma multidrug-resistant cell line SK-N-SH/MDR1 by low-intensity pulsed ultrasound. *Oncology Reports*, *29*(5), 1939–1945.

Sweet, D. H., Wolff, N. A., & Pritchard, J. B. (1997). Expression cloning and characterization of ROAT1. The basolateral organic anion transporter in rat kidney. *The Journal of Biological Chemistry*, *272*(48), 30088–30095.

Szaflarski, W., Sujka-Kordowska, P., Januchowski, R., Wojtowicz, K., Andrzejewska, M., Nowicki, M., et al. (2013). Nuclear localization of P-glycoprotein is responsible for protection of the nucleus from doxorubicin in the resistant LoVo cell line. *Biomedicine and Pharmacotherapy*, *67*(6), 497–502.

Takada, T., Suzuki, H., Gotoh, Y., & Sugiyama, Y. (2005). Regulation of the cell surface expression of human BCRP/ABCG2 by the phosphorylation state of Akt in polarized cells. *Drug Metabolism and Disposition*, *33*(7), 905–909.

Takayanagi, S., Kataoka, T., Ohara, O., Oishi, M., Kuo, M. T., & Ishikawa, T. (2004). Human ATP-binding cassette transporter ABCC10: Expression profile and p53-dependent upregulation. *Journal of Experimental Therapeutics and Oncology*, *4*, 239–246.

Tanaka, T., Kai, S., Matsuyama, T., Adachi, T., Fukuda, K., & Hirota, K. (2013). General anesthetics inhibit LPS-induced IL-1beta expression in glial cells. *PLoS One*, *8*(12), e82930.

Thal, D. R., Griffin, W. S., & Braak, H. (2008). Parenchymal and vascular Abeta-deposition and its effects on the degeneration of neurons and cognition in Alzheimer's disease. *Journal of Cellular and Molecular Medicine*, *12*(5B), 1848–1862.

Thiebaud, N., Menetrier, F., Belloir, C., Minn, A. L., Neiers, F., Artur, Y., et al. (2011). Expression and differential localization of xenobiotic transporters in the rat olfactory neuro-epithelium. *Neuroscience Letters*, *505*(2), 180–185.

Thompson, B. J., Sanchez-Covarrubias, L., Slosky, L. M., Zhang, Y., Laracuente, M. L., & Ronaldson, P. T. (2014). Hypoxia/reoxygenation stress signals an increase in organic anion transporting polypeptide 1a4 (Oatp1a4) at the blood-brain barrier: Relevance to CNS drug delivery. *Journal of Cerebral Blood Flow and Metabolism*, *34*(4), 699–707.

Tishler, D. M., Weinberg, K. I., Hinton, D. R., Barbaro, N., Annett, G. M., & Raffel, C. (1995). MDR1 gene expression in brain of patients with medically intractable epilepsy. *Epilepsia*, *36*, 1–6.

Tulpule, K., Schmidt, M. M., Boecker, K., Goldbaum, O., Richter-Landsberg, C., & Dringen, R. (2012). Formaldehyde induces rapid glutathione export from viable oligodendroglial OLN-93 cells. *Neurochemistry International*, *61*(8), 1302–1313.

Unkruer, B., Pekcec, A., Fuest, C., Wehmeyer, A., Balda, M. S., Horn, A., et al. (2009). Cellular localization of Y-box binding protein 1 in brain tissue of rats, macaques, and humans. *BMC Neuroscience*, *10*, 28.

van Assema, D. M., Lubberink, M., Bauer, M., van der Flier, W. M., Schuit, R. C., Windhorst, A. D., et al. (2012). Blood-brain barrier P-glycoprotein function in Alzheimer's disease. *Brain*, *135*(Pt 1), 181–189.

VanDuyn, N., & Nass, R. (2014). The putative multidrug resistance protein MRP-7 inhibits methylmercury-associated animal toxicity and dopaminergic neurodegeneration in Caenorhabditis elegans. *Journal of Neurochemistry*, *128*(6), 962–974.

Vautier, S., Lacomblez, L., Chacun, H., Picard, V., Gimenez, F., Farinotti, R., et al. (2006). Interactions between the dopamine agonist, bromocriptine and the efflux protein, P-glycoprotein at the blood-brain barrier in the mouse. *European Journal of Pharmaceutical Sciences*, *27*, 167–174.

van Vliet, E. A., Redeker, S., Aronica, E., Edelbroek, P. M., & Gorter, J. A. (2005). Expression of multidrug transporters MRP1, MRP2, and BCRP shortly after status epilepticus, during the latent period, and in chronic epileptic rats. *Epilepsia*, *46*, 1569–1580.

Vialou, V., Amphoux, A., Zwart, R., Giros, B., & Gautron, S. (2004). Organic cation transporter 3 (Slc22a3) is implicated in salt-intake regulation. *Journal of Neuroscience*, *24*(11), 2846–2851.

Vialou, V., Balasse, L., Callebert, J., Launay, J. M., Giros, B., & Gautron, S. (2008). Altered aminergic neurotransmission in the brain of organic cation transporter 3-deficient mice. *Journal of Neurochemistry*, *106*(3), 1471–1482.

Virgintino, D., Robertson, D., Errede, M., Benagiano, V., Girolamo, F., Maiorano, E., et al. (2002). Expression of P-glycoprotein in human cerebral cortex microvessels. *Journal of Histochemistry and Cytochemistry*, *50*, 1671–1676.

Vogelgesang, S., Kunert-Keil, C., Cascorbi, I., Mosyagin, I., Schroder, E., Runge, U., et al. (2004). Expression of multidrug transporters in dysembryoplastic neuroepithelial tumors causing intractable epilepsy. *Clinical Neuropathology*, *23*, 223–231.

Vogelgesang, S., Warzok, R. W., Cascorbi, I., Kunert-Keil, C., Schroeder, E., Kroemer, H. K., et al. (2004). The role of P-glycoprotein in cerebral amyloid angiopathy; implications for the early pathogenesis of Alzheimer's disease. *Current Alzheimer Research*, *1*, 121–125.

Volk, H. A., Potschka, H., & Loscher, W. (2004). Increased expression of the multidrug transporter P-glycoprotein in limbic brain regions after amygdala-kindled seizures in rats. *Epilepsy Research*, *58*, 67–79.

von Wedel-Parlow, M., Wolte, P., & Galla, H. J. (2009). Regulation of major efflux transporters under inflammatory conditions at the blood-brain barrier in vitro. *Journal of Neurochemistry*, *111*, 111–118.

Wang, T., Li, J., Chen, F., Zhao, Y., He, X., Wan, D., et al. (2007). Choline transporters in human lung adenocarcinoma: Expression and functional implications. *Acta Biochimica et Biophysica Sinica*, *39*(9), 668–674.

Wang, Z., Pekarskaya, O., Bencheikh, M., Chao, W., Gelbard, H. A., Ghorpade, A., et al. (2003). Reduced expression of glutamate transporter EAAT2 and impaired glutamate transport in human primary astrocytes exposed to HIV-1 or gp120. *Virology*, *312*, 60–73.

Warren, M. S., Zerangue, N., Woodford, K., Roberts, L. M., Tate, E. H., Feng, B., et al. (2009). Comparative gene expression profiles of ABC transporters in brain microvessel endothelial cells and brain in five species including human. *Pharmacological Research*, *59*, 404–413.

Warriner, E. M., Rourke, S. B., Rourke, B. P., Rubenstein, S., Millikin, C., Buchanan, L., et al. (2010). Immune activation and neuropsychiatric symptoms in HIV infection. *The Journal of Neuropsychiatry and Clinical Neurosciences*, *22*, 321–328.

Westerlund, M., Belin, A. C., Olson, L., & Galter, D. (2008). Expression of multi-drug resistance 1 mRNA in human and rodent tissues: Reduced levels in Parkinson patients. *Cell and Tissue Research*, *334*, 179–185.

Westerlund, M., Hoffer, B., & Olson, L. (2010). Parkinson's disease: Exit toxins, enter genetics. *Progress in Neurobiology*, *90*, 146–156.

Wilson, M. C., Kraus, M., Marzban, H., Sarna, J. R., Wang, Y., Hawkes, R., et al. (2013). The neuroplastin adhesion molecules are accessory proteins that chaperone the monocarboxylate transporter MCT2 to the neuronal cell surface. *PLoS One*, *8*(11), e78654.

Xiang, J., Hu, Y., Smith, D. E., & Keep, R. F. (2006). PEPT2-mediated transport of 5-aminolevulinic acid and carnosine in astrocytes. *Brain Research*, *1122*(1), 18–23.

Xiong, H., Callaghan, D., Jones, A., Bai, J., Rasquinha, I., Smith, C., et al. (2009). ABCG2 is upregulated in Alzheimer's brain with cerebral amyloid angiopathy and may act as a gatekeeper at the blood-brain barrier for Abeta(1-40) peptides. *Journal of Neuroscience*, *29*, 5463–5475.

Yamamoto, A., Shofuda, T., Islam, M. O., Nakamura, Y., Yamasaki, M., Okano, H., et al. (2009). ABCB1 is predominantly expressed in human fetal neural stem/progenitor cells at an early development stage. *Journal of Neuroscience Research*, *87*(12), 2615–2623.

Yamashita, T., Shimada, S., Guo, W., Sato, K., Kohmura, E., Hayakawa, T., et al. (1997). Cloning and functional expression of a brain peptide/histidine transporter. *The Journal of Biological Chemistry*, *272*(15), 10205–10211.

Yoshikawa, T., Naganuma, F., Iida, T., Nakamura, T., Harada, R., Mohsen, A. S., et al. (2013). Molecular mechanism of histamine clearance by primary human astrocytes. *Glia*, *61*(6), 905–916.

Young, J. D., Yao, S. Y., Sun, L., Cass, C. E., & Baldwin, S. A. (2008). Human equilibrative nucleoside transporter (ENT) family of nucleoside and nucleobase transporter proteins. *Xenobiotica*, *38*, 995–1021.

Yousif, S., Chaves, C., Potin, S., Margaill, I., Scherrmann, J. M., & Decleves, X. (2012). Induction of P-glycoprotein and Bcrp at the rat blood-brain barrier following a subchronic morphine treatment is mediated through NMDA/COX-2 activation. *Journal of Neurochemistry*, *123*(4), 491–503.

Yousif, S., Marie-Claire, C., Roux, F., Scherrmann, J. M., & Decleves, X. (2007). Expression of drug transporters at the blood-brain barrier using an optimized isolated rat brain microvessel strategy. *Brain Research*, *1134*, 1–11.

Yousif, S., Saubamea, B., Cisternino, S., Marie-Claire, C., Dauchy, S., Scherrmann, J. M., et al. (2008). Effect of chronic exposure to morphine on the rat blood-brain barrier: Focus on the P-glycoprotein. *Journal of Neurochemistry*, *107*, 647–657.

Zastre, J. A., Chan, G. N., Ronaldson, P. T., Ramaswamy, M., Couraud, P. O., Romero, I. A., et al. (2009). Up-regulation of P-glycoprotein by HIV protease inhibitors in a human brain microvessel endothelial cell line. *Journal of Neuroscience Research*, *87*, 1023–1036.

Zelcer, N., Reid, G., Wielinga, P., Kuil, A., van der Heijden, I., Schuet, J. D., et al. (2003). Steroid and bile acid conjugates are substrates of human multidrug-resistance protein (MRP) 4 (ATP-binding cassette C4). *Biochemical Journal*, *371*(Pt 2), 361–367.

Zhang, Y., Han, H., Elmquist, W. F., & Miller, D. W. (2000). Expression of various multidrug resistance-associated protein (MRP) homologues in brain microvessel endothelial cells. *Brain Research*, *876*, 148–153.

Zhang, W., Mojsilovic-Petrovic, J., Andrade, M. F., Zhang, H., Ball, M., & Stanimirovic, D. B. (2003). The expression and functional characterization of ABCG2 in brain endothelial cells and vessels. *The FASEB Journal*, *17*, 2085–2087.

Zhang, Y., Schuetz, J. D., Elmquist, W. F., & Miller, D. W. (2004). Plasma membrane localization of multidrug resistance-associated protein homologs in brain capillary endothelial cells. *The Journal of Pharmacology and Experimental Therapeutics*, *311*, 449–455.

Zhong, Y., Hennig, B., & Toborek, M. (2010). Intact lipid rafts regulate HIV-1 Tat protein-induced activation of the Rho signaling and upregulation of P-glycoprotein in brain endothelial cells. *Journal of Cerebral Blood Flow and Metabolism*, *30*, 522–533.

Zhou, S. F., Wang, L. L., Di, Y. M., Xue, C. C., Duan, W., Li, C. G., et al. (2008). Substrates and inhibitors of human multidrug resistance associated proteins and the implications in drug development. *Current Medicinal Chemistry*, *15*, 1981–2039.

Zhu, H. J., Wang, J. S., Markowitz, J. S., Donovan, J. L., Gibson, B. B., Gefroh, H. A., et al. (2006). Characterization of P-glycoprotein inhibition by major cannabinoids from marijuana. *The Journal of Pharmacology and Experimental Therapeutics*, *317*(2), 850–857.

CHAPTER FOUR

Blood–Brain Barrier Na Transporters in Ischemic Stroke

Martha E. O'Donnell[1]
Department of Physiology and Membrane Biology, School of Medicine, University of California, Davis, California, USA
[1]Corresponding author: e-mail address: meodonnell@ucdavis.edu

Contents

Abstract

Blood–brain barrier (BBB) endothelial cells form a barrier that is highly restrictive to passage of solutes between blood and brain. Many BBB transport mechanisms have been described that mediate transcellular movement of solutes across the barrier either into or out of the brain. One class of BBB transporters that is all too often overlooked is that of the ion transporters. The BBB has a rich array of ion transporters and channels that carry

Advances in Pharmacology, Volume 71
ISSN 1054-3589
http://dx.doi.org/10.1016/bs.apha.2014.06.011

Na, K, Cl, HCO_3, Ca, and other ions. Many of these are asymmetrically distributed between the luminal and abluminal membranes, giving BBB endothelial cells the ability to perform vectorial transport of ions across the barrier between blood and brain. In this manner, the BBB performs the important function of regulating the volume and composition of brain interstitial fluid. Through functional coupling of luminal and abluminal transporters and channels, the BBB carries Na, Cl, and other ions from blood into brain, producing up to 30% of brain interstitial fluid in healthy brain. During ischemic stroke cerebral edema forms by processes involving increased activity of BBB luminal Na transporters, resulting in "hypersecretion" of Na, Cl, and water into the brain interstitium. This review discusses the roles of luminal BBB Na transporters in edema formation in stroke, with an emphasis on Na–K–Cl cotransport and Na/H exchange. Evidence that these transporters provide effective therapeutic targets for reduction of edema in stroke is also discussed, as are recent findings regarding signaling pathways responsible for ischemia stimulation of the BBB Na transporters.

ABBREVIATIONS

ADC apparent diffusion coefficient
AMPK AMP-activated protein kinase
CMEC cerebral microvascular endothelial cells
DWI diffusion weighted imaging
ERK1/2 extracellular signal-regulated kinase
JNK Jun N-terminal kinase
MAPK mitogen-activated protein kinase
MCAO middle cerebral artery occlusion
NBC Na–HCO_3 cotransport
NHE Na/H exchange
NKCC Na–K–Cl cotransport
NMR nuclear magnetic resonance
TTC 2,3,5-triphenyltetrazolium chloride

1. INTRODUCTION

Blood–brain barrier (BBB) endothelial cells, joined together by extensive tight junction complexes, form a barrier that is highly restrictive to paracellular passage of solutes between blood and brain (Bradbury, 1984; Engelhardt, 2011; Fenstermacher & Rapoport, 1984; Hawkins & Davis, 2005; Huber, Egleton, & Davis, 2001; Petty & Lo, 2002). This barrier is not static but rather, functions as a dynamic interface between blood and brain, actively regulating transcellular movement of solutes between the vascular and extravascular brain compartments (Neuwelt et al., 2011). Studies conducted in recent years using a variety of *in vitro* and *in vivo* experimental models have provided an increasingly clear picture of the processes underlying BBB transport of many solutes. These include, e.g., nutrients, metabolites, peptides, proteins, and many xenobiotics (Neuwelt et al., 2011). An important class of BBB transporters that has received relatively little attention is that of ion transport systems. Endothelial cells of the BBB have an array of ion transporters and channels, many of which are asymmetrically distributed between the luminal and abluminal plasma membranes (as depicted in Fig. 1). This polarized arrangement of channels and transporters gives BBB endothelial cells the ability to perform vectorial transport of ions (with osmotically obliged water following) between blood and brain, much like vectorial ion transport occurring across tight epithelia of kidney and intestine. In this manner, the BBB participates in regulation of brain interstitial fluid volume and composition (Betz, 1986; Betz & Goldstein, 1986; Bradbury, 1984), producing up to 30% of brain interstitial fluid (Cserr, DePasquale, Patlak, & Pullen, 1989; Keep, 1993). Recent studies have shown that alteration of ion transport across the BBB is a major contributing factor to brain edema formation in ischemic stroke. In particular,

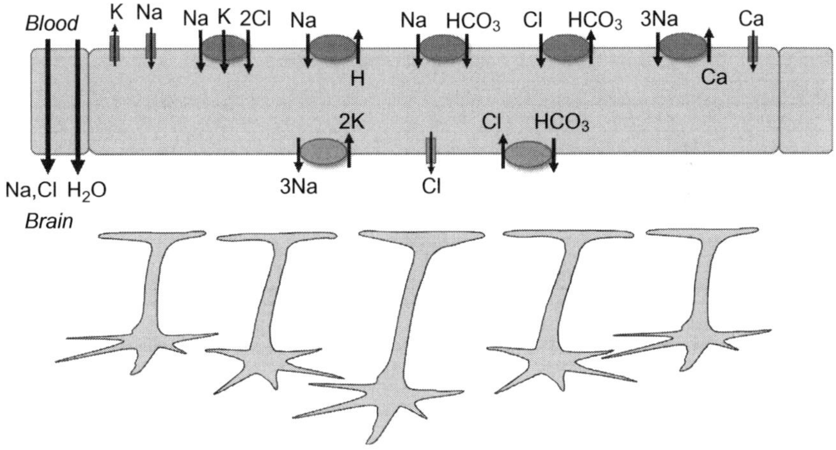

Figure 1 BBB ion transporters and channels. Several Na transporters have been documented in BBB endothelial cells. The Na/K pump is known to be primarily abluminal, while Na–K–Cl cotransport and Na/H exchange are predominantly luminal. While Na–HCO_3 cotransport and Na/Ca exchange are known to be present in the cells, their luminal/abluminal membrane distributions have not yet been established. Cl/HCO_3 exchange is also present and may functionally couple with Na/H exchange to bring Na and Cl into the cells for secretion of those ions at the abluminal membrane. A variety of ion channels are also present in BBB endothelial cells albeit less well studied.

BBB Na transporters, most notably Na–K–Cl cotransport and Na/H exchange, are stimulated by factors present during ischemia to increase secretion of Na, Cl, and water into brain during ischemic stroke, facilitating cytotoxic edema as astrocytes take up the ions and water presented to them. This chapter will focus primarily on the evidence that BBB Na–K–Cl cotransport and Na/H exchange participate in ischemia-induced brain edema formation and provide effective therapeutic targets for reducing edema and infarct in stroke.

2. ION TRANSPORTERS AND CHANNELS OF THE BBB

BBB endothelial cells express many types of ion transporters (depicted in Fig. 1). These include Na/K ATPase (Na/K pump), a primary active transporter that hydrolyzes ATP to pump Na out of the cell and K into the cell against their concentration gradients. The Na/K pump, which has been shown to reside in the abluminal BBB plasma membrane (Betz, 1986; Betz, Firth, & Goldstein, 1980; Betz & Goldstein, 1986), creates the all-important inwardly directed Na concentration gradient that powers many Na-dependent secondary active transport systems. Among the secondary active Na transporters present in BBB endothelial cells are a Na–K–Cl cotransporter (Kawai, Yamamoto, Yamamoto, McCarron, & Spatz, 1995; O'Donnell, Brandt, & Curry, 1995; Vigne, Farre, & Frelin, 1994), a Na/H exchanger (Betz, 1983b; Bronner, Kanter & Manson, 1995; Lam, Wise, & O'Donnell, 2009; Vigne, Ladoux, & Frelin, 1991), a Na–HCO_3 cotransporter (Nicola, Taylor, Wang, Barrand, & Hladky, 2008; Taylor, Nicola, Wang, Barrand, & Hladky, 2006), and a Na/Ca exchanger (Dömötör, Abbott, & Adam-Vizi, 1999). Evidence has also been provided for a Cl/HCO_3 exchanger in the cells (Nicola et al., 2008; Taylor et al., 2006). Although less information is available about the ion channels present in BBB endothelial cells we know that they exhibit inward rectifier K_{ir} channels (Hoyer, Popp, Meyer, Galla, & Gögelein, 1991), and ATP-sensitive K channels (Janigro, West, Gordon, & Winn, 1993). They also express an amiloride-sensitive Na channel (Vigne et al., 1989) and L-type voltage-dependent Ca channels (Yakubu & Leffler, 2002). Cation channels that mediate flux of Na and/or Ca have also been described, including a transient receptor potential C (TRPC) cation channel (Hicks, O'Neil, Dubinsky, & Brown, 2010) and a stretch-activated cation channel (Popp, Hoyer, Meyer, Galla, & Gögelein, 1992). A sulfonylurea receptor 1-regulated Ca- and ATP-sensitive cation channel (SUR-1 $NC_{Ca\text{-}ATP}$)

has also been shown to be expressed *de novo* in BBB following ischemia (Simard et al., 2006). Together, these transporters and channels perform a variety of functions, from regulating intracellular volume, pH, and [Ca] to performing vectorial transport of ions across the barrier. Two examples of the latter are transport of K from brain into blood to maintain appropriately low concentrations of K in the brain interstitial fluid, as well as transport of Na and Cl from blood into brain for BBB generation of brain interstitial fluid.

2.1. Na–K–Cl cotransport of BBB endothelial cells

The presence of Na–K–Cl cotransport (NKCC) in BBB endothelial cells is well documented. In early studies using *in vivo* methods Betz and coworkers showed that furosemide, an inhibitor of K–Cl and Na–K–Cl cotransporters reduced Cl-dependent Na uptake into the brain, leading them to hypothesize that a luminal Na-Cl cotransporter participates in secreting Na, Cl, and water from blood into brain (Betz, 1983a, 1983b). Other studies using isolated rat cerebral microvessels demonstrated a furosemide-sensitive, Na- and Cl-dependent K influx, further suggesting the presence of NKCC activity these cells (Lin, 1985, 1988). Subsequent studies using the more potent and specific NKCC inhibitor bumetanide provided more direct evidence for the presence of this transporter in BBB endothelial cells. Our group demonstrated NKCC activity, assessed as bumetanide-sensitive, Na- and Cl-dependent K influx, in cultured bovine cerebral microvascular endothelial cells (CMEC), freshly isolated rat microvessels (O'Donnell, Brandt and Curry, 1995; O'Donnell, Martinez, & Sun, 1995a, 1995b; Sun, Lytle, & O'Donnell, 1995) and human CMEC (O'Donnell, Duong, Suvatne, Foroutan, & Johnson, 2005). Other studies have also provided evidence for NKCC activity in rat and human BBB endothelial cells (Spatz, Merkel, Bembry, & McCarron, 1997; Vigne et al., 1994). The form of NKCC present in BBB is NKCC1, a finding not surprising given that of the two known forms of NKCC, NKCC1 has a widespread distribution and NKCC2 is found almost exclusively in kidney (Payne & Forbush, 1995; Pedersen, O'Donnell, Anderson, & Cala, 2006; Yerby, Vibat, Sun, Payne, & O'Donnell, 1997). In this regard, Western blot studies have demonstrated abundant NKCC1 protein in bovine and human BBB endothelial cell cultures as well as freshly isolated rat microvessels (O'Donnell, 2009; O'Donnell et al., 2005; O'Donnell, Martinez, & Sun, 1995a, 1995b; Sun et al., 1995). If BBB endothelial cell NKCC participates in vectorial transport of ions across the barrier from blood into brain, one would expect it to have a luminal location. In this manner, functional coupling of luminal NKCC with abluminal Na/K pump and an abluminal Cl efflux pathway would enable secretion of Na and Cl (with osmotically obliged water following) from blood into brain. Immunoelectron microscopy studies of perfusion-fixed rat brain that examined the cellular location of NKCC1 in BBB endothelial cells *in situ* using NKCC1 antibodies and immunogold labeling have shown that the transporter is indeed found predominantly in the luminal membrane with a minor component in the abluminal membrane (O'Donnell, Tran, Lam, Liu, & Anderson, 2004). This is consistent with a role for the cotransporter in secretion of Na, Cl, and water into the brain, contributing to the BBB generation of brain interstitial fluid (Fig. 2).

2.2. Na/H exchange of BBB endothelial cells

Early evidence of BBB Na/H exchange (NHE) activity was provided by studies that showed an amiloride-sensitive Na flux in isolated rat brain

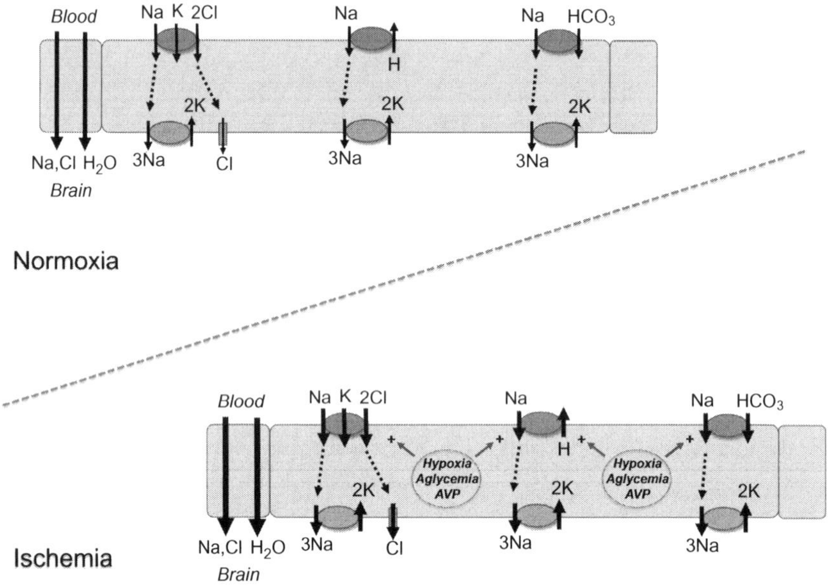

Figure 2 BBB Na transporters in secretion of Na, Cl, and water from blood into brain. (A) Role of BBB Na transporters in secretion of brain interstitial fluid normoxia. (B) Ischemic factor-stimulated BBB Na transporter activity contributes to "hypersecretion" of Na, Cl, and water into to brain during ischemia, contributing to edema formation.

capillaries (Betz, 1983b). Subsequent studies using more potent and selective NHE inhibitors, including EIPA and HOE642 (Masereel, Pochet, & Laeckmann, 2003), have demonstrated the presence of NHE activity in CMEC of rat (Kawai, McCarron, & Spatz, 1995; Sipos, Törocsik, Tretter, & Adam-Vizi, 2005; Vigne et al., 1991) as well as pig (Hsu, Haffner, Albuquerque, & Leffler, 1996) and bovine (Lam et al., 2009). Studies of bovine CMEC and freshly isolated rat microvessels have shown that both NHE1 and NHE2 forms of Na/H exchange are present in the cells (Chang, O'Donnell & Barakat, 2008; Lam et al., 2009; O'Donnell, 2009; O'Donnell, Yuen, Chen, & Anderson, 2013). Immunoelectron microscopy studies using antibodies that specifically recognize either NHE1 or NHE2 also demonstrated that both forms of Na/H exchange proteins are present in BBB *in situ* and that they reside predominantly in the luminal membrane (Lam et al., 2009;)O'Donnell et al., 2013. This suggests that, like NKCC, NHE is asymmetrically configured in the BBB in a manner that will support functional coupling with abluminal Na/K pump to perform vectorial transport of Na from blood into brain (Fig. 2).

3. BBB Na–K–Cl COTRANSPORT AND Na/H EXCHANGE IN ISCHEMIC STROKE AND CEREBRAL EDEMA

Alteration of BBB ion transporter and channel function is often a significant contributing factor to brain damage in pathophysiological states. In this regard, several studies have provided evidence that BBB Na transporters contribute to formation of cerebral edema during ischemic stroke. Edema is a major cause of morbidity and mortality in stroke (Bronner et al., 1995; Gartshore, Patterson, & Macrae, 1997; Klatzo, 1994) and despite the high cost of stroke in terms of dollars and human suffering there are only very limited therapies available to reduce stroke damage. Previous studies have shown that during the early hours of ischemic stroke edema forms by processes involving stimulation of BBB ion transporters and increased secretion of Na, Cl, and water from blood into brain across an intact BBB (Betz, 1996; Menzies, Betz, & Hoff, 1993; Menzies, Hoff, & Betz, 1990; Schielke, Moises, & Betz, 1991; Fig. 2), with breakdown of the barrier not occurring until 4–6 h after the start of ischemia (Kimelberg, 1995; Menzies et al., 1993). Perivascular astrocyte ion transporters are also stimulated during ischemic stroke, causing the cells to take up the ions and water presented to them by BBB secretion (Bourke et al., 1980; Gotoh, Asano, Koide, & Takakura, 1985; Iadecola, 1999; Kempski et al., 1991; Kimelberg, 1995;

Kimelberg, 1999). Early studies reported that luminal BBB Na transporters appeared to be rate-limiting in the process (Betz, Keep, Beer, & Ren, 1994; Kato, Kogure, Sakamoto, & Watanabe, 1987; Menzies et al., 1993; Menzies et al., 1990; Schielke et al., 1991), although little was known about the transporters responsible. More recent studies have focused on identifying BBB Na transporters that may contribute to ischemia-induced edema formation and determining whether they present effective therapeutic targets for reduction of edema and its consequent brain damage in stroke. These studies, discussed in the remainder of this section, have revealed that two BBB Na transporters, Na–K–Cl cotransport and Na/H exchange, appear to be major contributors to ischemia-induced brain edema and that preventing their stimulation during stroke can significantly reduce edema.

3.1. Effects of ischemic factors on BBB Na–K–Cl cotransporter activity

Several studies have tested the effects of factors present during cerebral ischemia on CMEC NKCC activity (as depicted in Fig. 2, lower panel). Three prominent ischemic factors are hypoxia, aglycemia, and arginine vasopressin (AVP). Reduction of cerebral blood flow rapidly reduces available O_2 resulting in severe to moderate hypoxia (as found in the core and surrounding penumbra, respectively, of the ischemic tissue). Glucose is also reduced causing hypoglycemia to aglycemia, depending on the severity and duration of the blood flow reduction. A third factor, AVP, is released during ischemia from extrahypothalamic neuronal processes terminating on brain microvessels (Dóczi, 1993; Jójárt, Joó, Siklós, & László, 1984; Landgraf, 1992; Sorensen, Gjerris, & Hammer, 1985). Exposing bovine CMEC to hypoxia levels ranging from moderate to severe (e.g., 7–0.5%) over a 120 min time course has been found to significantly increase NKCC activity, assessed as bumetanide-sensitive K influx (Foroutan, Brillault, Forbush, & O'Donnell, 2005). Na/K pump activity, assessed as ouabain-sensitive K influx is also increased by hypoxia (Foroutan et al., 2005), consistent with functional coupling of the luminal and abluminal transporters for secretion of Na from blood into brain. Exposing the cells to media lacking glucose causes a substantial (>2.5-fold) increase in NKCC activity and further, combined hypoxia and aglycemia produces an even more robust increase in activity (Foroutan et al., 2005). Representative studies showing hypoxia and aglycemia effects on CMEC NKCC activity are shown in Fig. 3. AVP also stimulates the transporter in both bovine and human CMEC, causing a nearly twofold increase in CMEC NKCC activity after

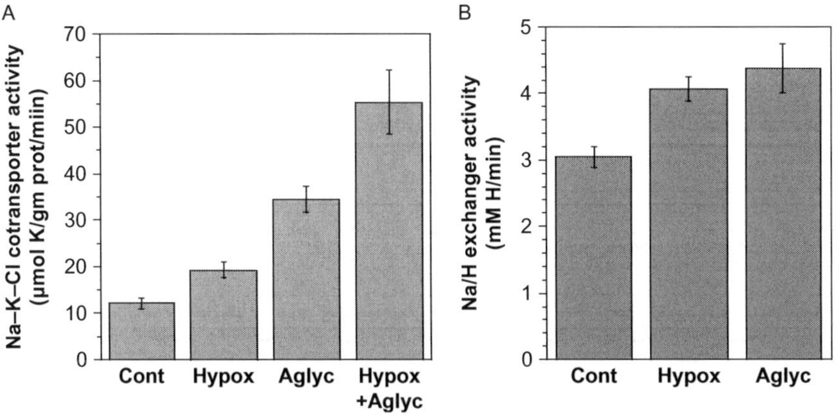

Figure 3 Ischemic factor stimulation of BBB Na–K–Cl cotransporter and Na/H exchanger activities. (A) Hypoxia- and aglycemia-induced increases in cerebral microvascular endothelial Na–K–Cl cotransporter activity. (B) Hypoxia- and aglycemia-induced increases in cerebral microvascular endothelial cell Na/H exchanger activity.

just 5 min (Foroutan et al., 2005; O'Donnell et al., 2005). Unlike aglycemia, however, AVP effects are not additive with hypoxia. Immunoelectron microscopy studies evaluating the presence of NKCC in BBB *in situ* have shown that NKCC resides predominantly in the luminal membrane in ischemic brain as well as normoxic brain (Brillault, Lam, Rutkowsky, Foroutan, & O'Donnell, 2008), consistent with its role in secretion of Na into the brain during ischemia. Other studies have shown that endothelin-1, another factor present during cerebral ischemia, also stimulates rat and human CMEC NKCC activity (Kawai, McCarron, & Spatz, 1996, 1997; Kawai, Yamamoto, et al., 1995; Spatz et al., 1997; Vigne et al., 1994), providing additional evidence that this BBB Na transporter is stimulated to participate in edema formation during ischemia. Thus, it appears that BBB NKCC activity is quite sensitive to several factors all increased in the brain during ischemic stroke.

3.2. *In vivo* studies: Effects of bumetanide on middle cerebral artery occlusion-induced edema and brain Na uptake

Studies using the rodent middle cerebral artery occlusion (MCAO) model of ischemic stroke have provided additional evidence that NKCC contributes to ischemia-induced cerebral edema formation. Nuclear magnetic resonance (NMR) diffusion weighted imaging (DWI) of rats subjected to permanent MCAO (pMCAO) can be used to evaluate cerebral edema formation in the living rats. By this method, DWI-derived apparent diffusion coefficients (ADCs) provide an established index of cytotoxic edema, with reduction of ADC indicating the presence of cytotoxic edema (O'Donnell et al., 2004; Fig. 4). Using pMCAO rather than the transient MCAO model of ischemia and reperfusion allows investigation of ischemia without the complicating effects of reperfusion. By this approach, it has been found that rats given intravenous bumetanide to inhibit BBB NKCC activity show a significant and sustained attenuation of edema formation compared to vehicle-treated rats. This suggests that inhibition of BBB NKCC activity does not simply delay formation of edema during the early hours of stroke. Studies using NMR Na spectroscopy chemical shift imaging (CSI) methods have further shown that rats subjected to MCAO exhibit a linear increase in brain Na uptake that is significantly reduced by intravenous bumetanide (O'Donnell et al., 2013). This is as expected because it is the secretion of Na from blood into brain that is the driving force for increased brain water. Further, bumetanide significantly reduces infarct following pMCAO, assessed by 2,3,5-triphenyltetrazolium chloride (TTC) staining (O'Donnell et al., 2013). In studies evaluating neurological outcome following pMCAO intravenous bumetanide was also found to significantly improve performance in both the 14 pt. sensorimotor test (DeRyck, Van Reempts, Borgers, Wauquier, & Janssen, 1989) and the Rotarod test (Hamm, Rice, O'Dell, Lyeth, & Jenkins, 1994) at 1 and 2 days after pMCAO induction (O'Donnell et al., 2013). These findings indicate the BBB Na–K–Cl cotransporter, positioned in the luminal membrane, stimulated by ischemic factors and readily accessible for inhibition by intravenous bumetanide, appears to be an effective target for reducing edema in ischemic stroke.

3.3. Effects of ischemic factors on BBB Na/H exchanger activity

Ischemic factors have also been found to stimulate BBB Na/H exchanger activity. As with NKCC, hypoxia, aglycemia, and AVP have all been shown to increase CMEC NHE activity (as depicted in Fig. 2). Exposing bovine CMEC to hypoxia, aglycemia, or AVP has been shown to cause rapid and significant increases in NHE activity, assessed as HOE642-sensitive H flux (Lam et al., 2009), with the increases in NHE activity sustained for at least 5 h (Yuen et al., 2014). Representative studies showing hypoxia and aglycemia effects on CMEC NHE activity are shown in Fig. 3. Studies evaluating the effects of ischemic factors on the expression of NHE1 and

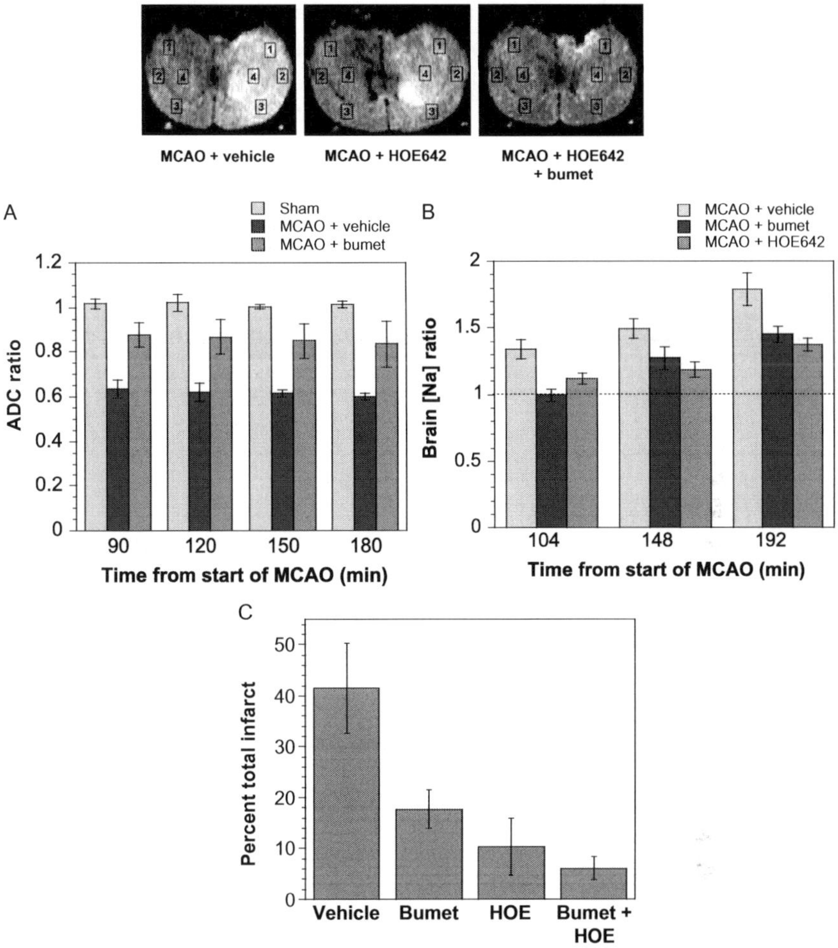

Figure 4 Bumetanide and HOE642 reduction of edema, brain Na uptake, and infarct in rat middle cerebral artery occlusion-induced cerebral ischemia. (A) IV administration of the Na–K–Cl cotransporter inhibitor bumetanide significantly reduces middle cerebral artery occlusion (MCAO)-induced cerebral edema, assessed as DWI-derived ADC values. DWI images in the upper panel show the ipsilateral and contralateral regions of interest (ROI) evaluated. (B) Reduction of brain Na uptake during MCAO in rats given IV bumetanide or the Na/H exchange inhibitor HOE642. (C) Bumetanide and HOE642 reduction of infarct as defined by TTC staining.

NHE2 Na/H exchangers present have revealed that CMEC exposed to hypoxia, aglycemia or AVP exhibit significantly elevated abundance of NHE1 protein with no change in NHE2 protein abundance. This raises the possibility that NHE1 plays a more prominent role in ischemia effects on BBB Na/H exchange. Additional studies are needed to further address this question, e.g., through separate knockdown of NHE1 and NHE2 proteins by siRNA. In addition to hypoxia, aglycemia, and AVP, endothelin-1 has also been shown to stimulate CMEC NHE activity (Kawai, McCarron, et al., 1995; Vigne et al., 1991), further supporting a role for BBB NHE in stroke-induced edema formation. Immunoelectron microscopy evaluation of NHE protein *in situ* location in BBB of ischemic brains has revealed that both NHE1 and NHE2 remain predominantly in the luminal membrane during ischemia as they are in normoxic brain (O'Donnell et al., 2013), consistent with one or both of these NHE forms participating in increased blood to brain secretion of Na during stroke.

3.4. *In vivo* studies: Effects of HOE642 on MCAO-induced edema and brain Na uptake

Investigation of HOE642 effects on cerebral edema in the pMCAO model of ischemic stroke has provided further evidence for a role of BBB NHE in stroke-induced edema formation (Fig. 4). IV administration of HOE642 to inhibit BBB NHE activity significantly attenuates cerebral edema formation, as determined by DWI-derived ADC values. As with bumetanide inhibition of BBB NKCC, HOE642 causes a sustained reduction of edema formation throughout the early hours of pMCAO (O'Donnell et al., 2013). Brain Na uptake, as determined by NMR Na CSI, and the TTC-defined infarct are also significantly reduced by HOE642 (O'Donnell et al., 2013). In a manner similar to bumetanide, neurological outcome following pMCAO, assessed by 14 pt. sensorimotor and Rotarod tests, is significantly improved by HOE642 (O'Donnell et al., 2013). If both NKCC and NHE serve as effective therapeutic BBB targets for reduction of edema and infarct in ischemia, then an important consideration is whether an even better outcome can be attained through inhibiting both Na transporters. This appears to be the case, as rats given a combination of bumetanide and HOE642 show further improved reduction of edema and infarct (O'Donnell et al., 2013). These findings are consistent with an earlier report that dimethylamiloride inhibition of Na/H exchange reduces infarct following MCAO in spontaneously hypertensive rats (Hom et al., 2007). Other studies have examined the effects of HOE642 in rodent models of ischemia/reperfusion induced by transient (reversible) MCAO. In this regard, HOE642 has been reported to reduce reperfusion injury in mice, evaluated by MRI methods (Ferrazzano et al., 2011). A related study evaluating the effects of intravenous HOE642 administered to mice subjected to 2 h of ischemia and 24 h reperfusion by reversible MCAO showed that the inhibitor reduces brain infarct, leading to the conclusion that inhibition of astrocyte and neuronal Na/H exchange reduces brain damage in stroke (Luo, Chen, Kintner, Shull, & Sun, 2005). However, in those studies, it was not determined whether HOE642 sufficiently penetrated into the brain to reach its intended brain parenchyma targets in the ischemia/reperfusion model. Thus, one must consider that the neuroprotective effects observed could have been due in part or in whole to inhibition of BBB Na/H exchange activity. This is an important consideration that will need to be addressed in future studies because the chemical structure and properties of HOE642 predict that it will not penetrate the BBB. This is also true for bumetanide and further, HPLC studies have shown that bumetanide penetration into the brain is very poor to negligible (Töllner et al., 2014).

3.5. Ischemia-induced BBB endothelial cell swelling: Roles of Na–K–Cl cotransport and Na/H exchange

NKCC and NHE are both well known for their roles in cell volume regulation of a variety of cell types (Eveloff & Warnock, 1987). Previous studies have provided evidence that both NKCC and NHE participate in cell volume regulation of aortic endothelial cells and brain microvascular endothelial cells (Behmanesh & Kempski, 2000; Kempski, Spatz, Valet, & Baethmann, 1985; O'Donnell, 1993; O'Donnell, Brandt, & Curry, 1995; O'Donnell, Martinez, & Sun, 1995a, 1995b). Under certain conditions, increased NKCC and NHE activities can also drive endothelial cell swelling (Behmanesh & Kempski, 2000; O'Donnell, 1993; Pedersen, 2006). In this regard, increases in BBB NKCC and NHE activities, if not effectively coupled to abluminal Na/K pump-mediated Na efflux, are predicted to cause swelling of the cells. This can occur, for example, as cell ATP levels fall in the continued presence of ischemia such that the Na/K pump no longer keeps pace with luminal NKCC and NHE activities, causing an increase in cell Na content and consequent cell swelling. Studies evaluating the possibility that NKCC and/or NHE might contribute to BBB endothelial cell swelling during ischemic stroke have shown that hypoxia (both moderate and severe) causes an increase in CMEC intracellular volume that develops over hours as compared to the very rapid hypoxia-induced increase in NKCC and NHE activities (Fig. 5; Brillault et al., 2008; Foroutan et al., 2005). Further, bumetanide and HOE642 treatment of the cells significantly reduces hypoxia-induced swelling and in combination,

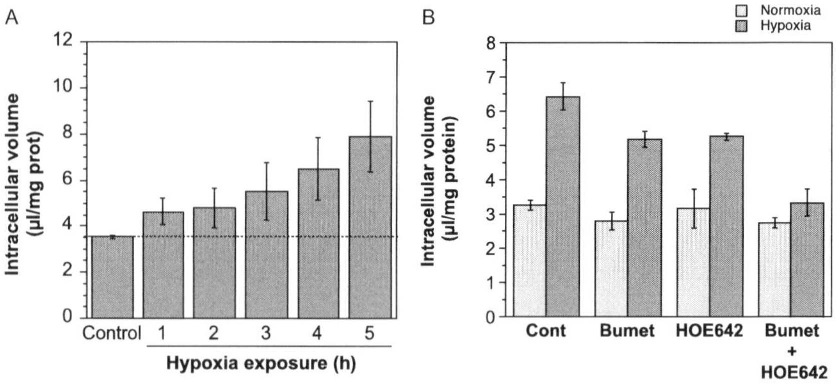

Figure 5 Time course of hypoxia-induced BBB endothelial cell swelling. (A) Cerebral microvascular endothelial cells (CMEC) exposed to hypoxia (7% O_2) show significant increases in intracellular volume after 4 and 5 h exposures. (B) Bumetanide and HOE642 significantly reduce CMEC swelling observed after 5 h hypoxia exposures.

the inhibitors nearly abolish swelling. Hypoxia also causes a slow onset increase in Na content of the cells (Brillault et al., 2008). These findings are consistent with NKCC and NHE both contributing to vectorial transport of Na across the BBB early in ischemia and, at later hours, also contributing to swelling of the cells. Because BBB endothelial cells also have a Na/Ca exchanger, elevation of intracellular [Na] can cause a rise in intracellular [Ca] via the exchanger operating in reverse mode (Murphy, Cross, & Steenbergen, 2002). Alteration of tight junctions leading to increased BBB paracellular permeability has been shown to occur in the presence of elevated intracellular [Ca] (Abbott & Revest, 1991; Hawkins & Davis, 2005). Thus, one might predict that NKCC- and NHE-driven increases in BBB endothelial intracellular [Na] following prolonged exposure to hypoxia will promote breakdown of the BBB. In this regard, the time course of the observed hypoxia-induced increase in CMEC cell volume is consistent with the time course of BBB breakdown in ischemic stroke.

4. SIGNALING MECHANISMS: ROLES OF AMP KINASE AND p38, JNK AND ERK MAP KINASES

Identifying the signaling pathways by which ischemic factors stimulate BBB Na–K–Cl cotransporter and Na/H exchanger activities has the potential of leading to therapies aimed at preventing ischemia stimulation of the Na transporters in patients at risk for stroke. While there are many possible signaling pathways that could be involved, perhaps the most likely are kinase pathways known to participate in cell stress responses. Previous studies have shown that increases in Na–K–Cl cotransporter activity are associated with increased phosphorylation of the cotransporter (Flemmer, Giménez, Dowd, Darman, & Forbush, 2002; Foroutan et al., 2005; O'Donnell, Martinez, & Sun, 1995a, 1995b). Similarly, an increase in Na/H exchanger phosphorylation occurs with increased exchanger activity (Noël & Pouysségur, 1995; Pedersen, 2006; Pedersen et al., 2006). In recent years, there has been increasing attention on the role of "stress" kinases in cellular responses to hypoxia, ischemia, and other stresses. These include AMP-activated protein kinase (AMPK) and three kinases belonging to the family of mitogen-activated protein kinases (MAPK), p38 MAPK, Jun N-terminal kinase (JNK) MAPK, and extracellular signal-regulated kinase (ERK1/2) MAPK (Fig. 6). AMPK is a key mediator of cell responses to stress. It is a downstream component of a protein kinase cascade that is switched on by a variety of stresses, including hypoxia, glucose deprivation, and ischemia (Carling, Sanders, & Woods, 2008; Hardie, 2003, 2004). AMPK is exquisitely sensitive to elevation of the intracellular AMP/ATP ratio and can be activated even when ATP levels have not detectably fallen (Carling, 2004; Hardie, 2003). A heterotrimer with α, β, and γ subunits, AMPK is activated by phosphorylation of thr172 on the α subunit by one or more upstream kinases (Hardie, 2004; Hawley et al., 1996; Kemp et al., 2003) in response to a variety of stresses that include hypoxia, glucose deprivation, and ischemia (Carling, 2004; Hardie, 2003, 2004). Activated AMPK is known to regulate anabolic and catabolic processes, e.g., glycolysis and glycogenolysis, with the

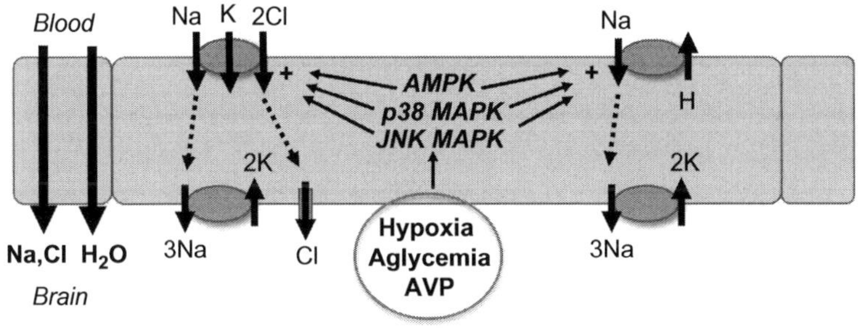

Figure 6 Role of AMP kinase and the p38 and JNK MAP kinases in ischemic factor-induced stimulation of BBB Na–K–Cl cotransporter and Na/H exchanger activities. Mounting evidence indicates that the "stress" kinases AMPK, p38 MAPK, and JNK MAPK, as well as ERK MAPK (not depicted here) are involved in mediating hypoxia, aglycemia, and AVP stimulation of BBB Na transporter activities.

effect of maintaining cell ATP levels even during stresses such as ischemia that tend to reduce ATP (Carling, 2004; Hardie, 2003, 2004). However, AMPK has also been shown to target transport proteins, including GLUT1 and GLUT4 glucose transporters, K and Cl channels (CFTR Cl channel and KCa3.1 channel) in epithelia (Hallows, Kobinger, Wilson, Witters, & Foskett, 2003; Klein et al., 2009), and the NKCC2 Na–K–Cl cotransporter (Fraser et al., 2007). While AMPK acts as a sensor of energy balance in cells, it can also be activated by hypoxia independently of changes in AMP/ATP ratio. Previous studies have provided evidence that AMPK activity is increased by MCAO-induced ischemia in rat brain (Li & McCullough, 2010; McCullough et al., 2005). Further, Compound C, a highly selective inhibitor of AMPK, was found in those studies to significantly reduce cerebral infarct in MCAO (Li, Zeng, Viollet, Ronnett, & McCullough, 2007; McCullough et al., 2005). There are two isoforms of the AMPK catalytic subunit, α1 and α2. Previous studies have reported both that both AMPK subunits are present in neurons and astrocytes (Li & McCullough, 2010; McCullough et al., 2005; Turnley et al., 1999) and that endothelial cells of the peripheral vasculature express the α1 subunit (Davis, Xie, Viollet, & Zou, 2006; Fisslthaler & Fleming, 2009; Zou et al., 2003). Studies aimed at addressing the question of whether AMPK participates in ischemic factor stimulation of BBB NKCC activity have evaluated the effects of hypoxia, aglycemia, and AVP on activation of AMPK in bovine CMEC. Using Western blot methods and antibodies that specifically recognize the phosphorylated, active form of AMPK (p-AMPK) as well as antibodies that recognize both phosphorylated and nonphosphorylated AMPK (total AMPK) these studies have shown that moderate or severe hypoxia (7 or 2% O_2) significantly increases p-AMPKα1 abundance (Wallace, Foroutan, & O'Donnell, 2011). The hypoxia-induced activation of AMPK in these cells is rapid and transient, with p-AMPK increased at 5 and 30 min then decreasing again at 60 through 120 min (Fig. 7). In contrast to p-AMPK, total AMPK abundance does not change in the presence of hypoxia, indicating that AMPK activity increases only by activation of the kinase and not through synthesis of new protein, as predicted given the rapidity of the response. Exposing CMEC to AVP or aglycemia also causes rapid transient increases in AMPK activity (Wallace et al., 2011). Studies have also shown that the AMPK inhibitor Compound C significantly reduces CMEC NKCC activity stimulated by hypoxia, aglycemia, or AVP, although the degree of inhibition varies with ischemic factor, such that Compound C abolishes hypoxia and aglycemia stimulation of NKCC activity but only

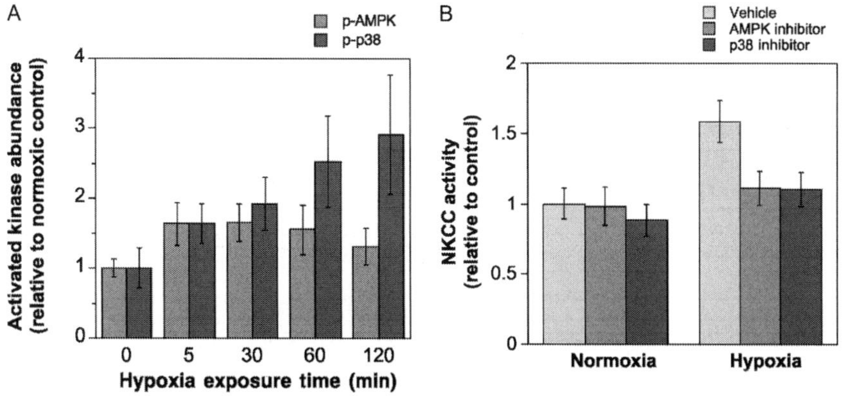

Figure 7 Activation of BBB AMPK and p38 MAPK by ischemic factors: effects on BBB Na–K–Cl cotransporter activity. (A) Hypoxia-induced activation of CMEC AMPK and p38 MAPK, evaluated as increased abundance of phosphorylated kinase. Both kinases are activated by 5 min. However, p38 activation is more prolonged than that of AMPK. (B) Inhibition of either AMPK or p38 activity by Compound C and SB239063, respectively) abolishes hypoxia stimulation of CMEC Na–K–Cl cotransporter activity.

reduces AVP stimulation of the cotransporter (Wallace et al., 2011). Confocal immunofluorescence microscopy of perfusion-fixed rat brain has further demonstrated that AMPKα1, both total and p-AMPKα1, are detected in BBB endothelial cells *in situ* of normoxic as well as ischemic brain (Wallace et al., 2011). Here, AMPKα1 and p-AMPKα1 are observed in both astrocytes (identified by an antibody to GFAP) and BBB endothelial cells (identified by the SMI71 antibody, specific for brain microvessel endothelial cells). Future studies are needed to determine whether AMPKα2 is also present in BBB and contributes to ischemic factor effects on NKCC. In addition, whether AMPK also mediates ischemic factor effects on BBB NHE activity has yet to be investigated.

p38 MAPK (often referred to simply as p38, the size of the protein band observed in Western blots) has also been reported to be a key mediator of cell responses to stress and, like AMPK, is also a downstream component of a protein kinase cascade that can be activated by a variety of stresses including ischemia, as well as osmotic and oxidative stresses (Cowan & Storey, 2003; Irving & Bamford, 2002; Kyriakis & Avruch, 2001). p38 MAPK belongs to a family of MAP kinases that also includes JNK MAPK and ERK1/2 MAPK (Irving & Bamford, 2002). Previous studies have demonstrated that p38 MAPK is activated by dual phosphorylation of thr180 and tyr182 by upstream kinases in response to hypoxia or ischemia in a variety of cell types including perfused rat heart (Bogoyevitch et al., 1996; Zhu, Mao, Sun, Xia, & Greenberg, 2002), cultured cortical neurons, and CMEC (Lee & Lo, 2003; Zhu et al., 2003). In addition, p38 MAPK activity has been shown to be increased in rat cerebral cortex within 15 min from the start of MCAO (Barone, Irving, Ray, Lee, Kassis, Kumar, et al., 2001a; Tian, Litvak, & Lev, 2000). Further, the highly selective p38 MAPK inhibitor SB239063 reduces infarct and improves neurological outcome following rat MCAO (Barone, Irving, Ray, Lee, Kassis, Kumar, et al., 2001b; Barone et al., 2000). JNK MAPK (often called JNK) has also been found to mediate cell responses to hypoxia and ischemia in several cell types (Cowan & Storey, 2003; Irving & Bamford, 2002; Yatsushige, Ostrowski, Tsubokawa, Colohan, & Zhang, 2007). JNK MAPK is activated by dual phosphorylation of thr183 and tyr185 by upstream kinases (Cowan & Storey, 2003; Irving & Bamford, 2002; Kyriakis & Avruch, 2001). Previous studies have shown that JNK, like p38, is activated by hypoxia and ischemia in several cell types (Cowan & Storey, 2003; Irving & Bamford, 2002; Kyriakis & Avruch, 2001). Further, inhibition of JNK activity was found to reduce infarct in rodent models of both transient and permanent ischemia (Borsello et al., 2003; Guo et al., 2005; Yatsushige et al., 2007). Studies conducted to assess the possible contributions of p38 and JNK to ischemic factor stimulation of BBB endothelial cell NKCC activity have revealed that exposing CMEC to moderate or severe hypoxia (7% or 2% O_2), aglycemia, or AVP causes rapid increases in p-p38 abundance (by 5 min) that are sustained through at least 120 min (Wallace, Jelks, & O'Donnell, 2012). As with AMPK, these increases in p-p38 occur without any change in total p38, indicating that the increased activity occurs through activation of the kinase, not increased expression of the kinase (Fig. 7). Ischemic conditions also increase JNK activity in CMEC with hypoxia causing transient increases but both aglycemia and AVP causing slower onset, more sustained increases in p-JNK (Wallace et al., 2012). Studies evaluating the effects of the highly selective p38 and JNK inhibitors SB239063 (Barone et al., 2001a, 2001b) and SP600125 (Bennett et al., 2001; Guo et al., 2005), respectively, have revealed that inhibiting either of these kinases reduces hypoxia, aglycemia, and AVP stimulation of CMEC NKCC activity (Wallace et al., 2012). Representative studies illustrating the effects of AMPK and p38 inhibition on hypoxia-stimulated CMEC NKCC activity are shown in Fig. 7. Complementary confocal immunofluorescence microscopy studies have shown that p-38 (both p-p38 and total p38) and JNK (both p-JNK and total JNK) are detected in BBB *in situ* as well as astrocytes of perfusion-fixed rat brain, using

GFAP and SMI71 antibodies to identify astrocytes and BBB endothelial cells, respectively (Wallace et al., 2012).

Other studies have implicated ERK1/2 MAPK (also known as simply ERK and sometimes referred to as p44/p42 for the size of the double bands in Western blots) in the response of many cells to stress (Cowan & Storey, 2003; Irving & Bamford, 2002; Kyriakis & Avruch, 2001). While ERK was recognized early on as a kinase activated by growth factors, it is also activated by hypoxia and ischemia (Cowan & Storey, 2003; Irving & Bamford, 2002; Kyriakis & Avruch, 2001). ERK activation has been demonstrated in brains of mice and rats subjected to MCAO (Sawe, Steinberg, & Zhao, 2008; Wu, Ye, Che, & Yang, 2000) as well as in human brain following acute ischemia (Slevin et al., 2000). Further, ischemia-induced activation of ERK has been reported to increase NHE activity in rat myocardium (Moore, Gan, Karmazyn, & Fliegel, 2001), astrocytes, and neurons (Kintner, Look, Shull, & Sun, 2005; Luo et al., 2005). Recent studies investigating a possible role for ERK in ischemic factor stimulation of BBB NKCC activity and NHE activity (Yuen et al., 2014) have shown that CMEC p-ERK abundance is increased in response to moderate or severe hypoxia (7% or 2% O_2), aglycemia, and AVP, although the response varies with ischemic factor (Yuen et al., 2014) in a manner similar to activation of the other MAP kinases. In this case, hypoxia and AVP cause rapid transient increases in p-ERK, while aglycemia induces a rapid and sustained increase in p-ERK. Further, FR180204, a highly selective ERK inhibitor (Ohori et al., 2005; Patnaik, Dietz, Zheng, Austin, & Marugan, 2009), significantly reduces hypoxia-stimulated NKCC activity and abolishes aglycemia-stimulated CMEC NKCC activity. FR180204 also abolishes hypoxia-, aglycemia-, and AVP-stimulated NHE activity (Yuen et al., 2014). As with AMPK, p38 and JNK, ERK is also present in BBB endothelial cells *in situ*, demonstrated by confocal immunofluorescence studies of perfusion fixed rat brain (Yuen et al., 2014). Here again, p-ERK and ERK are both detected in astrocytes (identified by GFAP) and BBB endothelial cells (identified by SMI71) in both normoxic and ischemic brain.

While inhibiting any one of these four kinases reduces or abolishes ischemic factor effects on NKCC and/or NHE activity, the time course profiles of activation differ with both the kinase and the ischemic factor. The rapid and transient activation of AMPK observed under all ischemic conditions as well as that of JNK and ERK for some conditions suggests that AMPK and JNK by themselves cannot account for sustained Na transporter activity occurring throughout the early hours of stroke when edema continues to form through BBB ion secretion. In contrast, increases in p38 activity are sustained during this time, suggesting that the p38 may participate directly in sustaining the elevated BBB Na transporter activities. It is possible, if not likely, that these signaling pathways do not act independently of each other during ischemia such that, e.g., early AMPK activation may lead to the more sustained increases in p38 activity observed. Future investigations are needed to clarify the relationship of these kinase pathways during ischemia.

Earlier studies investigating signaling pathways mediating AVP effects on CMEC NKCC activity revealed that AVP acts via a V1 AVP receptor, elevating intracellular [Ca] ([Ca_i]) and stimulating NKCC activity in a [Ca_i]-dependent manner (O'Donnell et al., 2005). This is consistent with other studies showing that AVP V1 receptors are present in brain microvasculature (Ostrowski et al., 1992; Ostrowski, Lolait, & Young, 1994). It is also consistent with the observation that ischemia causes increases in [Ca_i] in many cells and that severe hypoxia increases [Ca_i] in CMEC (Ikeda, Nagashim, Wu, Yamaguchi, & Tamaki, 1997; Kimura, Oike, & Ito, 2000). The relationship of this V1 receptor – and, [Ca_i]-dependent pathway to AMPK, p38, JNK, and ERK pathways remains to be clarified. However, it has been reported that elevation of [Ca_i] can lead to activation of AMPK via a Ca-calmodulin-dependent protein kinase direct activation of AMPK in some cells (Hurley, Anderson, Franzone, & Kemp, 2005; Woods et al., 2003) and possibly also p38 MAPK (Capano & Crompton, 2006; Li, Miller, Ninomiya-Tsuji, & Young, 2005).

5. HORMONAL AND METABOLIC FACTOR EFFECTS ON BBB NA TRANSPORTER EXPRESSION AND ACTIVITIES

Both NKCC and NHE activities of other cell types are well known to be modulated by many neurotransmitters, cytokines, growth factors, and hormones, the response depending on the type of cell (Pedersen et al., 2006) (Chipperfield, 1996; Haas & Forbush, 1998; Mahnensmith & Aronson, 1985; Noël & Pouysségur, 1995; Pedersen et al., 2003; Wakabayashi et al., 1992). The effects of these agents on BBB Na transporter activities, however, are less well studied than in other cell types. We do know that in addition to the observed AVP and endothelin stimulatory effects on BBB NKCC and NHE activities, bradykinin stimulates BBB NKCC activity, while atrial natriuretic peptide decreases BBB NKCC activity (O'Donnell, Martinez, & Sun, 1995a, 1995b). Other studies have shown that NKCC activity is decreased by the cytokine interleukin 1

(Vigne et al., 1994) and increased or decreased by interleukin 6 (low and high doses, respectively) (Sun, Lytle, & O'Donnell, 1997). Included among the hormones that can alter NKCC and/or NHE activities in BBB endothelial cells is estrogen (17β-estradiol). This will be addressed in more detail in Section 5.1.

5.1. Estradiol effects on CMEC Na transporters

Studies have shown that estradiol is yet another factor capable of regulating BBB NKCC and NHE activities (Chang et al., 2008; Lam et al., 2009). This is an important effect to consider given that estradiol (17β-estradiol) has been demonstrated to exert neuroprotective effects in stroke. In human males and postmenopausal females, stroke outcome is worse than in premenopausal females and postmenopausal females taking hormone replacement therapy (Dubal et al., 1998; Hurn & Macrae, 2000; Zhang, Shi, Rajakumar, Day, & Simpkins, 1998). In rodent experimental models of ischemic stroke both acute and chronic estrogen treatment reduced brain damage (Dubal et al., 1998; Hurn & Macrae, 2000; Rusa, Alkayad, Crain, Traystman, & Kimes, 1999; Yang, Shi, Day, & Simpkins, 2000; Zhang et al., 1998). Previous studies have also provided evidence that estradiol reduces the DWI-defined lesion volume in rats subjected to cerebral ischemia/reperfusion (Shi, Zhang, & Simpkins, 1997). Despite these findings, the mechanisms have not been fully understood. Studies evaluating estradiol effects in the rat pMCAO model of cerebral ischemia have found that intravenous 17β-estradiol given either 7 days or 30 min before occlusion result in significantly reduced edema and infarct (O'Donnell, Lam, Tran, Foroutan, & Anderson, 2006). Further, acute 17β-estradiol treatments (5 min or 3 h) reduce CMEC basal NKCC activity and abolish stimulation of the cotransporter by oligomycin, a form of chemical hypoxia, as well as stimulation by AVP (O'Donnell et al., 2006). Estradiol treatments of 1 h to 7 days also significantly reduce abundance of NKCC protein in CMEC in a manner inhibited by the estrogen receptor antagonist ICI 181-780 (O'Donnell et al., 2006). Similarly, estradiol treatment (1 day) reduces basal NHE activity and abolishes AVP-stimulated NHE activity in bovine CMEC (Lam et al., 2009). Thus, it appears that inhibition of ischemia-stimulated BBB NKCC and NHE activities accounts for at least some of estradiol neuroprotective effects in ischemic stroke, further supporting the value of targeting these BBB Na transporters for therapies to reduce edema and infarct in stroke.

5.2. Hyperglycemia effects on CMEC Na transporters

Metabolic changes can also alter BBB Na transporter activities. Decreased intracellular pH is a well-known activator of Na/H exchange (Mahnensmith & Aronson, 1985; Noël & Pouysségur, 1995; Pedersen et al., 2006; Wakabayashi et al., 1992) and thus increases in lactate resulting from anaerobic glycolysis during ischemia can stimulate NHE activity (Behmanesh & Kempski, 2000; Pedersen et al., 2006). Metabolic derangements in diabetes can also alter NKCC and NHE activities. For example, the ketoacids acetoacetate and β-hydroxybutyrate stimulate CMEC NKCC activity (Lam, Anderson, Glaser, & O'Donnell, 2005), an event that may underlie the increased brain edema formation observed in diabetic ketoacidosis (Glaser et al., 2000, 2012; Glaser, Yuen, Anderson, Tancredi, & O'Donnell, 2010). Further, patients with hyperglycemia during cerebral ischemia exhibit significantly increased edema and infarct and worsened neurological outcome (Baird et al., 2002; Berger & Hakim, 1986; Capes, Hunt, Malmberg, Pathak, & Gerstein, 2001; Ergul, Li, Elgebaly, Bruno, & Fagan, 2009; Ribo et al., 2007; Tureyen, Bowen, Linag, Dempsey, & Venuganti, 2010). This is true whether hyperglycemic patients have type I or type II diabetes or other causes of hyperglycemia. The reasons for hyperglycemia exacerbation of stroke damage are not well understood. However, previous studies have shown that hyperglycemia can alter expression and/or activity of NKCC and NHE in a variety of tissues. High glucose increases NHE activity of vascular smooth muscle (Williams & Howard, 1994) and both NHE expression and activity in glomerular mesangial cells (Ganz, Hawkins, & Reilly, 2000). Increased NKCC activity is found in aorta and choroid plexus of rats with streptozotocin (STZ)-induced diabetes (Egleton, Campos, Huber, Brown, & Davis, 2003; Michea, Irribarra, Goecke, & Marusic, 2001). Ongoing studies by our group have provided evidence that 6 h to 7 day exposures of CMEC to high glucose (30 mM compared to 5 mM glucose, comparable to ~550 mg/dl plasma glucose) increases activity of both NKCC and NHE in bovine CMEC and also increases abundance of NKCC and NHE1 but not NHE2 protein in the cells. When high glucose-treated CMEC are subsequently exposed to hypoxia, aglycemia, or AVP the resulting NKCC and NHE activities are significantly greater than in cells treated with high glucose or ischemic factors alone (Chechneva et al., 2014; Yuen et al., 2011). Ongoing *in vivo* MCAO studies suggest that rats with STZ-induced hyperglycemia have exacerbated edema, brain Na uptake, and infarct compared to normoglycemic rats. In addition, administration of intravenous bumetanide or HOE642 to the hyperglycemic rats effectively attenuates MCAO-induced edema, brain Na uptake, and infarct (Chechneva et al., 2014; Yuen et al., 2011). This suggests that targeting luminal BBB Na transporters is a therapeutic avenue worth pursing for hyperglycemic stroke as well as normoglycemic stroke.

6. FUTURE DIRECTIONS

Given that inhibiting ischemia-induced stimulation of BBB Na–K–Cl cotransport and Na/H exchange activities effectively reduces edema and infarct in stroke, an important task will be to determine whether there are additional BBB luminal membrane Na transporters that might be targeted to reduce edema in stroke. One promising candidate is Na–HCO_3 cotransport. A family of Na–HCO_3 cotransporters (NBCs), including electroneutral NBCn and electrogenic NBCe has been described in brain (Boedtkjer, Bunch, & Pedersen, 2012; Romero, Fulton, & Boron, 2004) and a variety of epithelial tissues (Boedtkjer et al., 2012; Choi, Hu, Rojas, Schmitt, & Boron, 2002; Damkler, Nielsen, & Praetorius, 2007; Pushkin & Kurtz, 2006; Romero et al., 2004). Both NBCs transport Na into the cell coupled to HCO_3 and these transporters are known to function in vectorial ion transport across epithelia (Boedtkjer et al., 2012; Romero et al., 2004). Of the two known NBCn proteins (NBCn1 and 2) and NBCe proteins (NBCe1 and 2), NBCn1 and NBCe1 are both found in brain (Boedtkjer et al., 2012; Boedtkjer, Praetorius, Füchtbauer, & Aalkjaer, 2008; Damkler, Brown, & Praetorius, 2010; Damkler, Nielsen, & Praetorius, 2006; Damkler et al., 2007; Praetorius & Nielsen, 2006) and respond to hypoxia/ischemia (Chen, Choi, Haddad, & Boron, 2007; Jung, Choi, & Kwon, 2007; Park et al., 2010). Studies have also shown that prominent NBC activity is observed in brain microvascular endothelial cells (Nicola et al., 2008; Taylor et al., 2006). In ongoing studies, our group has found evidence for the presence of both NBCn1 and NBCe1 proteins in bovine and rat CMEC (Chechneva et al., 2014). Prominent NBC activity is also observed in bovine, rat, and human CMEC and further, exposure of the cells to hypoxia, aglycemia, or AVP causes a robust increase in NBC activity. These findings suggest the promising possibility that BBB Na–CO_3 cotransport represents a third BBB Na transporter that can be targeted to improve outcome in ischemic stroke.

7. CONCLUSION

Accumulating evidence indicates that a luminal facing BBB Na–K–Cl cotransporter, Na/H exchanger, and possibly also Na–HCO_3 cotransporter, provide effective therapeutic targets for reducing edema and infarct in ischemic stroke. The simple fact that these Na transporters are at the luminal BBB membrane and thus readily targeted by intravenously administered agents makes them ideal therapeutic candidates. Given that a majority of drugs shown to reduce neuronal damage in *in vitro* studies have been later found to inadequately cross the BBB and reach their parenchymal cell targets, the opportunity to explore therapies that reduce damage by acting on the luminal BBB Na transporters is one that should not be missed.

CONFLICTS OF INTEREST

The author declares no conflict of interest

ACKNOWLEDGMENTS

The author's work presented in this chapter was supported by National Institutes of Health NINDS, the American Heart Association and the American Diabetes Association. The investigations were conducted in part in a facility constructed with support from Research Facilities Improvement Program Grant Number C06 RR17348-01 from the National Center for Research Resources, National Institutes of Health.

REFERENCES

Abbott, N. J., & Revest, P. A. (1991). Control of brain endothelial permeability. *Cerebrovascular and Brain Metabolism Reviews*, *3*, 39–72.

Baird, T. A., Parsons, M. W., Barber, A., Butcher, K. S., Desmond, P. M., Tress, B. M., et al. (2002). The influence of diabetes mellitus and hyperglycaemia on stroke incidence and outcome. *Journal of Clinical Neuroscience*, *9*, 618–626.

Barone, F. C., Irving, E. A., Ray, A. M., Lee, J. C., Kassis, S., Kumar, S., et al. (2001a). SB239063, a second-generation p38 mitogen-activated protein kinase inhibitor, reduces brain injury and neurological deficits in cerebral focal ischemia. *The Journal of Pharmacology and Experimental Therapeutics*, *296*, 312–321.

Barone, F. C., Irving, E. A., Ray, A. M., Lee, J. C., Kassis, S., Kumar, S., et al. (2001b). Inhibition of p38 mitogen-activated protein kinase provides neuroprotection in cerebral focal ischemia. *Medicinal Research Reviews*, *21*, 129–145.

Barone, F. C., Ohlstein, E. H., Hunter, A. J., Campbell, C. A., Hadingham, S. H., Parsons, A. A., et al. (2000). Selective antagonism of endothelin-A-receptors improves outcome in both head trauma and focal stroke in rat. *Journal of Cardiovascular Pharmacology*, *36*, S357–S361.

Behmanesh, S., & Kempski, O. (2000). Mechanisms of endothelial cell swelling from lactacidosis studied in vitro. *American Journal of Physiology. Heart and Circulatory Physiology*. *279*, H512–H517.

Bennett, B. L., Sasaki, D. T., Murray, B. W., O'Leary, E. C., Sakata, S. T., Xu, W., et al. (2001). SP600125, an anthrapyrazolone inhibitor of Jun N-terminal kinase. *Proceedings of the National Academy of Science*, *98*(24), 13681–13686. http://dx.doi.org/10.1073/pnas.251194298, 98/24/13681 [pii].

Berger, L., & Hakim, A. M. (1986). The association of hyperglycemia with cerebral edema in stroke. *Stroke*, *17*, 865–871.

Betz, A. L. (1983a). Sodium transport from blood to brain: Inhibition by furosemide and amiloride. *Journal of Neurochemistry*, *41*, 1158–1164.

Betz, A. L. (1983b). Sodium transport in capillaries isolated from rat brain. *Journal of Neurochemistry*, *41*, 1150–1157.

Betz, A. L. (1986). Transport of ions across the blood-brain barrier. *Federation Proceedings*, *45*, 2050–2054.

Betz, A. L. (1996). Alterations in cerebral endothelial cell function in ischemia. *Advances in Neurology*, *71*, 301–313 (Cellular and Molecular Mechanisms of Ischemic Brain Damage).

Betz, A. L., Firth, J. A., & Goldstein, G. W. (1980). Polarity of the blood-brain barrier: Distribution of enzymes between the luminal and antiluminal membranes of the brain capillary endothelial cells. *Brain Research*, *192*, 17–28.

Betz, A. L., & Goldstein, G. W. (1986). Specialized properties and solute transport in brain capillaries. *Annual Review of Physiology*, *48*, 241–250.

Betz, A. L., Keep, R. F., Beer, M. E., & Ren, X. (1994). Blood-brain barrier permeability and brain concentration of sodium, potassium, and chloride during focal ischemia. *Journal of Cerebral Blood Flow and Metabolism*, *14*, 29–37.

Boedtkjer, E., Bunch, L., & Pedersen, S. F. (2012). Physiology, pharmacology and pathophysiology of the pH regulatory transport proteins NHE1 and NBCn1: Similarities, differences, and implications for cancer therapy. *Current Pharmaceutical Design*, *18*, 1345–1371.

Boedtkjer, E., Praetorius, J., Füchtbauer, E.-M., & Aalkjaer, C. (2008). Antibody-independent localization of the electroneutral Na^+-HCO_3-cotransporter NBCn1 (slc4a7) in mice. *American Journal of Physiology. Cell Physiology*, *294*, C591–C603.

Bogoyevitch, M. A., Gillespie-Brown, J., Ketterman, A. J., Fuller, S. J., Ben-Levy, R., Ashworth, A., et al. (1996). Stimulation of the stress-activated mitogen-activated protein kinase subfamilies in perfused heart. *Circulation Research*, *79*, 162–173.

Borsello, T., Clarke, P. G. H., Hirt, L., Vercelli, A., Repici, M., Schorderet, D. F., et al. (2003). A peptide inhibitor of c-Jun N-terminal kinase protects against excitotoxicity and cerebral ischemia. *Nature Medicine*, *9*, 1180–1186.

Bourke, R. S., Kimelberg, H. K., Nelson, L. R., Barron, K. D., Auen, E. L., Popp, A. J., et al. (1980). Biology of glial swelling in experimental brain edema. *Advances in Neurology: Brain Edema*, *28*, 99–109.

Bradbury, M. W. B. (1984). The structure and function of the blood-brain barrier. *Federation Proceedings*, *43*, 186–190.

Brillault, J., Lam, T. I., Rutkowsky, J. M., Foroutan, S., & O'Donnell, M. E. (2008). Hypoxia effects on cell volume and ion uptake of cerebral microvascular endothelial cells. *American Journal of Physiology. Cell Physiology*, *294*(1), C88–C96. http://dx.doi.org/10.1152/ajpcell.00148.2007 [Research Support, N.I.H., Extramural Research Support, Non-U.S. Gov't].

Bronner, L. L., Kanter, D. S., & Manson, J. E. (1995). Primary prevention of stroke. *New England Journal of Medicine*, *333*, 1392–1400.

Capano, M., & Crompton, M. (2006). Bax translocates to mitochondria of heart cells during simulated ischaemia: Involvement of AMP-activated and p38 mitogen-activated protein kinases. *Biochemical Journal*, *395*, 57–64.

Capes, S. E., Hunt, D., Malmberg, P., Pathak, P., & Gerstein, H. C. (2001). Stress hyperglycemia and prognosis of stroke in nondiabetic and diabetic patients: A systematic overview. *Stroke*, *32*, 26–32.

Carling, D. (2004). The AMP-activated protein kinase cascade—A unifying system for energy control. *Trends in Biochemical Sciences*, *29*, 18–24.

Carling, D., Sanders, M. J., & Woods, A. (2008). The regulation of AMP-activated protein kinase by upstream kinases. *International Journal of Obesity*, *32*(Suppl. 4), S55–S59. http://dx.doi.org/10.1038/ijo.2008.124, ijo2008124 [pii].

Chang, E., O'Donnell, M. E., & Barakat, A. I. (2008). Shear stress and 17b-estradiol modulate cerebral microvascular endothelial Na-K-Cl cotransporter and Na/H exchanger protein levels. *American Journal of Physiology Cell Physiology*, *294*(1), C363–C371. http://dx.doi.org/10.1152/ajpcell.00045.2007, 00045.2007 [pii].

Chechneva, O. V., Yuen, N. Y., Tsai, Y.-C., Chen, Y.-J., Anderson, S. E., & O'Donnell, M. E. (2014). Evidence for blood-brain barrier Na-K-Cl cotransport, Na/H exchange and Na-HCO3 cotransport involvement in hyperglycemia exacerbation of cerebral edema formation in ischemic stroke. *The FASEB Journal*, *27*, A222.

Chen, L.-M., Choi, I., Haddad, G. G., & Boron, W. F. (2007). Chronic continuous hypoxia decreases the expression of SLCA7 (NBCn1) and SLC410 (NCBE) in mouse brain. *American Journal of Physiology. Regulatory, Integrative and Comparative Physiology*, *293*, R2412–R2420.

Chipperfield, A. R. (1996). The (Na^+-K^+-Cl^-) co-transport system. *Clinical Science*, *71*, 465–476.

Choi, I., Hu, L., Rojas, J. D., Schmitt, B. M., & Boron, W. F. (2002). Role of glycosylation in the renal electrogenic Na^+-HCO_3^- cotransporter (NBCe1). *American Journal of Physiology Renal Physiology*, *284*, F1199–F1206.

Cowan, K. J., & Storey, K. B. (2003). Mitogen-activated protein kinases: New signaling pathways functioning in cellular responses to environmental stress. *The Journal of Experimental Biology*, *206*, 1107–1115.

Cserr, H. F., DePasquale, M., Patlak, C. S., & Pullen, R. G. L. (1989). Convection of cerebral interstitial fluid and its role in brain volume regulation. *Annals of the New York Academy of Sciences*, *481*, 123–134.

Damkler, H. H., Brown, P. D., & Praetorius, J. (2010). Epithelial pathways in choroid plexus electrolyte transport. *Physiology*, *25*, 239–249.

Damkler, H. H., Nielsen, S., & Praetorius, J. (2006). An anti-NH_2-terminal antibody localizes NBCn1 to heart endothelia and skeletal and vascular smooth muscle cells. *American Journal of Physiology. Renal Physiology*, *290*, H172–H180.

Damkler, H. H., Nielsen, S., & Praetorius, J. (2007). Molecular expression of SLC4-derived Na^+-dependent anion transporters in selected human tissues. *American Journal of Physiology. Regulatory, Integrative and Comparative Physiology*, *293*, R2136–R2146.

Davis, B. J., Xie, Z., Viollet, B., & Zou, M.-H. (2006). Activation of the AMP-activated kinase by antidiabetes drug metformin stimulates nitric oxide synthesis in vivo by promoting the association of heat shock protein 90 and endothelial nitric oxide synthase. *Diabetes*, *55*, 496–505.

DeRyck, M., Van Reempts, J., Borgers, M., Wauquier, A., & Janssen, P. A. J. (1989). Photochemical stroke model: Flunarizine prevents sensorimotor deficits after neocortical infarcts in rats. *Stroke*, *20*, 1383–1390.

Dóczi, T. (1993). Volume regulation of the brain tissue—A survey. *Acta Neurochirurgica*, *121*, 1–8.

Dömötör, E., Abbott, N. J., & Adam-Vizi, V. (1999). Na+/Ca2+ exchange and its implications for calcium homeostasis in primary cultured rat brain microvascular endothelial cells. *Journal of Physiology*, *515*(1), 147–155.

Dubal, D. B., Kashon, M. L., Pettigrew, L. C., Ren, J. M., Finkelstein, S. P., Rau, S. W., et al. (1998). Estradiol protects against ischemic injury. *Journal of Cerebral Blood Flow and Metabolism*, *18*, 1253–1258.

Egleton, R. D., Campos, C. C., Huber, J. D., Brown, R. C., & Davis, T. P. (2003). Differential effects of diabetes on rat choroid plexus ion transporters. *Diabetes, 52*, 1496–1501.

Engelhardt, B. (2011). b1-Integrin/matrix interactions support blood-brain barrier integrity. *Journal of Cerebral Blood Flow and Metabolism, 31*, 1969–1971.

Ergul, A., Li, W., Elgebaly, M. M., Bruno, A., & Fagan, S. C. (2009). Hyperglycemia, diabetes and stroke: Focus on the cerebrovasculature. *Vascular Pharmacology, 51*, 44–49.

Eveloff, J. L., & Warnock, D. G. (1987). Activation of ion transport systems during cell volume regulation. *American Journal of Physiology, 252*, F1–F10.

Fenstermacher, J. D., & Rapoport, S. I. (1984). Blood-brain barrier. In E. M. Rankin, & C. C. Michel (Eds.), *The microcirculation: Vol. IV. Hand-book of physiology. Section 2: The cardiovascular system* (pp. 969–1000). Bethesda: American Physiological Society, Chapter 21.

Ferrazzano, P., Shi, Y., Manhas, N., Wang, Y., Hutchinson, B., Chen, X., et al. (2011). Inhibiting the Na+/H+ exchanger reduces reperfusion injury: A small animal MRI study. *Frontiers in Bioscience, 3*, 81–88.

Fisslthaler, B., & Fleming, I. (2009). Activation and signaling by the AMP-activated protein kinase in endothelial cells. *Circulation Research, 105*, 114–127.

Flemmer, A. W., Giménez, I., Dowd, B. F. X., Darman, R. B., & Forbush, B. (2002). Activation of the Na-K-Cl cotransporter NKCC1 detected with a phospho-specific antibody. *The Journal of Biological Chemistry, 277*, 37551–37558.

Foroutan, S., Brillault, J., Forbush, B., & O'Donnell, M. E. (2005). Moderate to severe ischemic conditions increase activity and phosphorylation of the cerebral microvascular endothelial cell Na-K-Cl cotransporter. *American Journal of Physiology. Cell Physiology, 289*, C1492–C1501.

Fraser, S. A., Giminez, I., Cook, N., Jennings, I., Katerelos, M., Katsis, F., et al. (2007). Regulation of the renal-specific Na+-K+-2Cl- co-transporter NKCC2 by AMP-activated protein kinase (AMPK). *Biochemical Journal, 405*, 85–93.

Ganz, M. B., Hawkins, K., & Reilly, R. F. (2000). High glucose induces the activity and expression of Na+/H+ exchange in glomerular mesangial cells. *American Journal of Physiology Renal Physiology, 278*, F91–F96.

Gartshore, G., Patterson, J., & Macrae, I. M. (1997). Influence of ischemia and reperfusion on the course of brain tissue swelling and blood-brain barrier permeability in a rodent model of transient focal cerebral ischemia. *Experimental Neurology, 147*, 353–360.

Glaser, N., Barnett, P., McCaslin, I., Nelson, D., Trainor, J., Louie, J., et al. (2000). Risk factors for cerebral edema in children with diabetic ketoacidosis. *New England Journal of Medicine, 344*, 264–269.

Glaser, N., Ngo, C., Anderson, S. E., Yuen, N., Trifu, A., & O'Donnell, M. E. (2012). Effects of hyperglycemia and ketosis on cerebral perfusion, cerebral water distribution and cerebral metabolism. *Diabetes, 61*, 1831–1837.

Glaser, N., Yuen, N., Anderson, S. E., Tancredi, D. J., & O'Donnell, M. E. (2010). Cerebral metabolic alterations in rats with diabetic ketoacidosis. Effects of treatment with insulin and intravenous fluids and effects of bumetanide. *Diabetes, 59*, 702–709.

Gotoh, O., Asano, T., Koide, T., & Takakura, K. (1985). Ischemic brain edema following occlusion of the middle cerebral artery in the rat. I: The time course of the brain water, sodium and potassium contents and blood-brain barrier permeability to 125I-albumin. *Stroke, 16*, 101–109.

Guo, Y., Signore, A. P., Yin, W., Cao, G., Yin, X. M., Sun, F., et al. (2005). Neuroprotection against focal ischemic brain injury by inhibition of c-Jun N-terminal kinase and attenuation of the mitochondrial apoptosis-signaling pathway. *Journal of Cerebral Blood Flow and Metabolism, 25*, 694–712.

Haas, M., & Forbush, B., III (1998). The Na-K-Cl cotransporter. *Journal of Bioenergetics and Biomembranes*, *30*(2), 161–172.
Hallows, K. R., Kobinger, G. P., Wilson, J. M., Witters, L. A., & Foskett, J. K. (2003). Physiological modulation of CFTR activity by AMP-activated protein kinase in polarized T84 cells. *American Journal of Physiology. Cell Physiology*, *284*, C1297–C1308.
Hamm, R. J., Rice, B. R., O'Dell, D. M., Lyeth, B. G., & Jenkins, L. W. (1994). The rotarod test: An evaluation of its effectiveness in assessing motor deficits following traumatic brain injury. *Journal of Neurotrauma*, *11*, 187–196.
Hardie, D. G. (2003). Minireview: The AMP-activated protein kinase cascade: The key sensor of cellular energy status. *Endocrinology*, *144*, 5179–5183.
Hardie, D. G. (2004). The AMP-activated protein kinase pathway—New players upstream and downstream. *Journal of Cell Science*, *117*, 5479–5487.
Hawkins, B. T., & Davis, T. P. (2005). The blood-brain barrier/neurovascular unit in health and disease. *Pharmacological Reviews*, *57*, 173–185.
Hawley, S. A., Davison, M., Woods, A., Davies, S. P., Beri, R. K., Carling, D., et al. (1996). Characterization of the AMP-activated protein kinase kinase from rat liver and identification of threonine 172 as the major site at which it phosphorylates AMP-activated protein kinase. *The Journal of Biological Chemistry*, *271*, 27879–27887.
Hicks, K., O'Neil, R. G., Dubinsky, W. S., & Brown, R. C. (2010). TRPC-mediated actin-myosin contraction is critical for BBB disruption following hypoxic stress. *American Journal of Physiology. Cell Physiology*, *298*, C1583–C1593.
Hom, S., Fleegal, M. A., Egleton, R. D., Campos, C. R., Hawkins, B. T., & Davis, T. P. (2007). Comparative changes in the blood-brain barrier and cerebral infarction of SHR and WKY rats. *American Journal of Physiology. Regulatory, Integrative and Comparative Physiology*, *292*, R1881–R1892.
Hoyer, J., Popp, R., Meyer, J., Galla, H.-J., & Gögelein, J. (1991). Angiotensin II, vasopressin and GTP[g-S] inhibit inward-rectifying K^+ channels in porcine cerebral capillary endothelial cells. *Journal of Membrane Biology*, *123*, 55–62.
Hsu, P., Haffner, J., Albuquerque, M. L., & Leffler, C. W. (1996). pHi in piglet cerebral microvascular endothelial cells: Recovery from an acid load. *Proceedings of the Society for Experimental Biology and Medicine*, *212*, 256–262.
Huber, J. D., Egleton, R. D., & Davis, T. P. (2001). Molecular physiology and pathophysiology of tight junctions in the blood-brain barrier. *Trends in Neurosciences*, *24*, 719–725.
Hurley, R. L., Anderson, D. A., Franzone, J. M., & Kemp, B. E. (2005). The Ca2+/calmodulin-dependent protein kinase kinases are AMP-activated protein kinase kinases. *The Journal of Biological Chemistry*, *280*, 29060–29066.
Hurn, P. D., & Macrae, I. M. (2000). Estrogen as a neuroprotectant in stroke. *Journal of Cerebral Blood Flow and Metabolism*, *20*, 631–652.
Iadecola, C. (1999). Mechanisms of cerebral ischemic damage. In W. Walz (Ed.), *Cerebral ischemia: Molecular and cellular pathophysiology* (pp. 3–34). Totowa, NJ: Humana Press.
Ikeda, K., Nagashim, T., Wu, S., Yamaguchi, M., & Tamaki, N. (1997). The role of calcium ion in anoxia/reoxygenation damage of cultured brain capillary endothelial cells. *Acta Neurochirurgica. Supplement*, *70*, 4–7.
Irving, E. A., & Bamford, M. (2002). Role of mitogen- and stress-activated kinases in ischemic injury. *Journal of Cerebral Blood Flow and Metabolism*, *22*, 631–647.
Janigro, D., West, G. A., Gordon, E. L., & Winn, H. R. (1993). ATP-sensitive K channels in rat aorta and brain microvascular endothelial cells. *American Journal of Physiology. Cell Physiology*, *265*, C812–C821.
Jójárt, I., Joó, F., Siklós, L., & László, F. A. (1984). Immunoelectronhistochemical evidence for innervation of brain microvessels by vasopressin-immunoreactive neurons in the rat. *Neuroscience Letters*, *51*, 259–264.

Jung, Y.-W., Choi, I.-J., & Kwon, R.-H. (2007). Altered expression of sodium transporters in ischemic penumbra after focal cerebral ischemia in rats. *Neuroscience Research, 59*, 152–159.

Kato, H., Kogure, K., Sakamoto, N., & Watanabe, T. (1987). Greater disturbance of water and ion homeostasis in the periphery of experimental focal cerebral ischemia. *Experimental Neurology, 96*, 118–126.

Kawai, N., McCarron, R. M., & Spatz, M. (1995). Endothelins stimulate sodium uptake into rat brain capillary endothelial cells through endothelin A-like receptors. *Neuroscience Letters, 190*, 85–88.

Kawai, N., McCarron, R. M., & Spatz, M. (1996). Effect of hypoxia on Na^+-K^+-Cl^- cotransport in cultured brain capillary endothelial cells of the rat. *Journal of Neurochemistry, 66*, 2572–2579.

Kawai, N., McCarron, R. M., & Spatz, M. (1997). The effect of endothelins on ion transport systems in cultured rat brain capillary endothelial cells. *Acta Neurochirurgica, 70*, 138–140.

Kawai, N., Yamamoto, T., Yamamoto, H., McCarron, R. M., & Spatz, M. (1995). Endothelin 1 stimulates Na+, K+-ATPase and Na+-K+-Cl- cotransport through ETA receptors and protein kinase C-dependent pathway in cerebral capillary endothelium. *Journal of Neurochemistry, 65*, 1588–1596.

Keep, R. F. (Ed.). (1993). *Potassium transport at the blood-brain and blood-CSF barriers*. New York: Plenum Press.

Kemp, B. E., Stapleton, D., Campbell, D. J., Chen, Z. P., Murthy, S., Walter, M., et al. (2003). AMP-activated protein kinase, super metabolic regulator. *Biochemical Society Transactions, 31*, 162–168.

Kempski, O., Spatz, M., Valet, G., & Baethmann, A. (1985). Cell volume regulation of cerebrovascular endothelium in vitro. *Journal of Cellular Physiology, 123*, 51–54.

Kempski, O., von Rosen, S., Weight, H., Staub, F., Peters, J., & Baethmann, A. (1991). Glial ion transport and volume control. In N. J. Abbott (Ed.), *Glial-neuronal interaction* (pp. 306–317). New York, NY: The New York Academy of Sciences.

Kimelberg, H. K. (1995). Current concepts of brain edema. Review of laboratory investigations. *Journal of Neurosurgery, 83*, 1051–1059.

Kimelberg, H. K. (1999). Cell Swelling in Cerebral Ischemia. In W. Walz (Ed.), *Cerebral Ischemia: Molecular and cellular pathophysiology* (pp. 45–68). Totowa, NJ: Humana Press.

Kimura, C., Oike, M., & Ito, Y. (2000). Hypoxia-induced alterations in Ca^{2+} mobilization in brain microvascular endothelial cells. *American Journal of Physiology Heart and Circulatory Physiology, 279*, H2310–H2318.

Kintner, D. B., Look, A., Shull, G. E., & Sun, D. (2005). Stimulation of astrocyte Na^+/H^+ exchange activity in response to in vitro ischemia depends in part on activation of ERK1/2. *American Journal of Physiology. Cell Physiology, 289*(4), C934–C945. http://dx.doi.org/10.1152/ajpcell.00092.2005 [Research Support, N.I.H., Extramural Research Support, Non-U.S. Gov't Research Support, U.S. Gov't, P.H.S.].

Klatzo, I. (1994). Evolution of brain edema concepts. *Acta Neurochirurgica. Supplement. 60*, 3–6.

Klein, H., Garneau, L., Trinh, N. T., Prive, A., Dionne, F., Goupil, E., et al. (2009). Inhibition of the KCa3.1 channels by AMP-activated protein kinase in human airway epithelial cells. *American Journal of Physiology. Cell Physiology, 296*, C285–C295.

Kyriakis, J. M., & Avruch, J. (2001). Mammalian mitogen-activated protein kinase signal transduction pathways activated by stress and inflammation. *Physiological Reviews, 81*, 807–869.

Lam, T. I., Anderson, S. E., Glaser, N., & O'Donnell, M. E. (2005). Bumetanide reduces cerebral edema formation in rats with diabetic ketoacidosis. *Diabetes, 54*, 510–516.

Lam, T. I., Wise, P. M., & O'Donnell, M. E. (2009). Cerebral microvascular endothelial cell Na/H exchange: Evidence for the presence of NHE1 and NHE2 isoforms and regulation by arginine vasopressin. *American Journal of Physiology. Cell Physiology*, *297*, C278–C289.

Landgraf, R. (1992). Central release of vasopressin: Stimuli, dynamics, consequences. *Progress in Brain Research*, *91*, 29–39.

Lee, S.-R., & Lo, E. H. (2003). Interactions between p38 mitogen-activated protein kinase and caspase-3 in cerebral endothelial cell death after hypoxia-reoxygenation. *Stroke*, *34*, 2704–2709.

Li, J., & McCullough, L. D. (2010). Effects of AMP-activated protein kinase in cerebral ischemia. *Journal of Cerebral Blood Flow and Metabolism*, *30*, 480–492.

Li, J., Miller, E. J., Ninomiya-Tsuji, J., Russell, R. R., III, & Young, L. H. (2005). AMP-activated protein kinase activates p38 mitogen-activated protein kinase by increasing its recruitment to TAB1 in the ischemic heart. *Circulation Research*, *97*, 872–879.

Li, J., Zeng, Z., Viollet, B., Ronnett, G. V., & McCullough, L. D. (2007). Neuroprotective effects of adenosine monophosphate-activated protein kinase inhibition and gene deletion in stroke. *Stroke*, *38*, 2992–2999.

Lin, J. D. (1985). Potassium transport is isolated cerebral microvessels from the rat. *Japanese Journal of Physiology*, *35*, 817–830.

Lin, J. D. (1988). Effect of osmolarity on potassium transport in isolated cerebral microvessels. *Life Sciences*, *43*, 325–333.

Luo, J., Chen, H., Kintner, D. B., Shull, G. E., & Sun, D. (2005). Decreased neuronal death in Na^+/H^+ exchanger isoform 1-null mice after in vitro and in vivo ischemia. *The Journal of Neuroscience*, *25*, 11256–11268.

Mahnensmith, R. L., & Aronson, P. S. (1985). The plasma membrane sodium-hydrogen exchanger and its role in physiological and pathophysiological processes. *Circulation Research*, *56*, 773–788.

Masereel, B., Pochet, L., & Laeckmann, D. (2003). An overview of inhibitors of Na^+/H^+ exchanger. *European Journal of Medicinal Chemistry*, *38*, 547–554.

McCullough, L. D., Zeng, Z., Li, H., Landree, L. E., McFadden, J., & Ronnett, G. V. (2005). Pharmacological inhibition of AMP-activated protein kinase provides neuroprotection in stroke. *The Journal of Biological Chemistry*, *280*, 20492–20502.

Menzies, S. A., Betz, A. L., & Hoff, J. T. (1993). Contributions of ions and albumin to the formation and resolution of ischemic brain edema. *Journal of Neurosurgery*, *78*, 257–266.

Menzies, S. A., Hoff, J. T., & Betz, A. L. (1990). Extravasation of albumin in ischaemic brain oedema. *Acta Neurochirurgica*, *51*(Suppl. 51), 220–222.

Michea, L., Irribarra, V., Goecke, I. A., & Marusic, E. T. (2001). Reduced Na-K pump but increased Na-K-2Cl cotransporter in aorta of streptozotocin-induced diabetic rat. *American Journal of Physiology. Heart and Circulatory Physiology*, *280*, H851–H858.

Moore, A. N., Gan, X. T., Karmazyn, M., & Fliegel, L. (2001). Activation of Na+/H+ exchanger-directed protein kinases in the ischemic and ischemic-reperfused rat myocardium. *Journal of Biological Chemistry*, *276*, 16113–16122.

Murphy, E., Cross, H. R., & Steenbergen, C. (2002). Is Na/Ca exchange during ishcemia and reperfusion beneficial or detrimental. *Annals of the New York Academy of Sciences*, *976*, 421–430.

Neuwelt, E. A., Bauer, B., Fahlke, C., Fricker, G., Iadecola, C., Janigro, D., et al. (2011). Engaging neuroscience to advance translational research in brain barrier biology. *Nature Reviews Neuroscience*, *12*, 169–182.

Nicola, P. A., Taylor, C. J., Wang, S., Barrand, M. A., & Hladky, S. B. (2008). Transport activities involved in intracellular pH recovery following acid and alkali challenges in rat brain microvascular endothelial cells. *Pflugers Archives—European Journal of Physiology*, *456*, 801–812.

Noël, J., & Pouysségur, J. (1995). Hormonal regulation, pharmacology, and membrane sorting of vertebrate Na^+/H^+ exchanger isoforms. *American Journal of Physiology. Cell Physiology*, *268*, C283–C296.

O'Donnell, M. E. (2009). Ion and water transport across the blood-brain barrier. In F. J. Alvarez-Leefmans, & E. Delpire (Eds.), *From molecules to diseases. Physiology and pathophysiology of chloride transporters and channels in the nervous system* (pp. 585–606). London: Elsevier.

O'Donnell, M. E., Yuen, N. Y., Chen, Y.-J., & Anderson, S. E. (2013). Blood-brain barrier Na-HCO3 cotransport: Evidence for a role in diabetic ischemic stroke. In *OHSU Blood-Brain Barrier Consortium Meeting*.

O'Donnell, M. E. (1993). Role of Na-K-Cl cotransport in vascular endothelial cell volume regulation. *American Journal of Physiology*, *264*, C1316–C1326.

O'Donnell, M. E., Brandt, J. D., & Curry, F.-R. E. (1995). Na-K-Cl cotransport regulates intracellular volume and monolayer permeability of trabecular meshwork cells. *American Journal of Physiology*, *268*, C1067–C1074.

O'Donnell, M. E., Chen, Y. J., Lam, T. I., Taylor, K. C., Walton, J. H., & Anderson, S. E. (2013). Intravenous HOE-642 reduces brain edema and Na uptake in the rat permanent middle cerebral artery occlusion model of stroke: Evidence for participation of the blood-brain barrier Na/H exchanger. *Journal of Cerebral Blood Flow and Metabolism*, *33*, 225–234.

O'Donnell, M. E., Duong, V., Suvatne, S., Foroutan, S., & Johnson, D. M. (2005). Arginine vasopressin stimulation of cerebral microvascular endothelial cell Na-K-Cl cotransport activity is V1 receptor- and [Ca]-dependent. *American Journal of Physiology. Cell Physiology*, *289*, C283–C292.

O'Donnell, M. E., Lam, T. I., Tran, L. Q., Foroutan, S., & Anderson, S. E. (2006). Estradiol reduces activity of the blood-brain barrier Na-K-Cl cotransporter and decreases edema formation in permanent middle cerebral artery occlusion. *Journal of Cerebral Blood Flow and Metabolism*, *26*, 1234–1249.

O'Donnell, M. E., Martinez, A., & Sun, D. (1995a). Cerebral microvascular endothelial cell Na-K-Cl cotransport: Regulation by astrocyte-conditioned medium. *American Journal of Physiology*, *268*, C747–C754.

O'Donnell, M. E., Martinez, A., & Sun, D. (1995b). Endothelial Na-K-Cl cotransport regulation by tonicity and hormones: Phosphorylation of cotransport protein. *American Journal of Physiology*, *269*, C1513–C1523.

O'Donnell, M. E., Tran, L., Lam, T., Liu, X. B., & Anderson, S. E. (2004). Bumetanide inhibition of the blood-brain barrier Na-K-Cl cotransporter reduces edema formation in the rat middle cerebral artery occlusion model of stroke. *Journal of Cerebral Blood Flow and Metabolism*, *24*, 1046–1056.

Ohori, M., Kinoshita, T., Okubo, M., Sato, K., Yamazaki, A., Arakawa, H., et al. (2005). Identification of a selective ERK inhibitor and structural determination of the inhibitor ERK-2 complex. *Biochemical and Biophysical Research Communications*, *336*, 357–363.

Ostrowski, N. L., Lolait, S. J., Bradley, D. J., O'Carroll, A.-M., Browstein, M. J., & Young, W. S. (1992). Distribution of V1a and V2 vasopressin receptor messenger ribonucleic acids in rat liver, kidney, pituitary and brain. *Endocrinology*, *131*, 533–535.

Ostrowski, N. L., Lolait, S. J., & Young, W. S. (1994). Cellular localization of vasopressin V1a receptor messenger ribonucleic acid in adult male rat brain, pineal and brain vasculature. *Endocrinology*, *135*, 1511–1528.

Park, H. J., Rajbhandari, I., Yang, H. S., Lee, S., Cucoranu, D., Cooper, D. S., et al. (2010). Neuronal expression of sodium/bicarbonate cotransporter NBCn1 (SLC4A7) and its response to chronic metabolic acidosis. *American Journal of Physiology. Cell Physiology*, *298*, C1018–C1028.

Patnaik, S., Dietz, H. C., Zheng, W., Austin, C., & Marugan, J. J. (2009). Multi-gra scale synthesis of FR180204. *Journal of Organic Chemistry*, *74*, 8870–8873.

Payne, J. A., & Forbush, B., III (1995). Molecular characterization of the epithelial Na-K-Cl cotransporter isoforms. *Current Opinion in Cell Biology*, 7, 493–503.

Pedersen, S. F. (2006). The Na+/H+ exchanger NHE1 in stress-induced signal transduction: Implications for cell proliferation and cell death. *Plugers Archives—European Journal of Physiology*, *452*, 249–259.

Pedersen, S. F., King, S. A., Rigor, R. R., Zhuang, S., Warren, J. M., & Cala, P. M. (2003). Molecular cloning of NHE1 from winter flounder RBCs: Activation by osmotic shrinkage, cAMP, and calyculin A. *American Journal of Physiology. Cell Physiology*, *284*, C1561–C1576.

Pedersen, S. F., O'Donnell, M. E., Anderson, S. E., & Cala, P. M. (2006). Physiology and pathophysiology of Na^{+}/H^{+} exchange and Na^{+}-K^{+}-$2Cl^{-}$ cotransporter in the heart, brain and blood. *American Journal of Physiology. Regulatory, Integrative and Comparative Physiology*, *291*, R1–R25.

Petty, M. A., & Lo, E. H. (2002). Junctional complexes of the blood-brain barrier: Permeability changes in neuroinflammation. *Progress in Neurobiology*, *68*, 311–323.

Popp, R., Hoyer, J., Meyer, J., Galla, H.-J., & Gögelein, H. (1992). Stretch-activated nonselective cation channels in the antiluminal membrane of porcine cerebral capillaries. *Journal of Physiology*, *454*, 435–449.

Praetorius, J., & Nielsen, S. (2006). Distribution of sodium transporters and aquaporin-1 in the human choroid plexus. *American Journal of Physiology. Cell Physiology*, *291*, C59–C67.

Pushkin, A., & Kurtz, I. (2006). SLC4 base (HCO_3^-, CO_3^{2-}) transporters: Classification, function, structure, genetic diseases, and knockout models. *American Journal of Physiology. Cell Physiology*, *290*, F580–F599.

Ribo, M., Molina, C. A., Delgado, P., Rubiera, M., Delgado-Mederos, R., Rovira, A., et al. (2007). Hyperglycemia during ischemia rapidly accelerates brain damage in stroke patients treated with tPA. *Journal of Cerebral Blood Flow and Metabolism*, *27*, 1616–1622.

Romero, M. F., Fulton, C. M., & Boron, W. F. (2004). The SLC4 family of HCO_3^- transporters. *Pflugers Archives—European Journal of Physiology*, *447*, 495–509.

Rusa, R., Alkayad, N. J., Crain, B. J., Traystman, R. J., & Kimes, A. S. (1999). 17-β estradiol reduces stroke injury in estrogen-deficient animals. *Stroke*, *30*, 1665–1670.

Sawe, N., Steinberg, G., & Zhao, H. (2008). Dual roles of the MAPK/ERK1/2 cell signalling pathway after stroke. *Journal of Neuroscience Research*, *86*, 1659–1669.

Schielke, G. P., Moises, H. C., & Betz, A. L. (1991). Blood to brain sodium transport and interstitial fluid potassium concentration during focal ischemia in the rat. *Journal of Cerebral Blood Flow and Metabolism*, *11*, 466–471.

Shi, J., Zhang, Y. Q., & Simpkins, J. W. (1997). Effects of 17β-estradiol on glucose transporter 1 expression and endothelial cell survival following focal ischemia in rats. *Experimental Brain Research*, *117*, 200–206.

Simard, J. M., Chen, M., Tarasov, K. V., Bhatta, S., Ivanova, S., Melnitchenko, L., et al. (2006). Newly expressed SUR1-regulated $NC_{Ca\text{-}ATP}$ channel mediates cerebral edema after ischemic stroke. *Nature Medicine*, *12*, 433–440.

Sipos, H., Törocsik, B., Tretter, L., & Adam-Vizi, V. (2005). Impaired regulation of pH homeostasis by oxidative stress in rat brain capillary endothelial cells. *Cellular and Molecular Neurobiology*, *25*, 141–151.

Slevin, N., Krupinski, J., Slowik, A., Rubio, F., Szczudlik, A., & Gaffney, J. (2000). Activation of MAP kinase (ERK-1/ERK-2), tryosine kinase and VEGF in the human brain following acute ischemic stroke. *NeuroReport*, *11*, 2759–2764.

Sorensen, P. S., Gjerris, A., & Hammer, M. (1985). Cerebrospinal fluid vasopressin in neurological and psychiatric disorders. *Journal of Neurology, Neurosurgery, and Psychiatry*, *48*, 50–57.

Spatz, M., Merkel, K. N., Bembry, J., & McCarron, R. M. (1997). Functional properties of cultured endothelial cells derived from large microvessels of human brain. *American Journal of Physiology, 272*, C231–C239.

Sun, D., Lytle, C., & O'Donnell, M. E. (1995). Astroglial cell-induced expression of Na-K-Cl cotransporter in brain microvascular endothelial cells. *American Journal of Physiology, 269*, C1506–C1512.

Sun, D., Lytle, C., & O'Donnell, M. E. (1997). IL-6 secreted by astroglial cells regulates Na-K-Cl cotransport in brain microvessel endothelial cells. *American Journal of Physiology, 272*, C1829–C1835.

Taylor, C. J., Nicola, P. A., Wang, S., Barrand, M. A., & Hladky, S. B. (2006). Transporters involved in regulation of intracellular pH (pHi) in primary cultured rat brain endothelial cells. *Journal of Physiology, 576*, 769–785.

Tian, D., Litvak, V., & Lev, S. (2000). Cerebral ischemia and seizures induce tyrosine phosphorylation of PYK2 in neurons and microglial cells. *The Journal of Neuroscience, 20*, 6478–6487.

Töllner, K., Brandt, C., Töpfer, M., Brunhofer, G., Erker, T., Gabriel, M., et al. (2014). A novel prodrug-based strategy to increase effects of bumetanide in epilepsy. *Annals of Neurology, 75*, 550–562.

Tureyen, K., Bowen, K., Linag, J., Dempsey, R. J., & Venuganti, R. (2010). Exacerbated brain damage, edema and inflammation in type-2 diabetic mice subjected to focal ischemia. *Journal of Neurochemistry, 116*, 499–507.

Turnley, A. M., Stapleton, D., Mann, R. J., Witters, L. A., Kemp, B. E., & Bartlett, P. F. (1999). Cellular distribution and developmental expression of AMP-activated protein kinase isoforms in mouse central nervous system. *Journal of Neurochemistry, 72*, 1707–1716.

Vigne, P., Champigny, G., Marsault, R., Barbry, P., Frelin, C., & Lazdunski, M. (1989). A new type of amiloride-sensitive cationic channel in endothelial cells of brain microvessels. *The Journal of Biological Chemistry, 264*, 7663–7668.

Vigne, P., Farre, A. L., & Frelin, C. (1994). Na^+-K^+-Cl^- cotransporter of brain capillary endothelial cells. Properties and regulation by endothelins, hyperosmolar solutions, calyculin A, and interleukin-1. *The Journal of Biological Chemistry, 269*, 19925–19930.

Vigne, P., Ladoux, A., & Frelin, C. (1991). Endothelins activate Na^+/H^+ exchange in brain capillary endothelial cells via a high affinity endothelin-3 receptor that is not coupled to phospholipase C. *The Journal of Biological Chemistry, 266*, 5925–5928.

Wakabayashi, S., Sardet, C., Fafournoux, P., Counillon, L., Meloche, S., Pages, G., et al. (1992). Structure function of the growth factor-activatable Na^+/H^+ exchanger (NHE1). *Reviews of Physiology, Biochemistry and Pharmacology, 119*, 157–186.

Wallace, B. K., Foroutan, S., & O'Donnell, M. E. (2011). Ischemia-induced stimulation of Na-K-Cl cotransport in cerebral microvascular endothelial cells involves AMP kinase. *American Journal of Physiology. Cell Physiology, 301*, C316–C326.

Wallace, B. K., Jelks, K. A., & O'Donnell, M. E. (2012). Ischemia-induced stimulation of cerebral microvascular endothelial cell Na-K-Cl cotransport involves p38 and JNK MAP kinases. *American Journal of Physiology. Cell Physiology, 302*, C505–C517.

Williams, B., & Howard, R. L. (1994). Glucose-induced changes in Na+/H+ antiport activity and gene expression in cultured bascular smooth muscle cells. *Journal of Clinical Investigation, 93*, 2623–2631.

Woods, A., Vertommen, D., Neumann, D., Turk, R., Bayliss, J., Schlattner, U., et al. (2003). Identification of phosphorylation sites in AMP-activated protein kinase (AMPK) for upstream AMPK kinases and study of their roles by site-directed mutagenesis. *The Journal of Biological Chemistry, 278*, 28434–28442.

Wu, D.-C., Ye, W., Che, X.-M., & Yang, G.-Y. (2000). Activation of mitogen-activated protein kinases after permanent cerebral artery occlusion in mouse brain. *Journal of Cerebral Blood Flow and Metabolism, 20*, 1320–1330.

Yakubu, M. A., & Leffler, C. W. (2002). L-type voltage-dependent Ca2+ channels in cerebral microvascular endothelial cells and ET-1 biosynthesis. *American Journal of Physiology. Cell Physiology*, *283*, C1687–C1695.
Yang, S., Shi, J., Day, A. L., & Simpkins, J. W. (2000). Estradiol exerts neuroprotective effects when administered after ischemic insult. *Stroke*, *31*, 745–749.
Yatsushige, H., Ostrowski, R. P., Tsubokawa, T., Colohan, A., & Zhang, J. H. (2007). Role of c-Jun N-terminal kinase in early brain injury after subarachnoid hemorrhage. *Journal of Neuroscience Research*, *85*, 1436–1448.
Yerby, T. R., Vibat, C. R. T., Sun, D., Payne, J. A., & O'Donnell, M. E. (1997). Molecular characterization of the Na-K-Cl cotransporter of bovine aortic endothelial cells. *American Journal of Physiology*, *273*, C188–C197.
Yuen, N., Lam, T. I., Wallace, B. K., Klug, N. R., Anderson, S. E., & O'Donnell, M. E. (2014). Ischemic factor-induced increases in cerebral microvascular endothelial cell Na/H exchange activity and abundance: Evidence for involvement of ERK1/2 MAP kinase. *American Journal of Physiology. Cell Physiology*, *306*.
Yuen, N., Wallace, B. K., Trifu, A., Glaser, N. S., Anderson, S. E., & O'Donnell, M. E. (2011). Hyperglycemia stimulates blood-brain barrier endothelial cell Na-K-Cl cotransporter and Na/H exchanger activities and induces cerebral edema in the rat. *The FASEB Journal*, *24*, A650.652.
Zhang, Y.-Q., Shi, J., Rajakumar, G., Day, A. L., & Simpkins, J. W. (1998). Effects of gender and estradiol treatment on focal brain ischemia. *Brain Research*, *784*, 321–324.
Zhu, Y., Mao, X. O., Sun, Y., Xia, Z., & Greenberg, D. A. (2002). p38 mitogen-activated protein kinase mediates hypoxic regulation of Mdm2 and p53 in neurons. *The Journal of Biological Chemistry*, *277*, 22909–22914.
Zhu, Y., Sun, Y., Xie, L., Jin, K., Sheibani, N., & Greenberg, D. A. (2003). Hypoxic induction of endoglin via mitogen-activated protein kinases in mouse brain microvascular endothelial cells. *Stroke*, *34*, 2483–2488.
Zou, M.-H., Hou, X.-Y., Shi, C.-M., Kirkpatick, S., Liu, F., Goldman, M. H., et al. (2003). Activation of 5'-AMP-activated kinase is mediated through c-src and phosphoinositide 3-kinase activity during hypoxia-reoxygenation of bovine aortic endothelial cells. *The Journal of Biological Chemistry*, *36*, 34003–34010.

CHAPTER FIVE

Transcytosis of Macromolecules at the Blood–Brain Barrier

Jane E. Preston, N. Joan Abbott, David J. Begley[1]
King's College London, Institute of Pharmaceutical Science, London, United Kingdom
[1]Corresponding author: e-mail address: david.begley@kcl.ac.uk

Contents

Abstract

The restrictive nature of the blood–brain barrier means that cellular machinery must be in place to deliver macromolecules to the brain. This is achieved by transcytosis which is more complex than initially supposed, both in terms of structure and regulation. Brain endothelial cells have relatively few pinocytotic vesicles compared to peripheral endothelia but can still deliver macromolecules via one of the three main types of vesicles: the most numerous clathrin-coated vesicles containing adaptor protein complex-2, the smaller caveolae formed from lipid raft domains of the plasma membrane, and the large fluid engulfing macropinocytotic vesicles. Both clathrin-coated vesicles and, to a lesser extent caveolae, endocytose plasma membrane receptors and their specific ligands which include insulin, transferrin, and lipoproteins. This receptor-mediated transcytosis (RMT) delivers the ligands to the brain and enables their receptors to be recycled back to the plasma membrane. However, once endocytosed, the ligands and/or receptors must be directed toward the correct plasma membrane and avoid degradation. How this is achieved has not been well studied although there is an important role for Rab GTPases in targeting vesicles to their correct location and enabling exocytosis. In this chapter, we discuss what is known about regulation of transcytosis in related cells such as the MDCK cell line and where are the gaps in our knowledge of brain endothelial transcytotic regulation. We discuss how RMT has been exploited to deliver therapeutic drugs to the brain and the importance of further investigation in this area to improve drug delivery.

Advances in Pharmacology, Volume 71
ISSN 1054-3589
http://dx.doi.org/10.1016/bs.apha.2014.06.001

ABBREVIATIONS

AP-1 clathrin adaptor protein complex-1
AP-2 clathrin adaptor protein complex-2
BBB blood–brain barrier
ICAM-1 intracellular adhesion molecule-1
Mct1 monocarboxylic acid transporter 1
RMT receptor-mediated transcytosis
TfR transferrin receptor

1. INTRODUCTION

Since the concept of a blood–brain barrier (BBB) first began to emerge in the early part of the twentieth century, our views of its structure and function have been constantly changing. The first crucial observations were made by Ehrlich (1885) at the turn of the century when he observed that, after intravenous injection, some dyes would enter and stain the brain and others would not. However, he attributed this phenomenon to differential affinity of the dyes for nervous tissue. Further experiments by Goldmann (1913) showed that trypan blue, when injected intravenously, did not stain the brain but when injected directly into the subarachnoid space was able to stain the tissue effectively. This was the first demonstration of a barrier between the CNS and the blood. It took many years and considerable argument and experimentation to finally establish that the mammalian BBB lies principally with the endothelium of the cerebral capillaries and was an endothelial barrier and that a secondary barrier was formed by the epithelium of the choroid plexus. It required the invention and application of electron microscopy to finally settle the dispute. Seminal in the resolution of this controversy were the studies of Reese and Karnovsky (1967), Brightman (1968), and Brightman and Reese (1969) who showed ultrastructurally that the BBB was at the level of the capillary endothelial cells (ECs) and that tight junctions between these cells effectively blocked the paracellular movement of both high and low molecular weight solutes from blood to brain. The BBB thus possesses the characteristics of the EC membranes, on both the brain- and blood-facing sides, and the transporters present and embedded in those membranes.

Reese and Karnovsky (1967) in their paper went a little further in their comment on the occurrence of endocytic vesicles that could be observed in the ECs of the barrier. They stated that "Micropinocytotic vesicles were few in number and did not appear to transport peroxidase while tight junctions between endothelial cells were probably responsible for preventing its intercellular passage." They went on to say "Since there is evidence that vesicles in the vascular endothelia in cardiac and skeletal muscle transport materials by filling on the luminal side of the endothelial cells and discharging their contents into the perivascular spaces, the paucity of similar vesicles in brain and their failure to discharge their peroxidase on the contraluminal side of the vessels could be regarded as another manifestation of a blood–brain barrier." This evidence has been clearly over-interpreted in the intervening years to imply that endocytosis and transcytosis at the BBB either do not occur or are insignificant. It is also unlikely that a mammalian BBB would transcytose a foreign plant protein, horse radish peroxidase, when many endogenous plasma proteins are not transported.

The picture began to change with the studies of Stewart (2000) who quantified the endocytic activity in a number of endothelial types and concluded that the cerebral endothelium exhibited approximately one-sixth of the observable endocytic profiles in, for example, cardiac and skeletal muscles. Endocytic profiles are clearly not absent in the BBB but less frequent than in other endothelia. Indeed, without some transcytosis mechanism being present for large molecules, the brain could not acquire these large molecules or smaller molecules transported in combination with them, without a synthesis in the brain itself. This is nowadays termed receptor-mediated transcytosis (RMT). Most endothelia exhibit this phenomenon; it is simply relatively downregulated in the BBB. Indeed, a number of receptors persist in the BBB which are capable of imitating RMT (Begley, 2007), for example, the transferrin receptor (TfR), the insulin receptor (InsR), and receptors responsible for lipoprotein transport. What seems to be happening at the BBB is that a number of receptors capable of imitating RMT are downregulated or not expressed, for example, albumin (Pardridge, Eisenberg, & Cefalu, 1985) and mannose-6-phosphate (Urayama, Grubb, Sly, & Banks, 2008), but a number persist and are capable of transporting large molecules, proteins, and constructs for drug delivery across the barrier. Hence, although the scale of this macromolecular transport is diminished in the BBB, it is crucial for CNS function and regulation. This review explores these processes further.

2. MECHANISMS OF MACROMOLECULE TRANSCYTOSIS

Unlike lipid soluble or small molecules, transport of macromolecules appears exclusive to the vesicular system. At least six different categories of endocytic vesicle have been described (Mayor & Pagano, 2007), but in brain endothelia only three major types have been definitively identified and defined. They are (Fig. 1):

(i) the most numerous clathrin-coated pits responsible for the majority of receptor-mediated endocytosis (RMT)
(ii) smaller, more flexible but much less numerous caveolae capable of mediating both nonselective adsorptive-mediated endocytosis of extracellular proteins and the trafficking of some membrane receptors
(iii) large, irregularly shaped macropinocytotic vesicles with a nonspecific cargo of extracellular components, but nonetheless regulated by inflammatory factors in particular (Table 1).

The clathrin-coated vesicles appear to be the most complex in their cargos and regulation. At the BBB, up to 20 receptors have been identified that can initiate RMT, and the majority use clathrin-coated vesicles to initiate transcytosis (Table 2). Despite the complexity and importance of RMT, brain endothelia have only 15% the number of vesicles of an equivalently size skeletal muscle capillary endothelium (Coomber & Stewart, 1986), and of those, only 1 in 10 are open to the plasma membrane at any given time. Perhaps because of the technical challenge of visualizing these infrequent events, relatively little is known about exactly how cargo destined for transcytosis actually gets from one side of the BBB EC to the other; what are the mechanics of endocytosis, intracellular trafficking, and exocytosis?

3. ENDOCYTOSIS IN BRAIN ENDOTHELIA

Recently, Gao, Yang, Zhang, Pang, and Jiang (2014) compared functionalized (receptor interacting) nanoparticle construct uptake in the mouse brain endothelia cell line bEND3, with that of rat C6 glioma cells. They observed clathrin-dependent internalization at the plasma membrane of both cell types which was inhibitable by chlorpromazine (which disrupts the formation of the clathrin coating of pits) and consistent with receptor-mediated endocytosis. Both cell types also demonstrated filipin-inhibitable, caveolae-dependent endocytosis. However, additional uptake mechanisms independent of clathrin or caveolae were apparent in C6 cells, but not seen

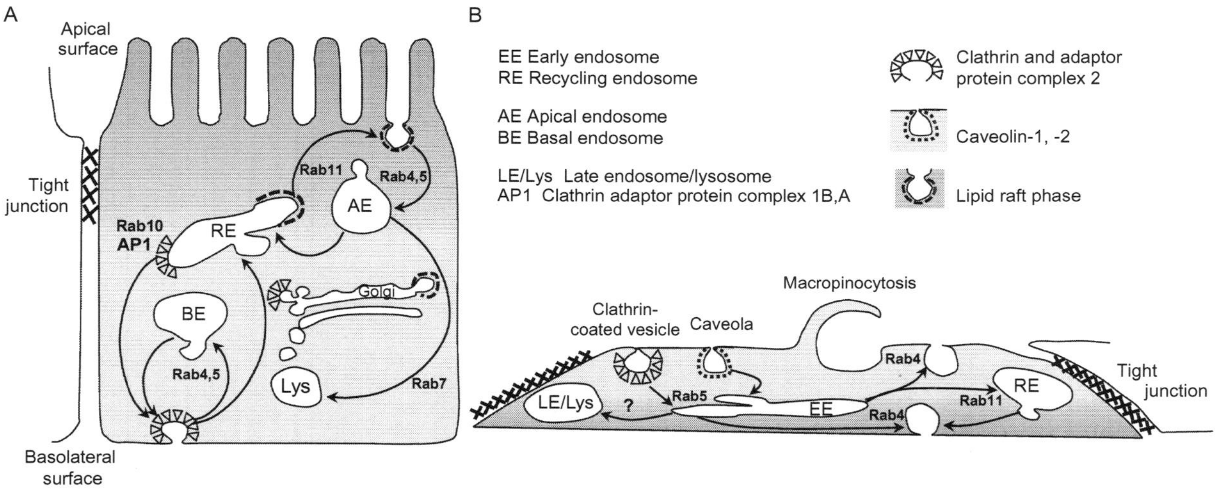

Figure 1 Regulation of transcytosis by Rab GTPases. A schematic diagram of proposed regulatory mechanisms directing transcytosis and intracellular trafficking in an MDCK (polarized epithelium) and HUVEC (endothelium) cell. The tight junctions prevent passage of macromolecules paracellularly, and in polarized cells, separate the apical and basal membrane domains. (A) In the polarized MDCK cell, endocytosed vesicles from basal and apical surfaces enter separate early sorting endosomes, AE (apical endosome) or BE (basal endosome). Carriers at the apical surface tend to be generated from lipid raft, cholesterol, and glycosphingolipid domains, and basolateral carriers are generated from adaptor protein-enriched coat domains. Rab4 and 5 control endocytic vesicle budding and fusion with the sorting endosome. Rab11 regulates entry to the recycling endosome (RE), which receives vesicles from both AE and BE. The RE has distinct domains which are either clathrin/AP-1-rich and destined for the basal membrane or lipid raft-rich and destined for the apical membrane, under the regulation of Rab11. Rab7 targets vesicles to the late endosome and lysosome for degradation. (B) In the endothelial cell, three vesicle types are clearly defined: the most frequently clathrin/AP-2-coated vesicle; the flask-shaped caveola formed from lipid raft material and caveolin1 and 2; and the large volume macropinocytotic vesicle. Little is known about control of vesicle trafficking in brain endothelia. In human umbilical vein endothelial cells (HUVECs), endocytosis is regulated by Rab4 and 5, as in epithelia. Rab4, when overexpressed, increases the fast recycling pathway from early endosome (EE) to the plasma membrane. Rab11 regulates entry into the RE, which is the slow pathway. Rab7 does not have an obvious function in these cells (Nayak, Keshava, Esmon, Pendurthi, & Rao, 2013). Note the cells are not to scale relative to each other: MDCK cell height in culture is 5–10 times greater than brain endothelial cells. *Panel (A): Adapted from Weisz and Rodriguez-Boulan (2009) and Bonifacino (2014).*

Table 1 Overview of endocytotic vesicles in brain endothelial cells

Vesicle	Size	Shape	Composition	Cargo	References
Caveolae	50–100 nm	Flask	Pit forms from plasma membrane cholesterol and sphingolipids (lipid raft components). Coated with flexible caveolin-1 and caveolin-2. Scission from the membrane requires the GTPase dynamin	Nonselective extracellular proteins. Receptors for folate, cholera and tetanus toxins, and alkaline phosphatase	Razani and Lisanti (2001), Humphries and Way (2013)
Clathrin coated	60–200 nm	Sphere	Pit forms from plasma membrane including protein components. Adaptor protein complex-2 (AP-2) and clathrin form a semi-rigid lattice network supporting the vesicle. Scission from the membrane requires the GTPase dynamin	Primary vesicle for receptor-mediated endocytosis. Wide range of plasma membrane receptors including LDL, LRP1, transferrin, insulin, and their ligands	Razani and Lisanti (2001), Vercauteren et al. (2010)
Macropinocytosis	0.2–5 μm	Irregular sphere → tubular	Ruffles of plasma membrane fold over to form an irregular invagination. Stimulated by inflammation/lipopolysaccharide	Nonspecific bulk engulfment of extracellular fluid, proteins, and macromolecules	Razani and Lisanti (2001), Lim and Gleeson (2011)

Table 2 Blood–brain barrier receptors initiating receptor-mediated endocytosis

Receptor	Ligand	References
Transferrin (TfR)	Fe–transferrin	Visser, Voorwinden, Crommelin, de Danhof, and Boer (2004)
Melanotransferrin (MTfR)	Melanotransferrin (p97)	Demeule et al. (2002)
Apolipoprotein E receptor 2 (ApoER2)	Lipoproteins	Hertz and Marchang (2003)
LDL receptor related protein 1 and 2 (LRP-1, LRP-2)	Lipoproteins Amyloid-β α-2-Macroglobulin Melanotransferrin (p97) Apolipoprotein E	Hertz and Marchang (2003)
Receptor for advanced glycation end-products (RAGE)	Amyloid-β, S-100, amphoterin Glycosylated proteins	Deane, Wu, and Zlokovic (2004) Stern, Yan, Yan, and Schmidt (2002)
Immunoglobulin G (Fcy-R)	IgG	Zlokovic et al. (1990)
Insulin (InsR)	Insulin	Banks (2004)
Leptin	Leptin	Banks, Niehoff, Martin, and Farrell (2002)
Insulin-like growth factor (IGFR)	IGF	Sly and Vogler (2013)
Tumor necrosis factor	TNFα	Pan and Kastin (2002)
Epidermal growth factor	EGF	Pan and Kastin (1999)
Heparin-binding epidermal growth factor (HB-EGF)	Diphtheria toxin	Gaillard, de Visser, and Boer (2005)
Scavenger receptors AI, BI (SR, SCAR)	Apolipoprotein A	Panzenboeck et al. (2002)

in endothelia, and would most probably include macropinocytosis since endocytosis in C6 cells was reduced by nocodazole, a known inhibitor of macropinocytosis. Despite this apparent lack of clathrin-independent and caveolae-independent endocytosis in brain endothelia, there are indications that it may be induced under certain circumstances when it could be useful to deliver larger cargos than those of the smaller coated vesicles in brain endothelia (~66–134 nm diameter) (Heymann et al., 2013). An example of this type of large-capacity vesicle formation is cell adhesion molecule (CAM)-mediated endocytosis, which involves the enrichment of ceramide in the plasma membrane regulating deformability and cytoskeleton rearrangement at the point of ICAM-1 interaction with the cell membrane, providing greater uptake capacity (Serrano, Bhowmick, Chadha, Garnacho, & Muro, 2012). During states of inflammation, ICAM-1 is upregulated, suggesting this mode of transport may be more important in pathological states and relevant for drug delivery exploitation. Hsu, Rappaport, and Muro (2014) tested anti-ICAM-1-coated 100-nm diameter FITC-polystyrene particles for uptake and distribution in human brain ECs, along with human astrocytes and pericytes. The anti-ICAM-1 nanocarriers were internalized by brain EC and this was enhanced fourfold under mock inflammatory conditions of TNF-α addition which correlated with an increase in ICAM-1 expression in the ECs. Astrocytes and pericytes also internalized the nanocarriers, but this was not augmented to the same extent by TNF-α. For the brain ECs, internalization was not reduced by inhibitors of clathrin- or caveolae-mediated endocytosis, confirming a distinct pathway for CAM-mediated endocytosis, comparable to gut epithelia (Ghaffarian, Bhowmick, & Muro, 2012; Hsu et al., 2014). Anti-ICAM-1 nanocarriers also transcytosed across brain ECs grown on filters and could enter astrocytes or pericytes grown in contact coculture below the endothelia. ICAM-1 has an endogenous role in leukocyte anchoring and extravasation (Millán et al., 2006) that may explain its capacity to transcytose larger-scale particles. These mechanisms also share properties with macropinocytosis (i.e., upregulated by inflammation, inhibited by proton exchanger antagonists; Lim & Gleeson, 2011).

4. VESICLE TRAFFICKING AND SUBCELLULAR LOCALIZATION IN BRAIN ENDOTHELIA

In bEND3 and C6 cells, subcellular localization of both functionalized and nonfunctionalized nanoparticles identified the endosome as a common distribution point (Gao et al., 2014). However, only in C6 cells were nanoparticles colocalized to the Golgi apparatus and lysosomes, suggesting that these subcellular organelles are not as important or as frequently used in brain endothelia for this particle. This has useful implication for designing nanoparticle drug delivery systems. Avoidance of lysosomes when traversing brain endothelia may prevent early degradation or release of the nanoparticle–drug complex, allowing deeper penetration to CNS target tissues, such as glioma, and release of the drug within glioma lysosomal systems.

Investigating the regulation of caveolae-mediated vesicle trafficking of the monocarboxylic acid transporter 1 (Mct1), Smith, Uhernik, Li, Liu, and Drewes (2012) identified β-adrenergic-stimulated, cAMP-dependent entry into early/sorting endosomes involving dephosphorylation of caveolin-1. Subsequent steps were suggested to involve the late endosome/lysosome compartments and presumed degradation. A clathrin-mediated pathway was also implicated, this time directing Mct1 to clathrin vesicles and Rab11-positive recycling endosomes (REs), and not to the lysosome. Mct1 contains a motif able to interact with clathrin-vesicle adaptor protein complex-2 (AP-2) (Smith et al., 2012) which is essential for assembly of clathrin-coated vesicles. This promotes internalization and trafficking to REs followed by recycling back to the plasma membrane. In HeLa cells, depletion of the AP-2 complex leads to increased routing of cargoes to late endosome- and lysosome-degradative compartments and reduces cargo recycling (Grant & Donaldson, 2009; Lau & Chou, 2008). It remains to be seen whether brain endothelia utilize the same sorting machinery to direct vesicle cargo for degradation or recycling, the latter being an essential requirement for successful drug delivery to brain across the BBB. The relative importance of clathrin-coated versus caveolae-mediated vesicular trafficking is illustrated by the fact that AP-2 knockout mice are unable to survive (Humphries & Way, 2013), unlike caveolae knockouts which are viable, though display some pathology (Razani & Lisanti, 2001).

5. RECYCLING OF VESICLES TO APICAL OR BASOLATERAL MEMBRANES

For successful transcytosis to occur, vesicle cargo and/or their receptors generated from one surface of a polarized cell must traverse the cell and be exocytosed at the opposite membrane. While there is no direct evidence for the mechanisms controlling this in brain endothelia, other polarized cells provide clues, at least for the mechanisms of receptor recycling. Trafficking back to the membrane can occur directly from early endosomes (EEs) (65% of recycled receptors) or via REs (35% of recycled receptors) (Thompson et al., 2007). In polarized epithelial cells, such as kidney-derived MDCK cells, there are separate EE compartments beneath the apical and basolateral surfaces (Bomsel, Parton, Kuznetsov, Schroer, & Gruenberg, 1990) that may then traffic into the same RE, where sorting occurs to return plasma membrane receptors to the correct location. Thompson et al. (2007) showed presorting of apical and basolateral proteins into separate membrane subdomains within an individual RE, but only after MDCK cells had been grown in culture sufficiently long to achieve polarization (from day 4 onward). This sorting was not seen in cells that do not normally polarize (Chinese hamster ovary cells) or in subconfluent MDCK cells. More recently, Hase et al. (2013) implicated clathrin adaptor protein complex (AP-1B) in protein sorting and basolateral targeting in intestinal cells in mice, and AP-1B is also required for lysosomal exocytosis to the basolateral membrane in MDCK cells (Xu et al., 2012). A role for AP-1A has also been described in MDCK cells mediating basolateral polarity (Gravotta et al., 2012) establishing AP-1 as a regulator of epithelial polarity, though its role in endothelia is unknown.

In a rare study of ECs, albeit umbilical vein (HUVECs), some of these regulatory pathways have been identified (Nayak et al., 2013). Tracing the movement of factor VIIa (FVIIa) which binds to the EC protein C receptor (EPCR), receptor-mediated internalization was shown to be regulated by the Rab GTPase, Rab5. At an early stage, VIIa also colocalized with Rab4, for targeting to the sorting endosomes. Interestingly, overexpression of Rab4 leads to increased accumulation in the RE, not the sorting endosome, and fast recycling back to the plasma membrane, although in this experiment the apical and basal membranes were not separated so the direction of transport was not assessed. It is suggested, however, that fast recycling may avoid lysosomal targeting. The role of Rab11 in transendothelial transport was investigated using dominant-negative Rab11, to reduce its expression. The entry of FVIIa into REs was reduced, as was transport of FVIIa across the entire endothelium when grown on transwell filters, strongly supporting a role for Rab11 in directing FV11a to the basal membrane in a similar way to that seen in epithelia (Weisz & Rodriguez-Boulan, 2009). However, there was still residual transcytosis, so other regulators must be invoked. The most likely candidate is a clathrin adaptor protein, since these are essential for epithelial cell polarization, and clathrin-coated vesicles are the main vesicle type in brain endothelia, but to our knowledge there have been no reports of AP-1-positive vesicles in endothelia and the essential component of polarized transport has not (yet) been identified.

Finally, the regulator of lysosomal targeting, Rab7, did not appear to play a role in HUVECs, leaving the molecular mechanisms for lysosomal targeting in endothelia still unclear (Nayak et al., 2013).

6. EXOCYTOSIS IN ENDOTHELIA

The final part in the process, vesicle fusion with the plasma membrane and exocytosis, is equally lacking in mechanistic detail for brain endothelia. Much work has been done with coronary, aortic, and lung endothelia which identify a family of soluble *N*-ethylmaleimide-sensitive factor attachment proteins and their receptors (SNAREs) as components in the tethering and exocytosis of vesicles (see Sehgal & Mukhopadhyay, 2007 for a review). In polarized epithelia, apical and basal membranes have different SNARE compositions, being rich in Syntaxin-3 apically and rich in Syntaxin-4 basally (Weisz & Rodriguez-Boulan, 2009). Given the fundamental similarities between endothelia from different organ systems, as well as parallels with epithelia, it is likely that equivalent protein complexes play a role in brain endothelia. We do know, however, the brain ECs generate exosomes or microvesicles that are released toward the brain. A recent paper by Haqqani et al. (2013) succeeded in isolating and characterizing extracellular microvesicles from human brain endothelia. In excess of 1000 proteins were identified contained within the microvesicles, but of particular interest was the presence of receptors which initiate RMT: TfR, InsR, low-density lipoprotein receptor (LDLR), and LDL-related proteins LRP1 and LRP2. These receptors have been shown to aid brain delivery of macromolecules across the BBB (discussed below) and so their release in vesicles from the basal/brain-facing membrane strongly points to transcytosis of the receptors, presumably along with their cargo. The authors also reported that stimulating RMT using the antibody FC5 resulted in a fourfold increase in the amount of EMVs being produced by human endothelium.

7. TARGETING RECEPTOR-MEDIATED TRANSPORT FOR DRUG DELIVERY TO BRAIN

In the 1990s, methods were being developed to enhance brain delivery of macromolecules using vectors, and notably by conjugation to antibodies raised against either the TfR (Granholm et al., 1994; Yoshikawa & Pardridge, 1992) or the insulin receptor (Wu, Yang, & Pardridge, 1997); the enhanced uptake of the cargo was attributed to RMT. Since then, the LRP1 receptor has been included as a target for CNS drug delivery, and strategies and techniques refined. A problem common for all studies investigating BBB delivery of therapeutics is quantifying whether the drug gets where it is needed in high enough concentrations to have an effect on CNS function. Recently, several groups have begun to show that these technologies can deliver drugs to modify CNS function *in vivo*. For example, Ulbrich, Knobloch, and Kreuter (2011) used an antibody against the mouse InsR (29B4) covalently attached to albumin nanoparticles to deliver loperamide to the mouse CNS. The CNS activity of loperamide was assessed based on its antinociceptive effect, which increased fourfold compared to giving loperamide alone. Interestingly, delivering the InsR antibody alone, before the nanoparticle/loperamide/antibody conjugate, completely prevented the antinociceptive effect. This could be explained by the high binding affinity of the antibody to the receptor which prevented later binding and/or transport of the drug conjugate. This illustrates a challenge faced by studies using antibodies that the therapy may block the receptor for transport and is then a problem for drug delivery, unless (i) the antibody-bound receptors can be replaced/resynthesized rapidly, or (ii) the dosing regimen needed is infrequent, or (iii) there is a way to reduce the affinity of the antibody for the receptor so it does not remain bound. The latter is the approach taken by Yu et al. (2011). They used an antibody against the TfR to access the brain, but initially found that the high affinity of binding meant the antibody did not detach from the receptor. By reducing the affinity of the anti-TfR antibody, they were able to show it detached on the brain side of the BBB and enhanced uptake into mouse brain. They then engineered a bispecific antibody to bind to both TfR and the enzyme β-secretase (BACE1) which is responsible for cleaving amyloid precursor protein into β-amyloid peptide, the fibrillar, neurotoxin found in Alzheimer's pathology. The bispecific antibody was able to target the TfR for transcytosis across the BBB and then bind and inhibit the BACE1 enzyme, so lowering CNS levels of β-amyloid (Yu et al., 2011). In a subsequent paper, the group investigated the intracellular fate of the high-affinity TfR bispecific antibody and the effect on brain levels of endogenous TfR. Mice given high-affinity bispecific antibody i.v. had less than half control levels of TfR in brain 4 days after the dosing. Using cell culture with bEND3 cells, intracellular high-affinity TfR antibody was visualized using quantum dot conjugated to an antimurine TfR Fab fragment (a different epitope to the TfR-binding site). This study revealed enhanced trafficking of the TfR antibody to the lysosomes and increased degradation compared to the low-affinity antibody (Bien-Ly et al., 2014). This underlines the importance of understanding the intracellular trafficking machinery in order to design successful drug delivery systems. In order to increase transcytosis to the brain, Niewoehner et al. (2014) designed a bispecific antibody, but with just one binding site for TfR (single anti-TfR Fab) rather than the usual double Fab, but still with a second therapeutic antibody fused, an anti-β-amyloid antibody. With this approach, they found the single anti-TfR Fab escaped the brain microvessels and entered brain considerably faster than the double Fab, and in cell culture, found the double Fab present in 50% of lysosomes, whereas the single Fab was seen in 20% of lysosomes.

Another major approach for drug delivery via receptor-mediated endocytosis is using the LRP1 receptor, but now making use of some of the many ligands that exist for LRP1, rather than using antibodies. The designed peptides, Angiopep and Angiopep-2, have been widely used since their introduction (Demeule et al., 2008), either conjugated directly to the drug of interest (for example, paclitaxel for treatment of brain tumors; Régina et al., 2008) or as a coating for nanoparticles to enhance delivery to the brain of a wide range of drugs and more recently gene therapy (Huang et al., 2011). Recently Angiopep conjugated to a gene-delivery vector, dendrigraft poly-L-lysine, was used to deliver the glial cell line-derived neurotrophic factor gene (hGDNF) to rats with Parkinsonism induced by rotenone (Huang et al., 2013). The rats demonstrated most improvement in movement after five doses, spread over 8 days, and preservation of dopaminergic neurons, demonstrating very promising biological outcomes.

8. CONCLUSION

The detailed mechanics of how the BBB enables transcytosis still remains something of a black box, but the mechanisms are being dissected out at an increasing rate, compared to the early studies postulating pores and paracellular movement and that absolutely no protein could cross the barrier. Understanding the role of the endocytotic protein complexes and receptors would help fill the gaps in our knowledge of intracellular trafficking specifically in brain endothelia in health and disease, which may differ in subtle ways to those of other cell types. It would also help us more intelligently design strategies to traverse the BBB. Using receptor- or adsorptive-mediated endocytosis mechanics, it may then be possible to control the rate of receptor recycling and vesicle transcytosis and bypass the lysosomal compartment while targeting the basal membrane. This would allow us to predict which strategies would be most likely to deliver intact cargo every time to the brain parenchyma.

CONFLICT OF INTEREST

The authors have no conflicts of interest to declare.

REFERENCES

Banks, W. A. (2004). The source of cerebral insulin. *European Journal of Pharmacology, 490*, 5–12.

Banks, W. A., Niehoff, M. L., Martin, D., & Farrell, C. L. (2002). Leptin transport across the blood–brain barrier of the Koletsky rat is not mediated by a product of the leptin receptor gene. *Brain Research, 950*, 130–136.

Begley, D. J. (2007). Structure and function of the blood–brain barrier. In E. Touitou, & B. W. Barry (Eds.), *Enhancement in drug delivery* (pp. 575–591). Boca Raton: CRC Press.

Bien-Ly, N., Yu, Y. J., Bumbaca, D., Elstrott, J., Boswell, C. A., Zhang, Y., et al. (2014). Transferrin receptor (TfR) trafficking determines brain uptake of TfR antibody affinity variants. *Journal of Experimental Medicine, 211*(2), 233–244.

Bomsel, M., Parton, R., Kuznetsov, S. A., Schroer, T. A., & Gruenberg, J. (1990). Microtubule- and motor-dependent fusion in vitro between apical and basolateral endocytic vesicles from MDCK cells. *Cell, 62*(4), 719–731.

Bonifacino, J. S. (2014). Adaptor proteins involved in polarized sorting. *Journal of Cell Biology, 204*(1), 7–17.

Brightman, M. W. (1968). The intracerebral movement of proteins injected into blood and cerebrospinal fluid of mice. *Progress in Brain Research, 29*, 19–37.

Brightman, M. W., & Reese, T. S. (1969). Junctions between intimately apposed cell membranes in the vertebrate brain. *Journal of Cell Biology, 40*, 648–677.

Coomber, B. L., & Stewart, P. A. (1986). Three-dimensional reconstruction of vesicles in endothelium of blood–brain barrier versus highly permeable microvessels. *The Anatomical Record, 215*, 256–261.

Deane, R., Wu, Z., & Zlokovic, B. V. (2004). RAGE (Yin) versus LRP (Yang) balance regulates Alzheimer amyloid β-peptide clearance through transport across the blood–brain barrier. *Stroke, 35*, 2628–2631.

Demeule, M., Poirier, J., Jodoin, J., Berttrand, Y., Desrosiers, R. R., Dagenais, C., et al. (2002). High transcytosis of melanotransferrin (P97) across the blood–brain barrier. *Journal of Neurochemistry, 83*, 924–933.

Demeule, M., Régina, A., Ché, C., Poirier, J., Nguyen, T., Gabathuler, R., et al. (2008). Identification and design of peptides as a new drug delivery system for the brain. *Journal of Pharmacology and Experimental Therapeutics, 324*(3), 1064–1072.

Ehrlich, P. (1885). *Das Sauerstoffbedürfnis des organismus*. Berlin: Eine Farbenanalytische Studie.

Gaillard, P., de Visser, C. C., & Boer, A. G. (2005). Targeted delivery across the blood–brain barrier. *Expert Opinion on Drug Delivery, 2*, 299–309.

Gao, H., Yang, Z., Zhang, S., Pang, Z., & Jiang, X. (2014). Internalization and subcellular fate of aptamer and peptide dual-functioned nanoparticles. *Journal of Drug Targeting, 22*(5), 450–459.

Ghaffarian, R., Bhowmick, T., & Muro, S. (2012). Transport of nanocarriers across gastrointestinal epithelial cells by a new transcellular route induced by targeting ICAM-1. *Journal of Controlled Release, 163*(1), 25–33.

Goldmann, E. (1913). Vitalfarbung am zentralnervensystem. *Abhandlungen der Preussischen Akademie der Wissenschaften, 1*, 1–60.

Granholm, A. C., Bäckman, C., Bloom, F., Ebendal, T., Gerhardt, G. A., Hoffer, B., et al. (1994). NGF and anti-transferrin receptor antibody conjugate: Short and long-term effects on survival of cholinergic neurons in intraocular septal transplants. *Journal of Pharmacology and Experimental Therapeutics, 268*(1), 448–459.

Grant, B. D., & Donaldson, J. G. (2009). Patways and mechanisms of endocytic recycling. *Nature Reviews Molecular and Cell Biology*, *10*(9), 597–608.
Gravotta, D., Carvajal-Gonzalez, J. M., Mattera, R., Deborde, S., Banfelder, J. R., Bonifacino, J. S., et al. (2012). The clathrin adaptor AP-1A mediates basolateral polarity. *Developmental Cell*, *22*(4), 811–823.
Haqqani, A. S., Delaney, C. E., Tremblay, T. L., Sodja, C., Sandhu, J. K., & Stanimirovic, D. B. (2013). Method for isolation and molecular characterization of extracellular microvesicles released from brain endothelial cells. *Fluids and Barriers of the CNS*, *10*(1), 4.
Hase, K., Nakatsu, F., Ohmae, M., Sugihara, K., Shioda, N., Takahashi, D., et al. (2013). AP-1B-mediated protein sorting regulates polarity and proliferation of intestinal epithelial cells in mice. *Gastroenterology*, *145*(3), 625–635.
Hertz, J., & Marchang, P. (2003). Coaxing the LDL receptor family into the fold. *Cell*, *112*, 289–292.
Heymann, J. B., Winkler, D. C., Yim, Y. I., Eisenberg, E., Greene, L. E., & Steven, A. C. (2013). Clathrin-coated vesicles from brain have small payloads: A cryo-electron tomographic study. *Journal of Structural Biology*, *184*(1), 43–51.
Hsu, J., Rappaport, J., & Muro, S. (2014). Specific binding, uptake and transport of ICAM-1 targeted nanocarriers across endothelial and subendothelial cell components of the blood–brain barrier. *Pharmaceutical Research*, *31*, 1855–1866.
Huang, S., Li, J., Han, L., Liu, S., Ma, H., Huang, R., et al. (2011). Dual targeting effect of Angiopep-2-modified, DNA-loaded nanoparticles for glioma. *Biomaterials*, *32*(28), 6832–6838.
Huang, R., Ma, H., Guo, Y., Liu, S., Kuang, Y., Shao, K., et al. (2013). Angiopep-conjugated nanoparticles for targeted long-term gene therapy of Parkinson's disease. *Pharmaceutical Research*, *30*(10), 2549–2559.
Humphries, A. C., & Way, M. (2013). The non-canonical roles of clathrin and actin in pathogen internalization, egress and spread. *Nature Reviews. Microbiology*, *11*(8), 551–560.
Lau, A. W., & Chou, M. M. (2008). The adaptor complex AP-2 regulates post-endocytic trafficking through the nonclathrin Arf6-dependent endocytic pathway. *Journal of Cell Science*, *121*, 4008–4017.
Lim, J. P., & Gleeson, P. A. (2011). Macropinocytosis: An endocytic pathway for internalising large gulps. *Immunology and Cell Biology*, *89*(8), 836–843. http://dx.doi.org/10.1038/icb.2011.20.
Mayor, S., & Pagano, R. E. (2007). Pathways of clathrin-independent endocytosis. *Nature Reviews Molecular Cell Biology*, *8*(8), 603–612.
Millán, J., Hewlett, L., Glyn, M., Toomre, D., Clark, P., & Ridley, A. J. (2006). Lymphocyte transcellular migration occurs through recruitment of endothelial ICAM-1 to caveola- and F-actin-rich domains. *Nature Cell Biology*, *8*(2), 113–123.
Nayak, R. C., Keshava, S., Esmon, C. T., Pendurthi, U. R., & Rao, L. V. (2013). Rab GTPases regulate endothelial cell protein C receptor-mediated endocytosis and trafficking of factor VIIa. *PLoS One*, *8*(3), e59304.
Niewoehner, J., Bohrmann, B., Collin, L., Urich, E., Sade, H., Maier, P., et al. (2014). Increased brain penetration and potency of a therapeutic antibody using a monovalent molecular shuttle. *Neuron*, *81*(1), 49–60.
Pan, W., & Kastin, A. (1999). Entry of EGF into brain is rapid and saturable. *Peptides*, *20*, 1091–1098.
Pan, W., & Kastin, A. (2002). TNFα transport across the blood–brain barrier is abolished in receptor knockout mice. *Experimental Neurology*, *174*, 193–200.
Panzenboeck, U., Balazs, Z., Sovic, A., Hrzenjak, A., Levak-Frank, S., Wintersperger, A., et al. (2002). ABCA1 and scavenger receptor class B, type 1, are modulators of reverse

sterol transport at an in vitro blood–brain barrier constituted of porcine capillary endothelial cells. *The Journal of Biological Chemistry, 277*, 42781–42789.

Pardridge, W. M., Eisenberg, J., & Cefalu, W. T. (1985). Absence of albumin receptor on brain capillaries in vivo or vitro. *The American Journal of Physiology, 249*, E264–E267.

Razani, B., & Lisanti, M. P. (2001). Caveolins and caveolae: Molecular and functional relationships. *Experimental Cell Research, 271*, 36–44.

Reese, T. S., & Karnovsky, M. J. (1967). Fine structural localization of a blood–brain barrier to exogenous peroxidase. *Journal of Cell Biology, 34*, 207–217.

Régina, A., Demeule, M., Ché, C., Lavallée, I., Poirier, J., Gabathuler, R., et al. (2008). Antitumour activity of ANG1005, a conjugate between paclitaxel and the new brain delivery vector Angiopep-2. *British Journal of Pharmacology, 155*(2), 185–197.

Sehgal, P. B., & Mukhopadhyay, S. (2007). Pulmonary arterial hypertension: A disease of tethers, SNAREs and SNAPs? *American Journal of Physiology. Heart and Circulatory Physiology. 293*(1), H77–H85.

Serrano, D., Bhowmick, T., Chadha, R., Garnacho, C., & Muro, S. (2012). Intercellular adhesion molecule 1 engagement modulates sphingomyelinase and ceramide, supporting uptake of drug carriers by the vascular endothelium. *Arteriosclerosis, Thrombosis, and Vascular Biology, 32*(5), 1178–1185.

Sly, W. S., & Vogler, C. (2013). The final frontier-crossing the blood-brain barrier. *EMBO Molecular Medicine, 5*, 655–657.

Smith, J. P., Uhernik, A. L., Li, L., Liu, Z., & Drewes, L. R. (2012). Regulation of Mct1 by cAMP-dependent internalization in rat brain endothelial cells. *Brain Research, 1480*, 1–11.

Stern, D., Yan, S. D., Yan, S. F., & Schmidt, A. M. (2002). Receptor for advanced glycation endproducts: A multiligand receptor magnifying cell stress in diverse pathologic settings. *Advanced Drug Delivery Reviews, 54*, 1615–1625.

Stewart, P. A. (2000). Endothelial vesicles in the blood–brain barrier: Are they related to permeability? *Cellular and Molecular Neurobiology, 20*, 149–163.

Thompson, A., Nessler, R., Wisco, D., Anderson, E., Winckler, B., & Sheff, D. (2007). Recycling endosomes of polarized epithelial cells actively sort apical and basolateral cargos into separate subdomains. *Molecular Biology of the Cell, 18*(7), 2687–2697.

Ulbrich, K., Knobloch, T., & Kreuter, J. (2011). Targeting the insulin receptor: Nanoparticles for drug delivery across the blood–brain barrier (BBB). *Journal of Drug Targeting, 19*(2), 125–132.

Urayama, A., Grubb, J. H., Sly, W. S., & Banks, W. A. (2008). Mannose 6-phosphate receptor-mediated transport of sulfamidase across the blood-brain barrier in the new born mouse. *Molecular Therapy, 16*(7), 1261–1265.

Vercauteren, D., Vandenbroucke, R. E., Jones, A. T., Rejman, J., Demeester, J., De Smedt, S. C., et al. (2010). The use of inhibitors to study endocytic pathways of gene carriers: Optimization and pitfalls. *Molecular Therapy, 18*(3), 561–569.

Visser, C. C., Voorwinden, H., Crommelin, D. J. A., de Danhof, M., & Boer, A. G. (2004). Characterisation of the transferrin receptor on brain capillary endothelial cells. *Pharmaceutical Research, 21*, 761–769.

Weisz, O. A., & Rodriguez-Boulan, E. (2009). Apical trafficking in epithelial cells: Signals, clusters and motors. *Journal of Cell Science, 122*(Pt. 23), 4253–4266.

Wu, D., Yang, J., & Pardridge, W. M. (1997). Drug targeting of a peptide radiopharmaceutical through the primate blood–brain barrier in vivo with a monoclonal antibody to the human insulin receptor. *Journal of Clinical Investigation, 100*(7), 1804–1812.

Xu, J., Toops, K. A., Diaz, F., Carvajal-Gonzalez, J. M., Gravotta, D., Mazzoni, F., et al. (2012). Mechanism of polarized lysosome exocytosis in epithelial cells. *Journal of Cell Science, 125*(Pt. 24), 5937–5943.

Yoshikawa, T., & Pardridge, W. M. (1992). Biotin delivery to brain with a covalent conjugate of avidin and a monoclonal antibody to the transferrin receptor. *Journal of Pharmacology and Experimental Therapeutics*, *263*(2), 897–903.
Yu, Y. J., Zhang, Y., Kenrick, M., Hoyte, K., Luk, W., Lu, Y., et al. (2011). Boosting brain uptake of a therapeutic antibody by reducing its affinity for a transcytosis target. *Science Translational Medicine*, *3*, 84ra44.
Zlokovic, B. V., Skundric, D. S., Segal, M. B., Lipovac, M. N., Makic, J. B., & Davson, H. A. (1990). Saturable mechanism for transport of immunoglobulin G across the blood–brain barrier of the guinea pig. *Experimental Neurology*, *107*, 263–270.

CHAPTER SIX

Drug Delivery to the Ischemic Brain

Brandon J. Thompson*, Patrick T. Ronaldson†,1
*Department of Physiology, University of Arizona College of Medicine, Tucson, Arizona, USA
†Department of Pharmacology, University of Arizona College of Medicine, Tucson, Arizona, USA
[1]Corresponding author: e-mail address: pronald@email.arizona.edu

Contents

Abstract

Cerebral ischemia occurs when blood flow to the brain is insufficient to meet metabolic demand. This can result from cerebral artery occlusion that interrupts blood flow, limits CNS supply of oxygen and glucose, and causes an infarction/ischemic stroke. Ischemia initiates a cascade of molecular events in neurons and cerebrovascular endothelial cells including energy depletion, dissipation of ion gradients, calcium overload, excitotoxicity, oxidative stress, and accumulation of ions and fluid. Blood–brain barrier (BBB) disruption is associated with cerebral ischemia and leads to vasogenic edema, a primary cause of stroke-associated mortality. To date, only a single drug has received US Food and Drug Administration (FDA) approval for acute ischemic stroke treatment, recombinant tissue plasminogen activator (rt-PA). While rt-PA therapy restores perfusion to ischemic brain, considerable tissue damage occurs when cerebral blood flow is reestablished. Therefore, there is a critical need for novel therapeutic approaches that can "rescue" salvageable brain tissue and/or protect BBB integrity during ischemic stroke. One class of drugs that may enable neural cell rescue following cerebral

Advances in Pharmacology, Volume 71
ISSN 1054-3589
http://dx.doi.org/10.1016/bs.apha.2014.06.013

ischemia/reperfusion injury is the HMG-CoA reductase inhibitors (i.e., statins). Understanding potential CNS drug delivery pathways for statins is critical to their utility in ischemic stroke. Here, we review molecular pathways associated with cerebral ischemia and novel approaches for delivering drugs to treat ischemic disease. Specifically, we discuss utility of endogenous BBB drug uptake transporters such as organic anion transporting polypeptides and nanotechnology-based carriers for optimization of CNS drug delivery. Overall, this chapter highlights state-of-the-art technologies that may improve pharmacotherapy of cerebral ischemia.

ABBREVIATIONS

ALK activin receptor-like kinase
BBB blood–brain barrier
CNS central nervous system
DPDPE [D-penicillamine2,5]-enkephalin
ETC electron transport chain
H/R hypoxia/reoxygenation
LDL low-density lipoprotein
NO nitric oxide
NOS nitric oxide synthase
OATP/Oatp organic anion transporting polypeptide
PARP poly(ADP-ribose) polymerase
PEG polyethylene glycol
PLGA poly(lactic acid-*co*-glycolic acid)
RES reticuloendothelial system
ROS reactive oxygen species
rt-PA recombinant tissue plasminogen activator
SOD superoxide dismutase
TEMPOL 4-hydoxy-2,2,6,6-tetramethylpiperidine-*N*-oxyl
TGF-β transforming growth factor-β

1. INTRODUCTION

Pharmacological treatment of cerebral ischemia requires a detailed understanding of pathophysiological changes that occur in the brain and in the cerebral microvasculature following ischemia/reperfusion injury. Cerebral hypoxia and subsequent reoxygenation is a central component of several diseases, including traumatic brain injury, acute respiratory distress syndrome, obstructive sleep apnea, high-altitude cerebral edema and acute mountain sickness, cardiac arrest, and ischemic stroke (Ronaldson & Davis, 2013). Stroke is the fourth leading cause of death and is a major cause of long-term morbidity in the United States (Feng & Belagaje, 2013). Of all stroke cases, 87% are ischemic (Roger et al., 2011). Ischemic stroke results from restricted blood flow to a portion of the brain that causes an irreversibly damaged ischemic core and a surrounding region of potentially viable, yet functionally impaired brain tissue known as the penumbra (Astrup, Siesjo, & Symon, 1981; Liu, Levine, & Winn, 2010). A complex cascade of molecular events initiated by cerebral ischemia is responsible for the widespread necrosis observed in the ischemic core and apoptosis detected in the penumbra. Theoretically, the penumbra can be salvaged if reperfusion therapy and/or pharmacotherapy are administered early during the course of disease (Shah & Abbruscato, 2014). This therapeutic objective is underscored by challenges in delivering drugs to the ischemic brain. Here, we discuss pathological mechanisms associated with cerebral ischemia and associated hypoxia and how detailed knowledge of such processes can lead to cutting-edge approaches to deliver drugs to ischemic brain. In particular, we focus on targeting endogenous blood–brain barrier (BBB) uptake transporters and utilization of nanoparticle delivery systems, two non-invasive chemical-based approaches that are highly promising for effective central nervous system (CNS) drug delivery.

2. PATHOPHYSIOLOGY OF ISCHEMIA

Physiologically, energy requirements of the CNS are met by brain uptake of glucose and oxygen, which are incorporated into metabolic pathways to enable phosphorylation of ADP to ATP. Cerebral ischemia results in reduction of molecular oxygen delivery to all CNS cell types within the core of the infarct zone. Lack of oxygen availability halts molecular shuttling of electrons in oxidative phosphorylation, which is essential for ATP generation. Most ATP generated within the brain is used for maintenance of intracellular homeostasis and transmembrane gradients for monovalent and divalent ions (i.e., Na^+, K^+, Ca^{2+}) (Adibhatla & Hatcher, 2008). Energy depletion in neuronal cells causes ion gradient failure via cessation of ATP-dependent Na^+/K^+-ATPase and Ca^{2+}-ATPase activity. When energy dependent ion extrusion is impeded, cations in extracellular fluid (i.e., Na^+) follow a strong inwardly directed electrochemical gradient and accumulate within the cell. Uptake of Na^+ is accompanied by influx of monovalent anions (i.e., Cl^-). Extracellular fluid then follows this net movement of ions resulting in cytotoxic edema. Additionally, Na^+ ion uptake causes extensive plasma membrane depolarization, leading to opening of voltage-gated cation channels and reverses the direction of the Na^{+}/Ca^{2+} exchanger, bringing additional Ca^{2+} into the cell (Kiedrowski, 2007; Luo et al., 2008). The widespread depolarization seen in ischemic neurons thwarts plasma membrane hyperpolarization, which is required to close and reactivate these cation channels.

Influx of Ca^{2+} prompts intracellular vesicles, containing glutamate or dopamine, to fuse with the neuronal presynaptic bouton membrane, releasing the neurotransmitters into the synapse. This uncontrolled increase in glutamate and dopamine concentrations is neurotoxic and leads to neuronal cell death and development of an infarction (i.e., ischemic stroke) (Adibhatla & Hatcher, 2008). Glutamate excitotoxicity coupled with cellular depolarization is particularly deleterious to the CNS due to overstimulation of metabotropic glutamate receptors as well as extensive activation of AMPA and NMDA receptors, resulting in disruption of CNS calcium homeostasis (Adibhatla, Hatcher, & Dempsey, 2006; Adibhatla, Hatcher, Larsen, et al., 2006; Arai et al., 2011). Energy reserves are quickly depleted in an effort to sequester increasing intracellular Ca^{2+} concentrations (Pundik, Xu, & Sundararajan, 2012). Inadvertent activation of inositol trisphosphate and ryanodine receptors, a process linked to mitochondrial reactive oxygen species (ROS) generation, can liberate intracellular Ca^{2+} stores (Camello-Almaraz, Gomez-Pinilla, Pozo, & Camello, 2006). Calcium overload also causes excessive stimulation of Ca^{2+}/calmodulin-dependent enzymes such as nitric oxide synthase (i.e., eNOS, nNOS, and mtNOS), as well as a host of Ca^{2+}-dependent enzymes such as proteases, phospholipases, and endonucleases (Fellman & Raivio, 1997). Overactivation of such catalytic enzymes can cause protein degradation, phospholipid hydrolysis, and DNA damage as well as a disruption of cellular signaling and enzymatic reactions. ROS generation increases dramatically during ischemia due to high Ca^{2+}-induced mitochondria dysfunction and impairment of ROS defense enzymes, and superoxide anion is released into the cytosol in increasing amounts. Neurons in the ischemic core that have died via necrotic processes release cytotoxic elements into the interstitial space that can penetrate adjacent neurons through damaged plasma membranes caused by lipid peroxidation and activity of phospholipases. In addition to ROS generation, cerebral ischemia is accompanied by widespread inflammation demarcated by cytokines, adhesion molecules, and other inflammatory mediators (Iadecola & Alexander, 2001).

2.1. ROS generation

Oxidative stress is observed in the CNS at early time points following ischemic injury and is well known to contribute to neuronal injury and cell death in the ischemic core (Candelario-Jalil, 2009). The CNS is especially sensitive to oxidative stress because it consumes substantial amounts of oxygen, contains large amounts of polyunsaturated fatty acids, accrues redox metal ions, and possesses relative low levels of endogenous antioxidants (Aksenova, Aksenov, Mactutus, & Booze, 2005). ROS have been recognized as central mediators of neuroinflammation and cytotoxicity in ischemia/reperfusion injury (Singhal, Morris, Labhasetwar, & Ghorpade, 2013). Furthermore, evidence of improved stroke outcome following clinical trials of antioxidant therapy underscores the critical role of ROS generation and oxidative stress in CNS pathology following cerebral ischemia/hypoxia (Lutsep & Clark, 2001).

Superoxide anion is the principal ROS generated when molecular oxygen is reduced by only one electron. This reaction occurs spontaneously and nonenzymatically through activity of electron transport systems in mitochondria. Briefly, electrons are donated by NADH, the reduced form of the coenzyme essential to all living cells, initiating a shuttling of electrons involving NADH–ubiquinone oxidoreductase or complex I, succinate dehydrogenase or complex II, ubiquinol–cytochrome *c* oxidoreductase or complex III, and cytochrome *c* oxidase or complex IV, ending with electron acceptance by molecular oxygen. Small amounts of superoxide (i.e., 1–4%) are regularly generated during this process, as the majority of reactions within the electron transport chain (ETC) involve single electron transfers (Turrens, 2003). In particular, complex I as well as both sides of complex III (i.e., Qi and Qo sites) are the most common sources of mitochondrial superoxide (Murphy, 2009). Superoxide generated within the intermembrane space of mitochondria can reach the cytosol through voltage-dependent mitochondrial anion channels (Zhang & Gutterman, 2007). Additionally, superoxide is produced by NADPH oxidases in endothelial cells, macrophages, microglia, and granular leukocytes, as well as by cytochrome P450-dependent oxygenases and cyclooxygenases (i.e., COX-2) (Pacher, Beckman, & Liaudet, 2007; Turrens, 2003). Furthermore, epithelial and neuronal nitric oxide synthase (eNOS/nNOS) directly produce superoxide when required cofactors, such as arginine or tetrahydrobiopterin, are deficient (i.e., uncoupled NOS) (Fang, Yang, & Wu, 2002), as occurs during cerebral ischemia.

Under normal physiological conditions, superoxide is scavenged by the cellular ROS defense system. However, due to activation of degradative enzymes and proteases, ROS defense enzymes (i.e., superoxide dismutases (SODs)) can become compromised and overwhelmed by high ROS concentrations. ROS induce mutations in mitochondrial DNA and damage enzymes and cytochrome complexes involved in the ETC. This leads to dysfunction of oxidative phosphorylation and further generation of ROS (Schild & Reiser, 2005). Superoxide levels steadily rise during ischemia in both microvascular endothelial cells and neurons (Fabian, DeWitt, & Kent, 1995; Pacher et al., 2007). This paradoxical increase of superoxide despite low oxygen concentrations has been well described (Guzy & Schumacker, 2006; Murphy, 2009). It is possible that physiological levels of nitric oxide (NO) can outcompete oxygen for binding to cytochrome oxidase in the setting of cerebral ischemia/hypoxia. NO binding can cause these cytochrome complexes to facilitate production of superoxide as well as increase the apparent K_m of this enzyme for NO, events that further interfere with oxidative phosphorylation (Murphy, 2009).

Peroxynitrite ($ONOO^-$), a potent cytotoxic and proinflammatory molecule, is formed rapidly and non-enzymatically from the combination of NO with superoxide and causes extensive damage to neurons and cerebral microvessels through lipid peroxidation, consumption of endogenous antioxidants (i.e., reduced glutathione), DNA fragmentation, and induction of mitochondrial failure (Pacher et al., 2007). Figure 1 illustrates ROS generation in cerebrovascular endothelial cells during ischemia/reperfusion, including peroxynitrite formation. Peroxynitrite causes cellular damage via its ability to nitrosylate tyrosine residues, leading to functional modifications of critical proteins (Salvemini, Doyle, & Cuzzocrea, 2006). Breakdown of peroxynitrite into nitrogen dioxide and hydroxyl radicals also leads to endothelial cell dysfunction and BBB disruption during cerebral ischemia (Heo, Han, & Lee, 2005). Administration of peroxynitrite decomposition catalysts 5,10,15,20-tetrakis(*N*-methyl-4′-pyridyl)porphyrinato iron III (FeTMPyP) and 5,10,15,20-tetrakis(4-sulphonatophenyl) porphyrinato iron (FeTPPS) during reperfusion, or even up to 6 h following reperfusion, have shown effectiveness in mitigating neuronal damage and reducing infarct size in rats subjected to transient middle cerebral artery occlusion (MCAO), an *in vivo* model of focal ischemic stroke. Additionally, brain edema was drastically reduced (i.e., up to 70%) in these studies, implying that peroxynitrite is a major contributor to BBB breakdown in ischemic brain (Pacher et al., 2007). Peroxynitrite formation in BBB endothelial cells

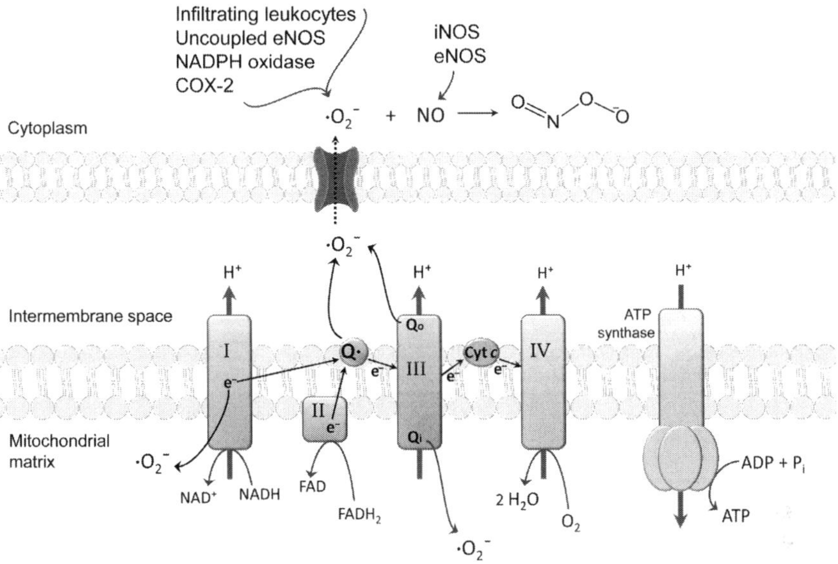

Figure 1 Generation of reactive oxygen species (ROS) in cerebrovascular endothelial cells. During ischemia, mitochondrial superoxide levels increase via NO inhibition of cytochrome complexes and oxidation of reducing equivalents in the electron transport chain (ETC). Complex I as well as both sides of complex III (i.e., Qi and Qo sites) are the most common sources of mitochondrial superoxide. Superoxide generated within the intermembrane space of mitochondria can reach the cytosol through voltage-dependent mitochondrial anion channels (Zhang et al., 2007). Superoxide levels further increase via cyclooxygenase-2, NADPH oxidase, uncoupled eNOS, and infiltrating leukocytes. The resulting high levels of superoxide coupled with the activation of NO-producing eNOS/iNOS, increases the likelihood of peroxynitrite formation. Peroxynitrite-induced cellular damage includes protein oxidation, tyrosine nitration, DNA damage and poly(ADP-ribose) polymerase (PARP) activation, lipid peroxidation, and mitochondrial dysfunction.

and neurons becomes more likely with activation of epithelial NOS (eNOS) and inducible NOS (iNOS) because NO diffuses easily through membranes and readily reacts with superoxide anion (Pacher et al., 2007).

2.2. Poly(ADP-ribose) polymerase

Recent evidence suggests that deleterious effects of peroxynitrite involve direct DNA damage and subsequent activation of poly(ADP-ribose) polymerases (PARPs). PARPs are a family of nuclear enzymes involved in DNA repair, programmed cell death, and necrotic tissue damage. PARP-1 is the dominant member of the PARP family and is critical in detection and repair of damaged DNA. PARP-1 binding to specific

DNA motifs such as single- and double-strand breaks, supercoils, cruciforms, and crossovers activates its catalytic domain. Activated PARP then utilizes NAD^+ to poly(ADP-ribosyl)ate itself, as well as other transcription-related factors (i.e., p53, nuclear factor-κB (NF-κB), activator protein 1, E2F-1) and DNA repair machinery (Chaitanya, Steven, & Babu, 2010; Kim, Zhang, & Kraus, 2005). Neurons with extensive DNA damage, such as is observed during cerebral ischemia, will experience depletion of nuclear and cytosolic pools of NAD^+ due to PARP-1 overactivation (M. Y. Kim et al., 2005). To prevent energy-failure-induced necrosis, activated caspases-3 and -7 will cleave PARP between aspartic acid 214 and glycine 215, yielding protein fragments of 24 and 89 kDa (Chaitanya et al., 2010). This cleavage effectively terminates PARP's ability to initiate DNA repair, an event that leads to DNA fragmentation and subsequent apoptosis. Therefore, pharmacological interventions that decrease PARP activation and cleavage in the brain are indicative of a potentially protective therapy that can attenuate neural apoptosis. Pharmacological compounds that inhibit PARP activation (i.e., 3-aminobenzamide, INO-1001, PJ-34) bestow neuroprotection against ischemia/reperfusion injury, even if administered several hours after hypoxic insult and, therefore, are potential candidates for clinical use (Pacher et al., 2007). Indeed, genetic deletion of PARP has protected animal subjects against DNA damage associated with pathophysiological conditions such as ischemia-reperfusion injury, neuroinflammatory stress, and glutamate excitotoxicity (Kim et al., 2005). Significant reductions (i.e., up to 80%) in infarct volume and brain tissue damage have also been observed in PARP knock-out mice following transient MCAO (Pacher et al., 2007).

In vivo, hypoxic-ischemic insult and/or hypoxia/reoxygenation (H/R) stress results in increased PARP cleavage in the brain (Martinez-Romero et al., 2009; Thompson et al., 2014; Tu, Lu, Huang, Ho, & Chou, 2012). The ratio of cleaved-to-uncleaved PARP is an established early indicator of end-stage cell death (Chaitanya et al., 2010; Thompson et al., 2014). Moreover, poly(ADP-ribose), the negatively charged polymer that results from PARP activity, has been shown to accumulate in neural tissue following global cerebral hypoxia (Pacher et al., 2007). Consistent with previous findings (Ghosh, Sarkar, Mandal, & Das, 2013), our laboratory found elevated cleaved-to-uncleaved PARP ratios in whole brain lysates prepared from animals subjected to hypoxic insult (1 h, 6% O_2) and reoxygenated for 10 min, 30 min, and 1 h as compared to these same ratios in brain lysates from normoxic animals (Thompson et al., 2014). We showed that a single dose of the 3-hydroxy-3-methylglutaryl coenzyme A (HMG-CoA) reductase inhibitor atorvastatin administered prior to hypoxic insult attenuated the H/R-induced increase in the cleaved-to-uncleaved PARP ratio at these early reoxygenation time points (Thompson et al., 2014). Recent evidence, including our own data, suggests that PARP cleavage is a critical factor in postischemic brain injury and represents a useful biomarker for neuroprotective drug efficacy in pharmacotherapy of diseases with an H/R component. Therefore, our data with atorvastatin suggest that pretreatment with statins may limit hypoxic injury and reduce the incidence of associated neurological deficits, as can occur following coronary artery bypass grafting (Kuhn et al., 2013; Kulik & Ruel, 2009).

2.3. Reperfusion and immune response

Reperfusion is known to cause large increases in ROS generation within the penumbra (Fabian et al., 1995; Zhao, Patzer, Herdegen, Gohlke, & Culman, 2006). Specifically, superoxide levels increase in both cerebrovascular endothelial cells and neurons during the early reoxygenation phase (Pacher et al., 2007). NO-inhibited cytochrome oxidases coupled with free radical-induced damage to the ETC machinery can further enhance production of superoxide, when molecular oxygen is reintroduced to the ischemic brain. Inhibition of ubiquinol–cytochrome *c* oxidoreductase or complex III of the ETC has been shown to reverse these reoxygenation-induced increases in superoxide *in vitro* (Therade-Matharan et al., 2005). Ceramide, which has been found to increase upon the onset of hypoxia, is also positively correlated with ROS generation during reoxygenation (Therade-Matharan et al., 2005).

A major contributor to reperfusion injury is the inflammatory response initiated by the uncontrolled release of cytotoxic chemicals and cellular debris into the interstitial space within damaged brain tissue. H/R is associated with activation of hypoxia-sensitive transcription factors such as NF-κB, hypoxia-inducible factor-1 (HIF-1), and signal transducer and activator of transcription 3 (STAT3) (Lochhead et al., 2010; Pacher et al., 2007; Witt, Mark, Huber, & Davis, 2005). Consequently, proinflammatory molecules and cytokines such as tumor necrosis factor-α (TNFα), interferon-γ, interleukin-1β (IL-1β), IL-6, and IL-18 are produced and secreted (Pacher et al., 2007). Endothelial cell adhesion molecules like P-selectins and E-selectins and intercellular adhesion molecule-1 (ICAM-1) are activated (Pacher et al., 2007), which allow leukocytes and macrophages to flood the infarcted area upon reperfusion. TNFα has also been linked to excitotoxicity and both TNFα and interferon-γ have been shown to increase expression of inducible nitric oxide synthase (iNOS) (Pundik et al., 2012). Enzymes activated by the inflammatory response include iNOS and COX-2, which produce substantial quantities of NO and $\cdot O_2^-$, respectively (Pacher et al., 2007). Additionally, reactive nitrogen species production in ischemic brain is enhanced due to activated macrophages and neutrophils releasing copious amounts of NO and $\cdot O_2^-$ in the penumbra. NO and superoxide rapidly form peroxynitrite, an effect that escalates peroxynitrite-induced cellular damage. As reperfusion proceeds, neuroinflammation and apoptosis become more prevalent and dramatically affect viability of salvageable brain tissue within the penumbra (Candelario-Jalil, 2009).

2.4. ROS and changes to the BBB

Cerebral ischemia is a complex insult that not only involves deprivation of oxygen and essential nutrient delivery (del Zoppo & Hallenbeck, 2000) but is also associated with increased microvascular permeability (Kempski, 2001; Petty & Wettstein, 2001). The BBB has developed as both a physical and metabolic barrier that is critical for survival. It is well established that disruption of the BBB during ischemia/reperfusion leads to vasogenic brain edema, a primary cause of stroke-associated mortality (Vibbert & Mayer, 2010); however, the majority of edema formation occurs across an intact BBB. Detectable BBB breakdown is not observed until approximately 5 h after onset of ischemia in experimental stroke models (O'Donnell, Lam, Tran, Foroutan, & Anderson, 2006; Shah & Abbruscato, 2014). Increased blood-to-brain net movement of Na^+ mediated by BBB Na^+ transporters appears to have a critical role in edema formation (Shah et al., 2013; Wallace, Foroutan, & O'Donnell, 2011). For example, O'Donnell and colleagues have demonstrated that increased activity of the luminal Na^+–K^+–$2Cl^-$ cotransporter in BBB endothelial cells contributes to development of cerebral edema following ischemia (O'Donnell, Tran, Lam, Liu, & Anderson, 2004). Furthermore, Na^+–K^+–Cl^- cotransporter inhibition reduces edema and infarct volume in a rat permanent MCAO model (O'Donnell et al., 2004; Wallace et al., 2011). Additionally, estradiol reduces both activity of the Na^+–K^+–Cl^- cotransporter and edema formation, suggesting that estrogens play a prominent neuroprotective role during stroke (O'Donnell et al., 2006). Integrity of BBB transport pathways during and after ischemic stroke is crucial, as perturbations in these processes can have significant effects on BBB permeability and therefore can exacerbate vasogenic edema.

BBB permeability is controlled by tight junction protein complexes localized between endothelial cells, which act to limit paracellular diffusion. Tight junctions are dynamic complexes of multiple protein constituents including junctional adhesion molecules, occludin, claudins (i.e., claudin-1, -3, and -5), and membrane-associated guanylate kinase-like proteins (i.e., ZO-1, -2, and -3) (Sanchez-Covarrubias, Slosky, Thompson, Davis, & Ronaldson, 2014). Production of ROS and subsequent oxidative stress alters expression and molecular organization of critical tight junction proteins claudin-5 and occludin at the BBB, leading to increased paracellular solute leak (Lochhead et al., 2010; Schreibelt et al., 2007). Reorganization of tight junction complexes and associated leak across the BBB following focal ischemia enables considerable movement of vascular fluid across the microvascular endothelium and development of vasogenic edema (Heo et al., 2005; Pillai et al., 2009; Sandoval & Witt, 2008). Reductions in post-ischemic edema and injury have been shown *in vivo* by vascular endothelial growth factor antagonism (van Bruggen et al., 1999), which has been identified as a possible mechanism that controls tight junction integrity (Fischer et al., 2007); these data indicate that tight junction disruption is involved in progression of ischemic brain injury.

Decreased expression of occludin is directly associated with increased BBB permeability as shown by an *in vivo* rodent model of H/R (Witt, Mark, Hom, & Davis, 2003; Witt et al., 2005). Additionally, H/R causes trafficking of occludin away from BBB tight junction protein complexes (Lochhead et al., 2010; McCaffrey et al., 2009). This occludin relocalization can be prevented *in vivo* by 4-hydoxy-2,2,6,6-tetramethylpiperidine-*N*-oxyl (TEMPOL) treatment, a superoxide scavenging antioxidant that readily crosses the BBB (Cuzzocrea et al., 2000; Deng-Bryant, Singh, Carrico, & Hall, 2008; Kwon et al., 2003; Lochhead et al., 2012; Rak et al., 2000; Saito, Takeshita, Ueda, & Ozawa, 2003; Zhelev et al., 2009). Specifically, TEMPOL prevents breakage of disulfide bonds on occludin thereby blocking disruption of occludin oligomeric assemblies and subsequent blood-to-brain leak of circulating solutes (Lochhead et al., 2010). Similarly, SOD-mimetics such as metalloporphyrin catalytic antioxidants and ceria nanoparticles have also been successful in protecting against ischemic damage to the BBB in *in vivo* rodent model systems (Kim et al., 2012; Pacher et al., 2007).

The increase in BBB permeability observed during ischemic stroke involves changes to transcellular transport pathways in addition to tight junction modifications. For example, Yeh et al. demonstrated in immortalized rat brain endothelial cells that hypoxia upregulates glucose transporters (GLUT1) (Yeh, Lin, & Fu, 2008). Functional expression of the sodium glucose cotransporter-1 (SGLT1) was also increased after ischemia/reperfusion (Elfeber et al., 2004). Vemula et al. showed that SGLT plays a significant role along with GLUT1 in glucose uptake across the BBB and cerebral edema formation during ischemia (Vemula et al., 2009). Recently, our own laboratory discovered that the endogenous transporter, organic anion transporting polypeptide (OATP in humans; Oatp in rodents) 1a4 (Oatp1a4), also increases at the rodent BBB and is capable of promoting transcellular xenobiotic transport (Thompson et al., 2014). Specifically, Oatp1a4 contributes to blood-to-brain flux of therapeutic drugs following H/R, some of which show considerable potential as neuroprotectants (Thompson et al., 2014). Increases in nonspecific vesicular transport and pinocytosis within BBB endothelial cells have also been reported (Cipolla, Crete, Vitullo, & Rix, 2004; Plateel, Teissier, & Cecchelli, 1997).

Ischemic stroke is an amalgamation of a vascular disorder and a neuronal disease. Central to the pathogenesis of ischemic damage is the neurovascular unit, a cohesive organization of endothelial cells, pericytes, neurons, and astrocytes as well as extracellular matrix. Cell-to-cell interactions and signaling occur in a coordinated manner between these multiple cell types and matrix constituents, events required for physiological and pathological functioning of the BBB. For example, chemical destruction of perivascular astrocytes has been shown to cause increased BBB permeability that is characterized by decreased occludin protein expression (Willis, Leach, Clarke, Nolan, & Ray, 2004). Focal loss of astrocytes both in the necrotic core and in the apoptotic penumbra contributes to increased BBB permeability during cerebral ischemia. Similarly, pericyte association with the microvasculature endothelium is critical to vascular integrity and loss of this relationship may lead to vascular leakage and induction of edema (Bonkowski, Katyshev, Balabanov, Borisov, & Dore-Duffy, 2011). Perturbation of the neurovascular unit generally leads to compromised BBB integrity and increased permeability. Such BBB permeabilization enables bloodborne substances that are normally restricted, such as excitatory amino acids, kinins, prostaglandins, metals, and proteins to enter the brain (Plateel et al., 1997). Pharmacological interventions aimed at preservation of the neurovascular unit and protection of neurons within the penumbra would clearly prevent exacerbation of brain tissue damage during cerebral ischemia/reperfusion.

2.5. Therapeutic approaches

Mechanisms of cell injury and/or death in the ischemic core occur extremely rapidly (i.e., within minutes), thereby rendering this region difficult to protect using traditional pharmacological approaches. In contrast, cells within the penumbra die more slowly by active cell death mechanisms (Arai et al., 2011). Residual and collateral blood flow to neurons within the penumbra allow preservation of brain tissue for up to 6 h following ischemic stroke, thus rendering therapeutic interventions theoretically possible (Arai et al., 2011). The primary goal of drug therapy for acute ischemic stroke is to salvage the penumbra as much as possible and as early as possible to prevent continued growth of the ischemic core and progressively worsening neurological outcomes (Liu et al., 2010). Throughout ischemia/reperfusion brain injury, the biophysical ramifications from changes in cerebral blood flow create unique challenges to drug delivery. Differences in these changes may occur between ischemic core and penumbra, or between ipsilateral and contralateral ischemic hemispheres. For example, decreased blood flow to the penumbra will likely decrease drug CNS bioavailability, reducing the ability of a drug to attain efficacious concentrations at its target site. Additionally, increased BBB permeability, a key determinant of blood-to-brain drug uptake, is not a static phenomenon during cerebral ischemia/reperfusion injury. Following transient focal ischemia in experimental stroke models, enhanced BBB permeability has been observed at approximately 5 h after ischemic insult, with a secondary increase at 72 h (Ronaldson & Davis, 2012; Shah et al., 2013). However, in the clinic, stroke patients have been reported to experience BBB opening only during early reperfusion (Barr et al., 2010; Henning, Latour, & Warach, 2008; Kastrup et al., 2008). Focal ischemic stroke, which causes lesions in discrete brain regions, results in regional BBB permeability differences between the ipsilateral and contralateral hemispheres (Cui et al., 2010; Hatashita & Hoff, 1990). However, within the affected hemisphere, recent studies have found no significant difference in BBB permeability between the ischemic core and the penumbra in human patients with acute hemispheric stroke as assessed by first-pass perfusion computed tomography (Dankbaar et al., 2008; Nguyen et al., 2013). Given the similarities in pathophysiological damage between the core and the penumbra, BBB permeability and therefore blood-to-brain movement of drugs and fluid is likely comparable between these two brain regions during ischemia/reperfusion injury.

Currently, there is only one therapeutic agent that has been approved by the US Food and Drug Administration for acute ischemic stroke treatment, recombinant tissue plasminogen activator (rt-PA) (Jahan & Vinuela, 2009). The objective of rt-PA therapy is to restore blood flow and oxygen supply to ischemic brain tissue. However, considerable brain cellular damage occurs when cerebral perfusion is reestablished (i.e., reoxygenation). Additionally, rt-PA therapy has a narrow therapeutic window, high risk of intracerebral bleeding, and other adverse effects (Messe et al., 2012; Shah et al., 2013). Among hospitals participating in the Get With The Guidelines (GWTG)-Stroke program, only 24.7% of ischemic stroke patients that presented themselves within 3 h were even eligible to receive rt-PA (Messe et al., 2012). Additionally, aspirin is included in the clinical standard of care for ischemic stroke because its anticoagulant properties may prevent against recurrent strokes during the high-risk period immediately after the initial ischemic insult (Chen et al., 2000). Aspirin treatment is exclusively preventative and does not confer any protection and/or rescue of ischemic brain tissue. Therefore, there is a critical need in stroke therapy for neuroprotective and/or antioxidant drugs that can be effectively delivered to the brain for "rescue" of salvageable tissue.

Currently, there is considerable interest in neuroprotective/antioxidant properties of HMG-CoA reductase inhibitors (i.e., statins). Recent evidence suggests that statins can act as free-radical scavengers independent of their well-documented effects on cholesterol biosynthesis (Barone et al., 2011; Butterfield et al., 2012; Kassan, Montero, & Sevilla, 2010). For example, *in vivo* studies in dogs demonstrated that high-dose atorvastatin reduced markers of oxidative and nitrosative stress (i.e., protein carbonyls, 4-hydroxy-2-nonenal, 3-nitrotyrosine) and increased the ratio of GSH to reduced GSH in the brain but not in the periphery, suggesting that this drug has efficacy as a neuroprotectant and CNS antioxidant (Barone et al., 2011). Studies in an *in vivo* rodent model of subarachnoid hemorrhage showed that atorvastatin reduced brain caspase-3 activity and DNA fragmentation, implying an ability to attenuate neuronal apoptosis (Cheng, Wei, Zhi-Dan, Shi-Guang, & Xiang-Zhen, 2009; Pan et al., 2010). In addition, rosuvastatin has been shown to protect neurons from stress induced by oxygen-glucose deprivation in rat cerebrocortical neuronal cultures, perhaps by decreasing ROS levels (Domoki et al., 2009). Similarly, simvastatin, a lipophilic HMG-CoA reductase inhibitor, has shown neuroprotective effects against oxygen-glucose deprivation and subsequent reoxygenation by inhibiting production of 4-hydroxy-2*E*-nonenal (HNE), a cytotoxic product of lipid peroxidation, and directly reducing HNE toxicity (Lim et al., 2006). In addition to these preclinical studies, statin treatment has been shown to reduce cerebral expression of oxidative stress markers (i.e., nitrotyrosine and F2-isoprostanes) in clinical investigations (Davignon, Jacob, & Mason, 2004; Shishehbor et al., 2003).

To date, the exact mechanism for statin-induced neuroprotection has not been elucidated. It has been proposed that neuroprotective effects of atorvastatin may be due to targeting and subsequent upregulation of biliverdin reductase-A, a pleiotropic enzyme known to be involved in cellular stress responses (Barone et al., 2012). Of particular note, Barone et al. (2012) reported that increased activity of biliverdin reductase-A induced by atorvastatin was inversely correlated with indices of oxidative stress, which points towards an antioxidant mechanism for statins. It has also been suggested that statins can exert neuroprotective effects through enhancement of eNOS expression in the CNS (Endres et al., 1998; Sironi et al., 2003), thereby improving collateral blood flow to the ischemic penumbra.

3. DRUG DELIVERY TO THE HYPOXIC/ISCHEMIC BRAIN

The ability of drugs such as statins to be effective neurotherapeutics following cerebral hypoxia/ischemia requires efficient and precise CNS delivery. A recent comparative *in vitro* study that evaluated efficacy of statins as neuroprotectants by assessing their chemical structure, theoretical lipophilicity, and ability to protect against neuronal cell death induced by okadaic acid, concluded that both atorvastatin and rosuvastatin were effective in mitigating neuronal cell death (Sierra et al., 2011). However, both of these drugs had CNS permeability values close to zero and BBB penetration estimates of less than 5% (Sierra et al., 2011). This study illustrates the critical importance of identifying and characterizing endogenous transport mechanisms that can be utilized to facilitate CNS statin delivery. Here, we describe two strategies for optimizing CNS statin delivery: targeting endogenous BBB uptake transport systems (i.e., OATPs/Oatps) and nanoparticle-based drug delivery technologies.

3.1. Organic anion transporting polypeptides

Brain uptake and distribution of currently marketed drugs such as statins are governed by transport systems that are endogenously expressed at the microvascular endothelium. Of these transport systems, some are unidirectional (i.e., facilitate either blood-to-brain or brain-to-blood peptide transport) and others are bidirectional. One family of transporters that may have utility in brain delivery (i.e., blood-to-brain transport) of statins is the OATPs/Oatps. OATPs/Oatps are a group of sodium-independent transporters classified within the larger solute carrier (SLC) superfamily (Ronaldson et al., 2013). The concept of focusing on influx processes (i.e., OATP) at the BBB as opposed to inhibition of efflux processes (i.e., P-gp) represents a highly promising approach to optimizing CNS drug delivery.

In rodent brain, expression of Oatp1a4, Oatp1c1, and Oatp2a1 have been reported in capillary enriched fractions, capillary endothelial cells, and brain microvessels (Kis et al., 2006; Ronaldson & Davis, 2011; Westholm, Stenehjem, Rumbley, Drewes, & Anderson, 2009). Oatp1c1 primarily transports thyroxine and conjugated sterols (Westholm et al., 2009), while Oatp2a1 regulates BBB transport of prostaglandins (Kis et al., 2006). In contrast, Oatp1a4 is the primary drug transporting Oatp isoform expressed at the rat BBB (Ronaldson & Davis, 2013). As shown in Fig. 2, studies in Oatp1a4(−/−) mice have demonstrated reduced blood-to-brain transport of pitavastatin and rosuvastatin as compared to wild-type controls, which suggests involvement of Oatp1a4 in statin transport across the BBB (Ose et al., 2010). The human orthologue of Oatp1a4 is OATP1A2, which exhibits an enrichment of mRNA expression in the brain as compared with other tissues including liver, kidney, and gastrointestinal tract (Kullak-Ublick et al., 1995; Steckelbroeck et al., 2004). Immunofluorescence staining of human brain frontal cortex demonstrated OATP1A2 localization at both the apical and basolateral sides of the microvascular endothelium (Gao et al., 2000). Although not directly studied at the BBB, OATP1A2 has been shown to transport rosuvastatin in isolated human hepatocytes and atorvastatin in human embryonic kidney cells (HEK293) stably transfected with OATP1A2 (Ho et al., 2006; Mandery et al., 2011). Localization and substrate profiles of OATP/Oatp isoforms known to be present at BBB are summarized in Table 1. Recently, we reported for the first time increased functional expression of Oatp1a4 at the BBB in rats subjected to H/R (Thompson et al., 2014). Evidence for increased Oatp1a4 transport at the BBB included increased brain accumulation of both

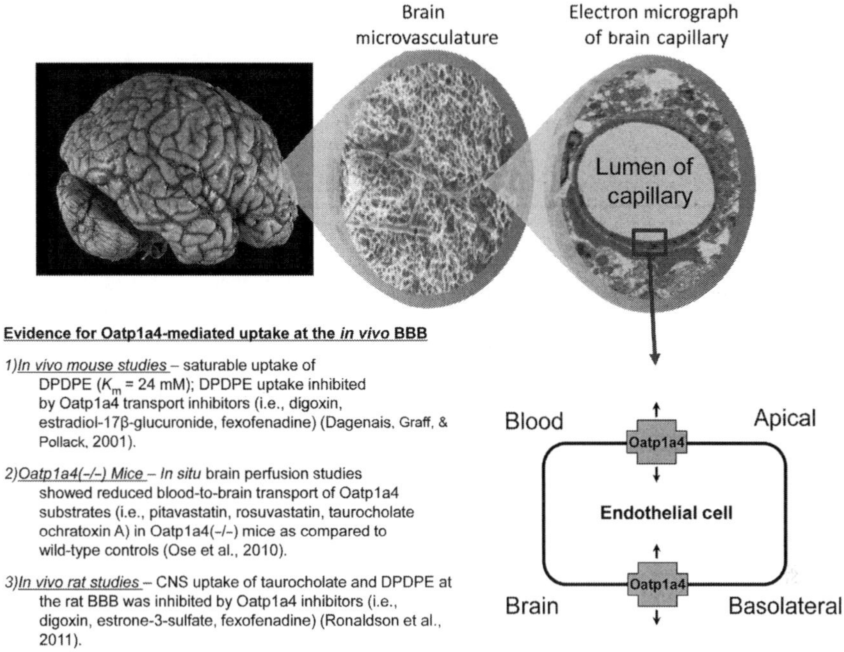
Brain microvasculature
Electron micrograph of brain capillary
Lumen of capillary
Evidence for Oatp1a4-mediated uptake at the in vivo BBB
1)In vivo mouse studies – saturable uptake of DPDPE (K_m = 24 mM); DPDPE uptake inhibited by Oatp1a4 transport inhibitors (i.e., digoxin, estradiol-17β-glucuronide, fexofenadine) (Dagenais, Graff, & Pollack, 2001).
2)Oatp1a4(-/-) Mice – In situ brain perfusion studies showed reduced blood-to-brain transport of Oatp1a4 substrates (i.e., pitavastatin, rosuvastatin, taurocholate ochratoxin A) in Oatp1a4(-/-) mice as compared to wild-type controls (Ose et al., 2010).
3)In vivo rat studies – CNS uptake of taurocholate and DPDPE at the rat BBB was inhibited by Oatp1a4 inhibitors (i.e., digoxin, estrone-3-sulfate, fexofenadine) (Ronaldson et al., 2011).
Blood
Apical
Oatp1a4
Endothelial cell
Oatp1a4
Brain
Basolateral

Figure 2 Evidence for blood-to-brain drug transport mediated by Oatp1a4 at the blood–brain barrier (BBB). Previous *in vivo* studies have shown that CNS uptake of drugs such as opioid peptide analgesics (i.e., DPDPE) and HMG-CoA reductase inhibitors (i.e., pitavastatin, rosuvastatin) is determined by functional expression of Oatp1a4 at the luminal and abluminal plasma membrane of the brain microvascular endothelium. *Adapted from Ronaldson and Davis (2013).*

Table 1 Localization and substrate profiles of OATP/Oatp isoforms known to be present at the blood–brain barrier (BBB)

Human Oatp isoform	BBB expression	Rodent ortholog	BBB expression	Potential substrate drugs
OATP1A2	Apical and basolateral	Oatp1a4	Apical and basolateral	HMG-CoA reductase inhibitors (e.g., atorvastatin, cerivastatin, fluvastatin, pitavastatin, pravastatin, rosuvastatin, simvastatin acid); opioid analgesic peptides (e.g., DPDPE)
OATP1C1	Localization not confirmed	Oatp1c1	Apical	Thyroid hormones and conjugated sterols
OATP2A1	Localization not confirmed	Oatp2a1	Apical	Prostaglandins

taurocholate and atorvastatin, two known Oatp substrates, and attenuation of taurocholate and atorvastatin uptake by Oatp transport inhibitors (i.e., estrone-3-sulfate, fexofenadine). Oatp1a4-mediated delivery of atorvastatin across the brain microvascular endothelium was demonstrated by our laboratory under normoxic conditions, hypoxic conditions, and following H/R stress (Thompson et al., 2014).

OATP/Oatp isoforms are also known to be involved in blood-to-brain transport of opioid analgesic peptides such as deltorphin II and [D-penicillamine2,5]-enkephalin (DPDPE) (Gao et al., 2000; Ose et al., 2010; Ronaldson, Finch, Demarco, Quigley, & Davis, 2011). This is highly significant due to preclinical evidence that such opioid peptides may have efficacy in treatment of ischemic stroke, particularly in the context of cerebral edema. For example, opioid peptides that selectively bind to the μ-opioid receptor (e.g., [Tyr-D-Ala, N-CH, -Phe4, Glyol]-enkephalin [DAMGO]), δ-opioid receptor (e.g., DPDPE), and κ-opioid receptor (e.g., U50,488) reduced water uptake in rat hippocampal slices *in situ* (Yang, Shah, Wang, Karamyan, & Abbruscato, 2011; Yang, Wang, Shah, Karamyan, & Abbruscato, 2011). However, the utility of these drugs as stroke therapeutics is dependent on their effective CNS delivery. Our group (Ronaldson et al., 2011) and others (Dagenais et al., 2004; Ose et al., 2010) have shown that opioid peptides (i.e., DPDPE) are Oatp1a4 substrates, further emphasizing the need to evaluate this SLC transporter as a facilitator of CNS drug delivery. Such an understanding of Oatp-mediated transport mechanisms at the BBB involved in CNS delivery of peptides will undoubtedly aid in development of these compounds as potential therapeutics.

3.1.1 Regulation of Oatp1a4

Although pathophysiological stressors can modulate endogenous BBB transporters, such changes must be effectively controlled in order to provide optimal CNS drug delivery. For example, studies in our *in vivo* inflammatory pain model demonstrated increased BBB functional expression of Oatp1a4 only between 1 and 6 h after induction of pain/inflammation (Ronaldson et al., 2011). We also observed Oatp1a4 upregulation at the BBB in our H/R model only following reoxygenation time points up to 1 h (Thompson et al., 2014). Therefore, if Oatps are to be utilized for effective delivery of therapeutics (i.e., statins, opioid peptides) for treatment of diseases with an H/R component, its functional expression must be controlled over a more desirable time course than is possible by only relying on pathophysiological processes. This objective can be accomplished by pharmacological targeting of signaling pathways that regulate Oatp functional expression such as the transforming growth factor-β (TGF-β) system (Ronaldson et al., 2011). TGF-β signaling is well known to regulate multiple cellular processes including vascular remodeling (Pepper, 1997). The TGF-βs are a family of pleiotropic cytokines that signal by binding to a heterotetrameric complex of type I and type II serine/threonine kinase receptors (Derynck & Zhang, 2003). The type I receptors, also known as activin receptor-like kinases (ALKs), propagate intracellular signals through phosphorylation of receptor-specific Smad proteins (i.e., receptor-regulated (R)-Smads). Phosphorylated (R)-Smads form complexes with the common Smad (i.e., Smad4), enabling nuclear translocation and subsequent changes in target gene transcription (Derynck et al., 2003). At the BBB, only two ALK receptors (i.e., ALK1, ALK5) have been identified (Ronaldson, Demarco, Sanchez-Covarrubias, Solinsky, & Davis, 2009). TGF-β regulates the endothelial cell activation state and angiogenesis through a precise balance between ALK1 and ALK5 signaling processes (Goumans et al., 2002; Wu, Ma, Han, Wang, & Chen, 2006). Whereas the ALK1 pathway leads to endothelial activation characterized by increased permeability, ALK5-mediated signaling promotes vascular resolution that is demarcated by decreased permeability (Lebrin, Deckers, Bertolino, & Ten Dijke, 2005; Wu et al., 2006). Such effects on vascular permeability have been attributed to the ability of TGF-β signaling to alter expression of tight junction constituent proteins (Ishihara et al., 2008; Ronaldson et al., 2009; Watabe et al., 2003).

Recently, our laboratory demonstrated that pharmacological inhibition of TGF-β signaling led to increased microvascular expression and activity of Oatp1a4 at the BBB (Ronaldson et al., 2011; Thompson et al., 2014). Of particular interest was the observation that this blockade of TGF-β/ALK5 signaling using the specific ALK5 antagonist, SB431542, enhanced Oatp1a4 transport activity in saline-treated control animals as indicated by increased delivery to the brain of Oatp substrates such as taurocholate and atorvastatin (Ronaldson et al., 2011; Thompson et al., 2014). Since TGF-β1 expression (i.e., the natural ligand for ALK5) is increased in the brain and in the periphery following cerebral hypoxia (Doyle, Cekanaviciute, Mamer, & Buckwalter, 2010), pharmacological blockade of TGF-β/ALK5 signaling may be critical in targeting Oatps for CNS drug delivery. A crucial consideration in interpretation of our data is the contribution of paracellular diffusion to brain uptake of Oatp substrate drugs. Our laboratory has previously reported that inhibition of TGF-β/ALK5 signaling with SB431542 increased paracellular BBB permeability for solutes such as sucrose by altering tight junction integrity (Ronaldson et al., 2009). The molecular weight of taurocholate (537.7 Da) and atorvastatin (558.6 Da) are greater than that of sucrose (342 Da), suggesting a lesser degree of paracellular diffusion. As our data showed no statistical difference in taurocholate or atorvastatin uptake in the presence of Oatp1a4 inhibitors in animals administered SB431542, we conclude that paracellular diffusion was not a significant factor in CNS uptake of taurocholate or atorvastatin. Nonetheless, it is critical to correct for paracellular transport in any study examining the effect of targeting TGF-β signaling for optimization of CNS drug delivery. Our work on TGF-β/ALK5 signaling is highly novel and significant because we showed that this pathway can regulate permeability at the BBB by increasing functional expression of an influx transporter. Furthermore, these studies highlight the potential of the TGF-β/ALK5 pathway as a pharmacological target that can be used for optimization of drug delivery to the CNS, particularly for treatment of cerebral ischemia.

3.1.2 Transporter/substrate interactions at the BBB

The ability of a pharmacological agent to cross the BBB endothelium and achieve efficacious concentrations within the CNS is dependent on multiple mechanisms of transport. Such mechanisms include uptake into the brain via an influx transporter and/or extrusion from the CNS mediated by an efflux transporter. For many drugs, it is this discrete balance between influx and efflux that determines whether a pharmacological agent will accumulate within the brain extracellular milieu and, therefore, elicit a therapeutic effect. The complexity of drug transporter biology at the BBB is further underscored by the observation that functional expression of such transport proteins may be dramatically altered by pathophysiological stressors (Hayashi et al., 2006; Ronaldson et al., 2011; Seelbach, Brooks, Egleton, & Davis, 2007; Yeh et al., 2008). A thorough understanding of regulation and functional expression of endogenous BBB transporters in both health and disease is critical for optimization of pharmacotherapy. Furthermore, such information will enable more effective targeting of transporters and/or transporter regulatory mechanisms, thus allowing endogenous BBB transport systems to be specifically exploited for improvement of CNS drug delivery.

OATP/Oatp family members are multispecific transporters capable of transporting a vast array of structurally diverse drugs, metabolites, and physiologic substrates. However, a full comprehension of how such transporters can be targeted to promote CNS delivery of therapeutics requires an appreciation that substrates transported by OATP/Oatp family members may also be transport substrates for organic anion transporters (OATs), P-gp, MRP/Mrp isoforms, and breast cancer resistance protein (BCRP in humans; Bcrp in rodents). At the BBB, organic anion transporter 3 (OAT3) (Miyajima, Kusuhara, Fujishima, Adachi, & Sugiyama, 2011; Ohtsuki et al., 2005), P-gp (Bendayan, Ronaldson, Gingras, & Bendayan, 2006; Hawkins, Sykes, & Miller, 2010; Seelbach et al., 2007), and several MRP/Mrp isoforms (Dallas, Miller, & Bendayan, 2006; Hawkins, Ocheltree, Norwood, & Egleton, 2007) are expressed and contributed to brain-to-blood (i.e., efflux) substrate transport. Many drug substrates of OATP/Oatp substrates are also transported by at least one additional transporter such as OAT1, OAT3, P-gp, MRP/Mrp isoforms, or BCRP/Bcrp. For example, DPDPE is a P-gp substrate as well as an Oatp1a4 substrate (Ose et al., 2010; Ronaldson et al., 2011). Additionally, rosuvastatin is a substrate for OAT3 (Windass, Lowes, Wang, & Brown, 2007), Bcrp (Huang, Wang, & Grimm, 2006), and Mrp2 (Abe, Bridges, Yue, & Brouwer, 2008). Therefore, it is highly possible that drugs that enter the brain microvascular endothelium or choroid plexus epithelium via one class of transporter may exit by another. Understanding how changes in expression of a specific transporter might affect brain uptake of a given drug will depend upon a thorough assessment of all competing transporters.

Previous research has attempted to overcome drug efflux transport by pharmacological targeting of transporters such as P-gp. P-gp is a major obstacle to CNS delivery of therapeutics, having almost an inexhaustible substrate profile of small, lipophilic drugs and a strong presence at the BBB. Reducing P-gp activity to allow enhanced passage of therapeutics across the BBB is an attractive prospect. However, translation of direct P-gp inhibition from animal models to the clinic has been unsuccessful, due mostly to systemic toxicity of the P-gp inhibitors themselves (Cannon, Peart, Hawkins, Campos, & Miller, 2012). As an alternative, identification and targeting of molecular signaling pathways that control basal P-gp activity have recently been done by Miller et al. Sphingosine-1-phosphate (S1P), a bioactive lipid metabolite, acting through its receptor (S1PR1) was shown to rapidly and reversibly reduce P-gp transport activity in rats, thereby enhancing brain uptake of drugs such as verapamil, loperamide and paclitaxel (Cannon et al., 2012). S1P signaling was found to be a downstream link to TNFα signaling through TNFR1, endothelin, iNOS and PKCβ1, a pathway previously outlined by Cannon et al. (2012). Speculation as to the mechanism of this P-gp manipulation includes covalent modification or changes to the microenvironment of the transporter. Further investigation into such a signaling pathway may lead to control of BBB efflux transport without sacrificing the neuroprotection afforded by P-gp. Theoretically, such control of P-gp-mediated transport at the molecular level may enhance the ability of influx transporters (i.e., OATPs/Oatps) to optimally deliver drugs to the brain.

3.2. Nanoparticles

Development of new drug delivery technologies is an area of intense research and scientific interest. Common flaws that plague conventional drug treatments include problems with accurate dosing, rapid drug metabolism or degradation, and unwanted distribution profiles. Nanotechnology-based delivery vehicles (i.e., nanoparticles) have emerged as a promising solution to such drug delivery issues. Nanocarriers can give new hope to existing therapeutics that suffer from inefficient delivery or problems with drug-tissue distribution. For example, cytidine 5′ diphosphocholine, found to be neuroprotective in the context of cerebral ischemia/reperfusion injury, is rapidly metabolized by the liver, rendering it incapable of reaching the brain if administered via the systemic circulation (Ghosh, Das, Mandal, Dungdung, & Sarkar, 2010). Encapsulation of cytidine 5′ diphosphocholine into nanoparticle liposomes has been shown to reduce hepatic hydrolysis and enabled this drug to attain therapeutic concentrations in brain parenchyma (Ghosh et al., 2010; Pinzon-Daza et al., 2013).

The term "nanoparticle" is used broadly to describe various nanosystems including liposomes, polymeric particles, hydrogels, micelles, inorganic/solid particles, dendrimers, nanotubes, and quantum dots (Marrache et al., 2013; Singh & Lillard, 2009). Therapeutic agents are typically encapsulated, entrapped, adsorbed, or chemically attached to the nanoparticle surface (Denora, Trapani, Laquintana, Lopedota, & Trapani, 2009). The most widely used and successful nanoparticle systems for delivery of bioactive compounds have been liposomes and polymeric nanoparticles or polymer–drug conjugates (Marrache et al., 2013; Singh & Lillard, 2009). The composition of biodegradable polymeric nanoparticles along with their degradation to biocompatible components can be seen in Fig. 3. In order for nanoparticles to be therapeutically effective, they must exhibit (i) prolonged circulation in the bloodstream (i.e., not immediately filtered

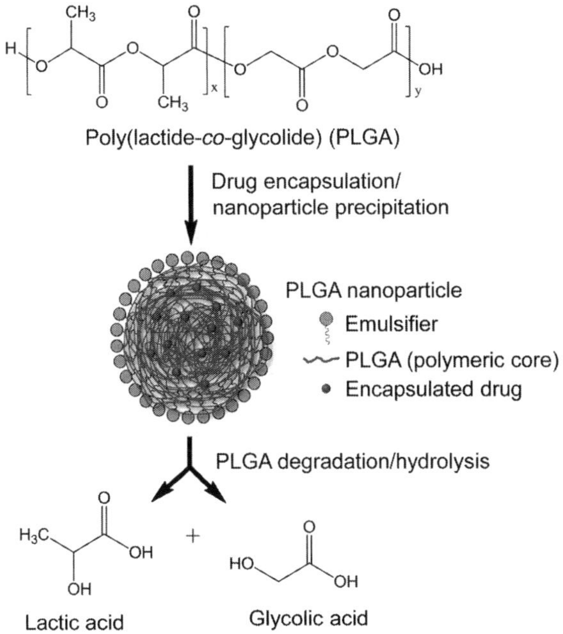

Figure 3 Schematic representation of the synthesis and degradation of poly(lactide-*co*-glycolide) (PLGA) nanoparticles.

or metabolized), (ii) specificity for adequate accumulation in a target tissue, (iii) selective cellular uptake by target endothelial cells, and (iv) controlled release of medicinal drugs. Nanoparticles are generally defined as ranging from 10 to 1000 nm in diameter. Typically, nanoparticles >200 nm are not commonly synthesized because smaller nanoparticles are more readily taken up into cells and/or tissues (Singh & Lillard, 2009). In comparison with microparticles of 1 μm in size, 100 nm particles showed a 2.5-fold greater cellular uptake in Caco-2 cells (Desai, Labhasetwar, Walter, Levy, & Amidon, 1997). Due to their small size and mobility, nanoparticles are able to access a wide variety of "druggable" targets, both extracellular and intracellular. As the smallest capillaries in the body have a diameter of approximately 5–6 μm (Hans & Lowman, 2002), administration of nanoparticles through the microcirculation is a viable approach for facilitation of CNS drug delivery.

Nanoparticle size, solubility, lipophilicity, and surface charge are all critical parameters to consider for efficient CNS drug delivery. Nanoparticle surface modifications are necessary to increase biocompatibility and usually involve a coating or specific attachment of hydrophilic or amphiphilic polymers/surfactants (Pinzon-Daza et al., 2013; Singh & Lillard, 2009). Without such surface modifications, nanoparticles introduced into systemic circulation are quickly cleared from the blood by the reticuloendothelial system (RES) at organs such as the liver, spleen, and lungs. Additionally, blood components (i.e., opsonins) bind to and mark the particle for destruction by phagocytic cells via a process known as opsonization. The degree of opsonization *in vivo* has been shown to correlate with the hydrophobicity of the nanoparticle (Singh & Lillard, 2009). For nanoparticles to be used effectively to deliver therapeutics to the CNS, they must be retained in the systemic circulation long enough to distribute to the desired target. Polysorbate, polyethylene glycol (PEG), polyethylene oxide (PEO), poloxamine, poloxamer, and pluronic polymers are commonly used to coat the surface of nanoparticles for this purpose (Pinzon-Daza et al., 2013; Singh & Lillard, 2009). PEGylation of drug-loaded liposomes has been particularly effective in enhancing the longevity of the particles in systemic circulation. The chemical nature of PEG allows liposomes to circulate in the bloodstream longer, avoiding collection by the RES in the liver and spleen (Hans & Lowman, 2002; Pinzon-Daza et al., 2013; Xie et al., 2012).

3.2.1 Targeting and delivery across the BBB

In addition to increasing the half-life of the encapsulated drug, nanoparticle surface coatings and covalent modifications also present an opportunity to enhance specificity, allowing nanoparticles to cross biological membranes, such as the BBB endothelium. For many nanoparticle delivery systems, PEG is used for this purpose because it has minimal effects on drug–matrix interactions (Singh & Lillard, 2009). PEG is often used as a linker, providing the chemical moieties or functional groups necessary for conjugation. Once incorporated onto the surface of the nanoparticle, the PEG "arms" of a specified length could then be conjugated with antibodies, peptide sequences, or ligands for targeting specific tissues. The adaptability of nanoparticle drug delivery systems suggests that specific transcellular transport routes can be targeted (i.e., adsorptive-mediated transcytosis, receptor-mediated transcytosis, carrier-mediated transcytosis) for CNS drug delivery (Alyautdin, Khalin, Nafeeza, Haron, & Kuznetsov, 2014). Paracellular diffusion of nanoparticles has also been achieved after administration of hyperosmotic mannitol (Avgoustakis et al., 2002), which causes "shrinkage" of microvascular endothelial cells, thereby mechanically stretching tight junction protein complexes (Denora et al., 2009; Ikeda, Bhattacharjee, Kondoh, Nagashima, & Tamaki, 2002). However, such a nonselective increase in paracellular diffusion also allows potentially neurotoxic blood-borne substances to accumulate in the brain. A more efficient approach is targeting of receptor-mediated endocytosis for delivery of drug-loaded nanoparticles through the BBB (Pinzon-Daza et al., 2013). Insulin, transferrin, lactoferrin, glutathione, peptides, and apolipoproteins are among the ligands successfully utilized to achieve receptor-mediated transcytosis of nanoparticles and drug delivery to the CNS (Alyautdin et al., 2014; Pinzon-Daza et al., 2013).

The biopolymer polysorbate has been especially successful in delivering therapeutics to brain parenchyma. Polysorbate coated nanoparticles are thought to permeate the BBB through receptor-mediated endocytosis by binding to low-density lipoprotein (LDL) receptors (Hans et al., 2002). Apolipoprotein E (ApoE), found in blood plasma, has been shown to adsorb on the surface of the polysorbate 20-, 40-, 60-, or 80-coated nanoparticles and likely mimics LDL, allowing receptor binding (Kreuter, 2001). Polysorbate 80 in particular has been shown to successfully cross the BBB as demonstrated by Kreuter et al. using polybutylcyanoacrylate nanoparticles (Beletsi, Leontiadis, Klepetsanis, Ithakissios, & Avgoustakis, 1999; Kreuter et al., 2003; Ramge et al., 2000). PLGA-b-PEG nanoparticles loaded with atorvastatin and coated in polysorbate 80 have been characterized and shown to accumulate in the rat brain *in vivo* (Simsek, Eroglu, Kurum, & Ulubayram, 2013). Similar to polysorbate-coated particles, poly(methoxy-PEG-cyanoacrylate-*co*-hexadecyl cyanoacrylate) (PEG-PHDCA) nanoparticles incubated in rat serum also adsorbed ApoE and ApoB100 on their surface and were delivered across the BBB into the CNS with greater success than apolipoprotein-lacking nanoparticles (Kim et al., 2007). However, dependence on whole protein adsorption on nanoparticle surfaces may not be the most efficient method for delivery of therapeutics across the BBB. Only a fraction of the nanoparticles will have adsorbed whole protein in the correct conformation to bind to and initiate endocytosis. Additionally, maximal efficacy of receptor-mediated endocytosis has been observed when smaller, targeting peptides for a specific endogenous receptor, such as transferrin, were employed in place of the whole protein as shown by Prades et al. (2012) using gold nanoparticles. To date, utility of nanoparticle-mediated delivery of neuroprotective drugs (i.e., statins) has not been studied in the context of cerebral hypoxia and/or ischemia.

Specific endogenous BBB transporters have also been targeted as means of nanoparticle drug release into the CNS. For example, Xie and colleagues synthesized liposomes modified by PEGs of varying lengths, covalently linking cholesterol with glucose. The glucose molecule was then recognized by the GLUT1 transporter in BBB endothelial cells and the liposomes were successful in delivering their drug load into the CNS. The length of the PEG chain was also found to affect BBB crossing as PEG-modified liposomes with a relative long chain length (i.e., PEG1000) maximized drug transport across the BBB barrier and subsequent uptake into brain parenchyma. However, the PEG linker between the ligand (i.e., glucose molecule for GLUT1) and liposome can be too long (i.e., PEG > 2000) and may result in self-folding and insufficient exposure of the covalently attached ligand (Xie et al., 2012).

3.2.2 Drug release

Nanoparticles composed of biodegradable polymers such as poly(lactic acid-*co*-glycolic acid) (PLGA) are perhaps the most accepted and widely used nanoparticle material. PLGA and related polymers PGA and PLA have been approved by the FDA as biocompatible and biodegradable drug delivery systems (Marrache et al., 2013; Singhal et al., 2013). The success of these polymeric nanoparticles is largely due to their aptitude for controlled drug release, which is perhaps the most critical parameter in nanoparticle formulation. The rate of drug release from nanoparticles is dependent on interactions between drug molecules and nanoparticle materials, the solubility of the drug, the diffusion rate of the drug through the nanoparticle matrix, and the degradation rate of the nanoparticle (Singh & Lillard, 2009). Nanoparticle drug delivery systems tend to exhibit an initial burst of drug release followed by a slower, sustained release. For example, Suh et al. demonstrated *in vitro* that 40% of loaded drug (i.e., paclitaxel) was released from PEO–PLGA nanoparticles within the first 3 days (Suh, Jeong, Rathi, & Kim, 1998). Afterward, drug release abated but continued, liberating a total of 85% of paclitaxel in 4 weeks. This initial burst observed is ascribed to drug molecules being weakly adsorbed to the nanoparticle matrix (Singh & Lillard, 2009), leading to rapid dissociation. Particle size has a significant effect on drug loading and unloading. Specifically, particles that are larger in size have a reduced surface area-to-volume ratio compared to smaller particles, and therefore exhibit a smaller initial burst of drug release followed by a longer sustained release. Smaller particles, conversely, have smaller cores and therefore the majority of the drug molecules are either at or near the nanoparticle surface. This leads to an enhanced initial burst of drug release (Hans & Lowman, 2002; Singh & Lillard, 2009). Regardless, the utility of nanoparticle carriers as drug delivery mechanisms has been well demonstrated and shows considerable potential for targeted drug delivery to the brain (Hans & Lowman, 2002; Marrache et al., 2013; Singh & Lillard, 2009).

4. CONCLUSION

Cerebral ischemia involves a dynamic pathophysiology that comprises a multiplicity of processes, including excitotoxicity, disruption of Ca^{2+} homeostasis, ROS generation, cerebral inflammation, and neuronal apoptosis. A detailed understanding of such pathways offers immense opportunities to design novel treatment strategies for cerebral ischemia, a condition with few viable therapeutic options. Successful pharmacotherapy of cerebral ischemia requires that drugs achieve effective concentrations in the CNS, a therapeutic goal that is hindered by the BBB. It was originally believed that microvascular endothelial cells in the brain represented a static barrier to administered therapeutics and that drug delivery across the BBB largely depended on physiochemical properties of the drug (i.e., lipophilicity, charge, size) and passive diffusion. However, many lipophilic drugs have limited or no efficacy in treatment of neurological diseases due to a clear inability to cross the BBB. This observation emphasizes involvement of ATP-binding cassette drug efflux transporters, which are key determinants of the ability of a therapeutic agent to accumulate within the brain. Such efflux transporters are a formidable obstacle; however, recent studies have shown that small-molecule drug delivery can be facilitated by targeting endogenous uptake transporters (i.e., OATPs/Oatps) at the BBB. Furthermore, molecular mechanisms that regulate the activity of OATPs/Oatps (i.e., TGF-β/ALK5 signaling) have been uncovered, offering an opportunity to "control" OATP/Oatp functional expression in order to provide optimal drug delivery to the CNS (Fig. 4). Additionally, drug-loaded nanoparticles represent a highly adaptable delivery system that offers significant advantages in drug stability and controlled release to the CNS (Fig. 4). A better understanding of mechanisms that regulate endocytosis-mediated uptake at the BBB will allow greater control of drug permeation and/or transport across the BBB via nanoparticles. Perhaps such drug delivery approaches will prove "paradigm shifting" for treatment of cerebral ischemia by enabling precise delivery of therapeutics with neuroprotective properties such as statins. Future work will continue to provide more insight on therapeutic targeting of the BBB via endogenous uptake transport systems and drug-loaded nanoparticles. Ultimately, data derived from these studies will allow achievement of more precise and more effective drug concentrations within the brain, thereby improving treatment of cerebral ischemia.

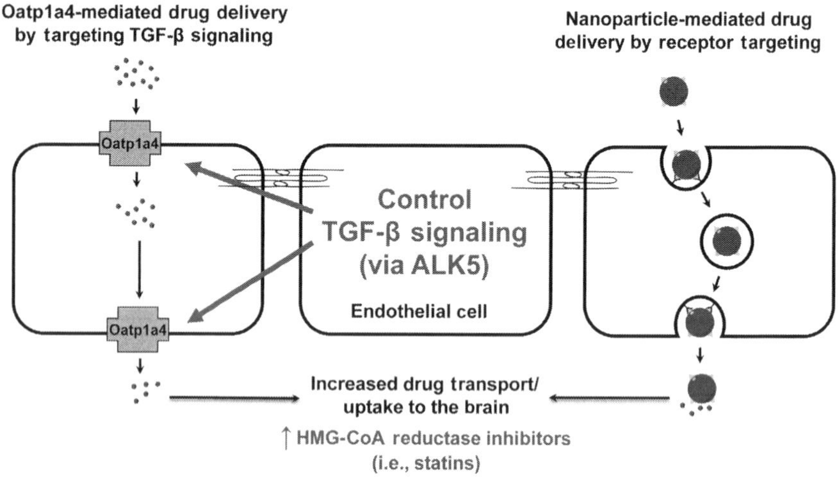

Figure 4 Summary. Data from our laboratory show that organic anion-transporting polypeptide 1a4 (Oatp1a4) facilitates brain delivery of drugs that may exhibit neuroprotective efficacy in treatment of cerebral hypoxia/ischemia. The transforming growth factor-β (TGF-β) signaling pathway regulates Oatp1a4 functional expression and may offer an opportunity to "control" Oatp1a4 expression/activity via small-molecule inhibition of activin receptor-like kinase 5 (ALK5). We also propose that nanotechnology-based delivery vehicles may offer unique advantages in the CNS penetration of therapeutics. Blood–brain barrier (BBB) endothelial cell receptors can be targeted for transcytosis of nanoparticles via attachment of specific ligands (i.e., transferrin).

CONFLICT OF INTEREST

The authors have no conflicts of interest to declare.

REFERENCES

Abe, K., Bridges, A. S., Yue, W., & Brouwer, K. L. (2008). In vitro biliary clearance of angiotensin II receptor blockers and 3-hydroxy-3-methylglutaryl-coenzyme A reductase inhibitors in sandwich-cultured rat hepatocytes: Comparison with in vivo biliary clearance. *The Journal of Pharmacology and Experimental Therapeutics*, *326*(3), 983–990. http://dx.doi.org/10.1124/jpet.108.138073.

Adibhatla, R. M., & Hatcher, J. F. (2008). Tissue plasminogen activator (tPA) and matrix metalloproteinases in the pathogenesis of stroke: Therapeutic strategies. *CNS & Neurological Disorders Drug Targets*, 7(3), 243–253.

Adibhatla, R. M., Hatcher, J. F., & Dempsey, R. J. (2006). Lipids and lipidomics in brain injury and diseases. *The AAPS Journal*, *8*(2), E314–E321. http://dx.doi.org/10.1208/aapsj080236.

Adibhatla, R. M., Hatcher, J. F., Larsen, E. C., Chen, X., Sun, D., & Tsao, F. H. (2006). CDP-choline significantly restores phosphatidylcholine levels by differentially affecting phospholipase A2 and CTP: Phosphocholine cytidylyltransferase after stroke. *The Journal of Biological Chemistry*, *281*(10), 6718–6725. http://dx.doi.org/10.1074/jbc.M512112200.

Aksenova, M. V., Aksenov, M. Y., Mactutus, C. F., & Booze, R. M. (2005). Cell culture models of oxidative stress and injury in the central nervous system. *Current Neurovascular Research*, *2*(1), 73–89.

Alyautdin, R., Khalin, I., Nafeeza, M. I., Haron, M. H., & Kuznetsov, D. (2014). Nanoscale drug delivery systems and the blood-brain barrier. *International Journal of Nanomedicine*, *9*, 795–811. http://dx.doi.org/10.2147/ijn.s52236.

Arai, K., Lok, J., Guo, S., Hayakawa, K., Xing, C., & Lo, E. H. (2011). Cellular mechanisms of neurovascular damage and repair after stroke. *Journal of Child Neurology*, *26*(9), 1193–1198. http://dx.doi.org/10.1177/0883073811408610.

Astrup, J., Siesjo, B. K., & Symon, L. (1981). Thresholds in cerebral ischemia—The ischemic penumbra. *Stroke*, *12*(6), 723–725.

Avgoustakis, K., Beletsi, A., Panagi, Z., Klepetsanis, P., Karydas, A. G., & Ithakissios, D. S. (2002). PLGA-mPEG nanoparticles of cisplatin: In vitro nanoparticle degradation, in vitro drug release and in vivo drug residence in blood properties. *Journal of Controlled Release*, *79*(1–3), 123–135.

Barone, E., Cenini, G., Di Domenico, F., Martin, S., Sultana, R., Mancuso, C., et al. (2011). Long-term high-dose atorvastatin decreases brain oxidative and nitrosative stress in a pre-clinical model of Alzheimer disease: A novel mechanism of action. *Pharmacological Research*, *63*(3), 172–180. http://dx.doi.org/10.1016/j.phrs.2010.12.007.

Barone, E., Mancuso, C., Di Domenico, F., Sultana, R., Murphy, M. P., Head, E., et al. (2012). Biliverdin reductase-A: A novel drug target for atorvastatin in a dog pre-clinical model of Alzheimer disease. *Journal of Neurochemistry*, *120*(1), 135–146. http://dx.doi.org/10.1111/j.1471-4159.2011.07538.x.

Barr, T. L., Latour, L. L., Lee, K. Y., Schaewe, T. J., Luby, M., Chang, G. S., et al. (2010). Blood-brain barrier disruption in humans is independently associated with increased matrix metalloproteinase-9. *Stroke*, *41*(3), e123–e128. http://dx.doi.org/10.1161/STROKEAHA.109.570515.

Beletsi, A., Leontiadis, L., Klepetsanis, P., Ithakissios, D. S., & Avgoustakis, K. (1999). Effect of preparative variables on the properties of poly(dl-lactide-co-glycolide)-methoxypoly(ethyleneglycol) copolymers related to their application in controlled drug delivery. *International Journal of Pharmaceutics*, *182*(2), 187–197.

Bendayan, R., Ronaldson, P. T., Gingras, D., & Bendayan, M. (2006). In situ localization of P-glycoprotein (ABCB1) in human and rat brain. *The Journal of Histochemistry and Cytochemistry*, *54*(10), 1159–1167. http://dx.doi.org/10.1369/jhc.5A6870.2006.

Bonkowski, D., Katyshev, V., Balabanov, R. D., Borisov, A., & Dore-Duffy, P. (2011). The CNS microvascular pericyte: Pericyte-astrocyte crosstalk in the regulation of tissue survival. *Fluids and Barriers of the CNS*, *8*(1), 8. http://dx.doi.org/10.1186/2045-8118-8-8.

Butterfield, D. A., Barone, E., Di Domenico, F., Cenini, G., Sultana, R., Murphy, M. P., et al. (2012). Atorvastatin treatment in a dog preclinical model of Alzheimer's disease leads to up-regulation of haem oxygenase-1 and is associated with reduced oxidative stress in brain. *The International Journal of Neuropsychopharmacology*, *15*(7), 981–987. http://dx.doi.org/10.1017/S1461145711001118.

Camello-Almaraz, C., Gomez-Pinilla, P. J., Pozo, M. J., & Camello, P. J. (2006). Mitochondrial reactive oxygen species and Ca2+ signaling. *American Journal of Physiology. Cell Physiology*, *291*(5), C1082–C1088. http://dx.doi.org/10.1152/ajpcell.00217.2006.

Candelario-Jalil, E. (2009). Injury and repair mechanisms in ischemic stroke: Considerations for the development of novel neurotherapeutics. *Current Opinion in Investigational Drugs*, *10*(7), 644–654.

Cannon, R. E., Peart, J. C., Hawkins, B. T., Campos, C. R., & Miller, D. S. (2012). Targeting blood-brain barrier sphingolipid signaling reduces basal P-glycoprotein activity and improves drug delivery to the brain. *Proceedings of the National Academy of Sciences of the United States of America*, *109*(39), 15930–15935. http://dx.doi.org/10.1073/pnas.1203534109.

Chaitanya, G. V., Steven, A. J., & Babu, P. P. (2010). PARP-1 cleavage fragments: Signatures of cell-death proteases in neurodegeneration. *Cell Communication and Signaling*, *8*, 31. http://dx.doi.org/10.1186/1478-811x-8-31.

Chen, Z. M., Sandercock, P., Pan, H. C., Counsell, C., Collins, R., Liu, L. S., et al. (2000). Indications for early aspirin use in acute ischemic stroke: A combined analysis of 40 000 randomized patients from the Chinese acute stroke trial and the international stroke trial. On behalf of the CAST and IST collaborative groups. *Stroke*, *31*(6), 1240–1249.

Cheng, G., Wei, L., Zhi-Dan, S., Shi-Guang, Z., & Xiang-Zhen, L. (2009). Atorvastatin ameliorates cerebral vasospasm and early brain injury after subarachnoid hemorrhage and inhibits caspase-dependent apoptosis pathway. *BMC Neuroscience*, *10*, 7. http://dx.doi.org/10.1186/1471-2202-10-7.

Cipolla, M. J., Crete, R., Vitullo, L., & Rix, R. D. (2004). Transcellular transport as a mechanism of blood-brain barrier disruption during stroke. *Frontiers in Bioscience*, *9*, 777–785.

Cui, L., Zhang, X., Yang, R., Wang, L., Liu, L., Li, M., et al. (2010). Neuroprotection of early and short-time applying atorvastatin in the acute phase of cerebral ischemia: Down-regulated 12/15-LOX, p38MAPK and cPLA2 expression, ameliorated BBB permeability. *Brain Research*, *1325*, 164–173. http://dx.doi.org/10.1016/j.brainres.2010.02.036.

Cuzzocrea, S., McDonald, M. C., Mota-Filipe, H., Mazzon, E., Costantino, G., Britti, D., et al. (2000). Beneficial effects of tempol, a membrane-permeable radical scavenger, in a rodent model of collagen-induced arthritis. *Arthritis and Rheumatism*, *43*(2), 320–328. http://dx.doi.org/10.1002/1529-0131(200002)43:2<320::AID-ANR11>3.0.CO;2-9.

Dagenais, C., Graff, C. L., & Pollack, G. M. (2004). Variable modulation of opioid brain uptake by P-glycoprotein in mice. *Biochemical Pharmacology*, *67*(2), 269–276.

Dallas, S., Miller, D. S., & Bendayan, R. (2006). Multidrug resistance-associated proteins: Expression and function in the central nervous system. *Pharmacological Reviews*, *58*(2), 140–161. http://dx.doi.org/10.1124/pr.58.2.3.

Dankbaar, J. W., Hom, J., Schneider, T., Cheng, S. C., Lau, B. C., van der Schaaf, I., et al. (2008). Dynamic perfusion CT assessment of the blood-brain barrier permeability: First pass versus delayed acquisition. *AJNR. American Journal of Neuroradiology*, *29*(9), 1671–1676. http://dx.doi.org/10.3174/ajnr.A1203.

Davignon, J., Jacob, R. F., & Mason, R. P. (2004). The antioxidant effects of statins. *Coronary Artery Disease*, *15*(5), 251–258.

del Zoppo, G. J., & Hallenbeck, J. M. (2000). Advances in the vascular pathophysiology of ischemic stroke. *Thrombosis Research*, *98*(3), 73–81.

Deng-Bryant, Y., Singh, I. N., Carrico, K. M., & Hall, E. D. (2008). Neuroprotective effects of tempol, a catalytic scavenger of peroxynitrite-derived free radicals, in a mouse traumatic brain injury model. *Journal of Cerebral Blood Flow and Metabolism*, *28*(6), 1114–1126. http://dx.doi.org/10.1038/jcbfm.2008.10.

Denora, N., Trapani, A., Laquintana, V., Lopedota, A., & Trapani, G. (2009). Recent advances in medicinal chemistry and pharmaceutical technology—Strategies for drug delivery to the brain. *Current Topics in Medicinal Chemistry*, *9*(2), 182–196.

Derynck, R., & Zhang, Y. E. (2003). Smad-dependent and smad-independent pathways in TGF-beta family signalling. *Nature*, *425*(6958), 577–584. http://dx.doi.org/10.1038/nature02006.

Desai, M. P., Labhasetwar, V., Walter, E., Levy, R. J., & Amidon, G. L. (1997). The mechanism of uptake of biodegradable microparticles in Caco-2 cells is size dependent. *Pharmaceutical Research*, *14*(11), 1568–1573.

Domoki, F., Kis, B., Gaspar, T., Snipes, J. A., Parks, J. S., Bari, F., et al. (2009). Rosuvastatin induces delayed preconditioning against oxygen-glucose deprivation in cultured cortical neurons. *American Journal of Physiology. Cell Physiology*, *296*(1), C97–C105. http://dx.doi.org/10.1152/ajpcell.00366.2008.

Doyle, K. P., Cekanaviciute, E., Mamer, L. E., & Buckwalter, M. S. (2010). TGFbeta signaling in the brain increases with aging and signals to astrocytes and innate immune cells in the weeks after stroke. *Journal of Neuroinflammation*, 7, 62. http://dx.doi.org/10.1186/1742-2094-7-62.

Elfeber, K., Kohler, A., Lutzenburg, M., Osswald, C., Galla, H. J., Witte, O. W., et al. (2004). Localization of the Na+-D-glucose cotransporter SGLT1 in the blood-brain barrier. *Histochemistry and Cell Biology*, *121*(3), 201–207. http://dx.doi.org/10.1007/s00418-004-0633-9.

Endres, M., Laufs, U., Huang, Z., Nakamura, T., Huang, P., Moskowitz, M. A., et al. (1998). Stroke protection by 3-hydroxy-3-methylglutaryl (HMG)-CoA reductase inhibitors mediated by endothelial nitric oxide synthase. *Proceedings of the National Academy of Sciences of the United States of America*, *95*(15), 8880–8885.

Fabian, R. H., DeWitt, D. S., & Kent, T. A. (1995). In vivo detection of superoxide anion production by the brain using a cytochrome c electrode. *Journal of Cerebral Blood Flow and Metabolism*, *15*(2), 242–247. http://dx.doi.org/10.1038/jcbfm.1995.30.

Fang, Y. Z., Yang, S., & Wu, G. (2002). Free radicals, antioxidants, and nutrition. *Nutrition*, *18*(10), 872–879.

Fellman, V., & Raivio, K. O. (1997). Reperfusion injury as the mechanism of brain damage after perinatal asphyxia. *Pediatric Research*, *41*(5), 599–606. http://dx.doi.org/10.1203/00006450-199705000-00001.

Feng, W., & Belagaje, S. R. (2013). Recent advances in stroke recovery and rehabilitation. *Seminars in Neurology*, *33*(5), 498–506. http://dx.doi.org/10.1055/s-0033-1364215.

Fischer, S., Gerriets, T., Wessels, C., Walberer, M., Kostin, S., Stolz, E., et al. (2007). Extracellular RNA mediates endothelial-cell permeability via vascular endothelial growth factor. *Blood*, *110*(7), 2457–2465. http://dx.doi.org/10.1182/blood-2006-08-040691.

Gao, B., Hagenbuch, B., Kullak-Ublick, G. A., Benke, D., Aguzzi, A., & Meier, P. J. (2000). Organic anion-transporting polypeptides mediate transport of opioid peptides across blood-brain barrier. *The Journal of Pharmacology and Experimental Therapeutics*, *294*(1), 73–79.

Ghosh, S., Das, N., Mandal, A. K., Dungdung, S. R., & Sarkar, S. (2010). Mannosylated liposomal cytidine 5' diphosphocholine prevent age related global moderate cerebral ischemia reperfusion induced mitochondrial cytochrome c release in aged rat brain. *Neuroscience*, *171*(4), 1287–1299. http://dx.doi.org/10.1016/j.neuroscience.2010.09.049.

Ghosh, A., Sarkar, S., Mandal, A. K., & Das, N. (2013). Neuroprotective role of nanoencapsulated quercetin in combating ischemia-reperfusion induced neuronal damage in young and aged rats. *PLoS One*, *8*(4), e57735. http://dx.doi.org/10.1371/journal.pone.0057735.

Goumans, M. J., Valdimarsdottir, G., Itoh, S., Rosendahl, A., Sideras, P., & ten Dijke, P. (2002). Balancing the activation state of the endothelium via two distinct TGF-beta type I receptors. *The EMBO Journal*, *21*(7), 1743–1753. http://dx.doi.org/10.1093/emboj/21.7.1743.

Guzy, R. D., & Schumacker, P. T. (2006). Oxygen sensing by mitochondria at complex III: The paradox of increased reactive oxygen species during hypoxia. *Experimental Physiology*, *91*(5), 807–819. http://dx.doi.org/10.1113/expphysiol.2006.033506.

Hans, M. L., & Lowman, A. M. (2002). Biodegradable nanoparticles for drug delivery and targeting. *Current Opinion in Solid State and Materials Science*, *6*(4), 319–327. http://dx.doi.org/10.1016/S1359-0286(02)00117-1.

Hatashita, S., & Hoff, J. T. (1990). Role of blood-brain barrier permeability in focal ischemic brain edema. *Advances in Neurology*, *52*, 327–333.

Hawkins, B. T., Ocheltree, S. M., Norwood, K. M., & Egleton, R. D. (2007). Decreased blood-brain barrier permeability to fluorescein in streptozotocin-treated rats. *Neuroscience Letters*, *411*(1), 1–5. http://dx.doi.org/10.1016/j.neulet.2006.09.010.

Hawkins, B. T., Sykes, D. B., & Miller, D. S. (2010). Rapid, reversible modulation of blood-brain barrier P-glycoprotein transport activity by vascular endothelial growth factor. *The Journal of Neuroscience*, *30*(4), 1417–1425. http://dx.doi.org/10.1523/JNEUROSCI.5103-09.2010.

Hayashi, K., Pu, H., Andras, I. E., Eum, S. Y., Yamauchi, A., Hennig, B., et al. (2006). HIV-TAT protein upregulates expression of multidrug resistance protein 1 in the blood-brain barrier. *Journal of Cerebral Blood Flow and Metabolism*, *26*(8), 1052–1065. http://dx.doi.org/10.1038/sj.jcbfm.9600254.

Henning, E. C., Latour, L. L., & Warach, S. (2008). Verification of enhancement of the CSF space, not parenchyma, in acute stroke patients with early blood-brain barrier disruption. *Journal of Cerebral Blood Flow and Metabolism*, *28*(5), 882–886. http://dx.doi.org/10.1038/sj.jcbfm.9600598.

Heo, J. H., Han, S. W., & Lee, S. K. (2005). Free radicals as triggers of brain edema formation after stroke. *Free Radical Biology & Medicine*, *39*(1), 51–70. http://dx.doi.org/10.1016/j.freeradbiomed.2005.03.035.

Ho, R. H., Tirona, R. G., Leake, B. F., Glaeser, H., Lee, W., Lemke, C. J., et al. (2006). Drug and bile acid transporters in rosuvastatin hepatic uptake: Function, expression, and pharmacogenetics. *Gastroenterology*, *130*(6), 1793–1806. http://dx.doi.org/10.1053/j.gastro.2006.02.034.

Huang, L., Wang, Y., & Grimm, S. (2006). ATP-dependent transport of rosuvastatin in membrane vesicles expressing breast cancer resistance protein. *Drug Metabolism and Disposition*, *34*(5), 738–742. http://dx.doi.org/10.1124/dmd.105.007534.

Iadecola, C., & Alexander, M. (2001). Cerebral ischemia and inflammation. *Current Opinion in Neurology*, *14*(1), 89–94.

Ikeda, M., Bhattacharjee, A. K., Kondoh, T., Nagashima, T., & Tamaki, N. (2002). Synergistic effect of cold mannitol and Na(+)/Ca(2+) exchange blocker on blood-brain barrier opening. *Biochemical and Biophysical Research Communications*, *291*(3), 669–674. http://dx.doi.org/10.1006/bbrc.2002.6495.

Ishihara, H., Kubota, H., Lindberg, R. L., Leppert, D., Gloor, S. M., Errede, M., et al. (2008). Endothelial cell barrier impairment induced by glioblastomas and transforming growth factor beta2 involves matrix metalloproteinases and tight junction proteins. *Journal of Neuropathology and Experimental Neurology*, *67*(5), 435–448. http://dx.doi.org/10.1097/NEN.0b013e31816fd622.

Jahan, R., & Vinuela, F. (2009). Treatment of acute ischemic stroke: Intravenous and endovascular therapies. *Expert Review of Cardiovascular Therapy*, 7(4), 375–387. http://dx.doi.org/10.1586/erc.09.13.

Kassan, M., Montero, M. J., & Sevilla, M. A. (2010). In vitro antioxidant activity of pravastatin provides vascular protection. *European Journal of Pharmacology*, *630*(1–3), 107–111. http://dx.doi.org/10.1016/j.ejphar.2009.12.037.

Kastrup, A., Groschel, K., Ringer, T. M., Redecker, C., Cordesmeyer, R., Witte, O. W., et al. (2008). Early disruption of the blood-brain barrier after thrombolytic therapy predicts hemorrhage in patients with acute stroke. *Stroke*, *39*(8), 2385–2387. http://dx.doi.org/10.1161/STROKEAHA.107.505420.

Kempski, O. (2001). Cerebral edema. *Seminars in Nephrology*, *21*(3), 303–307.

Kiedrowski, L. (2007). NCX and NCKX operation in ischemic neurons. *Annals of the New York Academy of Sciences*, *1099*, 383–395. http://dx.doi.org/10.1196/annals.1387.035.

Kim, H. R., Andrieux, K., Gil, S., Taverna, M., Chacun, H., Desmaele, D., et al. (2007). Translocation of poly(ethylene glycol-co-hexadecyl)cyanoacrylate nanoparticles into rat brain endothelial cells: Role of apolipoproteins in receptor-mediated endocytosis. *Biomacromolecules*, *8*(3), 793–799. http://dx.doi.org/10.1021/bm060711a.

Kim, C. K., Kim, T., Choi, I. Y., Soh, M., Kim, D., Kim, Y. J., et al. (2012). Ceria nanoparticles that can protect against ischemic stroke. *Angewandte Chemie International Edition in English*, *51*(44), 11039–11043. http://dx.doi.org/10.1002/anie.201203780.

Kim, M. Y., Zhang, T., & Kraus, W. L. (2005). Poly(ADP-ribosyl)ation by PARP-1: 'PAR-laying' NAD+ into a nuclear signal. *Genes & Development*, *19*(17), 1951–1967. http://dx.doi.org/10.1101/gad.1331805.

Kis, B., Isse, T., Snipes, J. A., Chen, L., Yamashita, H., Ueta, Y., et al. (2006). Effects of LPS stimulation on the expression of prostaglandin carriers in the cells of the blood-brain and blood-cerebrospinal fluid barriers. *Journal of Applied Physiology (1985)*, *100*(4), 1392–1399. http://dx.doi.org/10.1152/japplphysiol.01259.2005.

Kreuter, J. (2001). Nanoparticulate systems for brain delivery of drugs. *Advanced Drug Delivery Reviews*, *47*(1), 65–81.

Kreuter, J., Ramge, P., Petrov, V., Hamm, S., Gelperina, S. E., Engelhardt, B., et al. (2003). Direct evidence that polysorbate-80-coated poly(butylcyanoacrylate) nanoparticles deliver drugs to the CNS via specific mechanisms requiring prior binding of drug to the nanoparticles. *Pharmaceutical Research*, *20*(3), 409–416.

Kuhn, E. W., Liakopoulos, O. J., Stange, S., Deppe, A. C., Slottosch, I., Scherner, M., et al. (2013). Meta-analysis of patients taking statins before revascularization and aortic valve surgery. *The Annals of Thoracic Surgery*, *96*(4), 1508–1516. http://dx.doi.org/10.1016/j.athoracsur.2013.04.096.

Kulik, A., & Ruel, M. (2009). Statins and coronary artery bypass graft surgery: Preoperative and postoperative efficacy and safety. *Expert Opinion on Drug Safety*, *8*(5), 559–571. http://dx.doi.org/10.1517/14740330903188413.

Kullak-Ublick, G. A., Hagenbuch, B., Stieger, B., Schteingart, C. D., Hofmann, A. F., Wolkoff, A. W., et al. (1995). Molecular and functional characterization of an organic anion transporting polypeptide cloned from human liver. *Gastroenterology*, *109*(4), 1274–1282.

Kwon, T. H., Chao, D. L., Malloy, K., Sun, D., Alessandri, B., & Bullock, M. R. (2003). Tempol, a novel stable nitroxide, reduces brain damage and free radical production, after acute subdural hematoma in the rat. *Journal of Neurotrauma*, *20*(4), 337–345. http://dx.doi.org/10.1089/089771503765172291.

Lebrin, F., Deckers, M., Bertolino, P., & Ten Dijke, P. (2005). TGF-beta receptor function in the endothelium. *Cardiovascular Research*, *65*(3), 599–608. http://dx.doi.org/10.1016/j.cardiores.2004.10.036.

Lim, J. H., Lee, J. C., Lee, Y. H., Choi, I. Y., Oh, Y. K., Kim, H. S., et al. (2006). Simvastatin prevents oxygen and glucose deprivation/reoxygenation-induced death of cortical neurons by reducing the production and toxicity of 4-hydroxy-2E-nonenal. *Journal of Neurochemistry*, *97*(1), 140–150. http://dx.doi.org/10.1111/j.1471-4159.2006.03715.x.

Liu, S., Levine, S. R., & Winn, H. R. (2010). Targeting ischemic penumbra: Part I—From pathophysiology to therapeutic strategy. *Journal of Experimental Stroke & Translational Medicine*, *3*(1), 47–55.

Lochhead, J. J., McCaffrey, G., Quigley, C. E., Finch, J., DeMarco, K. M., Nametz, N., et al. (2010). Oxidative stress increases blood-brain barrier permeability and induces alterations in occludin during hypoxia-reoxygenation. *Journal of Cerebral Blood Flow and Metabolism*, *30*(9), 1625–1636. http://dx.doi.org/10.1038/jcbfm.2010.29.

Lochhead, J. J., McCaffrey, G., Sanchez-Covarrubias, L., Finch, J. D., Demarco, K. M., Quigley, C. E., et al. (2012). Tempol modulates changes in xenobiotic permeability and occludin oligomeric assemblies at the blood-brain barrier during inflammatory pain. *American Journal of Physiology Heart and Circulatory Physiology*, *302*(3), H582–H593. http://dx.doi.org/10.1152/ajpheart.00889.2011.

Luo, J., Wang, Y., Chen, H., Kintner, D. B., Cramer, S. W., Gerdts, J. K., et al. (2008). A concerted role of Na+−K+−Cl^- cotransporter and Na+/Ca2+ exchanger in ischemic damage. *Journal of Cerebral Blood Flow and Metabolism*, *28*(4), 737–746. http://dx.doi.org/10.1038/sj.jcbfm.9600561.

Lutsep, H., & Clark, W. (2001). An update of neuroprotectants in clinical development for acute stroke. *Current Opinion in Investigational Drugs*, *2*(12), 1732–1736.

Mandery, K., Sticht, H., Bujok, K., Schmidt, I., Fahrmayr, C., Balk, B., et al. (2011). Functional and structural relevance of conserved positively charged lysine residues in organic anion transporting polypeptide 1B3. *Molecular Pharmacology*, *80*(3), 400–406. http://dx.doi.org/10.1124/mol.111.071282.

Marrache, S., Pathak, R. K., Darley, K. L., Choi, J. H., Zaver, D., Kolishetti, N., et al. (2013). Nanocarriers for tracking and treating diseases. *Current Medicinal Chemistry*, *20*(28), 3500–3514.

Martinez-Romero, R., Canuelo, A., Martinez-Lara, E., Javier Oliver, F., Cardenas, S., & Siles, E. (2009). Poly(ADP-ribose) polymerase-1 modulation of in vivo response of brain hypoxia-inducible factor-1 to hypoxia/reoxygenation is mediated by nitric oxide and factor inhibiting HIF. *Journal of Neurochemistry*, *111*(1), 150–159. http://dx.doi.org/10.1111/j.1471-4159.2009.06307.x.

McCaffrey, G., Willis, C. L., Staatz, W. D., Nametz, N., Quigley, C. A., Hom, S., et al. (2009). Occludin oligomeric assemblies at tight junctions of the blood–brain barrier are altered by hypoxia and reoxygenation stress. *Journal of Neurochemistry*, *110*(1), 58–71. http://dx.doi.org/10.1111/j.1471-4159.2009.06113.x.

Messe, S. R., Fonarow, G. C., Smith, E. E., Kaltenbach, L., Olson, D. M., Kasner, S. E., et al. (2012). Use of tissue-type plasminogen activator before and after publication of the European cooperative acute stroke study III in get with the guidelines-stroke. *Circulation. Cardiovascular Quality and Outcomes*, *5*(3), 321–326. http://dx.doi.org/10.1161/circoutcomes.111.964064.

Miyajima, M., Kusuhara, H., Fujishima, M., Adachi, Y., & Sugiyama, Y. (2011). Organic anion transporter 3 mediates the efflux transport of an amphipathic organic anion, dehydroepiandrosterone sulfate, across the blood-brain barrier in mice. *Drug Metabolism and Disposition*, *39*(5), 814–819. http://dx.doi.org/10.1124/dmd.110.036863.

Murphy, M. P. (2009). How mitochondria produce reactive oxygen species. *The Biochemical Journal*, *417*(1), 1–13. http://dx.doi.org/10.1042/BJ20081386.

Nguyen, G. T., Coulthard, A., Wong, A., Sheikh, N., Henderson, R., O'Sullivan, J. D., et al. (2013). Measurement of blood-brain barrier permeability in acute ischemic stroke using standard first-pass perfusion CT data. *NeuroImage. Clinical*, *2*, 658–662. http://dx.doi.org/10.1016/j.nicl.2013.04.004.

O'Donnell, M. E., Lam, T. I., Tran, L. Q., Foroutan, S., & Anderson, S. E. (2006). Estradiol reduces activity of the blood-brain barrier Na-K-Cl cotransporter and decreases edema formation in permanent middle cerebral artery occlusion. *Journal of Cerebral Blood Flow and Metabolism*, *26*(10), 1234–1249. http://dx.doi.org/10.1038/sj.jcbfm.9600278.

O'Donnell, M. E., Tran, L., Lam, T. I., Liu, X. B., & Anderson, S. E. (2004). Bumetanide inhibition of the blood–brain barrier Na-K-Cl cotransporter reduces edema formation in the rat middle cerebral artery occlusion model of stroke. *Journal of Cerebral Blood Flow and Metabolism*, *24*(9), 1046–1056. http://dx.doi.org/10.1097/01.WCB.0000130867.32663.90.

Ohtsuki, S., Tomi, M., Hata, T., Nagai, Y., Hori, S., Mori, S., et al. (2005). Dominant expression of androgen receptors and their functional regulation of organic anion transporter 3 in·rat brain capillary endothelial cells; comparison of gene expression between the blood–brain and -retinal barriers. *Journal of Cellular Physiology*, *204*(3), 896–900. http://dx.doi.org/10.1002/jcp.20352.

Ose, A., Kusuhara, H., Endo, C., Tohyama, K., Miyajima, M., Kitamura, S., et al. (2010). Functional characterization of mouse organic anion transporting peptide 1a4 in the uptake and efflux of drugs across the blood–brain barrier. *Drug Metabolism and Disposition*, *38*(1), 168–176. http://dx.doi.org/10.1124/dmd.109.029454.

Pacher, P., Beckman, J. S., & Liaudet, L. (2007). Nitric oxide and peroxynitrite in health and disease. *Physiological Reviews*, *87*(1), 315–424. http://dx.doi.org/10.1152/physrev.00029.2006.

Pan, H. C., Yang, D. Y., Ou, Y. C., Ho, S. P., Cheng, F. C., & Chen, C. J. (2010). Neuroprotective effect of atorvastatin in an experimental model of nerve crush injury. *Neurosurgery*, *67*(2), 376–388. http://dx.doi.org/10.1227/01.neu.0000371729.47895.a0, discussion 388–379.

Pepper, M. S. (1997). Transforming growth factor-beta: Vasculogenesis, angiogenesis, and vessel wall integrity. *Cytokine & Growth Factor Reviews*, *8*(1), 21–43.

Petty, M. A., & Wettstein, J. G. (2001). Elements of cerebral microvascular ischaemia. *Brain Research. Brain Research Reviews*, *36*(1), 23–34.

Pillai, D. R., Dittmar, M. S., Baldaranov, D., Heidemann, R. M., Henning, E. C., Schuierer, G., et al. (2009). Cerebral ischemia-reperfusion injury in rats—A 3 T MRI study on biphasic blood-brain barrier opening and the dynamics of edema formation. *Journal of Cerebral Blood Flow and Metabolism*, *29*(11), 1846–1855. http://dx.doi.org/10.1038/jcbfm.2009.106.

Pinzon-Daza, M. L., Campia, I., Kopecka, J., Garzon, R., Ghigo, D., & Riganti, C. (2013). Nanoparticle- and liposome-carried drugs: New strategies for active targeting and drug delivery across blood-brain barrier. *Current Drug Metabolism*, *14*(6), 625–640.

Plateel, M., Teissier, E., & Cecchelli, R. (1997). Hypoxia dramatically increases the non-specific transport of blood-borne proteins to the brain. *Journal of Neurochemistry*, *68*(2), 874–877.

Prades, R., Guerrero, S., Araya, E., Molina, C., Salas, E., Zurita, E., et al. (2012). Delivery of gold nanoparticles to the brain by conjugation with a peptide that recognizes the transferrin receptor. *Biomaterials*, *33*(29), 7194–7205. http://dx.doi.org/10.1016/j.biomaterials.2012.06.063.

Pundik, S., Xu, K., & Sundararajan, S. (2012). Reperfusion brain injury: Focus on cellular bioenergetics. *Neurology*, *79*(13 Suppl. 1), S44–S51. http://dx.doi.org/10.1212/WNL.0b013e3182695a14.

Rak, R., Chao, D. L., Pluta, R. M., Mitchell, J. B., Oldfield, E. H., & Watson, J. C. (2000). Neuroprotection by the stable nitroxide tempol during reperfusion in a rat model of transient focal ischemia. *Journal of Neurosurgery*, *92*(4), 646–651. http://dx.doi.org/10.3171/jns.2000.92.4.0646.

Ramge, P., Unger, R. E., Oltrogge, J. B., Zenker, D., Begley, D., Kreuter, J., et al. (2000). Polysorbate-80 coating enhances uptake of polybutylcyanoacrylate (PBCA)-nanoparticles by human and bovine primary brain capillary endothelial cells. *The European Journal of Neuroscience*, *12*(6), 1931–1940.

Roger, V. L., Go, A. S., Lloyd-Jones, D. M., Adams, R. J., Berry, J. D., Brown, T. M., et al. American Heart Association Statistics Committee and Stroke Statistics Subcommittee (2011). Heart disease and stroke statistics–2011 update: A report from the American Heart Association. *Circulation*, *123*, e18–e209.

Ronaldson, P. T., & Davis, T. P. (2011). Targeting blood-brain barrier changes during inflammatory pain: An opportunity for optimizing CNS drug delivery. *Therapeutic Delivery*, *2*(8), 1015–1041. http://dx.doi.org/10.4155/tde.11.67.

Ronaldson, P. T., & Davis, T. P. (2012). Blood-brain barrier integrity and glial support: Mechanisms that can be targeted for novel therapeutic approaches in stroke. *Current Pharmaceutical Design*, *18*(25), 3624–3644.

Ronaldson, P. T., & Davis, T. P. (2013). Targeted drug delivery to treat pain and cerebral hypoxia. *Pharmacological Reviews*, *65*(1), 291–314. http://dx.doi.org/10.1124/pr.112.005991.

Ronaldson, P. T., Demarco, K. M., Sanchez-Covarrubias, L., Solinsky, C. M., & Davis, T. P. (2009). Transforming growth factor-beta signaling alters substrate permeability and tight junction protein expression at the blood-brain barrier during inflammatory pain. *Journal of Cerebral Blood Flow and Metabolism*, *29*(6), 1084–1098. http://dx.doi.org/10.1038/jcbfm.2009.32.

Ronaldson, P. T., Finch, J. D., Demarco, K. M., Quigley, C. E., & Davis, T. P. (2011). Inflammatory pain signals an increase in functional expression of organic anion transporting polypeptide 1a4 at the blood-brain barrier. *The Journal of Pharmacology and Experimental Therapeutics*, *336*(3), 827–839. http://dx.doi.org/10.1124/jpet.110.174151.

Saito, K., Takeshita, K., Ueda, J., & Ozawa, T. (2003). Two reaction sites of a spin label, TEMPOL (4-hydroxy-2,2,6,6-tetramethylpiperidine-N-oxyl), with hydroxyl radical. *Journal of Pharmaceutical Sciences*, *92*(2), 275–280. http://dx.doi.org/10.1002/jps.10304.

Salvemini, D., Doyle, T. M., & Cuzzocrea, S. (2006). Superoxide, peroxynitrite and oxidative/nitrative stress in inflammation. *Biochemical Society Transactions*, *34*(Pt. 5), 965–970. http://dx.doi.org/10.1042/BST0340965.

Sanchez-Covarrubias, L., Slosky, L. M., Thompson, B. J., Davis, T. P., & Ronaldson, P. T. (2014). Transporters at CNS barrier sites: Obstacles or opportunities for drug delivery? *Current Pharmaceutical Design*, *20*(10), 1422–1449.

Sandoval, K. E., & Witt, K. A. (2008). Blood-brain barrier tight junction permeability and ischemic stroke. *Neurobiology of Disease*, *32*(2), 200–219. http://dx.doi.org/10.1016/j.nbd.2008.08.005.

Schild, L., & Reiser, G. (2005). Oxidative stress is involved in the permeabilization of the inner membrane of brain mitochondria exposed to hypoxia/reoxygenation and low micromolar Ca2+. *The FEBS Journal*, *272*(14), 3593–3601. http://dx.doi.org/10.1111/j.1742-4658.2005.04781.x.

Schreibelt, G., Kooij, G., Reijerkerk, A., van Doorn, R., Gringhuis, S. I., van der Pol, S., et al. (2007). Reactive oxygen species alter brain endothelial tight junction dynamics via RhoA, PI3 kinase, and PKB signaling. *The FASEB Journal*, *21*(13), 3666–3676. http://dx.doi.org/10.1096/fj.07-8329com.

Seelbach, M. J., Brooks, T. A., Egleton, R. D., & Davis, T. P. (2007). Peripheral inflammatory hyperalgesia modulates morphine delivery to the brain: A role for P-glycoprotein. *Journal of Neurochemistry*, *102*(5), 1677–1690. http://dx.doi.org/10.1111/j.1471-4159.2007.04644.x.

Shah, K., & Abbruscato, T. (2014). The role of blood-brain barrier transporters in pathophysiology and pharmacotherapy of stroke. *Current Pharmaceutical Design*, *20*(10), 1510–1522.

Shishehbor, M. H., Aviles, R. J., Brennan, M. L., Fu, X., Goormastic, M., Pearce, G. L., et al. (2003). Association of nitrotyrosine levels with cardiovascular disease and modulation by statin therapy. *JAMA*, *289*(13), 1675–1680. http://dx.doi.org/10.1001/jama.289.13.1675.

Sierra, S., Ramos, M. C., Molina, P., Esteo, C., Vazquez, J. A., & Burgos, J. S. (2011). Statins as neuroprotectants: A comparative in vitro study of lipophilicity, blood-brain-barrier penetration, lowering of brain cholesterol, and decrease of neuron cell death. *Journal of Alzheimer's Disease*, *23*(2), 307–318. http://dx.doi.org/10.3233/JAD-2010-101179.

Simsek, S., Eroglu, H., Kurum, B., & Ulubayram, K. (2013). Brain targeting of Atorvastatin loaded amphiphilic PLGA-b-PEG nanoparticles. *Journal of Microencapsulation*, *30*(1), 10–20. http://dx.doi.org/10.3109/02652048.2012.692400.

Singh, R., & Lillard, J. W., Jr. (2009). Nanoparticle-based targeted drug delivery. *Experimental and Molecular Pathology*, *86*(3), 215–223. http://dx.doi.org/10.1016/j.yexmp.2008.12.004.

Singhal, A., Morris, V. B., Labhasetwar, V., & Ghorpade, A. (2013). Nanoparticle-mediated catalase delivery protects human neurons from oxidative stress. *Cell Death & Disease*, *4*, e903. http://dx.doi.org/10.1038/cddis.2013.362.

Sironi, L., Cimino, M., Guerrini, U., Calvio, A. M., Lodetti, B., Asdente, M., et al. (2003). Treatment with statins after induction of focal ischemia in rats reduces the extent of brain damage. *Arteriosclerosis, Thrombosis, and Vascular Biology*, *23*(2), 322–327.

Steckelbroeck, S., Nassen, A., Ugele, B., Ludwig, M., Watzka, M., Reissinger, A., et al. (2004). Steroid sulfatase (STS) expression in the human temporal lobe: Enzyme activity, mRNA expression and immunohistochemistry study. *Journal of Neurochemistry*, *89*(2), 403–417. http://dx.doi.org/10.1046/j.1471-4159.2004.02336.x.

Suh, H., Jeong, B., Rathi, R., & Kim, S. W. (1998). Regulation of smooth muscle cell proliferation using paclitaxel-loaded poly(ethylene oxide)-poly(lactide/glycolide) nanospheres. *Journal of Biomedical Materials Research*, *42*(2), 331–338.

Therade-Matharan, S., Laemmel, E., Carpentier, S., Obata, Y., Levade, T., Duranteau, J., et al. (2005). Reactive oxygen species production by mitochondria in endothelial cells exposed to reoxygenation after hypoxia and glucose depletion is mediated by ceramide. *American Journal of Physiology. Regulatory, Integrative and Comparative Physiology*, *289*(6), R1756–R1762. http://dx.doi.org/10.1152/ajpregu.00480.2004.

Thompson, B. J., Sanchez-Covarrubias, L., Slosky, L. M., Zhang, Y., Laracuente, M. L., & Ronaldson, P. T. (2014). Hypoxia/reoxygenation stress signals an increase in organic anion transporting polypeptide 1a4 (Oatp1a4) at the blood-brain barrier: Relevance to CNS drug delivery. *Journal of Cerebral Blood Flow and Metabolism*, *34*, 699–707. http://dx.doi.org/10.1038/jcbfm.2014.4.

Tu, Y. F., Lu, P. J., Huang, C. C., Ho, C. J., & Chou, Y. P. (2012). Moderate dietary restriction reduces p53-mediated neurovascular damage and microglia activation after hypoxic ischemia in neonatal brain. *Stroke*, *43*(2), 491–498. http://dx.doi.org/10.1161/STROKEAHA.111.629931.

Turrens, J. F. (2003). Mitochondrial formation of reactive oxygen species. *The Journal of Physiology*, *552*(Pt 2), 335–344. http://dx.doi.org/10.1113/jphysiol.2003.049478.

van Bruggen, N., Thibodeaux, H., Palmer, J. T., Lee, W. P., Fu, L., Cairns, B., et al. (1999). VEGF antagonism reduces edema formation and tissue damage after ischemia/reperfusion injury in the mouse brain. *The Journal of Clinical Investigation*, *104*(11), 1613–1620. http://dx.doi.org/10.1172/JCI8218.

Vemula, S., Roder, K. E., Yang, T., Bhat, G. J., Thekkumkara, T. J., & Abbruscato, T. J. (2009). A functional role for sodium-dependent glucose transport across the blood-brain barrier during oxygen glucose deprivation. *The Journal of Pharmacology and Experimental Therapeutics*, *328*(2), 487–495. http://dx.doi.org/10.1124/jpet.108.146589.

Vibbert, M., & Mayer, S. A. (2010). Early decompressive hemicraniectomy following malignant ischemic stroke: The crucial role of timing. *Current Neurology and Neuroscience Reports*, *10*(1), 1–3. http://dx.doi.org/10.1007/s11910-009-0081-y.

Wallace, B. K., Foroutan, S., & O'Donnell, M. E. (2011). Ischemia-induced stimulation of Na-K-Cl cotransport in cerebral microvascular endothelial cells involves AMP kinase. *American Journal of Physiology. Cell Physiology*, *301*(2), C316–C326. http://dx.doi.org/10.1152/ajpcell.00517.2010.

Watabe, T., Nishihara, A., Mishima, K., Yamashita, J., Shimizu, K., Miyazawa, K., et al. (2003). TGF-beta receptor kinase inhibitor enhances growth and integrity of embryonic stem cell-derived endothelial cells. *The Journal of Cell Biology*, *163*(6), 1303–1311. http://dx.doi.org/10.1083/jcb.200305147.

Westholm, D. E., Stenehjem, D. D., Rumbley, J. N., Drewes, L. R., & Anderson, G. W. (2009). Competitive inhibition of organic anion transporting polypeptide 1c1-mediated thyroxine transport by the fenamate class of nonsteroidal antiinflammatory drugs. *Endocrinology*, *150*(2), 1025–1032. http://dx.doi.org/10.1210/en.2008-0188.

Willis, C. L., Leach, L., Clarke, G. J., Nolan, C. C., & Ray, D. E. (2004). Reversible disruption of tight junction complexes in the rat blood-brain barrier, following transitory focal astrocyte loss. *Glia*, *48*(1), 1–13. http://dx.doi.org/10.1002/glia.20049.

Windass, A. S., Lowes, S., Wang, Y., & Brown, C. D. (2007). The contribution of organic anion transporters OAT1 and OAT3 to the renal uptake of rosuvastatin. *The Journal of Pharmacology and Experimental Therapeutics*, *322*(3), 1221–1227. http://dx.doi.org/10.1124/jpet.107.125831.

Witt, K. A., Mark, K. S., Hom, S., & Davis, T. P. (2003). Effects of hypoxia-reoxygenation on rat blood-brain barrier permeability and tight junctional protein expression. *American Journal of Physiology. Heart and Circulatory Physiology*, *285*(6), H2820–H2831. http://dx.doi.org/10.1152/ajpheart.00589.2003.

Witt, K. A., Mark, K. S., Huber, J., & Davis, T. P. (2005). Hypoxia-inducible factor and nuclear factor kappa-B activation in blood-brain barrier endothelium under hypoxic/reoxygenation stress. *Journal of Neurochemistry*, *92*(1), 203–214. http://dx.doi.org/10.1111/j.1471-4159.2004.02871.x.

Wu, X., Ma, J., Han, J. D., Wang, N., & Chen, Y. G. (2006). Distinct regulation of gene expression in human endothelial cells by TGF-beta and its receptors. *Microvascular Research*, *71*(1), 12–19. http://dx.doi.org/10.1016/j.mvr.2005.11.004.

Xie, F., Yao, N., Qin, Y., Zhang, Q., Chen, H., Yuan, M., et al. (2012). Investigation of glucose-modified liposomes using polyethylene glycols with different chain lengths as the linkers for brain targeting. *International Journal of Nanomedicine*, 7, 163–175. http://dx.doi.org/10.2147/IJN.S23771.

Yang, L., Shah, K., Wang, H., Karamyan, V. T., & Abbruscato, T. J. (2011). Characterization of neuroprotective effects of biphalin, an opioid receptor agonist, in a model of focal brain ischemia. *The Journal of Pharmacology and Experimental Therapeutics*, *339*(2), 499–508. http://dx.doi.org/10.1124/jpet.111.184127.

Yang, L., Wang, H., Shah, K., Karamyan, V. T., & Abbruscato, T. J. (2011). Opioid receptor agonists reduce brain edema in stroke. *Brain Research*, *1383*, 307–316. http://dx.doi.org/10.1016/j.brainres.2011.01.083.

Yeh, W. L., Lin, C. J., & Fu, W. M. (2008). Enhancement of glucose transporter expression of brain endothelial cells by vascular endothelial growth factor derived from glioma exposed to hypoxia. *Molecular Pharmacology*, *73*(1), 170–177. http://dx.doi.org/10.1124/mol.107.038851.

Zhang, D. X., & Gutterman, D. D. (2007). Mitochondrial reactive oxygen species-mediated signaling in endothelial cells. *American Journal of Physiology. Heart and Circulatory Physiology*, *292*(5), H2023–H2031. http://dx.doi.org/10.1152/ajpheart.01283.2006.

Zhao, Y., Patzer, A., Herdegen, T., Gohlke, P., & Culman, J. (2006). Activation of cerebral peroxisome proliferator-activated receptors gamma promotes neuroprotection by attenuation of neuronal cyclooxygenase-2 overexpression after focal cerebral ischemia in rats. *The FASEB Journal*, *20*(8), 1162–1175. http://dx.doi.org/10.1096/fj.05-5007com.

Zhelev, Z., Bakalova, R., Aoki, I., Matsumoto, K., Gadjeva, V., Anzai, K., et al. (2009). Nitroxyl radicals for labeling of conventional therapeutics and noninvasive magnetic resonance imaging of their permeability for blood-brain barrier: Relationship between structure, blood clearance, and MRI signal dynamic in the brain. *Molecular Pharmaceutics*, *6*(2), 504–512. http://dx.doi.org/10.1021/mp800175k.

CHAPTER SEVEN

Delivery of Chemotherapeutics Across the Blood–Brain Barrier: Challenges and Advances

Nancy D. Doolittle*, Leslie L. Muldoon*,†, Aliana Y. Culp*, Edward A. Neuwelt*,‡,§,1

*Department of Neurology, Oregon Health and Science University, Portland, Oregon, USA
†Department of Cell and Developmental Biology, Oregon Health and Science University, Portland, Oregon, USA
‡Department of Neurosurgery, Oregon Health and Science University, Portland, Oregon, USA
§Office of Research and Development, Department of Veterans Affairs Medical Center, Portland, Oregon, USA
[1]Corresponding author: e-mail address: neuwelte@ohsu.edu

Contents

Advances in Pharmacology, Volume 71
ISSN 1054-3589
http://dx.doi.org/10.1016/bs.apha.2014.06.002

Abstract

The blood–brain barrier (BBB) limits drug delivery to brain tumors. We utilize intraarterial infusion of hyperosmotic mannitol to reversibly open the BBB by shrinking endothelial cells and opening tight junctions between the cells. This approach transiently increases the delivery of chemotherapy, antibodies, and nanoparticles to brain. Our preclinical studies have optimized the BBB disruption (BBBD) technique and clinical studies have shown its safety and efficacy. The delivery of methotrexate-based chemotherapy in conjunction with BBBD provides excellent outcomes in primary central nervous system lymphoma (PCNSL) including stable or improved cognitive function in survivors a median of 12 years (range 2–26 years) after diagnosis. The addition of rituximab to chemotherapy with BBBD for PCNSL can be safely accomplished with excellent overall survival. Our translational studies of thiol agents to protect against platinum-induced toxicities led to the development of a two-compartment model in brain tumor patients. We showed that delayed high-dose sodium thiosulfate protects against carboplatin-induced hearing loss, providing the framework for large cooperative group trials of hearing chemoprotection. Neuroimaging studies have identified that ferumoxytol, an iron oxide nanoparticle blood pool agent, appears to be a superior contrast agent to accurately assess therapy-induced changes in brain tumor vasculature, in brain tumor response to therapy, and in differentiating central nervous system lesions with inflammatory components. This chapter reviews the breakthroughs, challenges, and future directions for BBBD.

ABBREVIATIONS

BAT brain around tumor
BBB blood–brain barrier
BBBD blood–brain barrier disruption
BDT brain distant to tumor
BTB blood–tumor barrier
CNS central nervous system
CR complete response
CSF cerebrospinal fluid
CT computed tomography
CTCAE Common Terminology Criteria for Adverse Events
DCE dynamic contrast-enhanced
DSC dynamic susceptibility-weighted contrast-enhanced
GBCA gadolinium-based contrast agent
IA intraarterial
IV intravenous
mAb monoclonal antibody
MRI magnetic resonance imaging
MTD maximum tolerated dose
MTX methotrexate
NAC *N*-acetylcysteine
OS overall survival

PCNSL primary central nervous system lymphoma
PFS progression-free survival
PNET primitive neuroectodermal tumor
rCBV relative cerebral blood volume
SPECT single photon emission computed tomography
STS sodium thiosulfate
WBRT whole brain radiotherapy

1. INTRODUCTION

The goal of blood–brain barrier disruption (BBBD) is maximizing the delivery of chemotherapy and antibodies to the brain while preserving neurocognitive function and quality of life and minimizing systemic toxicity. Taken together, preclinical and clinical blood–brain barrier (BBB) studies at Oregon Health & Science University (OHSU) evaluate (1) the toxicity of chemotherapeutics and chemoprotectants, (2) the potential for chemotherapy dose intensification in combination with chemoprotectants, and (3) the antitumor efficacy of chemotherapeutics in combination with chemoprotectants and/or monoclonal antibodies, in primary and metastatic brain tumors.

The BBB, consisting of tight junctions between endothelial cells of the cerebral vasculature, limits the access of blood-borne agents to the brain and brain tumor. The surrounding microenvironment plays a critical role in promoting the unique features of the BBB. The microenvironment (i.e., the neurovascular unit) consists of horizontal elements such as the endothelium, basal lamina, and astrocyte end-feet as well as vertical elements such as intervening astrocytes, neurons and their axons, and pericytes (Muldoon et al., 2013; Neuwelt et al., 2011). The barrier in malignant central nervous system (CNS) tumors can have extremely variable permeability, ranging from nearly the low permeability of normal BBB to nearly the high permeability of systemic vasculature. Low and inconsistent blood–tumor barrier (BTB) permeability is an effective impediment to drug entry. Blood–Brain Barrier Program preclinical and clinical research studies have focused on characterizing the role of the BBB in imaging, diagnosis, and therapy of brain tumors.

2. BLOOD–BRAIN BARRIER DISRUPTION

2.1. Delivering agents across the BBB: Preclinical studies

Delivery of agents across the BBB and the BTB in rats can be achieved by intracarotid infusion of hyperosmotic mannitol, resulting in transient shrinkage of cerebrovascular endothelial cells and opening of the BBB tight junctions (Fig. 1). Brightman et al. showed in the early 1970s that osmotic disruption of the BBB opened a clear channel between endothelial cells for the passage of agents from the blood to the brain (Brightman et al., 1973; Brightman & Reese, 1969; Rapoport & Robinson, 1986).

The maximum delivery and the time course for barrier opening vary depending on the size, charge, and protein and lipid binding characteristics of the agent delivered. Vascular permeability to water-soluble small molecular weight chemotherapeutics such as methotrexate (MTX) is increased maximally by 15 min after the infusion of 25% mannitol, after which it decreases to preinfusion levels within 2 h. We can measure 10- to 100-fold

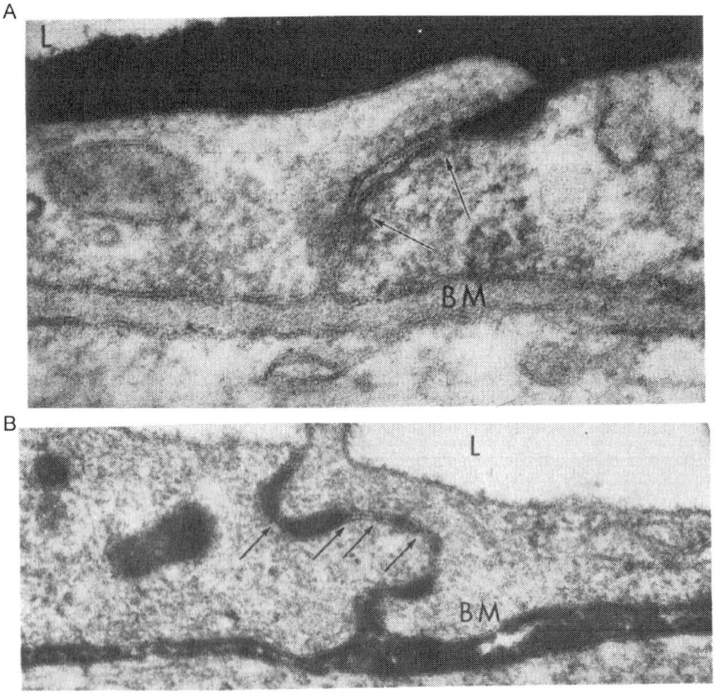

Figure 1 The anatomical basis of osmotic blood–brain barrier disruption. (A) Lanthanum passage from cerebral capillary lumen to neuropil prevented by a tight junction between two endothelial cells. (B) Opening of tight junction between endothelial cells to peroxidase tracer, by intracarotid perfusion of 3 M urea in the rabbit. Arrows indicate tight junctions; BM, basement membrane; L, lumen. *Panel (A) is reprinted with permission from Brightman and Reese (1969), © 1969 Rockefeller University Press. Panel (B) is reprinted with permission from Brightman, Hori, Rapoport, Reese, and Westergaard (1973).*

increases in the delivery of radiolabeled markers to intracerebral tumors and tumor-infiltrated brain, comparing intravenous (IV) administration to intraarterial (IA) administration with BBBD (Neuwelt, Barnett, et al., 1998; Remsen, Trail, Hellstrom, Hellstrom, & Neuwelt, 2000). Larger agents such as immunoconjugates (approximately 150 kDa), nanoparticles (30 nm diameter), or virus particles (200 nm diameter) have only a short window (15 min) of enhanced brain delivery.

We evaluated BBBD delivery of iron oxide nanoparticles magnetic resonance imaging (MRI) contrast agents as a model for visualizing the delivery of virus-sized particles to rat brain (Muldoon et al., 1999; Muldoon, Sandor, Pinkston, & Neuwelt, 2005; Fig. 2). Delivery of ferumoxytol nanoparticles across the BBB showed signal enhancement throughout the disrupted hemisphere that was maximal at 24 h and faded to baseline over 3 to 7 days. These particles, with a complete coating of modified carbohydrate that limits protein binding, disperse throughout the brain parenchyma after BBBD and are metabolized over time by brain cells (Muldoon et al., 2005). Ferumoxides iron oxide nanoparticles with an incomplete dextran coating cross through the endothelial tight junctions after osmotic BBBD

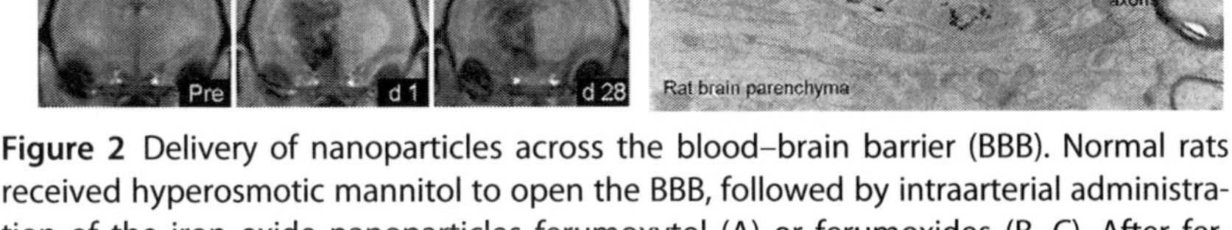

Figure 2 Delivery of nanoparticles across the blood–brain barrier (BBB). Normal rats received hyperosmotic mannitol to open the BBB, followed by intraarterial administration of the iron oxide nanoparticles ferumoxytol (A) or ferumoxides (B, C). After ferumoxytol administration, MRI signal intensity peaks by 24 h then fades over 3 to 7 days as the nanoparticles are metabolized (A, T1W indicates T1-weighted MRI). In contrast, ferumoxides induce signal dropout in the rat brain for over a month (B, T2* indicates T2*-weighted MRI). Electron microscopy shows that ferumoxides particles (Fe) are trapped between the vascular endothelial cells and the basement membrane after BBB disruption. *Panels (A) and (B) are adapted with permission from Lippincott Williams and Wilkins/Wolters Kluwer Health: Neurosurgery (Muldoon et al., 2005), ©2005. Panel (C) is modified with permission from Muldoon et al. (1999), © by American Society of Neuroradiology.*

but then bind to the basal lamina and do not actually enter the brain (Muldoon et al., 1999).

Drug delivery studies showed that BBBD was consistent in normal rat brain, with every animal attaining a good to excellent disruption, but was less consistent in rats with brain tumor xenografts, indicating that the BBBD procedure was not optimized when an intracerebral mass was present. We investigated pharmacologic and physiologic factors that may impact the quality and reproducibility of BBBD in implanted brain tumor xenograft models. Infusion flow rate and time, pCO_2, and osmotic agent (mannitol vs. arabinose or other sugars) were found to be important for BBBD. Anesthesia has a marked effect on cerebral blood flow and cerebral metabolic rate, and also impacts cardiac output and vascular tone. In rats with intracerebral tumors, propofol anesthesia was significantly superior to isoflurane for optimizing BBBD, yielding uniform Evans blue staining and enhanced drug delivery to tumor, brain around tumor (BAT), and brain distant to tumor (BDT) (Remsen et al., 1999).

2.2. Factors that impact chemotherapy delivery to brain tumors

Despite the rapid development of targeted therapeutics, chemotherapy remains the mainstay for brain tumor therapy, and our prediction is that it will remain widely used in adult and pediatric brain tumors. In fact, most of the new targeted therapies exclude primary brain tumors as an indication for their use. Therefore, it remains essential to maximize chemotherapy delivery and efficacy.

Numerous factors impact chemotherapy delivery to tumor including variable BBB permeability and drug concentrations achieved in the CNS. New vasculature within the tumor is often disordered and highly permeable, but infiltrating tumor makes use of the existing brain vasculature with a largely intact BBB. The magnitude of tumor vascular permeability varies within tumors both spatially and temporally, with the greatest permeability elevation in the tumor core and a relatively intact BBB at the proliferating edge of the tumor. The key to successful chemotherapy in brain tumors is drug delivery to the tumor-infiltrated BAT and the individual tumor cells and micrometastases distant from the main tumor mass in the BDT.

Chemotherapeutic drug concentrations within the CNS depend on multiple factors, including the permeability of the BBB to the chemotherapeutic agent, the extent to which the drug is actively transported out of the brain, and the drug volume of distribution in the brain parenchyma (Muldoon et al., 2007). Tissue concentrations of lipophilic agents are predominantly controlled by plasma protein binding, active efflux transport, and drug metabolism. Delivery of water-soluble drugs to brain tumors is more complex, and pharmacokinetic data in this issue are scarce. MTX is an example of a widely used hydrophilic chemotherapeutic agent in primary central nervous system lymphoma (PCNSL); however, very high doses must be administered to achieve therapeutic drug concentrations in the tumor and surrounding brain. In contrast, MTX delivery to the CNS is enhanced four- to sevenfold when administered IA after BBBD when compared with IA administration without BBBD. For a review of the pharmacokinetics of common chemotherapeutic drugs in the brain and in brain tumors, see Muldoon et al. (2007).

Drug concentration in brain tumors can vary by the route of drug delivery. For example, therapeutic concentrations of etoposide were found in glioblastomas and astrocytomas after IV delivery, but concentration decreased with increasing distance from the tumor (Zucchetti et al., 1991). The etoposide concentration was found to be four times higher after IA administration than IV administration (Savaraj, Lu, Feun, Burgess, & Loo, 1987). Route of delivery has been shown to impact brain delivery of cisplatin, with IA administration increasing delivery to glioma twofold compared with IV administration (Nakagawa et al., 1993). One study reported the results of brain pharmacokinetics of cytarabine, comparing different routes of administration (Groothuis et al., 2000). After IV administration of cytarabine, a diffuse pattern of low drug concentrations was detected throughout the brain (Groothuis et al., 2000).

Animal studies have also shown that antecedent cranial irradiation decreases agent delivery to the brain (Remsen, Marquez, Garcia, Thrun, & Neuwelt, 2001; Remsen et al., 1995). The studies evaluated long-term effects of various sequences of radiation therapy and BBBD chemotherapy in rodents. Drug delivery, acute toxicity, and long-term (1 year) neuropathological effects of MTX or carboplatin plus etoposide were evaluated. External beam whole brain radiotherapy (WBRT) of 2000 cGy as a single fraction using parallel opposed portals, either 30 days before or concurrent with BBBD, resulted in a statistically significant decrease in drug delivery compared to animals not receiving cranial irradiation. Seizures were observed in 26% of the animals that received irradiation before or concurrent with BBBD and MTX, but not carboplatin. The mortality rate for animals receiving radiotherapy 30 days prior to chemotherapy was significantly higher than the mortality rate for animals receiving only BBBD chemotherapy without irradiation (Remsen et al., 1997, 1995).

Increasing dose intensity with BBBD enhances antitumor efficacy in animal models. BBBD delivery of BR96–DOX, a tumor-specific monoclonal antibody (mAb)–doxorubicin immunoconjugate, significantly increased antitumor efficacy compared with IV or IA administration without BBBD (Remsen et al., 2000). We evaluated whether prior irradiation would decrease the dose intensity and efficacy of antibody-targeted chemotherapy given with BBBD. Results showed that BR96–DOX administered prior to WBRT significantly increased survival compared to rodents receiving irradiation prior to chemotherapy or compared to those receiving chemotherapy concurrently (Remsen et al., 2001). These findings were later supported in the clinic when subjects with PCNSL who received cranial irradiation before beginning BBBD chemotherapy had significantly decreased median survival time compared to those who received initial BBBD chemotherapy as first-line treatment (Dahlborg et al., 1996).

2.3. Preclinical BBBD chemotherapy neurotoxicity studies

The choice of chemotherapy agents is extremely important in the setting of BBBD for malignant brain tumors. The BBB preclinical team carefully conducts toxicity studies in rodents. Chemotherapy agents that can be safely administered with BBBD with acceptable toxicity are determined. Neurotoxicity can be caused by the chemotherapy itself or by agents such as detergents or strong salts in the diluent. Important knowledge was gained when laboratory studies showed severe neurotoxicity when doxorubicin (IA) (Neuwelt, Pagel, Barnett, Glassberg, & Frenkel, 1981), cisplatin (IA), or 5-FU (IA) (Neuwelt, Barnett, Glasberg, & Frenkel, 1983) was administered as single agents after BBBD. Fortin, McCormick, Remsen, Nixon, and Neuwelt (2000) reported unexpected neurotoxicity in the preclinical setting, when etoposide phosphate (IA) was administered in combination with melphalan (IA), MTX (IA), or carboplatin (IA) after BBBD, when propofol anesthesia was used. Neurotoxicity was minimized by appropriate timing of drug administration, with etoposide phosphate prior to BBBD, and carboplatin and melphalan immediately after BBBD (Fortin et al., 2000).

2.4. The clinical technique of osmotic BBB opening

The technique of clinical BBBD used by Neuwelt et al. is based on extensive preclinical toxicity and efficacy studies (Neuwelt, 2004). BBBD involves infusing hyperosmolar mannitol (25%, warmed) IA in the carotid or in the vertebral arteries. The infusion of mannitol is theorized to cause osmotic shrinkage of the endothelial cells which line CNS capillaries, with resultant separation of the tight junctions between the endothelial cells (Rapoport & Robinson, 1986). To date, BBBD has shown very promising clinical results especially as front-line treatment in chemosensitive brain tumors such as PCNSL (Angelov et al., 2009; Doolittle, Korfel, et al., 2013; Neuwelt et al., 1991).

The BBBD treatment is conducted on two consecutive days (24 h apart) every 4 weeks for 12 months. BBBD is performed under general anesthesia to ensure patient comfort and safety during the rapid (30 s) IA infusion of a large volume of mannitol. A femoral artery is catheterized, and a selected intracranial artery (either an internal carotid or a vertebral artery) is accessed. Mannitol is delivered IA via an infusion device at a predetermined flow rate of 3–12 cc/s into the cannulated artery for 30 s. The precise mannitol flow rate is determined by fluoroscopy, to just exceed cerebral blood flow. Following the administration of mannitol, chemotherapy is infused IA over 10 min. Immediately following the mannitol, nonionic contrast dye is administered IV.

Following completion of the chemotherapy infusion, patients undergo a computed tomography (CT) brain scan. Contrast enhancement in the disrupted territory of the brain is compared to the nondisrupted territory and graded using the results reported by Roman-Goldstein et al. (1994). During each monthly treatment, one of the intracranial arteries (right or left internal carotid or a vertebral) is infused on the first day of BBBD treatment and a different artery is infused on the second day, depending on the tumor type, extent, and location. Since many tumors such as PCNSL have widespread microscopic infiltration of the brain, infusion of the arteries is rotated such that during a year of BBBD treatment, each of the three intracranial arteries is infused eight times, thus providing global delivery to all cerebral hemispheres.

Chemotherapy agents used most frequently in conjunction with BBBD in the clinical setting are MTX (IA, 2500 mg/day × two consecutive days), carboplatin (IA, 200 mg/m^2/day × two consecutive days), melphalan (IA, a dose of 8 mg/m^2/day × two consecutive days is currently under study), cyclophosphamide (IV, 500 mg/m^2/day × two consecutive days when given with MTX; 330 mg/m^2/day × two consecutive days when given with carboplatin), etoposide and etoposide phosphate (IV, 150 mg/m^2/day × two consecutive days when given with MTX; 200 mg/m^2/day × two consecutive days when given with carboplatin). Depending on the brain tumor histology and according to the specific IRB-approved protocol, a combination of the above drugs is given with BBBD. These agents, infused by the respective routes and doses, have been routinely used in the clinical setting with minimal toxicity (Angelov et al., 2009; Dahlborg et al., 1996, 1998; Doolittle, Korfel, et al., 2013; Doolittle et al., 2000; McAllister et al., 2000; Tyson et al., 2003).

2.5. Safety of BBBD in a multicenter setting

Utilizing BBBD treatment and managing the care of patients treated with the BBBD procedure require a multidisciplinary team approach including a neurooncologist, neurosurgeon, pharmacist, neuroradiologist, anesthesiologist, nurse coordinator, audiologist, physical therapist, and social worker. Uniform guidelines for anesthesia, transfemoral arterial catheterization, IA infusion of mannitol and chemotherapy, radiographic assessment of disruption and tumor response, and patient care guidelines must be used by participating centers when performing BBBD. In the setting of rapidly progressing brain tumor with associated rapid neurological deterioration, there is a risk of increasing mass effect following BBBD. Thus, BBBD is safest before tumor burden becomes excessive (Doolittle et al., 2000).

As part of the treatment regimen, neuroimaging studies are performed before each monthly treatment course, after the final course, and at specified follow-up intervals depending on the type of tumor and tumor response. Routine follow-up includes complete blood counts and audiologic and neurologic examinations. Ophthalmologic evaluations and cerebrospinal fluid (CSF) cytopathology are conducted when clinically indicated. The frequency and severity of toxicities associated with BBBD treatment are well described (Angelov et al., 2009; Guillaume et al., 2010). Indeed the exceptional preservation of cognitive function in the long-term PCNSL survivors treated with BBBD as well as the preservation of hearing in brain tumor patients treated with carboplatin (IA) with BBBD and delayed high-dose sodium thiosulfate (STS) have formed the basis of numerous publications, ongoing studies, and future research (Doolittle, Korfel, et al., 2013; Doolittle, Muldoon, et al., 2001; Neuwelt, Brummett, et al., 1998; Neuwelt et al., 1991).

3. PRIMARY CNS LYMPHOMA

PCNSL is a generally diffuse, aggressive large B-cell lymphoma confined to the brain, leptomeninges, spinal cord, and eyes at the time of presentation, with a characteristic pattern of scattered and perivascular infiltration. High-dose MTX (IV) is the most widely used drug for PCNSL. In combination with WBRT, high-dose MTX improved survival rates over WBRT alone. However, delayed treatment-related neurotoxicity emerged as a significant disabling complication of the combined treatment especially in patients older than 60 years (Correa et al., 2012; Harder et al., 2004; Morris & Abrey, 2009; Thiel et al., 2010).

There is a trend toward more intensive first-line treatments for PCNSL such as dose-intensive chemotherapy and myeloablative chemotherapy followed by stem cell transplantation, as a strategy to achieve durable remissions while avoiding the neurotoxicity associated with WBRT. As treatment regimens intensify, durable remission rates and survival are expected to increase. However, reducing toxicity from intensive induction and high-dose chemotherapy regimens will be critical to achieving acceptable long-term outcomes.

Many clinical investigators have added the $CD20^+$ antibody rituximab to the first-line PCNSL regimens. Inclusion of this mAb is primarily based on the increased survival when rituximab was added to chemotherapy for patients with systemic $CD20^+$ diffuse large B-cell non-Hodgkin lymphoma (Coiffier et al., 2002), and on evidence of radiographic response to rituximab monotherapy in patients with recurrent PCNSL (Batchelor et al., 2011). Although initially thought to have poor CNS penetration because of its large molecular size, rituximab has a long plasma half-life with notable binding and accumulation at target B cells.

3.1. Development and characterization of a CNS lymphoma rat model

In order to evaluate PCNSL biology and new treatment approaches, we developed an animal model that closely mimics the clinical situation (Jahnke et al., 2009; Muldoon, Lewin, et al., 2011; Soussain et al., 2007). We implanted MC116 human B-cell lymphoma cells either intracerebrally or intracerebroventricularly in athymic rats. The intracerebral CNSL tumor model is inconsistent with ~25% of rats showing no tumors, and the tumors that grow are unpredictable, ranging in size from tiny (2 mm^3) to huge (175 mm^3) at 19–26 days after tumor implantation. In the intraventricular model, all rats ($n=4$) showed weight loss and behavioral changes such as agitation in response to noise.

In very large intracerebral tumors (>100 mm^3), T2/FLAIR signal changes at the inoculation site (caudate nucleus) and in the cortex and ventricles indicated tumor infiltration and edema throughout the inoculated hemisphere and also in the contralateral side along white matter tracts. Gadolinium enhancement was found primarily in the central region of large tumors, indicating relative low permeability in most of the tumor-infiltrated brain. In smaller tumors (2–50 mm^3), FLAIR sequences appeared to be the most sensitive in the delineation of the tumor-infiltrated brain and showed a good visual correlation with hematoxylin staining. After intraventricular cell implantation, FLAIR MRI showed large ventricles with periventricular enhancement suggesting tumor infiltration.

The MC116 CNSL model showed positive staining for a variety of human B-cell markers, including CD19, CD20, CD22, and CD45 (Fig. 3). Immunohistochemistry showed diffuse infiltration of the MC116 cells from the inoculation site spreading into the cortex, meninges, subarachnoid space, and tracking along the corpus callosum into the contralateral hemisphere. Perivascular infiltration was found in brain tissue up to 5 mm from the inoculation site. In the intraventricular model,

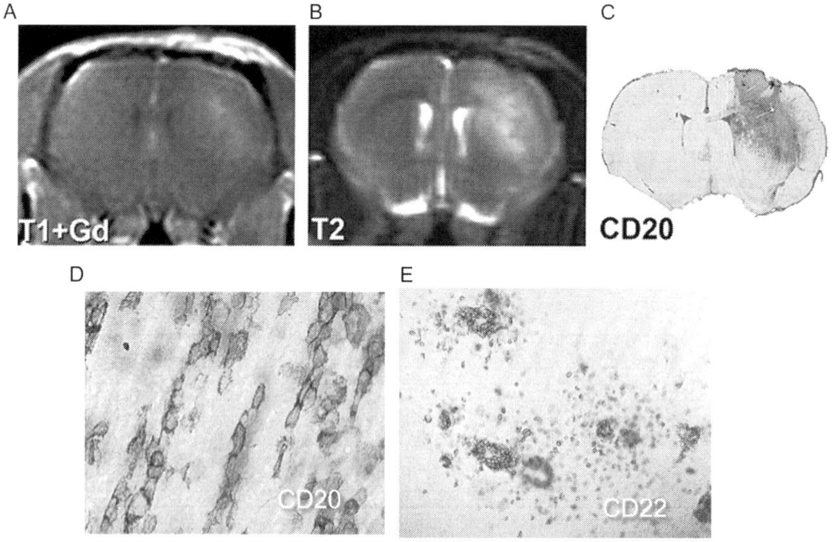

Figure 3 MRI and histology of the rat CNS lymphoma model. Intracerebral implantation of human MC116 B-lymphoma cells forms an infiltrative brain tumor that shows minimal leakage to gadolinium contrast on T1-weighted MRI (A). Prominent hyperintensity on T2-weighted MRI (B) correlates with tumor extent as determined by immunohistochemistry for CD20 (C). The tumor shows infiltration along fiber tracts and around blood vessels distant to the tumor mass (D and E). *Panels (A)–(C) are reprinted with permission from Jahnke et al. (2009) by the permission of Society for Neuro-Oncology. Panels (D) and (E) are reprinted from Soussain et al. (2007).*

immunocytochemistry for CD20 showed diffuse tumor cell infiltration into the brain parenchyma around both the right and left ventricles and in the subarachnoid space.

To replicate and confirm findings in the MC116 CNSL model, we are developing a second animal model utilizing intracerebral implantation of NALM-6 human pre-B cell line. This cell line forms a model of acute lymphoblastic leukemia when injected IV in immunocompromised mice.

3.2. Therapy studies in the rat CNS lymphoma model

MC116 cells were sensitive to radiation *in vitro*, with toxicity seen 3–4 days after a single treatment in the dose range of 2–10 Gy. *In vivo*, WBRT (20 Gy) was effective in five animals with MRI-confirmed tumor. One week after WBRT, histochemistry showed minimal tumor with scattered enlarged and necrotic CD45-positive cells near the inoculation site. Although radiation appeared effective, because of the short time frame in the pilot study, it remains unknown whether tumor regrowth could take place.

MC116 cells were also highly sensitive to MTX *in vitro*, with most cells killed by a clinically relevant dose of 0.1 μM within 5 days of treatment (Jahnke et al., 2009; Soussain et al., 2007). In contrast, three independent studies demonstrated a lack of responsiveness of the CNSL model to MTX *in vivo*. In the initial study, five rats with MRI-confirmed tumor received one dose of IV MTX (3 g/m^2). Immunocytochemistry demonstrated histologically infiltrative tumor in all five animals 1 week after treatment, including clusters of tumor cells throughout the inoculated hemisphere. The second study assessed MRI tumor volumetrics 1 week after treatment with a single dose of MTX (1 g/m^2 IV). MTX treatment appeared to reduce tumor growth compared to the control, but several animals showed an increase in the area of enhancement or no change in enhancement. Histology showed the presence of viable tumor infiltrated into the brain parenchyma. A third study assessing the impact of BBBD-enhanced delivery of MTX with or without rituximab on survival in the rat model is described below.

3.3. mAb delivery and efficacy in the preclinical setting

A study of IV rituximab with or without MTX chemotherapy was evaluated in the rat CNSL model. Both agents were given IV as a single dose and outcome was determined by MRI 1 week after treatment (Jahnke et al., 2009). Control tumors showed approximately a doubling of volume over the 1-week assessment period. Overall, rituximab-treated tumors did not grow compared to baseline, and included 60% of rats with an objective response (tumor shrinkage on MRI). We hypothesized that improving delivery would enhance the efficacy of rituximab in the brain tumor model.

To evaluate the effect of BBBD on the delivery of mAb to CNSL tumor mass and tumor-infiltrated rat brain, we used ^{90}Y-labeled mAb ibritumomab tiuxetan (Zevalin), which targets CD20 on B cells similar to rituximab (Muldoon, Lewin, et al., 2011; Fig. 4). BBBD improved ^{90}Y-ibritumomab delivery throughout the disrupted hemisphere compared with IV mAb administration. At 10 min after BBBD, there was a significant increase in mAb levels in tumor, tumor-infiltrated BAT, and BDT. Levels of mAb in brain were elevated at 10 min and 24 h after BBBD, but by 3 days mAb concentrations in brain were no different than IV infusion. IV mAb gave 10–20% increased concentration in tumor-infiltrated brain compared to the normal contralateral hemisphere, but the difference was not significant. We conclude that BBBD was effective for the delivery of high-molecular-weight agents such as mAbs, giving a rapid two- to fourfold increase in the delivery of mAb to brain tumor. However, elevated

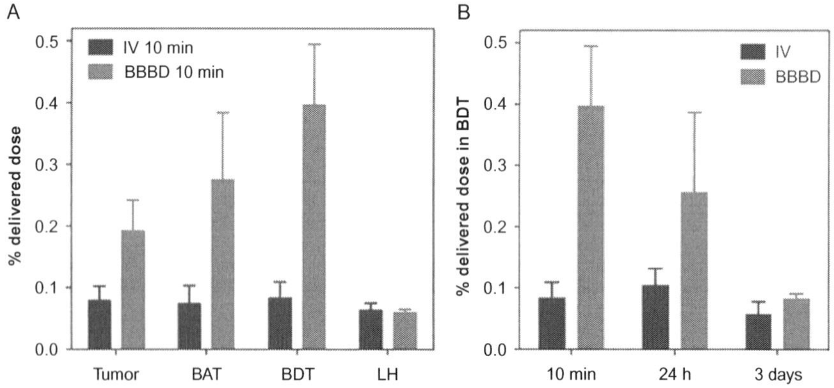

Figure 4 Blood–brain barrier disruption (BBBD) increases antibody delivery in the rat model of CNS lymphoma. Rats with intracerebral MC116 xenografts received ^{90}Y-ibritumomab intravenously with or without BBBD. (A) Radiolabel in tumor, brain around tumor (BAT), ipsilateral brain distant to tumor (BDT), and contralateral left hemisphere (LH), was determined at 10 min after antibody administration. There was a significant effect of BBBD in the repeated measures ANOVA model ($P = 0.0361$). (B) Radiolabel localized in BDT is shown at 10 min, 24 h, and 3 days after antibody administration. *Reprinted from Muldoon, Lewin, et al. (2011).*

localization of the mAb was not maintained compared to IV delivery over time. IV delivery alone gave slightly elevated mAb localization in tumor, BAT, and BDT, but this was not significantly different from the contralateral normal brain levels.

We tested the hypothesis that BBBD-enhanced delivery would improve the effectiveness of rituximab, MTX, or combination therapy. Five groups were evaluated: (1) BBBD control (IA saline); (2) MTX 1 g/kg IA with BBBD; (3) rituximab 375 mg/m^2 IV with BBBD; (4) rituximab plus MTX with BBBD; and (5) rituximab IV. Animals were followed for survival, with an interim outcome measure of MRI at 1 week after treatment, with follow-up MRI if possible. We found three patterns of response: (a) increased tumor size on MRI with short survival. Many control rats fit this phenotype; (b) increased tumor size on the 1-week MRI coupled with long survival. Some animals with this phenotype showed later tumor shrinkage on subsequent MRI; and (c) decreased tumor size and long survival. No rat showed decreased tumor size on MRI coupled with short survival. Control tumors grew by 201 ± 102% at the 1-week assessment period, and both the MTX and rituximab groups had significantly smaller tumors than control. The tumors treated with MTX had a reduced growth rate on MRI, with 70 ± 42% increase in volume, but this did not translate to improved survival (Fig. 5). Overall survival (OS) in the control group was 14 days (range: 6–33 days). Survival time after MTX was actually decreased (median: 7 days; range: 5–19 days), but this was not significantly different from controls ($P = 0.18$). The reasons for the lack of MTX efficacy in the rat CNSL model are not clear, given that the cells are chemosensitive. Possible reasons include the lower dose compared to humans, lack of delivery across the BBB, and that we are limited to a single dose in the rat model.

The impact of rituximab on early tumor volumetrics was inconsistent. Tumors in the combined rituximab groups showed both increased and decreased size on MRI, with an overall 32 ± 122% increase in volume at 1 week. In contrast, rituximab improved survival in all groups. Survival times ranged from 37.5 days (20–60 days, predetermined end of study) for rituximab BBBD, 42 days (27–60 days) for rituximab plus MTX BBBD, and undefined (26–60 days) for IV rituximab. The study lacks adequate power to determine whether there were differences between the three rituximab groups. Thus, this study demonstrated that a single dose of rituximab was effective at prolonging survival in the CNSL model, whether or not it was delivered with BBBD, and whether or not MTX was included. We conclude that the long slow leak of mAb across the minimally disrupted

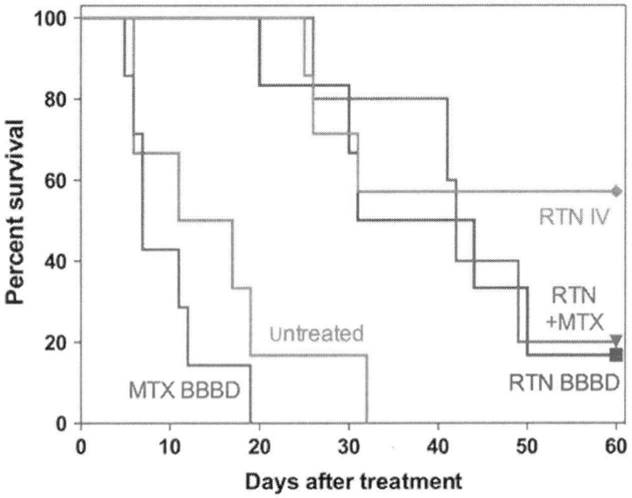

Figure 5 Rituximab increases survival in the rat model of CNS lymphoma. Rats with MRI-confirmed MC116 CNS lymphoma were randomized to treatment groups and followed for survival. The Kaplan–Meier survival curves show that methotrexate (MTX) was ineffective in this model ($P=0.18$), whereas all rituximab (RTN) groups improved survival compared with control (RTN BBBD [blood–brain barrier disruption], $P=0.013$; RTN +MTX BBBD, $P=0.0042$; RTN IV [intravenous], $P=0.0049$). *Reprinted from Muldoon, Lewin, et al. (2011).*

BBB of the brain tumor was sufficient to prove an effective dose. Of interest, many long-term survival rats showed tumor regression, even complete response (CR), at the inoculation site, with tumor growth in cortex or contralateral hemisphere. This tumor histology suggests that tumor was responsive where vasculature was leaky, but infiltrating tumor far from the initial mass was protected by a more normal BBB.

3.4. PCNSL: Clinical studies

The first PCNSL patients successfully treated with BBBD-enhanced delivery of MTX-based chemotherapy were reported by Neuwelt et al. in the early 1980s (Neuwelt, Balaban, Diehl, Hill, & Frenkel, 1983). Since then, excellent clinical outcomes have been obtained in PCNSL which is a highly chemosensitive brain tumor, using IA MTX in conjunction with BBBD without the use of WBRT (Angelov et al., 2009; Doolittle, Fu, et al., 2013; Doolittle, Korfel, et al., 2013; Neuwelt, Balaban, et al., 1983; Neuwelt et al., 1991). We reported our multi-institutional experience using BBBD in conjunction with IA MTX-based chemotherapy in 149 patients newly diagnosed with PCNSL (Angelov et al., 2009). The patients achieved an overall response rate of 82% (58% CR; 24% partial response). The median OS was 3.1 years (25% estimated survival at 8.5 years). The median progression-free survival (PFS) was 1.8 years, with 5-year and 7-year PFS of 31% and 25%, respectively. In low-risk patients (age <60 years and Karnofsky Performance Score [KPS] ≥70), median OS was approximately 14 years, with a survival plateau after approximately 8 years (Fig. 6). The BBBD procedures were generally well tolerated; peri-procedural focal seizures in 9.2% of the patients almost exclusively after MTX infusion were the most frequent side effect and lacked long-term sequelae. Durable remissions have been achieved with stable or improved cognitive function, a median of 12 years (range: 2–26 years) after diagnosis (Doolittle, Dosa, et al., 2013; Doolittle, Korfel, et al., 2013).

Isolated brain parenchyma relapse is a rare complication of systemic non-Hodgkin lymphoma. A large multinational retrospective analysis of isolated brain relapse cases was conducted by our group in collaboration with the International Primary CNS Lymphoma Collaborative Group (Doolittle

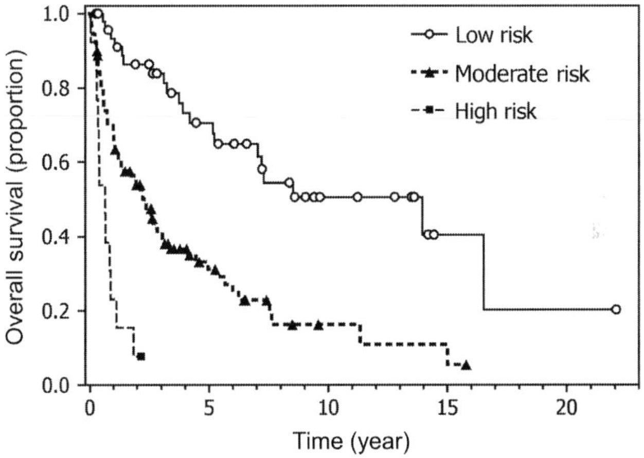

Figure 6 Overall survival (OS) in patients newly diagnosed with primary CNS lymphoma according to risk groups. OS is from the date of first intraarterial in conjunction with blood–brain barrier disruption treatment stratified by age and Karnofsky Performance Score (KPS). Low risk, age younger than 60 years with KPS ≥70 (47 patients); moderate risk, age older than 60 years with any KPS or age younger than 50 years with KPS <70 (89 patients); high risk, age 50 to less than 60 years with KPS <70 (13 patients) ($P > 0.0001$). In low-risk patients, median OS was approximately 14 years, with a survival plateau after approximately 8 years. Symbols on lines indicate censored observations. *Reprinted with permission from Angelov et al. (2009), © 2009 American Society of Clinical Oncology.*

et al., 2008). MTX was found to be the optimal treatment for isolated brain relapse. Although the number of patients treated with MTX (IA) in conjunction with BBBD included in the report was small, the majority of the patients treated with this approach were listed as long-term survivors.

3.5. mAb delivery to brain in the clinical setting

Data from anti-CD20 radioimmunotherapy support the idea that the BBB limits efficacy. Clinical studies of ^{90}Y-labeled anti-CD20 antibody ibritumomab tiuxetan provide evidence of target accumulation of the antibody within the brain as assessed by single photon emission computed tomography (SPECT) imaging with ^{111}In-labeled ibritumomab tiuxetan in recurrent PCNSL, in the absence of BBBD (Doolittle et al., 2007; Maza et al., 2009; Muldoon et al., 2007; Fig. 7). We studied ^{90}Y-ibritumomab tiuxetan in two patients with refractory PCNSL (Doolittle et al., 2007; Muldoon et al., 2007). SPECT imaging in one patient at 45 h and one patient at 48 h showed uptake of ^{111}In-ibritumomab localized at enhancing lesions, which were detected on brain MRI, providing evidence of mAb leakage across the BBB. The original lesions achieved CR to ^{90}Y-ibritumomab; however, recurrence was detected on brain MRI in multiple locations distant to the original lesions. An independent report showed ^{90}Y-ibritumomab efficacy in four of six PCNSL patients (Maza

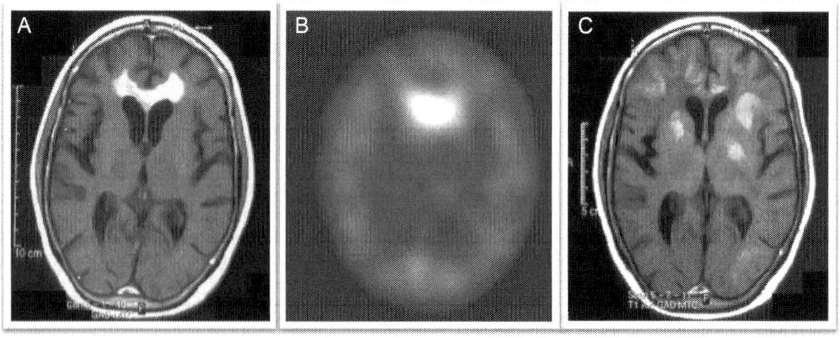

Figure 7 ^{111}In-ibritumomab to assess delivery and ^{90}Y-ibritumomab to assess efficacy in refractory primary CNS lymphoma. (A) Brain MRI, gadolinium-enhanced T1 axial view, 11 days prior to ^{111}In-ibritumomab showing large enhancing tumor in the genu of the corpus callosum. (B) Brain axial SPECT image, 48 h after 5.2 mCi of ^{111}In-ibritumomab showing uptake in the genu of the corpus callosum. (C) Brain MRI, gadolinium-enhanced T1 axial view, 8 weeks after 5.2 mCi of ^{111}In- and 23.1 mCi of ^{90}Y-ibritumomab showing progressive disease distant from the genu of the corpus callosum. *Reproduced with permission from Doolittle et al. (2007), © 2007 Informa Healthcare.*

et al., 2009). The ^{90}Y-ibritumomab study provides insight into the leakage and efficacy of rituximab in brain. At the original lesion, the BBB was leaky secondary to lymphomatous infiltration and ^{90}Y-ibritumomab provided local efficacy. However, the BBB was mostly intact at distant brain areas at the time of ^{90}Y-ibritumomab infusion and may have received less ^{90}Y--ibritumomab for efficacy. Impaired BBB integrity at the original lesion improved mAb delivery.

Based on the safety and efficacy using rituximab in combination with increased delivery to the CNS with BBBD in recurrent PCNSL as well as our translational laboratory studies including the development of a rodent model of human B-cell CNS lymphoma, we treated PCNSL patients with the first-line rituximab in combination with MTX-based chemotherapy and BBBD (Doolittle et al., 2007; Jahnke et al., 2009; Muldoon, Lewin, et al., 2011; Soussain et al., 2007). The rituximab was infused IV approximately 12 h prior to day 1 of monthly BBBD. The addition of rituximab safely improved the CR rate (74%) and median OS (61 months) in newly diagnosed PCNSL patients when compared with our previous series, with an acceptable toxicity profile (Doolittle, Fu, et al., 2013). Immunotherapy with rituximab improved clinical outcomes even in high-risk patients without escalating chemotherapy doses.

3.6. Neurocognitive outcomes in long-term PCNSL survivors

Since the goal of BBBD is enhanced CNS delivery while preserving neurocognitive function, BBBD clinical protocols include a standardized neuropsychological test battery, which is conducted at study entry and at follow-up. Long-term PCNSL survivors were prospectively evaluated to assess changes in neuropsychological scores and the association with pretreatment and long-term neuroimaging outcomes. Survivors who were a minimum of 2 years postdiagnosis and in complete remission after BBBD treatment were evaluated with neuropsychological tests and brain MRI or CT (Doolittle, Dosa, et al., 2013; Doolittle, Korfel, et al., 2013). Complete disease remission was required to assess neurotoxicity without the confounding presence of infiltrative, often multifocal CNS disease.

Neuropsychological scores obtained pretreatment and long-term were available on 23 of 26 long-term PCNSL survivors. The median interval from diagnosis to long-term evaluation was 12 years (min 2 years, max 26 years); eight survivors (35%) were evaluated 15 years or more after diagnosis. There was significant improvement in tests of attention/executive function from pretreatment to long-term. The majority of survivors showed stable or improved cognitive status at long term (Fig. 8). Of the eight survivors evaluated 15 years or more after diagnosis, five were working in high-level occupations as surgeon, attorney, registered nurse, law-enforcement agent, and optician. Three were retired (Doolittle, Dosa, et al., 2013).

On neuroimaging, the total T2 MRI hyperintensities or CT hypodensities decreased or resolved by the end of treatment in 75% of survivors. Total T2 MRI hyperintensities or CT hypodensities did not change from the end of treatment to long term. There was no association between neuropsychological scores and neuroimaging pretreatment and long term. We are not aware of studies that have evaluated cognition and neuroimaging with such lengthy follow-up, showing preserved or improved cognitive functioning in this rare cancer (Doolittle, Dosa, et al., 2013).

In addition, 80 PCNSL survivors from four MTX-based treatment groups (one group with WBRT and three groups without WBRT) who were a minimum of 2 years after diagnosis and in complete remission underwent prospective cognitive testing and brain MRI evaluation (Doolittle, Korfel, et al., 2013). The patients who had been treated with BBBD ($n=25$) showed long-term cognitive, quality of life, and imaging outcomes that were as good as if not better than the outcomes in the other three treatment groups (Fig. 9). The patients treated with BBBD were a median of 12 years (min 2 years, max 26 years) after diagnosis. This group had the longest median interval from diagnosis to long-term evaluation of the four treatment groups. Overall, the PCNSL patients treated with WBRT had significantly poorer cognitive performance when compared with the non-WBRT treatment groups ($P \leq 0.05$).

3.7. Anaplastic oligodendroglioma and CNS embryonal tumors: BBBD outcomes

Anaplastic oligodendroglioma and oligoastrocytoma, especially in patients demonstrating 1p and/or 19q deletion, are chemosensitive brain tumors, which respond well to alkylating agents. We have reported acceptable toxicity and encouraging efficacy in patients with anaplastic oligodendroglioma and oligoastrocytoma who were treated with melphalan (IA), carboplatin (IA), and etoposide phosphate (IV) in conjunction with BBBD (Guillaume et al., 2010). The patients had undergone prior treatment with temozolomide. During the completed phase I component of the study, 13 patients who had undergone 147 BBBD treatments were assessed.

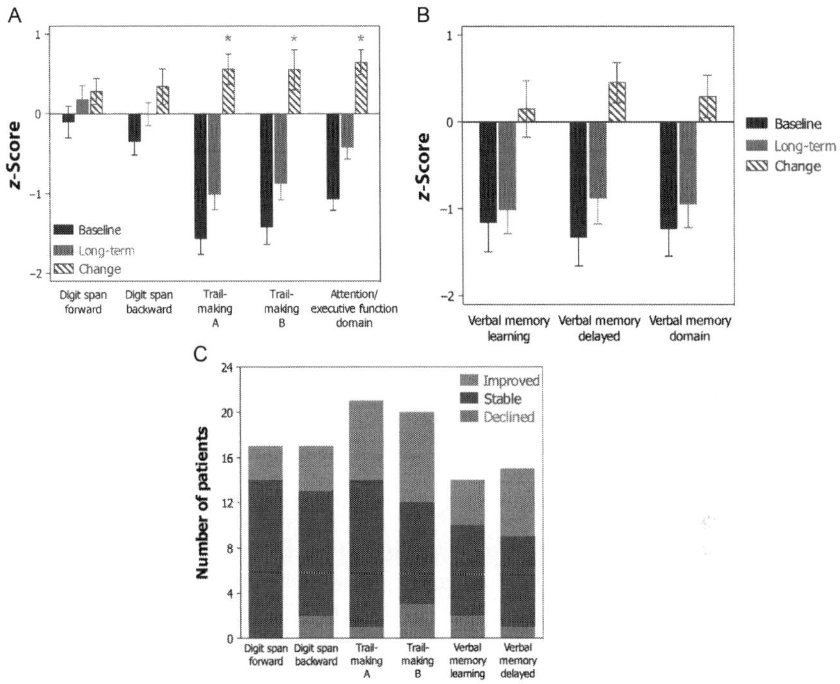

Figure 8 Long-term cognitive outcomes in patients treated with blood–brain barrier disruption (BBBD). Patients with newly diagnosed primary CNS lymphoma (PCNSL) were treated with intraarterial (IA) methotrexate-based chemotherapy with BBBD. The median time from diagnosis to long-term evaluation was 12 years (range: 2–26 years). (A) Raw cognitive test scores were converted to *z*-scores based on the normative values demographically adjusted to age. A z-score is the number of standard deviations above or below the mean for a population of similar age. A domain score was obtained by averaging all test *z*-scores in each domain, for each participant. The *z*-scores (mean, $\pm$SD) across survivors at baseline (pretreatment), long-term follow-up, and the change score are shown. The asterisks indicate statistical significance. There was improvement in Trail-making A, $P = 0.0085$; Trail-making B, $P = 0.0411$; and attention/executive function domain, $P < 0.001$. (B) The *z*-scores (mean, $\pm$SD) across the PCNSL survivors at baseline, long-term follow-up, and the change score for verbal memory, learning; verbal memory, delayed; and verbal memory domain are shown. There was no significant change from baseline to long-term follow-up. (C) Number of PCNSL patients declined (*z*-score declined one SD or more), stable (*z*-score remained within one SD of baseline score), and improved (*z*-score improved one SD or more) from baseline to long-term for the following tests: digit span forward, digit span backward, trail making a, trail making b, verbal memory learning, and verbal memory delayed. *Reprinted with permission from Doolittle, Dosa, et al. (2013), © 2013 American Society of Clinical Oncology.*

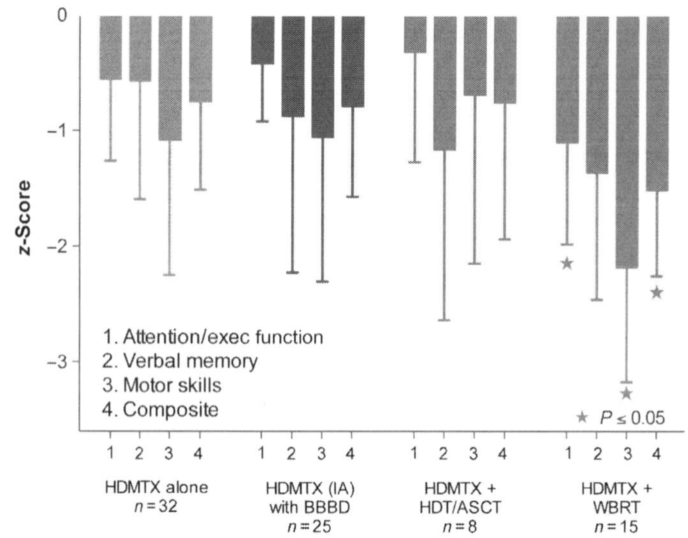

Figure 9 Long-term neuropsychological outcomes in primary CNS lymphoma survivors, according to the treatment type. Neuropsychological domain (attention/executive function, verbal memory, and motor skills) and neuropsychological composite *z*-score results (crude mean, SD) are shown, according to the following treatment groups: HDMTX (high-dose methotrexate) alone; HDMTX IA (intraarterial) with BBBD (blood–brain barrier disruption); HDMTX+HDT/ASCT (high-dose chemotherapy with autologous stem cell transplantation); and HDMTX+WBRT (whole brain radiotherapy) group. A *z*-score is the number of standard deviations above or below the mean for a population of similar age. Asterisks indicate a statistically significant difference ($P \leq 0.05$) between the WBRT group and the non-WBRT groups in attention/executive function, motor skills, and composite score. *Reprinted with permission from Doolittle, Korfel, et al. (2013).*

The most common grade 3 and grade 4 adverse events (graded according to Common Terminology Criteria for Adverse Events [CTCAE]) was thrombocytopenia in 20% and 12% of BBBD procedures, respectively. The maximum tolerated dose (MTD) of melphalan (IA) when administered in combination with carboplatin (IA, 200 mg/m^2/day) and etoposide phosphate (IV, 200 mg/m^2/day) was determined to be 4 mg/m^2. In terms of tumor response, 5 of 13 patients demonstrated complete or partial response, five patients remained stable, and three developed disease progression. The efficacy component of the study, using the MTD of melphalan (4 mg/m^2) determined during the phase I component, is ongoing.

We have reported outcomes in 54 patients with primitive neuroectodermal tumor (PNET), medulloblastoma, and germ cell tumor who were treated with MTX (IA)-based chemotherapy and carboplatin (IA)-based chemotherapy in conjunction with BBBD (Jahnke et al., 2008). Many of the patients had adverse prognostic factors and received IA/BBBD as salvage treatment. Nonetheless, the response, survival, and toxicity data are encouraging. A plateau in the survival curves in conjunction with the long median follow-up suggests possible cure for some patients with PNET and germinomas. Long-term survival may be achieved with focal or reduced dose radiotherapy in some IA/BBBD patients (Jahnke et al., 2008).

3.8. CNS metastases

The occurrence of CNS metastases of systemic cancers far exceeds the number of primary malignant brain tumors. Current therapies such as radiosurgery are effective for short-term palliation of CNS metastases, however often do not provide long-term disease control. The use of WBRT to treat CNS metastases has been associated with neurotoxicity. BBBD may offer a new treatment strategy for CNS metastases, since BBBD enables global delivery to all cerebral circulations. Based on the results of preclinical studies, preirradiation BBBD chemotherapy may provide improved drug penetration to CNS metastases in the clinic.

Metastasis of solid tumors from the periphery to the CNS requires a complex series of events, including extravasation of tumor cells from the primary site, travel through the blood stream, binding to and infiltrating through the cerebral vasculature, and growth in the foreign site. In the laboratory, we have investigated the hypothesis that cell adhesion proteins, particularly αv integrin, are involved in multiple steps in the metastatic process. The pan-αv integrin mAb intetumumab blocks integrin-mediated cell migration and signaling *in vitro* and *in vivo*. We used a hematogenous breast cancer brain metastasis model to test the impact of intetumumab as a preventive agent (Wu et al., 2012). Rats received human breast cancer cells into the internal carotid artery either alone or in combination with intetumumab. MRI at 5–7 weeks after tumor cell infusion showed multiple brain metastases in control animals (Fig. 10), while animals receiving IV intetumumab prior to tumor cell infusion showed few metastases even at 11 weeks after infusion. Intetumumab decreased the number of metastases on histology, with 32% of intetumumab-treated rats showing no metastases at 11 weeks. Rats given intetumumab had significantly longer survival compared to rats with untreated hematogenous metastases. Our results suggest that cancer patients at risk of metastases would benefit from early intetumumab treatment.

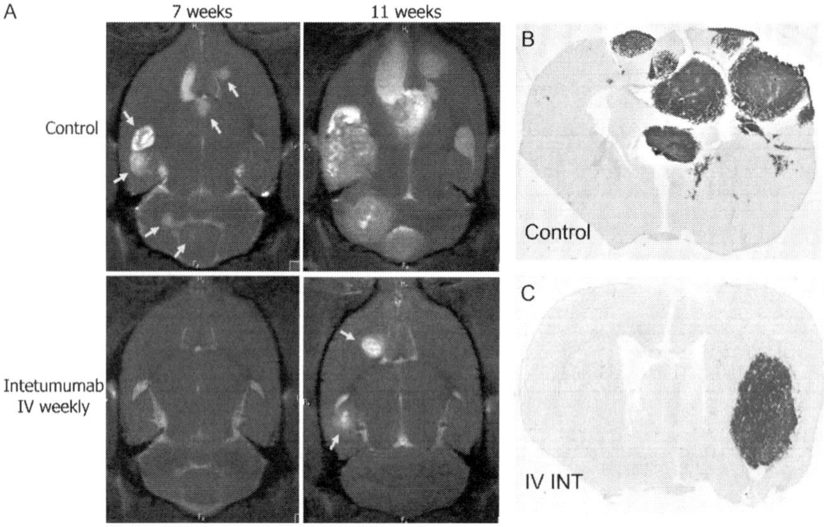

Figure 10 Effect of intetumumab anti-αv integrin mAb on breast cancer brain metastasis in the rat. (A) MRI shows that the control rat had multiple metastases at 7 weeks (top; arrows). The intetumumab-treated rat showed no metastases at 7 weeks and 2 lesions at 11 weeks (bottom; arrows). Histochemistry for human mitochondrial antigen showed 15 ± 9 metastases in control rats (B) and 4 ± 5 metastases in intetumumab-treated rats (IV INT, intravenous intetumumab) (C). *Material was originally published in Wu et al. (2012). Reprinted with kind permission from Springer Science and Business Media.*

4. CHEMOPROTECTION STUDIES

Platinum-based chemotherapy is associated with progressive and irreversible ototoxicity, and can also cause bone marrow toxicity, renal toxicity, and hepatotoxicity. Platinum-induced toxicities are mediated at least in part by free radical damage. Sulfur-containing thiol chemoprotective agents that mimic activities of the endogenous antioxidant glutathione can protect against free radical damage and chemotherapy toxicity. Our preclinical and clinical studies have evaluated chemoprotection using STS and *N*-acetylcysteine (NAC).

4.1. Preclinical chemoprotection studies with thiols

Early rat and guinea pig studies showed that STS (8 g/m^2 IV) blocked platinum-induced damage to the cochlea when administered as late as 8 h after carboplatin but not at 24 h after carboplatin (Dickey, Wu, Muldoon, & Neuwelt, 2005; Muldoon et al., 2000; Neuwelt et al., 1996;

Neuwelt, Pagel, Kraemer, Peterson, & Muldoon, 2004). In a rat model using IA infusion of cisplatin (6 mg/kg) to induce ototoxicity, NAC (400 mg/kg IV) protects against hearing loss when administered 15 or 30 min prior to chemotherapy or 4 h after chemotherapy (Dickey, Muldoon, Kraemer, & Neuwelt, 2004). NAC protects against cisplatin-induced weight loss (Dickey et al., 2004) suggesting that it may decrease mucositis. Pretreatment with high-dose NAC (1200 mg/kg) protected against bone marrow toxicity induced by a cocktail of chemotherapeutics (carboplatin, etoposide phosphate, and melphalan) (Neuwelt, Pagel, Hasler, Deloughery, & Muldoon, 2001). Rescue of white blood cells and platelets was found with NAC even if animals were pretreated with buthionine sulfoximine to lower glutathione synthesis (Neuwelt et al., 2001). The combination of NAC plus STS improved bone marrow chemoprotection (Neuwelt, 2004). STS alone did not protect against nephrotoxicity (Dickey et al., 2005). In contrast, pretreatment or 4 h posttreatment with NAC significantly decreased cisplatin-induced kidney damage as determined by measurement of the kidney blood urea nitrogen and creatinine and by pathological assessment (Dickey et al., 2005). We showed that NAC delivered IA in the descending aorta is more efficacious than IV NAC for kidney chemoprotection, while oral administration is ineffective (Dickey et al., 2008; Fig. 11). Nephroprotection correlated with blood concentrations of NAC, showing the importance of high dose and IV route of delivery.

Clinical use of chemoprotection has been limited by the possibility of protecting the cancer against chemotherapy toxicity. Our *in vitro* studies demonstrated that while both STS and NAC are protective to tumor cells if administered at the same time as chemotherapy, tumor cell protection was lost if the thiols were delayed by 2–4 h (Muldoon et al., 2001; Wu, Muldoon, & Neuwelt, 2005). STS was not tumor protective in a mouse model of neuroblastoma if delayed until 6 h after cisplatin (Harned et al., 2008). In a rat model of lung cancer brain metastasis, 8 h delayed STS, 1 h pretreatment with NAC, or the combination of NAC pretreatment plus STS postreatment did not impact the antitumor efficacy of carboplatin chemotherapy (Neuwelt et al., 2004). We further assessed the impact of the timing of NAC on the efficacy of cisplatin in rat models of pediatric tumors (Muldoon, Wu, Pagel, & Neuwelt, submitted for publication). We found that pretreatment with NAC significantly decreased cisplatin efficacy in both a systemic solid tumor model (neuroblastoma) and an intracerebral tumor model (medulloblastoma). In contrast, delay of NAC until 4 h after cisplatin did not decrease chemotherapy efficacy in either tumor model.

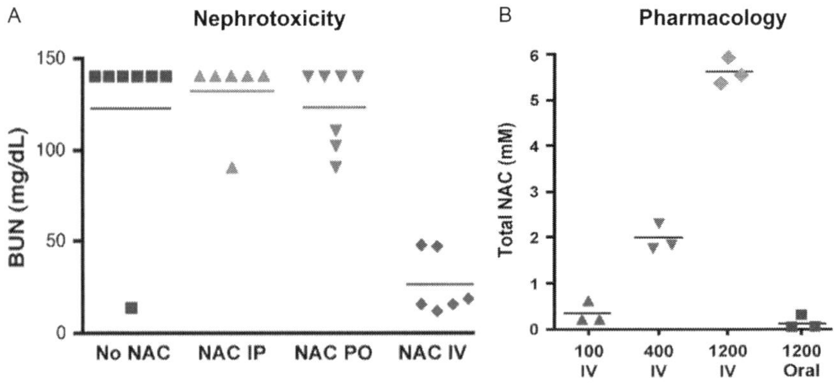

Figure 11 Effect of dose and route of administration on *N*-acetylcysteine (NAC) chemoprotection. (A) Nephroprotection. Rats received a nephrotoxic dose of cisplatin followed in 4 h by no NAC or NAC 400 mg/kg given by oral or IV route of administration. NAC significantly reduced cisplatin-induced kidney toxicity, when given by IV but not by oral route of administration. (B) NAC pharmacology. Serum NAC concentrations were measured by HPLC 15 min after IV or oral administration. Chemoprotective doses of NAC (400–1000 mg/kg) gave peak blood concentrations of 2 mM or greater only when administered IV and were not effective when administered intraperitoneal or oral. *Panels (A) and (B) were originally published in Dickey et al. (2008), © with kind permission of Springer Science and Business Media, adapted figure 4.*

4.2. Clinical chemoprotection studies with thiols

Dose intensive chemotherapy strategies for the treatment of malignant brain tumors necessitate minimizing CNS and systemic toxicities. Carboplatin has shown efficacy in malignant brain tumors. However, carboplatin causes myelosuppression including severe thrombocytopenia, often requiring platelet transfusions and dose reductions of subsequent carboplatin treatments. When administered in conjunction with BBBD, carboplatin (IA) causes irreversible hearing loss in a large proportion of subjects (Doolittle, Muldoon, et al., 2001; Neuwelt, Brummett, et al., 1998).

Clinical studies have shown hearing protection when high-dose STS (16–20 g/m^2) was administered as part of a two-compartment model in adult patients with malignant brain tumors (Doolittle, Muldoon, et al., 2001; Neuwelt, Brummett, et al., 1998; Fig. 12). Carboplatin was administered IA in conjunction with BBBD. High-dose STS was administered IV in a delayed fashion, 4 h (or 4 and 8 h) after carboplatin, thus providing spatial and temporal separations between chemotherapy and chemoprotectant. The study showed a protective effect against carboplatin-induced hearing loss. We later reviewed hematologic data from patients with malignant brain

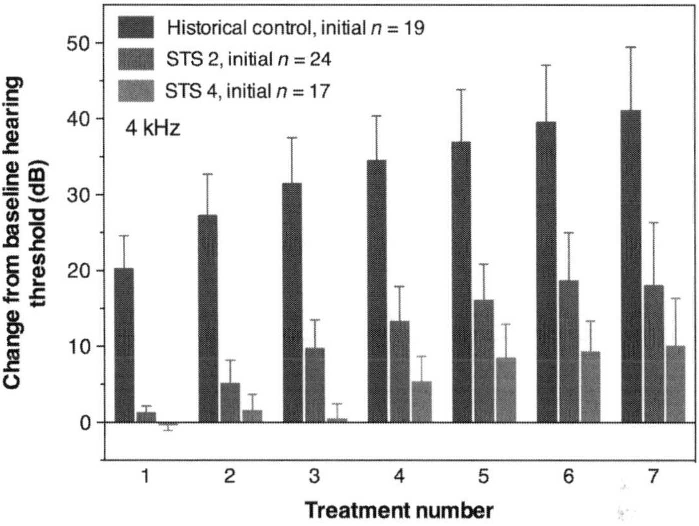

Figure 12 Sodium thiosulfate (STS) shows hearing protection in adults with malignant brain tumors. Comparison of hearing threshold shift against carboplatin treatment number, at 4000 Hz, in historical comparison brain tumor patients who were treated with carboplatin (intraarterial [IA]) with blood–brain barrier disruption (BBBD) without STS and brain tumor patients treated with delayed STS 2 h (STS2) or 4 h (STS4) after carboplatin (IA) with BBBD. There was a significant difference in hearing protection between the STS treatment groups and the historical comparison group ($P = 0.0075$). *Reprinted from Doolittle, Muldoon, et al. (2001).*

tumors treated with carboplatin IA with BBBD, with or without delayed high-dose STS for hearing protection. The rate of grade 3 or 4 platelet toxicity (CTCAE) without STS was 47.8% and with STS was 17.2%; there was a significant association of grade 3 or 4 platelet toxicity in patients without STS treatment ($P = 0.0018$). The rates of dose reduction of carboplatin, controlling for prior chemotherapy, were statistically significant between the two groups ($P = 0.0046$). These results suggest that STS may protect against severe thrombocytopenia, decreasing the number of platelet transfusions and dose reductions of carboplatin (Doolittle, Tyson, et al., 2001).

Our studies led to the implementation of two phase III trials of STS for protection against cisplatin-induced hearing loss. The Children's Oncology Group Study ACCL0431 evaluated the efficacy of STS treatment compared with observation in children diagnosed with childhood cancers typically treated with cisplatin therapy (Freyer 2014). The study is completed and concluded that STS protects against cisplatin-induced hearing loss in children. STS was not associated with a change in OS in patients with localized disease. However STS treatment was associated with lower OS in patients with disseminated disease. The COG study raised the bar for supportive hearing protection in children, while pointing out the role of disease extent (non-disemminated versus disseminated) in possible tumor protective effect when STS is administered on this dose and schedule. A second trial conducted by Societe Internationale d'Oncologie Pediatrique is continuing (Maibach 2014). In this trial, children with standard-risk hepatoblastoma (ie localized tumor) are treated with cisplatin monotherapy or cisplatin and STS. An Independent Data Monitoring Committee has periodically reviewed the efficacy results to assess any potential adverse impact of STS on cisplatin efficacy. To date, the periodic safety checks indicate no evidence of tumor protection. The expected end of accrual for this trial is December 2014.

A phase I clinical study of NAC in adult patients undergoing endovascular procedures is almost complete. Sixteen patients were randomized to receive IV or IA NAC in a standard dose escalation study. As the study nears completion, it appears that the NAC MTD is in the range of 300–450 mg/kg. A phase I NAC dose escalation study is underway in children with a variety of cancer diagnoses undergoing treatment with cisplatin-based chemotherapy.

5. ADVANCES IN NEUROIMAGING

Neuroimaging techniques are critical in assessing biologic and physiologic aspects of brain tumors as well as other neurologic diseases. The ability to accurately image infiltrative disease and to assess the true extent of disease and actual tumor volume is essential. Conventional MRI allows visualization of brain areas with abnormal BBB leakage but does not actually show tumor vasculature. New MRI techniques can characterize physiological changes in the vasculature in brain tumors and CNS lesions.

Dynamic MRI techniques use very rapid signal acquisition to track a bolus of contrast agent as it passes through the brain vasculature. Dynamic contrast-enhanced (DCE) MRI of CNS lesions with gadolinium-based contrast agents (GBCAs) provides a noninvasive mechanism to measure vascular permeability and pharmacokinetic properties, such as the contrast agent transfer rate constant (K^{trans}), with high spatial and temporal resolutions. A second technique is perfusion-weighted dynamic susceptibility-weighted contrast-enhanced (DSC) MRI, which can be used to noninvasively measure relative cerebral blood volume (rCBV) in brain lesions relative to normal-appearing white matter, providing a measure of blood vessel size and density. The high permeability of GBCA limits its use in rCBV measurements. Instead we use the ultrasmall superparamagnetic iron oxide nanoparticle ferumoxytol (Feraheme) as a blood pool contrast agent. Ferumoxytol is a virus-sized carbohydrate-coated particle with an iron oxide core, which serves not only as a contrast agent for MRI but can be identified histologically and ultrastructurally by electron microscopy (as shown in Fig. 2). It is FDA-approved for iron replacement therapy, and is safe for neuroimaging in both rats and patients.

5.1. Preclinical studies of dynamic MRI

Standard GBCAs have limitations in medical imaging involving inconsistent measurement of rCBV. In a landmark preclinical study, we investigated rCBV measurement with ferumoxytol in comparison to GBCA in order to evaluate the technique of contrast leakage correction that is used clinically with GBCA (Gahramanov, Muldoon, Li, & Neuwelt, 2011). We found that ferumoxytol improves the consistency of rCBV measurements in rats before and after treatment with the anti-VEGF mAb bevacizumab and does not require contrast preload or leakage correction. This rat study showed that the technical and mathematical manipulations necessary to use GBCA for vascular MRI are not necessary using ferumoxytol and demonstrated the utility of DSC-MRI in measuring vascular changes.

We have used both the DCE-MRI and DSC-MRI techniques to assess brain tumor vasculature and vascular-targeting agents in animal models. DCE-MRI permeability measurements showed that glyburide decreases edema in brain metastasis models, which may allow reduced doses of steroids and lessen the morbidity associated with steroids in brain tumor patients (Thompson, Pishko, Muldoon, & Neuwelt, 2013). In a glioma model, we showed that bevacizumab significantly decreased the blood volume and permeability of the brain tumor vasculature, analogous to high-dose dexamethasone (Varallyay et al., 2009). In a lung metastasis model, using intracerebral implantation of human LX-1 small cell lung carcinoma cells, bevacizumab decreased blood volume and vascular permeability on dynamic MRI, which correlated with a 10-fold decrease in microvessel density on histology (Muldoon, Gahramanov, et al., 2011; Fig. 13). The changes in vasculature correlated with a significantly increased volume of tumor necrosis, yet the brain metastases continued to grow over the week assessment period after bevacizumab treatment (Muldoon, Gahramanov, et al., 2011). In another study, we used DCE-MRI and DSC-MRI to evaluate the effects

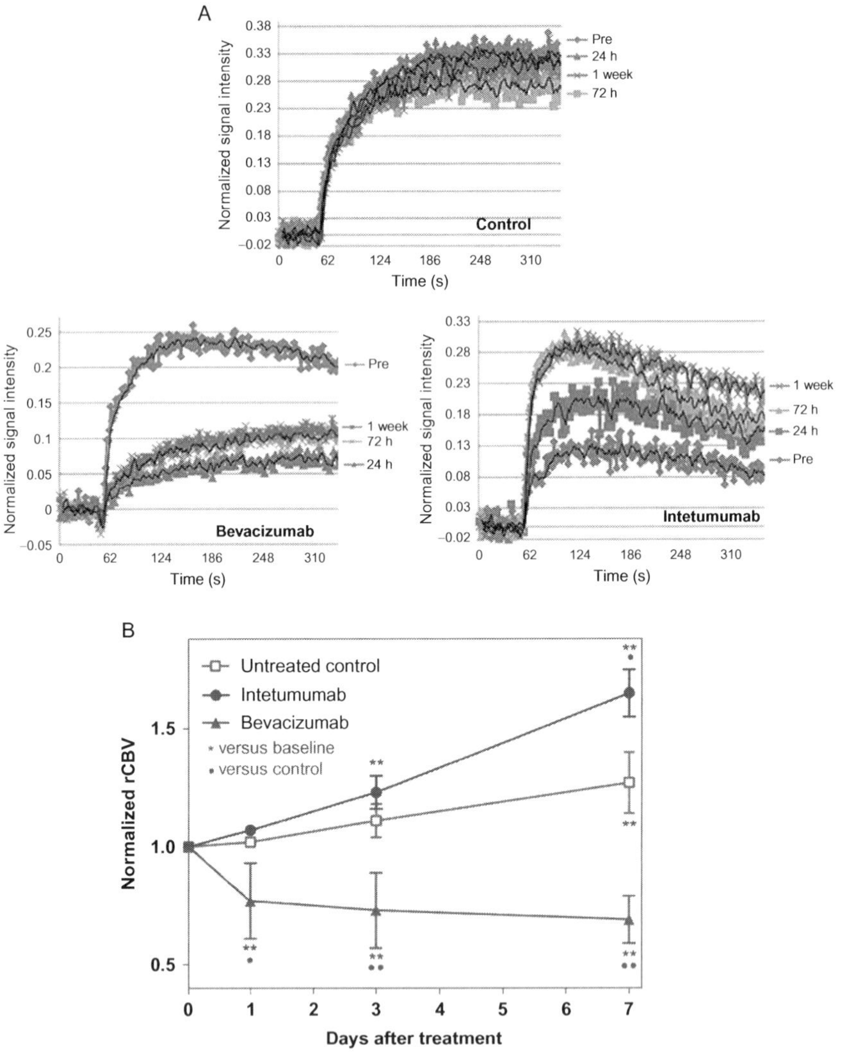

Figure 13 Effect of intetumumab and bevacizumab on brain tumor vasculature. Rats with intracerebral LX-1 SCLC xenografts were randomized to no treatment, intetumumab anti-αv integrin mAb, or bevacizumab anti-VEGF mAb. Rats underwent serial dynamic contrast-enhanced MRI with gadolinium-based contrast agent to evaluate vascular permeability (A) and dynamic susceptibility-weighted contrast-enhanced MRI with ferumoxytol to evaluate relative cerebral blood volume (rCBV) (B). Bevacizumab decreased vascular permeability and rCBV within 24 h, while intetumumab increased both permeability and rCBV over a week following treatment. *Reprinted from Muldoon, Gahramanov, et al. (2011) by the permission of Society for Neuro-Oncology.*

of the anti-αv integrin mAb intetumumab on tumor vasculature in the lung cancer brain metastasis model (Muldoon, Lewin, et al., 2011; Muldoon et al., 2005). Intetumumab increased tumor vascular permeability and blood volume on dynamic MRI and increased blood vessel size but not the number of vessels on histology. We hypothesize that alterations of tumor vasculature with intetumumab will increase the delivery of chemotherapy in brain tumors and may thus enhance chemotherapy efficacy. These results demonstrated the opposite effects of targeting brain tumor vasculature with differing agents and clearly show the interrelationship of vascular permeability and relevant tumor phenotype.

5.2. Clinical imaging studies using ferumoxytol

In the clinic, MRI using ferumoxytol shows good correlation with GBCA-enhanced scans 24 h postinjection and improves visualization of vasculature associated with malformations, tumors, inflammation, as well as rCBV measurements (Dosa, Guillaume, et al., 2011; Dosa, Tuladhar, et al., 2011; Hamilton et al., 2011). Our clinical findings of the use of ferumoxytol give both anatomic and physiologic information about the BBB and CNS vasculature parameters (Neuwelt et al., 2007, 2009; Weinstein et al., 2010). Ferumoxytol shows signal changes on T1W and T2W sequences in demyelinating disease as well as in PCNSL and lymphoproliferative disorders (Farrell et al., 2013). Different enhancement patterns compared to GBCA-enhanced scans have been observed in some patients. Such differences might distinguish patients with differing degrees of inflammation, a characteristic which has prognostic or therapeutic importance.

In patients with malignant brain tumors, radiographic worsening after radiation therapy can be caused by true tumor progression or by pseudoprogression. Unlike true tumor progression, MRI signal changes in pseudoprogression reflect treatment-induced inflammatory change with increased permeability of the BBB. These changes stabilize spontaneously and are associated with a favorable prognosis (Fig. 14). The inability to differentiate tumor progression from pseudoprogression can lead to the continuation of ineffective therapy or early discontinuation of chemotherapy; it can cause inclusion of patients with pseudoprogression in experimental protocols, with further false-positive response to experimental treatment. Two recent studies showed the benefit of perfusion MRI with ferumoxytol for CBV assessment in the differential diagnosis of true tumor progression and pseudoprogression (Gahramanov et al., 2013; Gahramanov, Raslan, et al., 2011). We introduced dual-contrast imaging during a single MRI

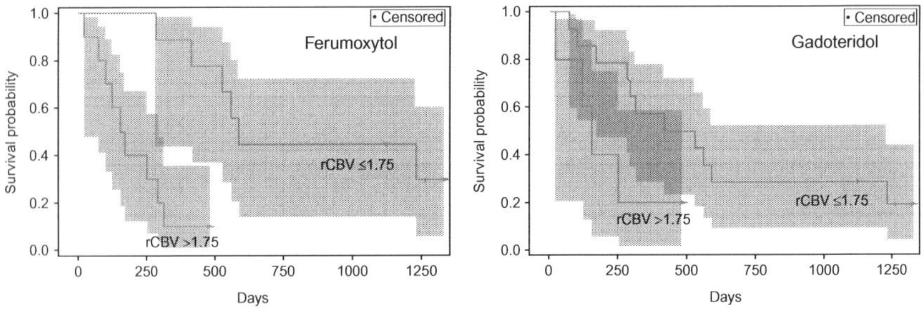

Figure 14 Survival of glioblastoma multiforme patients according to the relative cerebral blood volume (rCBV) cutoff value >1.75. Brain tumor rCBV was measured using ferumoxytol vs. gadoteridol. Kaplan–Meier survival curves show the best survival prediction by using rCBV values obtained with ferumoxytol ($P < 0.001$). By using gadoteridol, survival prediction is similar but not statistically significant. *Reprinted with permission from Gahramanov et al. (2013).*

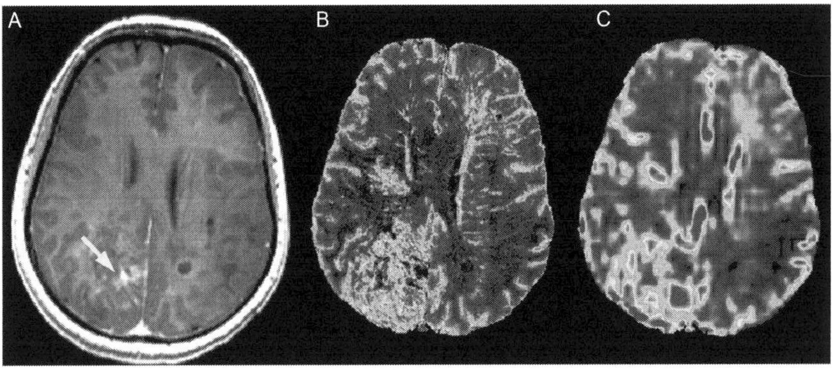

Figure 15 Comparison of steady-state-cerebral blood volume (SS-CBV) and dynamic susceptibility contrast (DSC)-CBV maps in a glioblastoma patient. (A) T1-weighted post-gadoteridol scan describes the multifocal signal abnormalities. In corresponding slices, the SS-CBV (B) and DSC-CBV (C) maps show increased areas of CBV referring to highly vascular tumor areas. Note the mismatch between the most enhancing region (arrow) and the highest CBV values. *Reprinted from Varallyay et al. (2013).*

session: GBCA for BBB integrity assessment and ferumoxytol for CBV assessment. Dual-contrast imaging may be the beginning of a multicontrast imaging era when different contrast agents are applied for specific purposes, to confirm or rule out certain tumor types, establish the presence and magnitude of inflammation, or evaluate angiogenesis (Gahramanov et al., 2013; Gahramanov, Raslan, et al., 2011).

Dynamic MRI with ferumoxytol is a major advance toward the goal of delineating tumor response, but the technique has significant limitations. Because the entire brain must be scanned in a very short time frame (2 s) the images are necessarily low resolution. We have utilized the strong susceptibility effect of ferumoxytol to develop a new steady-state technique for imaging the cerebrovasculature. Our aim is to improve CBV maps by substantially eliminating image distortion and increasing resolution. We found that high-resolution CBV maps can be achieved using clinically applicable doses of ferumoxytol and in comparison with DSC-CBV (Fig. 15). The high spatial resolution and distortion-free parametric maps will help differentiate active tumor from necrotic tissue and better localize most malignant tumor regions, therefore increasing accurate targeted biopsy (Christen et al., 2013; D'Arceuil et al., 2013; Varallyay et al., 2013).

6. CONCLUSION

Many important observations regarding BBBD have been made in animal studies. For example, (1) a marked increase in brain and CSF concentrations of MTX were documented after BBBD with IA chemotherapy administration (Kroll & Neuwelt, 1998; Neuwelt, 1989; Neuwelt, Frenkel, Rapoport, & Barnett, 1980), (2) disruption of the BBB provides global delivery throughout the disrupted hemisphere, but delivery is variable depending on the brain region and the type and size of tumor, (3) vascular permeability to small molecules such as MTX, as well as large molecules such as mAbs, is increased maximally by 15 min after mannitol infusion, and (4) BBB permeability rapidly decreases, returning to preinfusion levels within 2 h after BBBD.

Delivery of chemotherapy in conjunction with BBBD has provided excellent clinical outcomes especially in PCNSL. Long-term follow-up has shown that patients with this disease treated with enhanced chemotherapy delivery can maintain stable if not improved cognitive function and quality of life. The addition of rituximab to chemotherapy with BBBD treatment for PCNSL can be safely accomplished with excellent OS. The use of delayed high-dose STS has shown hearing protection in patients undergoing treatment with carboplatin-based chemotherapy when administered with BBBD. This approach laid the groundwork for chemoprotection studies using thiols such as STS and NAC to protect against cisplatin-based hearing loss in children.

Neuroimaging using, dynamic MRI techniques and the new steady-state MRI technique using ferumoxytol will have important implications for monitoring patient outcomes and response to therapy. These techniques improve the detection of pseudoprogression, a treatment-induced inflammatory response that is associated with markedly improved survival. The measurements of tumor blood volume clearly differentiate pseudoprogression from true tumor progression, and pseudoresponse (decreased tumor vascular permeability) from true response to therapy. One of the major implications is that patients with pseudoprogression will continue with their effective therapy and will not be placed in trials of experimental therapy. We anticipate that improved neuroimaging will be incorporated into standard of care for assessing therapy-induced changes in brain tumor vasculature, improving detection of brain tumor response to therapy, and differentiating CNS lesions with an inflammatory component.

BBBD treatment is not without challenges. The procedure should be undertaken only by trained multidisciplinary teams at centers where neuro-oncology, interventional neurosurgery/neuroradiology, neuroanesthesia, and experienced oncology nursing are available. Uniform chemotherapy protocols and comprehensive guidelines for anesthesia, transfemoral arterial cannulation, mannitol/chemotherapy infusion, pre- and post-BBBD procedure patient care, and follow-up cognitive and neuroimaging assessment must be followed by the trained teams. Nonetheless, BBBD has been safely conducted at several institutions, an active BBBD Consortium is in place, and scientific meetings are convened annually to discuss preclinical and clinical advances in delivering agents across the BBB. Regarding imaging, ferumoxytol has not yet received FDA approval for neuroimaging, and image analysis is not yet standardized. However, processes are currently well underway to turn these goals into reality.

Future directions include preclinical and clinical dose intensification of platinum-based chemotherapeutics with thiol chemoprotection and further development of steady-state MRI techniques with ferumoxytol that provide high-resolution images of CNS lesions to improve rCBV measurements and measure absolute CBV. In addition, further preclinical and clinical investigations of the role of mAbs (1) as first-line treatment for PCNSL, (2) as maintenance immunotherapy as a mechanism to improve clinical progression-free and OS in PCNSL, and (3) for the prevention of brain metastases are planned.

CONFLICT OF INTEREST

N. D. D., E. A. N., and A. Y. C. have no conflicts of interest to declare.

L. L. M., OHSU, Portland Veterans Affairs Medical Center (PVAMC), and the Department of Veterans Affairs have a significant financial interest in Adherex, a company that may have a commercial interest in the results of this research and technology. This potential conflict of interest was reviewed and managed by the OHSU Integrity Program Oversight Council and the PVAMC Conflict of Interest in Research Committee. Dr. Neuwelt, inventor of technology licensed to Adherex, has divested himself of all potential earnings.

ACKNOWLEDGMENTS

We thank the OHSU preclinical and clinical BBB team as well as our colleagues in blood-brain barrier disruption, primary central nervous system lymphoma, thiol chemoprotection, and neuroimaging for their commitment and ongoing collaboration. This work was supported by the National Institutes of Health R01 Grants CA137488, NS44687, and NS53468 from National Cancer Institute and from National Institute of Neurological Disorders and Stroke (E. A. N.); The Walter S. and Lucienne Driskill Foundation Grant (E. A. N.); and a Veterans Administration Merit Review Grant (E. A. N.).

REFERENCES

Angelov, L., Doolittle, N. D., Kraemer, D. F., Siegal, T., Barnett, G. H., Peereboom, D. M., et al. (2009). Blood–brain barrier disruption and intra-arterial methotrexate-based therapy for newly diagnosed primary CNS lymphoma: A multi-institutional experience. *Journal of Clinical Oncology*, *27*(21), 3503–3509.

Batchelor, T. T., Grossman, S. A., Mikkelsen, T., Ye, X., Desideri, S., & Lesser, G. J. (2011). Rituximab monotherapy for patients with recurrent primary CNS lymphoma. *Neurology*, *76*(10), 929–930.

Brightman, M. W., Hori, M., Rapoport, S. I., Reese, T. S., & Westergaard, E. (1973). Osmotic opening of tight junctions in cerebral endothelium. *Journal of Comparative Neurology*, *152*(4), 317–325.

Brightman, M. W., & Reese, T. S. (1969). Junctions between intimately apposed cell membranes in the vertebrate brain. *Journal of Cell Biology*, *40*(3), 648–677.

Christen, T., Ni, W., Qiu, D., Schmiedeskamp, H., Bammer, R., Moseley, M., et al. (2013). High-resolution cerebral blood volume imaging in humans using the blood pool contrast agent ferumoxytol. *Magnetic Resonance in Medicine*, *70*(3), 705–710. http://dx.doi.org/10.1002/mrm.24500.

Coiffier, B., Lepage, E., Briere, J., Herbrecht, R., Tilly, H., Bouabdallah, R., et al. (2002). CHOP chemotherapy plus rituximab compared with CHOP alone in elderly patients with diffuse large-B-cell lymphoma. *New England Journal of Medicine*, *346*(4), 235–242.

Correa, D. D., Shi, W., Abrey, L. E., Deangelis, L. M., Omuro, A. M., Deutsch, M. B., et al. (2012). Cognitive functions in primary CNS lymphoma after single or combined modality regimens. *Neuro-Oncology*, *14*(1), 101–108.

Dahlborg, S. A., Henner, W. D., Crossen, J. R., Tableman, C. M., Petrillo, A., Braziel, R., et al. (1996). Non-AIDS primary CNS lymphoma: First example of a durable response in a primary brain tumor using enhanced chemotherapy delivery without cognitive loss and without radiotherapy. *The Cancer Journal from Scientific American*, *2*(3), 166–174.

Dahlborg, S. A., Petrillo, A., Crossen, J. R., Roman-Goldstein, S., Doolittle, N. D., Fuller, K. H., et al. (1998). The potential for complete and durable response in nonglial primary brain tumors in children and young adults with enhanced chemotherapy delivery. *The Cancer Journal from Scientific American*, *4*(2), 110–124.

D'Arceuil, H., Coimbra, A., Triano, P., Dougherty, M., Mello, J., Moseley, M., et al. (2013). Ferumoxytol enhanced resting state fMRI and relative cerebral blood volume mapping in normal human brain. *NeuroImage*, *83*, 200–209.

Dickey, D. T., Dickey, D. T., Muldoon, L. L., Doolittle, N. D., Peterson, D. R., Kraemer, D. F., et al. (2008). Effect of N-acetylcysteine route of administration on chemoprotection against cisplatin-induced toxicity in rat models. *Cancer Chemotherapy and Pharmacology*, *62*(2), 235–241.

Dickey, D. T., Muldoon, L. L., Kraemer, D. F., & Neuwelt, E. A. (2004). Protection against cisplatin-induced ototoxicity by N-acetylcysteine in a rat model. *Hearing Research*, *193*(1–2), 25–30.

Dickey, D. T., Wu, Y. J., Muldoon, L. L., & Neuwelt, E. A. (2005). Protection against cisplatin-induced toxicities by N-acetylcysteine and sodium thiosulfate as assessed at the molecular, cellular, and in vivo levels. *Journal of Pharmacology and Experimental Therapeutics*, *314*(3), 1052–1058.

Doolittle, N. D., Abrey, L. E., Shenkier, T. N., Tali, S., Bromberg, J. E., Neuwelt, E. A., et al. (2008). Brain parenchyma involvement as isolated central nervous system relapse of systemic non-Hodgkin lymphoma: An International Primary CNS Lymphoma Collaborative Group report. *Blood*, *111*(3), 1085–1093.

Doolittle, N. D., Dosa, E., Fu, R., Muldoon, L. L., Maron, L. M., Lubow, M. A., et al. (2013). Preservation of cognitive function in primary CNS lymphoma survivors a median of 12 years after enhanced chemotherapy delivery. *Journal of Clinical Oncology*, *31*(31), 4026–4027.

Doolittle, N. D., Fu, R., Muldoon, L. L., Tyson, R. M., Lacy, C., & Neuwelt, E. A. (2013). Rituximab in combination with methotrexate-based chemotherapy with blood–brain barrier disruption in newly diagnosed primary CNS lymphoma. *Hematological Oncology*, *31*(S1), 179.

Doolittle, N. D., Jahnke, K., Belanger, R., Ryan, D. A., Nance, R. W., Jr., Lacy, C. A., et al. (2007). Potential of chemo-immunotherapy and radioimmunotherapy in relapsed primary central nervous system (CNS) lymphoma. *Leukemia and Lymphoma*, *48*(9), 1712–1720.

Doolittle, N. D., Korfel, A., Lubow, M. A., Schorb, E., Schlegel, U., Rogowski, S., et al. (2013). Long-term cognitive function, neuroimaging, and quality of life in primary CNS lymphoma. *Neurology*, *81*(1), 84–92.

Doolittle, N. D., Miner, M. E., Hall, W. A., Siegal, T., Jerome, E., Osztie, E., et al. (2000). Safety and efficacy of a multicenter study using intraarterial chemotherapy in conjunction with osmotic opening of the blood–brain barrier for the treatment of patients with malignant brain tumors. *Cancer*, *88*(3), 637–647.

Doolittle, N. D., Muldoon, L. L., Brummett, R. E., Tyson, R. M., Lacy, C., Bubalo, J. S., et al. (2001). Delayed sodium thiosulfate as an otoprotectant against carboplatin-induced hearing loss in patients with malignant brain tumors. *Clinical Cancer Research*, 7(3), 493–500.

Doolittle, N. D., Tyson, R. M., Lacy, C., Quipotla, J., Kraemer, D. F., Deloughery, T. G., et al. (2001). Potential role of delayed sodium thiosulfate as protectant against severe carboplatin-induced thrombocytopenia in patients with malignant brain tumors. *Blood*, *98*(11), 37a–38a.

Dosa, E., Guillaume, D. J., Haluska, M., Lacy, C. A., Hamilton, B. E., Njus, J. M., et al. (2011). Magnetic resonance imaging of intracranial tumors: Intra-patient comparison of gadoteridol and ferumoxytol. *Neuro-Oncology*, *13*(2), 251–260.

Dosa, E., Tuladhar, S., Muldoon, L. L., Hamilton, B. E., Rooney, W. D., & Neuwelt, E. A. (2011). MRI using ferumoxytol improves the visualization of central nervous system vascular malformations. *Stroke*, *42*(6), 1581–1588.

Farrell, B. T., Hamilton, B. E., Dosa, E., Rimely, E., Nasseri, M., Gahramanov, S., et al. (2013). Using iron oxide nanoparticles to diagnose CNS inflammatory diseases and PCNSL. *Neurology*, *81*(3), 256–263.
Fortin, D., McCormick, C. I., Remsen, L. G., Nixon, R., & Neuwelt, E. A. (2000). Unexpected neurotoxicity of etoposide phosphate administered in combination with other chemotherapeutic agents after blood–brain barrier modification to enhance delivery, using propofol for general anesthesia, in a rat model. *Neurosurgery*, *47*(1), 199–207.
Freyer, D. R. (2014). The effects of sodium thiosulfate (STS) on cisplatin-induced hearing loss: A report from the Children's Oncology Group. *Journal of Clinical Oncology*, *32*, 5s (suppl: abstr 10017).
Gahramanov, S., Muldoon, L. L., Li, X., & Neuwelt, E. A. (2011). Improved perfusion MR imaging assessment of intracerebral tumor blood volume and antiangiogenic therapy efficacy in a rat model with ferumoxytol. *Radiology*, *261*(3), 796–804.
Gahramanov, S., Muldoon, L. L., Varallyay, C. G., Li, X., Kraemer, D. F., Fu, R., et al. (2013). Pseudoprogression of glioblastoma after chemo- and radiation therapy: Diagnosis by using dynamic susceptibility-weighted contrast-enhanced perfusion MR imaging with ferumoxytol versus gadoteridol and correlation with survival. *Radiology*, *266*(3), 842–852.
Gahramanov, S., Raslan, A. M., Muldoon, L. L., Hamilton, B. E., Rooney, W. D., Varallyay, C. G., et al. (2011). Potential for differentiation of pseudoprogression from true tumor progression with dynamic susceptibility-weighted contrast-enhanced magnetic resonance imaging using ferumoxytol vs. gadoteridol: A pilot study. *International Journal of Radiation Oncology, Biology, Physics*, *79*(2), 514–523.
Groothuis, D. R., Benalcazar, H., Allen, C. V., Wise, R. M., Dills, C., Dobrescu, C., et al. (2000). Comparison of cytosine arabinoside delivery to rat brain by intravenous, intrathecal, intraventricular and intraparenchymal routes of administration. *Brain Research*, *856*(1–2), 281–290.
Guillaume, D. J., Doolittle, N. D., Gahramanov, S., Hedrick, N. A., Delashaw, J. B., & Neuwelt, E. A. (2010). Intra-arterial chemotherapy with osmotic blood-brain barrier disruption for aggressive oligodendroglial tumors: Results of a phase I study. *Neurosurgery*, *66*(1), 48–58, discussion 58.
Hamilton, B. E., Nesbit, G. M., Dosa, E., Gahramanov, S., Rooney, B., Nesbit, E. G., et al. (2011). Comparative analysis of ferumoxytol and gadoteridol enhancement using T1- and T2-weighted MRI in neuroimaging. *AJR. American Journal of Roentgenology*, *197*(4), 981–988.
Harder, H., Holtel, H., Bromberg, J. E., Poortmans, P., Haaxma-Reiche, H., Kluin-Nelemans, H. C., et al. (2004). Cognitive status and quality of life after treatment for primary CNS lymphoma. *Neurology*, *62*(4), 544–547.
Harned, T. M., Kalous, O., Neuwelt, A., Loera, J., Ji, L., Iovine, P., et al. (2008). Sodium thiosulfate administered six hours after cisplatin does not compromise antineuroblastoma activity. *Clinical Cancer Research*, *14*(2), 533–540.
Jahnke, K., Kraemer, D. F., Knight, K. R., Fortin, D., Bell, S., Doolittle, N. D., et al. (2008). Intraarterial chemotherapy and osmotic blood–brain barrier disruption for patients with embryonal and germ cell tumors of the central nervous system. *Cancer*, *112*(3), 581–588.
Jahnke, K., Muldoon, L. L., Varallyay, C. G., Lewin, S. J., Brown, R. D., Kraemer, D. F., et al. (2009). Efficacy and MRI of rituximab and methotrexate treatment in a nude rat model of CNS lymphoma. *Neuro-Oncology*, *11*(5), 503–513.
Kroll, R. A., & Neuwelt, E. A. (1998). Outwitting the blood–brain barrier for therapeutic purposes: Osmotic opening and other means. *Neurosurgery*, *42*(5), 1083–1099, discussion 1099–1100.

Maibach, R., Childs, M., Rajput, K., Neuwelt, E. A., Roebuck, D., Sullivan, M. J., et al. (2014). SIOPEL6: A multicenter open-label randomized phase III trial of the efficacy of sodium thiosulphate (STS) in reducing ototoxicity in patients receiving cisplatin (Cis) monotherapy for standard-risk hepatoblastoma (SR-HB). *Journal of Clinical Oncology*, *32*, 5s (suppl; asbtr TPS 10094).

Maza, S., Kiewe, P., Munz, D. L., Korfel, A., Hamm, B., Jahnke, K., et al. (2009). First report on a prospective trial with yttrium-90-labeled ibritumomab tiuxetan (Zevalin) in primary CNS lymphoma. *Neuro-Oncology*, *11*(4), 423–429.

McAllister, L. D., Doolittle, N. D., Guastadisegni, P. E., Kraemer, D. F., Lacy, C. A., Crossen, J. R., et al. (2000). Cognitive outcomes and long-term follow-up results after enhanced chemotherapy delivery for primary central nervous system lymphoma. *Neurosurgery*, *46*(1), 51–60, discussion 60–51.

Morris, P. G., & Abrey, L. E. (2009). Therapeutic challenges in primary CNS lymphoma. *Lancet Neurology*, *8*(6), 581–592.

Muldoon, L. L., Alvarez, J. I., Begley, D. J., Boado, R. J., Del Zoppo, G. J., Doolittle, N. D., et al. (2013). Immunologic privilege in the central nervous system and the blood–brain barrier. *Journal of Cerebral Blood Flow and Metabolism*, *33*(1), 13–21.

Muldoon, L. L., Gahramanov, S., Li, X., Marshall, D. J., Kraemer, D. F., & Neuwelt, E. A. (2011). Dynamic magnetic resonance imaging assessment of vascular targeting agent effects in rat intracerebral tumor models. *Neuro-Oncology*, *13*(1), 51–60.

Muldoon, L. L., Lewin, S. J., Dosa, E., Kraemer, D. F., Pagel, M. A., Doolittle, N. D., et al. (2011). Imaging and therapy with rituximab anti-CD20 immunotherapy in an animal model of central nervous system lymphoma. *Clinical Cancer Research*, *17*(8), 2207–2215.

Muldoon, L. L., Pagel, M. A., Kroll, R. A., Brummett, R. E., Doolittle, N. D., Zuhowski, E. G., et al. (2000). Delayed administration of sodium thiosulfate in animal models reduces platinum ototoxicity without reduction of antitumor activity. *Clinical Cancer Research*, *6*(1), 309–315.

Muldoon, L. L., Pagel, M. A., Kroll, R. A., Roman-Goldstein, S., Jones, R. S., & Neuwelt, E. A. (1999). A physiological barrier distal to the anatomic blood–brain barrier in a model of transvascular delivery. *American Journal of Neuroradiology*, *20*(2), 217–222.

Muldoon, L. L., Sandor, M., Pinkston, K. E., & Neuwelt, E. A. (2005). Imaging, distribution, and toxicity of superparamagnetic iron oxide magnetic resonance nanoparticles in the rat brain and intracerebral tumor. *Neurosurgery*, *57*(4), 785–796 discussion 785–796.

Muldoon, L. L., Soussain, C., Jahnke, K., Johanson, C., Siegal, T., Smith, Q. R., et al. (2007). Chemotherapy delivery issues in central nervous system malignancy: A reality check. *Journal of Clinical Oncology*, *25*(16), 2295–2305.

Muldoon, L. L., Walker-Rosenfeld, S. L., Hale, C., Purcell, S. E., Bennett, L. C., & Neuwelt, E. A. (2001). Rescue from enhanced alkylator-induced cell death with low molecular weight sulfur-containing chemoprotectants. *Journal of Pharmacology and Experimental Therapeutics*, *296*(3), 797–805.

Muldoon, L. L., Wu, Y. J., Pagel, M. A., Beeson, K. A., & Neuwelt, E. A. (2014). N-acetylcysteine chemoprotection without decreased cisplatin antitumor efficacy in pediatric tumor models. In *Proceedings of the 105th Annual Meeting of the American Association for Cancer Research; San Diego, CA*. Philadelphia.

Nakagawa, H., Fujita, T., Izumoto, S., Kubo, S., Nakajima, Y., Tsuruzono, K., et al. (1993). Cis-diamminedichloroplatinum (CDDP) therapy for brain metastasis of lung cancer. *Journal of Neuro-Oncology*, *16*(1), 61–67.

Neuwelt, E. A. (Ed.). *Implications of the blood–brain barrier and its manipulation: Vol. 2*. (1989) New York: Plenum Publishing Corporation.

Neuwelt, E. A. (2004). Mechanisms of disease: The blood–brain barrier. *Neurosurgery*, *54*(1), 131–140, discussion 141–132.

Neuwelt, E. A., Balaban, E., Diehl, J., Hill, S., & Frenkel, E. (1983). Successful treatment of primary central nervous system lymphomas with chemotherapy after osmotic blood–brain barrier opening. *Neurosurgery*, *12*(6), 662–671.

Neuwelt, E. A., Barnett, P. A., Glasberg, M., & Frenkel, E. P. (1983). Pharmacology and neurotoxicity of cis-diamminedichloroplatinum, bleomycin, 5-fluorouracil, and cyclophosphamide administration following osmotic blood–brain barrier modification. *Cancer Research*, *43*(11), 5278–5285.

Neuwelt, E. A., Barnett, P. A., McCormick, C. I., Remsen, L. G., Kroll, R. A., & Sexton, G. (1998). Differential permeability of a human brain tumor xenograft in the nude rat: Impact of tumor size and method of administration on optimizing delivery of biologically diverse agents. *Clinical Cancer Research*, *4*(6), 1549–1555.

Neuwelt, E. A., Bauer, B., Fahlke, C., Fricker, G., Iadecola, C., Janigro, D., et al. (2011). Engaging neuroscience to advance translational research in brain barrier biology. *Nature Reviews Neuroscience*, *12*(3), 169–182.

Neuwelt, E. A., Brummett, R. E., Doolittle, N. D., Muldoon, L. L., Kroll, R. A., Pagel, M. A., et al. (1998). First evidence of otoprotection against carboplatin-induced hearing loss with a two-compartment system in patients with central nervous system malignancy using sodium thiosulfate. *Journal of Pharmacology and Experimental Therapeutics*, *286*(1), 77–84.

Neuwelt, E. A., Brummett, R. E., Remsen, L. G., Kroll, R. A., Pagel, M. A., McCormick, C. I., et al. (1996). In vitro and animal studies of sodium thiosulfate as a potential chemoprotectant against carboplatin-induced ototoxicity. *Cancer Research*, *56*(4), 706–709.

Neuwelt, E. A., Frenkel, E. P., Rapoport, S., & Barnett, P. (1980). Effect of osmotic blood–brain barrier disruption on methotrexate pharmacokinetics in the dog. *Neurosurgery*, 7(1), 36–43.

Neuwelt, E. A., Goldman, D. L., Dahlborg, S. A., Crossen, J., Ramsey, F., Roman-Goldstein, S., et al. (1991). Primary CNS lymphoma treated with osmotic blood–brain barrier disruption: Prolonged survival and preservation of cognitive function. *Journal of Clinical Oncology*, *9*(9), 1580–1590.

Neuwelt, E. A., Hamilton, B. E., Varallyay, C. G., Rooney, W. R., Edelman, R. D., Jacobs, P. M., et al. (2009). Ultrasmall superparamagnetic iron oxides (USPIOs): A future alternative magnetic resonance (MR) contrast agent for patients at risk for nephrogenic systemic fibrosis (NSF)? *Kidney International*, *75*(5), 465–474.

Neuwelt, E. A., Pagel, M., Barnett, P., Glassberg, M., & Frenkel, E. P. (1981). Pharmacology and toxicity of intracarotid adriamycin administration following osmotic blood–brain barrier modification. *Cancer Research*, *41*(11 Pt. 1), 4466–4470.

Neuwelt, E. A., Pagel, M. A., Hasler, B. P., Deloughery, T. G., & Muldoon, L. L. (2001). Therapeutic efficacy of aortic administration of N-acetylcysteine as a chemoprotectant against bone marrow toxicity after intracarotid administration of alkylators, with or without glutathione depletion in a rat model. *Cancer Research*, *61*(21), 7868–7874.

Neuwelt, E. A., Pagel, M. A., Kraemer, D. F., Peterson, D. R., & Muldoon, L. L. (2004). Bone marrow chemoprotection without compromise of chemotherapy efficacy in a rat brain tumor model. *Journal of Pharmacology and Experimental Therapeutics*, *309*(2), 594–599.

Neuwelt, E. A., Varallyay, C. G., Manninger, S., Solymosi, D., Haluska, M., Hunt, M. A., et al. (2007). The potential of ferumoxytol nanoparticle magnetic resonance imaging, perfusion, and angiography in central nervous system malignancy: A pilot study. *Neurosurgery*, *60*(4), 601–611, discussion 611–602.

Rapoport, S. I., & Robinson, P. J. (1986). Tight-junctional modification as the basis of osmotic opening of the blood–brain barrier. *Annals of the New York Academy of Sciences*, *481*, 250–267.

Remsen, L. G., Marquez, C., Garcia, R., Thrun, L. A., & Neuwelt, E. A. (2001). Efficacy after sequencing of brain radiotherapy and enhanced antibody targeted chemotherapy delivery in a rodent human lung cancer brain xenograft model. *International Journal of Radiation Oncology, Biology, Physics*, *51*(4), 1045–1049.

Remsen, L. G., McCormick, C. I., Sexton, G., Pearse, H. D., Garcia, R., Mass, M., et al. (1997). Long-term toxicity and neuropathology associated with the sequencing of cranial irradiation and enhanced chemotherapy delivery. *Neurosurgery*, *40*(5), 1034–1040, discussion 1040–1032.

Remsen, L. G., McCormick, C. I., Sexton, G., Pearse, H. D., Garcia, R., & Neuwelt, E. A. (1995). Decreased delivery and acute toxicity of cranial irradiation and chemotherapy given with osmotic blood–brain barrier disruption in a rodent model: The issue of sequence. *Clinical Cancer Research*, *1*(7), 731–739.

Remsen, L. G., Pagel, M. A., McCormick, C. I., Fiamengo, S. A., Sexton, G., & Neuwelt, E. A. (1999). The influence of anesthetic choice, PaCO2, and other factors on osmotic blood–brain barrier disruption in rats with brain tumor xenografts. *Anesthesia and Analgesia*, *88*(3), 559–567.

Remsen, L. G., Trail, P. A., Hellstrom, I., Hellstrom, K. E., & Neuwelt, E. A. (2000). Enhanced delivery improves the efficacy of a tumor-specific doxorubicin immunoconjugate in a human brain tumor xenograft model. *Neurosurgery*, *46*(3), 704–709.

Roman-Goldstein, S., Clunie, D. A., Stevens, J., Hogan, R., Monard, J., Ramsey, F., et al. (1994). Osmotic blood–brain barrier disruption: CT and radionuclide imaging. *American Journal of Neuroradiology*, *15*(3), 581–590.

Savaraj, N., Lu, K., Feun, L. G., Burgess, M. A., & Loo, T. L. (1987). Comparison of CNS penetration, tissue distribution, and pharmacology of VP 16-213 by intracarotid and intravenous administration in dogs. *Cancer Investigation*, *5*(1), 11–16.

Soussain, C., Muldoon, L. L., Varallyay, C., Jahnke, K., DePaula, L., & Neuwelt, E. A. (2007). Characterization and magnetic resonance imaging of a rat model of human B-cell central nervous system lymphoma. *Clinical Cancer Research*, *13*(8), 2504–2511.

Thiel, E., Korfel, A., Martus, P., Kanz, L., Griesinger, F., Rauch, M., et al. (2010). High-dose methotrexate with or without whole brain radiotherapy for primary CNS lymphoma (G-PCNSL-SG-1): A phase 3, randomised, non-inferiority trial. *Lancet Oncology*, *11*(11), 1036–1047.

Thompson, E. M., Pishko, G. L., Muldoon, L. L., & Neuwelt, E. A. (2013). Inhibition of SUR1 decreases the vascular permeability of cerebral metastases. *Neoplasia*, *15*(5), 535–543.

Tyson, R. M., Siegal, T., Doolittle, N. D., Lacy, C., Kraemer, D. F., & Neutwelt, E. A. (2003). Current status and future of relapsed primary central nervous system lymphoma (PCNSL). *Leukemia and Lymphoma*, *44*(4), 627–633.

Varallyay, C. G., Muldoon, L. L., Gahramanov, S., Wu, Y. J., Goodman, J. A., Li, X., et al. (2009). Dynamic MRI using iron oxide nanoparticles to assess early vascular effects of antiangiogenic versus corticosteroid treatment in a glioma model. *Journal of Cerebral Blood Flow and Metabolism*, *29*(4), 853–860.

Varallyay, C. G., Nesbit, E., Fu, R., Gahramanov, S., Moloney, B., Earl, E., et al. (2013). High-resolution steady-state cerebral blood volume maps in patients with central nervous system neoplasms using ferumoxytol, a superparamagnetic iron oxide nanoparticle. *Journal of Cerebral Blood Flow and Metabolism*, *33*(5), 780–786.

Weinstein, J. S., Varallyay, C. G., Dosa, E., Gahramanov, S., Hamilton, B., Rooney, W. D., et al. (2010). Superparamagnetic iron oxide nanoparticles: Diagnostic magnetic resonance imaging and potential therapeutic applications in neurooncology and central nervous system inflammatory pathologies, a review. *Journal of Cerebral Blood Flow and Metabolism*, *30*(1), 15–35.

Wu, Y. J., Muldoon, L. L., Gahramanov, S., Kraemer, D. F., Marshall, D. J., & Neuwelt, E. A. (2012). Targeting alphaV-integrins decreased metastasis and increased survival in a nude rat breast cancer brain metastasis model. *Journal of Neuro-Oncology*, *110*(1), 27–36.

Wu, Y. J., Muldoon, L. L., & Neuwelt, E. A. (2005). The chemoprotective agent N-acetylcysteine blocks cisplatin-induced apoptosis through caspase signaling pathway. *Journal of Pharmacology and Experimental Therapeutics*, *312*(2), 424–431.

Zucchetti, M., Rossi, C., Knerich, R., Donelli, M. G., Butti, G., Silvani, V., et al. (1991). Concentrations of VP16 and VM26 in human brain tumors. *Annals of Oncology*, *2*(1), 63–66.

CHAPTER EIGHT

Delivery of Antihuman African Trypanosomiasis Drugs Across the Blood–Brain and Blood–CSF Barriers

Gayathri N. Sekhar[1], Christopher P. Watson[1], Mehmet Fidanboylu, Lisa Sanderson, Sarah A. Thomas[2]
King's College London, Institute of Pharmaceutical Sciences, London, United Kingdom
[1]These authors contributed equally to this work.
[2]Corresponding author: e-mail address: sarah.thomas@kcl.ac.uk

Contents

Advances in Pharmacology, Volume 71
ISSN 1054-3589
http://dx.doi.org/10.1016/bs.apha.2014.06.003

Abstract

Human African trypanosomiasis (HAT or sleeping sickness) is a potentially fatal disease caused by the parasite, *Trypanosoma brucei* sp. The parasites are transmitted by the bite of insect vectors belonging to the genus *Glossina* (tsetse flies) and display a life cycle strategy that is equally spread between human and insect hosts. *T.b. gambiense* is found in western and central Africa whereas, *T.b. rhodesiense* is found in eastern and southern Africa.

The disease has two clinical stages: a blood stage after the bite of an infected tsetse fly, followed by a central nervous system (CNS) stage where the parasite penetrates the brain; causing death if left untreated. The blood–brain barrier (BBB) makes the CNS stage difficult to treat because it prevents 98% of all known compounds from entering the brain, including some anti-HAT drugs. Those that do enter the brain are toxic compounds in their own right and have serious side effects.

There are only a few drugs available to treat HAT and those that do are stage specific. This review summarizes the incidence, diagnosis, and treatment of HAT and provides a close examination of the BBB transport of anti-HAT drugs and an overview of the latest drugs in development.

ABBREVIATIONS

BBB blood–brain barrier
CT combination therapy
CVOs circumventricular organs
HAPT1 adenosine-insensitive high-affinity pentamidine transporter 1
HAT human African trypanosomiasis
hOCTs human organic cationic transporters
LAPT1 adenosine-insensitive low-affinity pentamidine transporter 1
NMCT nifurtimox and melarsoprol combination therapy
P2 adenosine-sensitive pentamidine transporter
RMT receptor-mediated transcytosis
T.b. *Trypanosoma brucei*

1. INTRODUCTION

Human African trypanosomiasis (HAT) or more commonly called African sleeping sickness is a parasitic disease in humans that is endemic in rural parts of sub-Saharan Africa (Brun et al., 2010). It occurs as a result of infection by one of the two unicellular protozoan organisms: *Trypanosoma brucei gambiense* (*T.b. gambiense*) and *Trypanosoma brucei rhodesiense* (*T.b. rhodesiense*). They belong to the *Trypanosoma* genus and are classified as subspecies of *Trypanosoma brucei brucei* (http://www.who.int/trypanosomiasis_african/parasite/en/ - accessed on 14/07/2014.). *T.b. gambiense* infect only humans, *T.b. rhodesiense* infect humans and animals, whereas *Trypanosoma congolense*, *T. vivax*, and *T. brucei brucei* cause disease only in animals called *nagana* (meaning "in low spirits" in Zulu) which result in huge economic losses (Matovu, Seebeck, Enyaru, & Kaminsky, 2001).

Parasites such as *Trypanosoma brucei* require the help of vectors for their transmission and survival. They take advantage of the ability of these vectors to infect both animals and humans alike extending their reach across the different species. *Trypanosoma brucei* are transmitted by the bite of insect vectors belonging to the genus *Glossina* (tsetse flies) and display a life cycle strategy that is equally spread between human and insect hosts (Brun, Blum, Chappuis, & Burri, 2010). *T.b. gambiense* is found in western and central Africa, whereas *T.b. rhodesiense* is found in eastern and southern Africa.

There are currently below 10,000 new cases of HAT reported each year with a total of 48,000 deaths due to HAT in 2008, a drop of 63% since 2000. Out of the 10,000 new cases, 9689 were of the *gambiense* form and around 100 were of the *rhodesiense* form. This reduction in new cases is the result of improved diagnostics, active and passive case-finding, and improved health care facilities (Simarro, Diarra, Postigo, Franco, & Jannin, 2011). Furthermore, there is a substantial unreported burden of HAT—for example, around 40% of *rhodesiense* HAT in Uganda are not reported and is assumed untreated and 100% fatal, on the other hand, for the *gambiense* form, although it has not been directly estimated, a similar proportion of cases are thought to be not reported but only 50% fatal due to the long period of illness and the chances of subsequent detection (Hackett, Ford, Fèvre, & Simarro, 2014).

2. A BRIEF HISTORY OF HAT

It has been suggested that trypanosomes have played a major role in the evolution of hominids by selecting for hominids resistant to trypanosome infections. Even today, human beings are resistant to all subspecies of trypanosomes except for two that are infectious. Even better amongst primates are baboons who are resistant to all types of trypanosome infections (Lambrecht, 1985). The first historical account of HAT dates back to the twentieth century providing evidence of HAT epidemics occurring then.

By the nineteenth century, the disease was easily recognized; however, no one knew what caused it (Steverding, 2008).

In 1852, the explorer and missionary David Livingston first recognized that the bite of tsetse flies causes *nagana* in cattle. However, it was not until 1895 when David Bruce (1855–1931) discovered the parasite, named it *Trypanosoma brucei* (*T.b.*) after himself and identified it as the causative agent responsible for cattle trypanosomiasis. In 1901, Robert Michael Forde (1861–1948) observed these parasites in the human vascular system for the first time and later in 1902, Joseph Everett Dutton (1874–1905) recognized them as trypanosomes and named them *Trypanosoma gambiense* (now *T.b. gambiense*). Meanwhile, Aldo Castellani (1878–1971) observed trypanosomes in the cerebrospinal fluid of patients and the following year Bruce found evidence for the transmission of the parasites by tsetse flies. This led to an understanding of the cyclical transmission of *T. brucei* in these flies. The other trypanosome-affecting humans named *T.b. rhodesiense* (after then state Northern Rhodesia, now Zambia) was not discovered until 1910 by the parasitologists John William Watson Stephens (1865–1946) and Harold Benjamin Fantham (1876–1937) (Steverding, 2008).

3. CLINICAL PRESENTATION OF THE DISEASE

The clinical features of HAT arise from the two distinct stages of infection and disease progression. The first stage of HAT is known as the hemolymphatic stage and characterized by the presence of trypanosomes in the blood and lymphatic systems of patients (Priotto et al., 2007). Initially, stage 1 is asymptomatic, but once the parasite numbers increase patients can suffer from chronic and intermittent fever, pruritus, and lymphadenopathy (Brun et al., 2010). Having entered the circulation, trypanosomes have several effective strategies to avoid the host's immune system, including a wide repertoire of genes encoding variant surface glycoproteins (VSG) that coat their outer layer and can be interchanged and even intragenetically shuffled at will to avoid antibody binding (Donelson, Hill, & El-Sayed, 1998). These VSG genes are arranged on chromosomes 1–11. An array of 806 VSG genes that the parasite can use have been analyzed (Berriman et al., 2005).Only one VSG protein is expressed on the outer layer of the parasite at any given time, and since an antibody response to this protein is raised roughly once every 10 days, the parasite changes the VSG protein it expresses by antigenic variation (Cross, Wirtz, & Navarro, 1998; Turner, 1997). For this reason, it is impossible for a vaccine or chemoprophylactic to be developed against this parasite making tourists very susceptible to the disease. This change in VSG protein leads to characteristic waves of parasitemia, and eventually the disease progresses to stage 2—the meningoencephalitic or CNS phase. This can occur months (*T.b. rhodesiense*) or years (*T.b. gambiense*) after the initial infection (Checchi, Filipe, Haydon, Chandramohan, & Chappuis, 2008; Odiit, Kansiime, & Enyaru, 1997).

Stage 2 of HAT arises when the parasite leaves the circulation and lymphatic system to invade the CNS. The precise mechanism for how the parasite is able to do this is a subject of debate. One school of thought hypothesizes that the parasite crosses the blood–brain barrier (BBB) by transcytosis without affecting paracellular permeability and TJ protein expression (Mulenga, Mhlanga, Kristensson, & Robertson, 2001), or by another as yet unidentified mechanism involving the proinflammatory cytokine, interferon gamma (Masocha, Rottenberg, & Kristensson, 2007). Meanwhile, other groups theorize that trypanosomes are more opportunistic and require transient increases in BBB paracellular permeability to infect the CNS (Grab & Kennedy, 2008; Philip, Dascombe, Fraser, & Pentreath, 1994). Most recently, the choroid plexus has been put forward as the only site of entry for trypanosomes into the CNS, excluding the BBB, by virtue of the fact that parasites are consistently detected in the choroid plexus epithelium before the brain parenchyma (Wolburg et al., 2012).

The trypanosome invasion of the CNS in stage 2 gives rise to a variety of debilitating CNS disorders. The hallmark of stage 2 is insomnia and changes in sleeping cycle which give the disease its nickname "sleeping sickness." Other neurological symptoms include tremor, limb paralysis, motor weakness, and Parkinson-like movements due to muscular hypertension (Kristensson, Nygård, Bertini, & Bentivoglio, 2010). These conditions are not seen in stage 1 and increase in severity with the duration and progression of stage 2, until the patient falls into a coma with death following shortly afterward. The progression of stage 2 HAT varies depending on the parasite involved. Typically, *T.b. rhodesiense*-induced disease progresses more rapidly (Balasegaram et al., 2009).

HAT is mostly fatal if left untreated, which is of particular significance when considering not only the resource-poor setting of sub-Saharan Africa but also the initial asymptomatic disease manifestation meaning people do not seek medical intervention until the disease proper has manifested. It is lapses in disease surveillance that appear to be the main reasoning behind reemergence of HAT as it believed to be an eradicable disease by the WHO.

3.1. *T.b. gambiense*

HAT caused by *T.b. gambiense* results in a chronic form of the disease unlike the acute *T.b. rhodesiense* form. In the endemic population, most HAT cases (97%) found are of the *gambiense* form and only 3% is a result of *T.b. rhodesiense* infection. However, most tourists are infected by the *rhodesiense* form (Blum, Neumayr, & Hatz, 2012; Brun et al., 2010; Kennedy, 2013). The common course of illness, as mentioned above, begins at the hemolymphatic stage (stage 1) with nonspecific symptoms and progresses on to the meningoencephalitic stage (stage 2) when there is manifestation of severe neurological symptoms. The exact duration of each stage is debatable, although many have cited a period of months–years (Brun et al., 2010; Chretien & Smoak, 2005). Although it is widely accepted that untreated HAT is fatal, there is little empirical evidence for concluding so.

In their review, they have found evidence for the existence of HAT that is nonfatal, i.e., the infection is able to clear itself from the human body (Checchi, Filipe, et al., 2008). This is further highlighted by Jamonneau et al. (2012) who have found some evidence for trypano-tolerance in humans. However, such tolerant HAT cases could be caused by strains other than gambiense since their clinical presentation can be similar. For instance, there have been incidences where trypanosomes that are believed to not infect humans (*T.b. brucei*, *congolense*, and *vivax*) have caused illnesses possibly due to the absence of lytic factors in the human serum which usually eradicates them (Checchi, Filipe, et al., 2008). Despite the existence of the *gambiense* form HAT that takes an unusual course of progression, it is certain that most infections if left untreated will result in death. A survival analysis carried out by Checchi, Filipe, Barrett, and Chandramohan (2008) reports that the duration of stage 1 and stage 2 of the disease is roughly equal to 500 days each and the median duration of the illness is 3 years.

In terms of clinical presentation of HAT, there are differences between the gambiense and the *rhodesiense* form of HAT. The first definitive symptom of HAT regardless of the type is the appearance of a chancre. This is a skin lesion found at the site of the bite of a tsetse fly. It is usually 2–5 cm in diameter and occurs as a result of local immune response. This always occurs before the appearance of trypanosomes in the blood and therefore can be used as a diagnostic tool. The chancre is red, swollen, and edematous. The swelling is due to the huge invasion of polymorphonuclear cells at the site of the bite followed by an influx of lymphoid and macrophage cells (Chretien & Smoak, 2005).

It is important to note, however, that the chancre does not appear in all patients with HAT. The *rhodesiense* form is more likely to result in a chancre compared to the *gambiense* form. Also, African natives are rarely found with a chancre unlike Caucasian travellers. The chancre disappears within a few weeks followed by a febrile state in patients (Lejon, Boelaert, Jannin, Moore, & Büscher, 2003). Fever at this stage can be mistaken for malarial infection contributing to misdiagnosis. The fever is intermittent with intervals lasting days, weeks, or months until the disease progresses to stage 2 (Brun et al., 2010). Other symptoms can include pruritus, posterior cervical lymphadenopathy (or Winterbottom's sign—hallmark of *T.b. gambiense* HAT), and occasionally hepatosplenomegaly. Stage 2 symptoms of the disease are as mentioned above.

3.2. *T.b. rhodesiense*

The major difference between *T.b. gambiense* and *T.b. rhodesiense* infections is duration of the illness. While the *gambiense* form lasts roughly 3 years in an untreated person, the *rhodesiense* form will only last a few weeks to months with the person dying in both cases if not treated. The *rhodesiense* form progresses from stage 1 to stage 2 rapidly and therefore, correct diagnosis and efficient treatment is highly important (Gibson, 2002). A study conducted in Tororo, Uganda observed that within 3 weeks to 2 months of infection the disease had developed into the meningoencephalitic stage (Odiit et al., 1997). The symptoms are similar to the *gambiense* form of HAT with a few exceptions such as a higher likelihood of chancre occurring during stage 1 of the disease.

4. UNIQUE DIAGNOSTIC MARKERS

4.1. *T.b. gambiense*

Both parasite species cause a relatively similar clinical disease, but with differing degrees of virulence, and can be distinguished using molecular methods (Berberof, Pérez-Morga, & Pays, 2001; Picozzi, Carrington, & Welburn, 2008; Radwanska et al., 2002). It seems like there is evidence for a "receptor-like flagellar pocket glycoprotein" specific to *T.b. gambiense* responsible for its ability to infect humans. It is a truncated VSG protein named the TgsGP gene (47 kDa) which may confer resistance to parasites against the human lytic factor. It is transcribed as a 1.5-kb mRNA specific to the bloodstream stage *T.b. gambiense*. Surprisingly, this gene was present in parasites that lacked the antigen that is currently used for Card Agglutination Test for trypanosomiasis (CATT) (Berberof et al., 2001). Further analysis with polymerase chain reaction showed that TgsGP can be used to confirm the status of a patient through detecting *T.b. gambiense* in a blood sample regardless of geographic origins of the parasite (Picozzi et al., 2008).

However, these methods are often unavailable in the field, and the differential diagnosis of HAT often relies on the parasites' discrete geographical distributions, although there are concerns that the distributions may be blurring in recent years (Picozzi et al., 2005).

4.2. *T.b. rhodesiense*

T.b. rhodesiense is phenotypically different to *T.b. gambiense* due to its postero-nuclear form. They are also genetically different. A VSG-expression site-associated gene, the SRA gene, responsible for its resistance against the human lytic factor was discovered in 1994 and was found in all strains of *T.b. rhodesiense* across East Africa (De Greef & Hamers, 1994; Picozzi et al., 2008; Van Xong et al., 1998). Its function was confirmed when *T.b. brucei* which does not usually infect humans became resistant to human serum when the SRA gene was transfected into it. This SRA gene in *T.b. rhodesiense* corresponds to the TgsGP gene in *T.b. gambiense* both of which can be useful tools diagnostically.

Epidemiologically, *T.b. rhodesiense* stands out due to its unique ability to affect both humans and animals alike (zoonosis). It can be argued that this characteristic is due to the presence of the SRA gene. Efforts to identify the SRA gene in *T.b. brucei* were not successful (De Greef & Hamers, 1994).

5. VECTOR

The vector responsible for HAT is the tsetse fly of the genus *Glossina*. Although all tsetse flies can be infected by trypanosomes, only a few take the role of a vector due to its geographic distribution and contact with hosts. (http://apps.who.int/iris/bitstream/10665/95732/1/9789241209847_eng.pdf).

5.1. *T.b. gambiense*

T.b. gambiense found in central and West Africa is dependent on certain subtypes of tsetse flies for their transmission. These tsetse fly species belong to the riverine kind (Subgenus: *Nemorhina*) namely *Glossina fuscipes fuscipes*,

G. f. quanzensis, *G. palpalis gambiensis*, *G. p. palpalis* (http://apps.who.int/iris/bitstream/10665/95732/1/9789241209847_eng.pdf).

5.2. *T.b. rhodesiense*

T.b. rhodesiense found in southern and East Africa is transmitted by tsetse flies of the savannah species (Subgenus: *mortisans*) and also by *G. fuscipes* (of the *Nemorhina* subgenus) in Kenya and Uganda. (http://apps.who.int/iris/bitstream/10665/95732/1/9789241209847_eng.pdf).

6. DIAGNOSIS OF HAT

The initial clinical presentation of the disease often leads to misdiagnosis since symptoms are confused with other prevalent tropical diseases such as malaria, tuberculosis, and HIV. Therefore, the diagnosis of the disease is reliant on laboratory tests to check for the presence of trypanosomes (Brun et al., 2010). Systematic screening programme is in place for bringing the spread of HAT under control. This involves active case-finding, diagnosis, and treatment (Simarro et al., 2011). The most common diagnostic tool is the CATT which involves the detection of specific antigens related to the VSG such as the variable antigen type designated LiTat 1.3 (Dukes et al., 1992). This can be combined with the detection of a palpable lymph node. CATT can be carried out on capillary blood sample, serum, or blood from impregnated filter papers (Brun et al., 2010). CATT is fast and easy to use especially in rural areas where the disease is mostly prevalent. It allows for high-throughput screening which is useful when the whole population is involved. However, the positive predictive value of CATT is low (43–65% depending on the area) (Truc et al., 2002).

In addition, anti-HAT drugs are toxic to some extent and therefore treatment should be carefully considered. The second stage of diagnosis then is to confirm the presence of parasites in the blood or lymph aspirates using microscopy or the CSF using a lumbar puncture. This allows the determination of the stage of the disease. More sensitive blood detection methods such as quantitative buffy coat or miniature anion-exchange centrifugation technique can be used to test negative results with CATT (Brun et al., 2010).

7. TREATMENT OF HAT

A small number of drugs are available for the treatment HAT, depending on the stage of disease. Pentamidine and suramin are used for stage 1; and melarsoprol, eflornithine, and nifurtimox for stage 2 (see Fig. 1 for their respective chemical structures). All of these drugs are donated to the WHO by the manufacturers under a public–private partnership contract which was established in 2001 and is set to continue until the disease is eliminated (Brun et al., 2010) (WHO, 2013). Information on stage 1 and stage 2 acting drugs against *T.b. rhodesiense* or *T.b. gambiense* is described and summarized in Table 1.

7.1. Pentamidine

Pentamidine ($C_{19}H_{24}N_4O_2$ MW = 240.42 g/mol) is an aromatic diamidine ([1,5-bis(4-amidi-phenoxypentane]) and the current drug of choice for stage 1 HAT caused by *T.b. gambiense*. It was developed after a related compound, known as synthalin, was shown to have anti-trypanosomal activity (Sands, Kron, & Brown, 1985). It is the isethionate form of pentamidine (Pentacarinate) that is currently used therapeutically (Docampo & Moreno, 2003). Pentamidine is also used in the treatment of American cutaneous leishmaniasis and in the treatment and prophylaxis of *Pneumocystis jirovecii* pneumonia (the cause of death of many AIDS patients).

It is administered via intramuscular injection or by slow intravenous infusion (Docampo & Moreno, 2003) at a dose of 4 mg/kg of body weight about 7–10 times daily or on alternative days (Wang, 1995). There are a

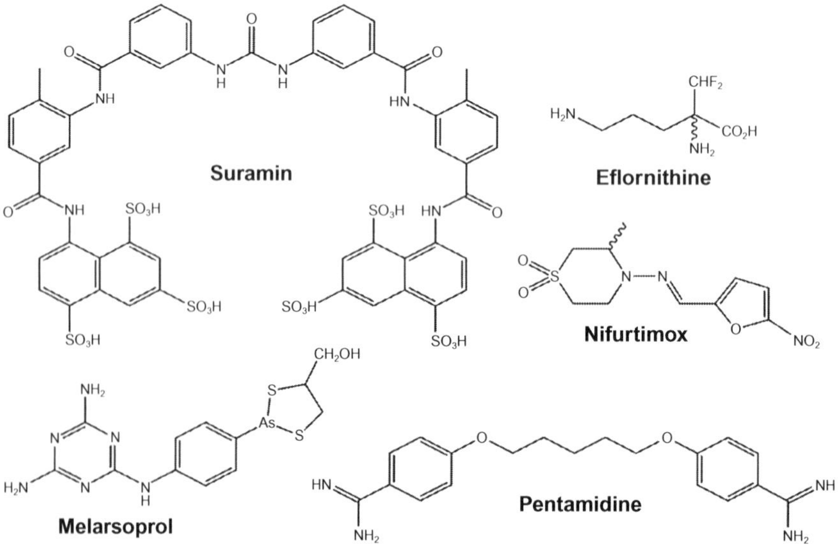

Figure 1 Drugs available for treatment of stage 1 and stage 2 HAT.

Table 1 Standard drugs used for the treatment of human African trypanosomiasis

Parasite species	Drug	HAT stage	Route of application	Dosing
Trypanosoma brucei gambiense	Pentamidine	1	Intramuscular	4 mg/kg body weight at 24 h intervals for 7 days
	Eflornithine	2	Intravenous	100 mg/kg body weight at 6 h intervals for 14 days
	Melarsoprol	2	Intravenous	2.2 mg/kg body weight at 24 h intervals for 10 days
Trypanosoma brucei rhodesiense	Suramin	1	Intravenous	Test dose of 4–5 mg/kg body weight at day 1, then five injections of 20 mg/kg body weight every 7 days; maximum dose per injection 1 g
	Melarsoprol	2	Intravenous	

number of putative mechanisms of action for its trypanocidal activity—namely through selective inhibition of Ca^{2+}-ATPase (Benaim, Lopez-Estrano, Docampo, & Moreno, 1993), nonspecific inhibition of tRNA aminoacylation in the trypanosomal mitochondria (Sun & Zhang, 2008), diskinetoplasty or by decreasing the mitochondrial membrane potential of trypanosomatids (Wang, 1995). While the exact mechanism of action for pentamidine trypanocidal activity is not clear (Calderano, De Melo Godoy, Da Cunha, & Elias, 2011), its success in the treatment of HAT has led to the development of other diamidine compounds (Sturk, Brock, Bagnell, Hall, & Tidwell, 2004; Wenzler et al., 2013). Previously, it was even used as a prophylactic by the French, Belgian, and Portuguese in the 1950s (Sands et al., 1985) and now, despite being historically viewed as a stage 1 HAT drug (Raseroka & Ormerod, 1986), pentamidine has been found to be effective in treating the very early stages of stage 2 HAT (Doua, Miezan, Sanon Singaro, Boa Yapo, & Baltz, 1996).

The initial impression of pentamidine indicates that it is a water-soluble molecule that is dicationic at physiological pH, and therefore poor at crossing biological membranes by diffusion. Yet it exhibits a slow anti-trypanosomal action against *T.b. gambiense* (Docampo & Moreno, 2003). This suggested that the drug must enter the parasite via facilitated diffusion. Consequentially, pentamidine accumulation within the trypanosome was

Table 2 Summary of known transporter interaction with anti-HAT drugs

Anti-HAT drug	Interacting transporters	References
Suramin	Unknown	
Pentamidine	Polyamine and adenosine transporters (e.g., adenosine-sensitive P2 transporter), HAPT1, LAPT1, OCT, MRPs, P-gp	Damper and Patton (1976a) and Damper and Patton (1976b) de Koning and Jarvis (2001) de Koning (2001), Sanderson et al. (2007), Sanderson et al. (2009), and Ming et al. (2009)
Melarsoprol	P2	Barrett, Boykin, Brun, and Tidwell (2007)
Eflornithine	Amino acid transporter 6 (AAT6)	Baker, Alsford, and Horn (2011)
Nifurtimox	BCRP, OATP	Watson et al. (2012)

found to involve multiple transporters (Table 2) including an adenosine-sensitive pentamidine transporter (or P2), an adenosine-insensitive high-affinity pentamidine transporter 1 (HAPT1), and an adenosine-insensitive low-affinity pentamidine transporter 1 (LAPT1) with K_m values of 0.26, 36, and 56 μM, respectively (de Koning, 2001; de Koning & Jarvis, 2001). In support of this evidence, drug resistance against pentamidine has also been identified with the loss of P2 function in trypanosomes (Matovu et al., 2001, 2003). Please see Gehrig and Efferth (2008) for a recent review of drug resistance amongst trypanosomes.

Considering this, it is inevitable that transporters are important for the cellular delivery of pentamidine for treatment against HAT (Basselin, Lawrence, & Robert-Gero, 1997; Sanderson, Dogruel, Rodgers, De Koning, & Thomas, 2009). In mammals, the human organic cationic transporters (hOCTs) were found to be involved in the uptake of pentamidine using hOCT-expressing Chinese hamster ovary cells (Ming et al., 2009).

Although pentamidine is generally considered to be one of the lesser toxic anti-HAT drugs, it causes peripheral side effects including hypoglycemia (incidence: 5–40%) and diabetes mellitus (incidence: occasional)—often dose-limiting factors that can lead to incomplete treatment (Brun et al., 2010).

7.2. Suramin

Suramin ($C_{51}H_{40}N_6O_{23}S_6$ MW = 1297.29 g/mol) is a symmetrical polysulfonated naphthylamine polyanionic compound that is the current first choice stage 1 treatment drug used in infections by *T.b. rhodesiense*. It is a potent anti-trypanosomal drug which has been in use since 1922 (Docampo & Moreno, 2003). The molecule carries six anionic charges at physiological pH making it extremely difficult for suramin to cross any biological membrane and therefore it is restricted to treating stage 1 of HAT (Sanderson, Khan, & Thomas, 2007). It is injected intravenously five times a day at a dose of 20 mg/kg body weight for 5–7 days (Wang, 1995). Suramin is unstable in air and must be rapidly solubilized in water before injection (Brun et al., 2010).

Since diffusion is not an option for suramin, it can be assumed that transporters and endocytosis might be key for its anti-trypanosomal action. Fairlamb and Bowman (1980) found that suramin when injected intravenously into *T.b. brucei*-infected rats, bound tightly to plasma proteins such as albumin. In trypanosomes, it was found in granules in lysosomes or ribosomal aggregates. The results of their experiments suggested that suramin was taken up into trypanosomes as a protein-bound complex via endocytosis.

Also, unlike other drugs such as pentamidine, suramin does not kill the trypanosomes off immediately. It is a slow-acting drug. What is known about the anti-trypanosomal activity of suramin is that it inhibits all the glycolytic enzymes in *T.b. brucei*. The positively charged enzymes are drawn toward the negatively charged suramin. However, the enzymes are enclosed in an organelle called glycosome that suramin has no access to. It has therefore been suggested that suramin does not act on these enzymes inside the organelle but interacts with them in the cytoplasm, while they are imported into the glycosomes which accounts for the slow anti-trypanosomal action of suramin (Wang, 1995).

As always, the potency of the drug gives patients severe adverse reactions that can include hypersensitivity reactions and peripheral neuropathy (Brun et al., 2010).

7.3. Melarsoprol

Melarsoprol ($C_{12}H_{15}AsN_6OS_2$ MW = 398.341 g/mol), first used in 1949, is the most widely used drug for stage 2 HAT induced by *T.b. rhodesiense* (Nok, 2003). The drug is poorly soluble in water, ether, or alcohol and must be dissolved in propylene glycol before intravenous administration, with the solvent causing pain upon injection (Docampo & Moreno, 2003; Nok, 2003).

Melarsoprol is believed to work not only by inhibiting glycolytic enzymes as with suramin but also by lysing the trypanosomes themselves, and it is believed this lysing action is a reason the drug is so toxic to patients (Balasegaram et al., 2006). It is also apparent that in some regions trypanosomes are developing resistance to melarsoprol, in which the trypanosome P2 adenosine transporter is implicated (Barrett, Boykin, Brun, & Tidwell, 2007; Table 2). Melarsoprol is also effective against *T.b. gambiense* but due to the toxicity of the drug in patients, eflornithine is the preferred alternative.

As an organoarsenic derivative, melarsoprol is highly toxic to patients and adverse reactions to its administration are common. In 5–10% of cases, melarsoprol induces severe encephalopathic syndrome which causes death in 50% of these patients (Kennedy, 2004). This encephalopathic syndrome itself requires careful management through labour intensive means and drug treatment.

7.4. Eflornithine

Eflornithine (DL-alpha-difluoromethylornithine or DFMO, $C_6H_{12}F_2N_2O_2$ MW = 182.2 g/mol), has been nicknamed the "resurrection drug" after its ability to revive comatose patients suffering from stage 2 HAT (Jennings et al., 1997). Initially synthesized as an anticancer drug, eflornithine has been used as a trypanocide since the 1980s as it inhibits the parasite's ornithine decarboxylase, a key enzyme in the synthesis of polyamines needed for cell proliferation and reduced production of the trypanosome specific redox active metabolite trypanothione (Brun et al., 2010). Due to the short half-life of the drug, treatment with eflornithine requires an extensive administration process—four infusions of 100 mg/kg body weight daily for up to 2 weeks is not uncommon (Burri & Brun, 2003).

Recently, it was found that eflornithine is taken up into the parasites via an amino acid transporter encoded by the gene *TbAAT6* (Table 2). The gene was found to be deleted in parasites resistant to eflornithine and when the gene was reintroduced the parasites gained sensitivity to the drug (Vincent et al., 2010).

Despite this intensive treatment regime of the drug and although several side effects are apparent, eflornithine is generally tolerated well by patients and so is now the recommended treatment choice for *T.b. gambiense*, being active against both stage 1 and stage 2 forms of the parasite. Unfortunately, it is ineffective against *T.b. rhodesiense* due to the parasites resilience to the drug through the parasites' high ornithine decarboxylase turnover (Iten et al., 1997). There have also been instances of eflornithine therapeutic failure with relapse rates of 8.1% reported, meaning eflornithine, along with melarsoprol, remain far from an ideal treatments for stage 2 HAT (Balasegaram et al., 2009).

7.5. Nifurtimox

Nifurtimox ($C_{10}H_{13}N_3O_5S$ MW=287.293 g/mol), currently licensed for treatment of the closely related American trypanosomiasis (Chagas disease) caused by *Trypanosoma cruzi*, was originally only used in HAT for compassionate melarsoprol refractory cases (Pepin et al., 1989) but due to the limitations of melarsoprol and eflornithine, the drug has recently come into the fray for fighting both stage 1 and stage 2 HAT. Nifurtimox is a trypanocidal nitrofuran and has several advantages compared to the intensive intravenous administration regimes of the current stage 2 drugs, which are often accompanied by adverse reactions. These advantages include the facts that nifurtimox is orally active and considerably cheaper than current stage 2 drugs (Lutje, Seixas, & Kennedy, 2010) and that it is also effective against *T.b. gambiense* and *T.b. rhodesiense* (albeit to a lesser extent) (Bouteille, Oukem, Bisser, & Dumas, 2003; Haberkorn & Gönnert, 1972; Lutje et al., 2010).

Despite these advantages, treatment with nifurtimox can also have toxic side effects which include neurological aggravations such as headaches, confusion, and sleep dysfunction as well nausea/vomiting and dyspepsia (Priotto et al., 2007). However, nifurtimox is generally better-tolerated than the other stage 2 HAT drugs, and many of the adverse conditions associated are dose and duration dependent (Priotto et al., 2009).

8. PARASITE RESISTANCE: IS COMBINATION THERAPY THE WAY FORWARD?

The limited availability of anti-HAT drugs has made it difficult to overcome parasite strains that are resistant to treatment. Initiatives to counter the emergence of drug-resistant parasite populations, while improving efficacy and reducing the toxic side effects of the anti-HAT drugs when used alone (monotherapy) have resulted in large-scale trials of combination therapy (CT). CT of suramin with the three S2-acting drugs has shown improved cure rates compared to monotherapy in rodent models (Clarkson et al., 1984; Jennings, 1993; Raseroka & Ormerod, 1986). Other results from human trials CT of melarsoprol with nifurtimox and eflornithine have demonstrated improved efficacy compared to melarsoprol monotherapy, but toxicity was still a major issue (Bouteille et al., 2003; Mpia & Pépin, 2002; Priotto et al., 2009). One large-scale trail started in 2003 and finishing in 2008 tested nifurtimox and eflornithine combination therapy (NECT) and concluded NECT had an improved toxicity profile and shortened treatment regime compared to eflornithine monotherapy. The authors argued that despite a more complicated logistic implementation, NECT represented the best form of treatment for S2 HAT (Priotto et al., 2009). As a result, NECT is now the treatment of choice for S2 HAT caused by *T.b. gambiense* and implemented by the WHO (Simarro et al., 2011).

Parasite resistance can occur due to several reasons. One of the common causes is the lack of a transporter or mutation of the gene encoding the transporter responsible for the uptake of the drug into trypanosomes. For instance, as mentioned earlier, the absence of the purine receptor P2 in trypanosomes led to small amounts of resistance to the drug pentamidine and melarsoprol (de Koning & Jarvis, 2001). Silent mutations of the gene also led to substrate specificity changes. Absence of both P2 and HAPT1 resulted in high levels of resistance to pentamidine and melarsoprol (Gehrig & Efferth, 2008).

Parasite resistance can also occur against eflornithine due to the loss of the gene *TbAAT6* that encodes an amino acid transporter in *T.b. brucei*. Reintroduction of this gene led to gain in sensitivity to the drug (Vincent et al., 2010).

Another common cause of resistance is the high expression of efflux transporters such as the TbMRPA which is present in *T. brucei*. Drugs that are taken up into the parasite being efficiently extruded back outside (Gehrig & Efferth, 2008).

Therefore, it is important to understand the mechanisms of drug action before the problems of parasite resistance can be solved.

9. BBB TRANSPORT OF ANTI-HAT DRUGS

9.1. Human BBB characteristics

The human BBB is a dynamic system which acts as a physical, metabolic, and transport barrier for substances that enter the brain. The cerebral microvessel endothelial cells form the BBB along with other entities such as the astrocytes and pericytes that help maintain the BBB. This complex unit is responsible for the constant regulation of the internal environment through selective uptake of molecules (Abbott, Patabendige, Dolman, Yusof, & Begley, 2010).

9.2. The physical barrier

The endothelial cells form a physical barrier by blocking the diffusion of molecules paracellularly (in between cells). This occurs due to the high transendothelial electrical resistance (TEER) of $>1000\,\Omega\,cm^2$ found between the endothelial cells owing to the presence of complex tight junctions (TJ) between the cells. These TJs are formed by proteins called claudins, occludins, and junctional adhesion molecules along with other cytoplasmic accessory proteins. It is the presence of these TJs that polarizes the cell membrane into apical and basolateral sides. Any damage to these TJs will decrease TEER and increase paracellular permeability of potentially toxic substances into the brain (Huber, Egleton, & Davis, 2001).

9.3. The metabolic barrier

Aside from being a physical barrier, the presence of several enzymes within the endothelial cell, such as acetylcholinesterase, alkaline phosphatase, gamma-glutamyl transpeptidase, monoamine oxidases, and other drug-metabolizing enzymes, form an enzymatic barrier that can break down several toxic compounds that may enter the brain (Wilhelm, Fazakas, & Krizbai, 2011).

9.4. The selective barrier

9.4.1 The ATP-binding cassette family

The ability of the cerebral microvessel endothelial cells to act as a barrier to blood-borne substances is critical in protecting the brain from harm. However, this barrier poses a challenge when therapeutic drugs are required to enter the brain to treat several diseases ranging from Alzheimer's disease to brain tumors. It is precisely this that results in many potentially efficacious drugs failing clinical trials (Pardridge, 2005). It is also important to note that even if the molecule is lipid soluble, they do not necessarily enter the brain transcellularly (i.e., across the plasma membranes) due to the efflux transporters present at the BBB—such is the case with stage 1 drug pentamidine which has been shown to enter the cerebral capillary endothelium but is effluxed by the ATP-binding cassette (ABC) transporters, P-glycoprotein

(P-gp), and multidrug-associated protein (MRP) present (Sanderson et al., 2009).

There are 48 known members in the superfamily of ABC transporters which are divided into seven subfamilies based on molecular sequencing data. As the name suggests, all of them use ATP to efflux molecules from the endothelial cell back into the blood. Many of these ABC transporters are present at the BBB (Dean, Rzhetsky, & Allikmets, 2001). Of the BBB significant ABC transporters, ABCB1 (P-gp) remains the most well known due to its ability to transport several drugs out of the brain. Structurally, it has 12-transmembrane domains that are divided into equal halves with an ATP-binding site. P-gp is thought to be very promiscuous in terms of accepting molecules to transport; it recognizes molecules of differing characteristics. Substrates for P-gp have been found to be hydrophobic in nature which results in many therapeutic drugs being effluxed from the brain (Aller et al., 2009).

Other ABC transporters at the BBB include ABCG2 (breast cancer-resistant protein or BCRP) and the ABCC family (MRPs) (Wilhelm et al., 2011). BCRP was initially found on breast cancer cell lines that were multidrug resistant. Like P-gp, it also has several substrates (Ni, Bikadi, Rosenberg, & Mao, 2010). It was found to be the most abundantly expressed efflux transporter at the human BBB (1.85-fold more than in mice). On the other hand, P-gp levels were found to be lower in humans compared to mice (Uchida et al., 2011). However, in the human blood–brain barrier cell line hCMEC/D3, P-gp expression was found to be higher than any other ABC transporter (Carl et al., 2010; Ohtsuki et al., 2013).

9.4.2 The solute carrier family

The solute carrier (SLC) family is composed of the different transporter families that include ion channels, exchangers, passive transporters (Abbott et al., 2010).

There are 52 SLC gene families consisting of around 400 transporter genes (http://www.bioparadigms.org/slc/intro.htm accessed on 18/04/2013). A list of all current SLC families can be found at http://slc.bioparadigms.org/.

At the BBB, there are several transporters that are part of the SLC family such as GLUT 1 that specifically transports glucose (Mueckler & Thorens, 2013), systems A, ASC and N that transport amino acids (O'Kane & Hawkins, 2003), system y^+ that transports cationic amino acids (Fotiadis, Kanai, & Palacín, 2013; O'Kane et al., 2006), system y^+L that transports cationic and neutral amino acids (Fotiadis et al., 2013; Kageyama et al., 2000), and the organic cation and anion transporter family (OCTs and OATs) (Koepsell, Lips, & Volk, 2007). However, it is still unclear if several of the others are found at the BBB.

9.5. BBB entry of anti-HAT drugs

Besides slowing trypanosome drug resistance, the precise reasoning why CT improves drug efficacy against stage 2 HAT is not yet completely understood and led to the hypothesis that perhaps CT improves drug delivery to the brain (Enanga, Keita, Chauvière, Dumas, & Bouteille, 1998). This is of particular significance for stage 2 as the parasites are in the host CNS and for the drugs to be effective they must be able to cross the BBB. However, the exact mechanisms of how stage 2 HAT-acting drugs cross the BBB has been under researched until fairly recently. This is even more alarming considering the fact that stage 2 HAT acting drugs are actively being used in the field. Much of what was known about the ability of the trypanocidal drugs to cross biological membrane has been deduced from their chemical structures and lipophilicity. Pentamidine, for instance, is hydrophilic and poor at crossing biological membranes, yet has been shown to accumulate in trypanosomes at concentrations in excess of 1 mM, which suggests there is a transporter for the drug (Damper & Patton, 1976a, 1976b). It has since been demonstrated that pentamidine requires the action of several polyamine and adenosine transporters in the outer membranes of parasites to enter and exhibit trypanocidal action including the adenosine-insensitive high-affinity and low-affinity pentamidine transporters and the adenosine P2 transporter already mentioned (see de Koning & Jarvis, 2001 for more details).

As with pentamidine, suramin is poor at crossing intact biological membranes and it is believed the ability of trypanosome transporters to take up the drug from plasma owes to its success as a potent anti-trypanosomal agent. Because of its charged nature, suramin is able to bind to many serum proteins and it was suggested that perhaps it was transported into trypanosomes by binding to LDL and proceeding through the receptor-mediated transcytosis RMT system and this was demonstrated in trypanosomes (Pal, Hall, & Field, 2002).

Due to their poor lipophilic properties, pentamidine and suramin are believed not to cross the BBB and as such are used in stage 1 treatment only, although this was not looked at directly until work by our group using *in situ* brain perfusion mouse models of late stage trypanosomiasis. For suramin, our group investigated the ability of the drug to cross the mouse BBB and the effects of CT on its brain distribution. It was discovered that suramin poorly crossed the BBB and was not affected by the presence of other trypanocidal drugs or by P-gp knockout animals, confirming the suspicion that it is not a suitable stage 2-acting drug (Sanderson et al., 2007). Conversely in similar experiments, it was discovered that pentamidine was able to cross the BBB, but a large proportion was retained in the mouse brain microvessel endothelial cells, meaning the concentration that reached the brain would be insufficient for effective parasite removal (Sanderson et al., 2009). It was also shown that pentamidine was a substrate for MRPs and P-gp as demonstrated using FVB-Mdr1a/1b (+/+) and FVB-Mdr1a/1b (−/−) mice (Table 2) and that CT with nifurtimox, suramin, and melarsoprol caused changes in brain distribution of pentamidine (increase, decrease, and decrease, respectively). These data demonstrated unequivocally that pentamidine (and possibly melarsoprol and nifurtimox) interacted with transport systems at the BBB and circumventricular organs (CVOs), particularly efflux systems. It is interesting to point out that several ABC transporter genes have been discovered in trypanosomes (Maser & Kaminsky, 1998), although it has not been demonstrated if trypanosomes are able to efflux drugs through these mechanisms. The results regarding suramin are more equivocal; however, as trail data have shown improved rodent cure rates with CT involving suramin (see Section 8). The *in situ* findings of Sanderson et al. (2007) suggest that it is unlikely that suramin interferes with transport mechanisms at the BBB to improve delivery (Sanderson et al., 2007) and so perhaps drug–drug interactions (DDI) reduced the toxicity of the stage 2-acting drugs which saw cure rate increases.

Studies on melarsoprol distribution have revealed that the presence of its arsenoxide group confers lipid solubility, enabling BBB traversal (Pepin & Milord, 1994; Pépin et al., 1994). Melarsoprol is also transported into trypanosomes by the P2 adenosine transporter as with pentamidine and it is believed mutations in the transporter confer drug resistance to trypanosomes, but the utilization of BBB transport mechanisms has not been demonstrated (de Koning, 2001). It therefore remains likely that it is the high lipophilicity of the drug allows it to cross the BBB to kill trypanosomes within the brain.

As a stage 2-acting drug, eflornithine was assumed to cross the BBB and has been shown to accumulate intracellularly to millimolar ranges in bloodstream forms of trypanosomes (Iten et al., 1997). The study by Iten and colleagues showed similar intracellular concentrations were reached at 4 and

26 °C, indicating that passive diffusion was the method as opposed to facilitated diffusion. However, the study only looked at 60 min time points and not early stage time points, which give better indications of facilitated diffusion via transporters. Intracellular levels of a charged molecule such as eflornithine are unlikely to reach such levels by passive diffusion alone. On the contrary, in an earlier study, it was shown that eflornithine uptake in trypanosomes was indeed temperature dependent, reminiscent of transport activity (Bellofatto, Fairlamb, Henderson, & Cross, 1987). Work by our group showed that eflornithine poorly traversed the murine BBB and perhaps this was an explanation as to why such an intensive treatment regime using this is necessary—to get sufficient quantities of eflornithine into the brain to exhibit trypanocidal effects (Sanderson, Dogruel, Rodgers, Bradley, & Thomas, 2008). The data here also showed no interaction between P-gp and eflornithine occurred but it did indicate that CT with suramin improved distribution of eflornithine into the brain, the mechanism of which is unknown, but may be evidence of RMT of LDL–suramin–eflornithine DDI complexes as earlier work by our group indicated evidence of interactions between suramin and plasma membranes (Sanderson et al., 2007). CT with excess eflornithine, pentamidine, melarsoprol, and nifurtimox caused no significant changes in brain distribution of eflornithine, suggesting a passive diffusion method of brain entry. However, perhaps a species difference in transporters could explain why eflornithine delivery to the brain is efficacious in humans but not mice, or that other transport systems are involved in eflornithine BBB transport that were not investigated.

As the name suggests, eflornithine is an analogue of the CAA ornithine and so this proposes that CAA transport systems could be involved in eflornithine transport at the BBB and in trypanosomes. Evidence for involvement of eflornithine in a CAA system was shown when ablation of the amino acid transporting gene *TbAAT6* in *T. brucei brucei* conferred them both viable and resistant to the action of eflornithine (Vincent et al., 2010). More recent evidence from genome-wide Rani screens revealed a loss-of-amino acid transporter 6 (AT) function, representing not only a method of eflornithine entry into parasites but also another method of drug resistance (Baker, Alford, & Horn, 2011).

With NECT becoming the treatment of choice for stage 2 HAT, our group also recently investigated the BBB-crossing abilities of nifurtimox, alone or in CT with other trypanocidal drugs. We showed that nifurtimox was highly lipophilic and able to cross the murine BBB, but was expelled by an unidentified efflux transport process not involving P-gp (Jeganathan et al., 2011; Watson et al., 2012). The research demonstrated that CT of nifurtimox with pentamidine increased the brain distribution of nifurtimox, which is interesting because not only was pentamidine previously demonstrated to be a P-gp substrate, but also P-gp-deficient mice caused no changes in the brain distribution of nifurtimox as seen in the *in situ* brain perfusion model. That nifurtimox caused an increase in pentamidine brain distribution suggests a different transport system is at work as well as P-gp. Research by our group using the human brain endothelial cell line (hCMEC/D3) has indicated that nifurtimox is a substrate of BCRP and possibly to a lesser extent, members of the OATP transport family (Watson et al., 2012; Table 2).

10. LATEST RESEARCH DEVELOPMENTS

Research has advanced in terms of identifying targets for new anti-HAT drugs and in trying to select drugs that have the potential to treat HAT. A few of those are under clinical trials currently. For example, fexinidazole, a two-substituted 5-nitroimidazole, entered Phase II/III clinical trials in October 2012 and is thought to be effective against both subtypes of HAT. The aim of the trial is to prove its safety and efficacy compared to NECT as the standard. The project which began in 2007 is conducted by the Drugs for Neglected Disease *initiative* (DND*i*) (http://www.dndi.org/diseases-projects/portfolio/fexinidazole.html accessed on 30/01/2014). In the preclinical phase, the drug displayed moderate efficacy *in vitro* against the parasites and oral administration of fexinidazole at doses of 100 mg/kg/day for 4 days or 200 mg/kg/day for 5 days cured mice with acute and chronic infection, respectively. The compound was also found to cross the BBB adequately to allow the killing of parasites within the brain (Torreele et al., 2010). This is promising since it seems active against both strains of HAT at both stages of the disease. In addition, since none of the drugs currently used are orally administered, fexinidazole, if successful, would greatly simplify the process of drug administration in remote areas of rural Africa.

Oxaboroles are another category of anti-HAT drugs currently under clinical trials. In 2010, during a preclinical trial, the compounds *N*-(1-hydroxy-1,3-dihydrobenzo[*c*][1,2]oxaborol-6-yl)-2-trifluoromethylbenzamide (AN3520) and 4-fluoro-*N*-(1-hydroxy-1,3-dihydrobenzo[*c*][1,2]oxaborol-6-yl)-2-trifluoromethylbenzamide (SCYX-6759) showed efficacy against the two strains of HAT-affecting humans. They also successfully cured stage 1 trypanosomiasis infection in mice when administered orally at 2.5–10 mg/kg of body weight for 4 consecutive days. They cured stage 2 HAT in infected mice with *T.b. brucei* when AN3520 or SCYX-6759 were administered intraperitoneally or orally (50 mg/kg) twice daily for 7 days. SCYX-6759 was ultimately selected for clinical trials considering its better pharmacokinetics in stage 2 of the mouse model. In addition, they were not found to interact with the P-gp transporter at the BBB aiding its uptake into the brain (Nare et al., 2010). The drug entered Phase I clinical trial in 2012 which is currently ongoing (http://www.dndi.org/diseases-projects/portfolio/oxaborole-scyx-7158.html accessed on 30/01/2014).

Another apparently promising drug candidate was DB289 or pafuramidine maleate which successfully went through Phases I–III clinical trials until an additional Phase I clinical trial conducted to assess its safety data for registration found that the compound led to hepatotoxicity and nephrotoxicity (http://apps.who.int/iris/bitstream/10665/95732/1/9789241209847_eng.pdf accessed on 30/01/2014).

Another drug candidate on the horizon is DB829, which displayed exceptional efficacy in mice infected with both *T.b. rhodesiense* and *T.b. gambiense*. The drug displayed no cross resistance with pentamidine and a single intraperitoneal injection of DB829 (20 mg/kg) cured mice with blood-stage parasites (Wenzler et al., 2013). A similar compound DB868 has been tested in a Vervet monkey model of HAT-oral administration of the drug being one of the advantages of it. The drug was found to be converted into the active compound DB829 and has been successful in treating first stage HAT monkey models (Thuita et al., 2013).

Keeping the existing anti-HAT drugs in mind, efforts have been also been directed toward the development of prodrugs of pentamidine and eflornithine. Several prodrugs of pentamidine were tested *in silico*, *in vitro*, and *in vivo* to finally choose *N,N'*-bis(succinyloxy)pentamidine with the best characteristics in terms of solubility, activation, permeability, oral bioavailability, and ultimately its ability to cross the BBB (Kotthaus et al., 2011). On the other hand, another study which looked at mono-, di-, and trisubstituted derivatives of eflornithine found that none of the prodrugs were able to deliver eflornithine into the plasma owing to not being absorbed into the gastrointestinal tract or not being metabolized into eflornithine (Cloete et al., 2011).

Another class of drugs that specifically target *N*-myristoyltransferase in *T. brucei* have been found to be promising. Both *in vitro* and *in vivo* experiments have shown that these compounds are able to kill the parasites and thus cure infection. The drug takes advantage of the fact that N-myristoylation of proteins occurs in all eukaryotic organisms and the inhibition of this process affects many proteins vital to the viability of the parasite (Frearson et al., 2010).

Recently, research into new anti-HAT drugs came across the substituted 2-phenylimidazopyridines. One of the analogues was found to have antiparasitic activity *in vitro* with an EC50 of 2 nM and was also found to be orally available in mice which led to a cure in infected mice (Tatipaka et al., 2014).

11. CONCLUSION

Many compounds have thus been identified as having the potential to treat HAT at both stages of the disease. For an antiparasitic compound to be successful in treating both stages of HAT, primarily, it has to have the ability to cross the BBB without being subjected to extrusion by the ABC transporters and at the same time have a good safety profile with an acceptable range of toxicity. In addition, its pharmacokinetic and physicochemical properties should ideally increase the oral bioavailability of the drug. Many fail due to their inability to cross the BBB or poor oral availability and even the ones that do can cause additional harm. Considering the lack of options for treating HAT it is imperative to develop new drugs immediately.

CONFLICT OF INTEREST

The authors have no conflicts of interest.

ACKNOWLEDGMENTS

The Thomas laboratory has received funding from The Wellcome Trust (Ref No.: 073542 and 080268), MRC (Ref No.: MR/K015451/1 and MR/K500811/1), BBSRC (Ref No.: BB/E527098/1), and EPSRC (Ref No.: EP503523/1).

REFERENCES

Abbott, N. J., Patabendige, A. A. K., Dolman, D. E. M., Yusof, S. R., & Begley, D. J. (2010). Structure and function of the blood-brain barrier. *Neurobiology of Disease*, *37*(1), 13–25. http://dx.doi.org/10.1016/j.nbd.2009.07.030.

Aller, S. G., Yu, J., Ward, A., Weng, Y., Chittaboina, S., Zhuo, R., et al. (2009). Structure of P-glycoprotein reveals a molecular basis for poly-specific drug binding. *Science*, *323*(5922), 1718–1722. http://dx.doi.org/10.1126/science.1168750.

Baker, N., Alsford, S., & Horn, D. (2011). Genome-wide RNAi screens in African trypanosomes identify the nifurtimox activator NTR and the eflornithine transporter AAT6.

Molecular and Biochemical Parasitology, 176(1), 55–57. http://dx.doi.org/10.1016/j.molbiopara.2010.11.010.

Balasegaram, M., Harris, S., Checchi, F., Ghorashian, S., Hamel, C., & Karunakara, U. (2006). Melarsoprol versus eflornithine for treating late-stage Gambian trypanosomiasis in the republic of the Congo. *Bulletin of the World Health Organization, 84*(10), 783–791. http://dx.doi.org/10.2471/BLT.06.031955.

Balasegaram, M., Young, H., Chappuis, F., Priotto, G., Raguenaud, M., & Checchi, F. (2009). Effectiveness of melarsoprol and eflornithine as first-line regimens for gambiense sleeping sickness in nine médecins sans frontières programmes. *Transactions of the Royal Society of Tropical Medicine and Hygiene, 103*(3), 280–290. http://dx.doi.org/10.1016/j.trstmh.2008.09.005.

Barrett, M. P., Boykin, D. W., Brun, R., & Tidwell, R. R. (2007). Human African trypanosomiasis: Pharmacological re-engagement with a neglected disease. *British Journal of Pharmacology, 152*(8), 1155–1171. http://dx.doi.org/10.1038/sj.bjp.0707354.

Basselin, M., Lawrence, F., & Robert-Gero, M. (1997). Altered transport properties of pentamidine-resistant leishmania donovani and L. amazonensis promastigotes. *Parasitology Research, 83*(5), 413–418. http://dx.doi.org/10.1007/s004360050274.

Bellofatto, V., Fairlamb, A. H., Henderson, G. B., & Cross, G. A. M. (1987). Biochemical changes associated with a-difluoromethylornithine uptake and resistance in Trypanosoma brucei. *Molecular and Biochemical Parasitology, 25*(3), 227–238.

Benaim, G., Lopez-Estrano, C., Docampo, R., & Moreno, S. N. J. (1993). A calmodulin-stimulated Ca^{2+} pump in plasma-membrane vesicles from Trypanosoma brucei; selective inhibition by pentamidine. *Biochemical Journal, 296*(3), 759–763.

Berberof, M., Pérez-Morga, D., & Pays, E. (2001). A receptor-like flagellar pocket glycoprotein specific to Trypanosoma brucei gambiense. *Molecular and Biochemical Parasitology, 113*(1), 127–138. http://dx.doi.org/10.1016/S0166-6851(01)00208-0.

Berriman, M., Ghedin, E., Hertz-Fowler, C., Blandin, G., Renauld, H., Bartholomeu, D. C., et al. (2005). The genome of the African trypanosome Trypanosoma brucei. *Science, 309*(5733), 416–422. http://dx.doi.org/10.1126/science.1112642.

Blum, J. A., Neumayr, A. L., & Hatz, C. F. (2012). Human African trypanosomiasis in endemic populations and travellers. *European Journal of Clinical Microbiology and Infectious Diseases, 31*(6), 905–913. http://dx.doi.org/10.1007/s10096-011-1403-y.

Bouteille, B., Oukem, O., Bisser, S., & Dumas, M. (2003). Treatment perspectives for human African trypanosomiasis. *Fundamental and Clinical Pharmacology, 17*(2), 171–181. http://dx.doi.org/10.1046/j.1472-8206.2003.00167.x.

Brun, R., Blum, J., Chappuis, F., & Burri, C. (2010). Human African trypanosomiasis. *The Lancet, 375*(9709), 148–159. http://dx.doi.org/10.1016/S0140-6736(09)60829-1.

Burri, C., & Brun, R. (2003). Eflornithine for the treatment of human African trypanosomiasis. *Parasitology Research, 90*(Suppl. 1), S49–S52.

Calderano, S. G., De Melo Godoy, P. D., Da Cunha, J. P. C., & Elias, M. C. (2011). Trypanosome prereplication machinery: A potential new target for an old problem. *Enzyme Research, 2011*(1), 8. http://dx.doi.org/10.4061/2011/518258.

Carl, S. M., Lindley, D. J., Couraud, P. O., Weksler, B. B., Romero, I., Mowery, S. A., et al. (2010). ABC and SLC transporter expression and pot substrate characterization across the human CMEC/D3 blood-brain barrier cell line. *Molecular Pharmaceutics, 7*(4), 1057–1068. http://dx.doi.org/10.1021/mp900178j.

Checchi, F., Filipe, J. A. N., Barrett, M. P., & Chandramohan, D. (2008a). The natural progression of gambiense sleeping sickness: What is the evidence? *PLoS Neglected Tropical Diseases, 2*(12), e303. http://dx.doi.org/10.1371/journal.pntd.0000303.

Checchi, F., Filipe, J. A. N., Haydon, D. T., Chandramohan, D., & Chappuis, F. (2008b). Estimates of the duration of the early and late stage of gambiense sleeping sickness. *BMC Infectious Diseases, 8*, 16. http://dx.doi.org/10.1186/1471-2334-8-16.

Chretien, J. P., & Smoak, B. L. (2005). African trypanosomiasis: Changing epidemiology and consequences. *Current Infectious Disease Reports*, 7(1), 54–60.
Clarkson, A. B., Jr., Bienen, E. J., Bacchi, C. J., McCann, P. P., Nathan, H. C., Hutner, S. H., et al. (1984). New drug combination for experimental late-stage African trypanosomiasis: DL-a-difluoromethylornithine (DFMO) with suramin. *American Journal of Tropical Medicine and Hygiene*, *33*(6), 1073–1077.
Cloete, T. T., Johansson, C. C., N'Da, D. D., Vodnala, S. K., Rottenberg, M. E., Breytenbach, J. C., et al. (2011). Mono-, di- and trisubstituted derivatives of eflornithine: Synthesis for in vivo delivery of DL-a-difluoromethylornithine in plasma. *Arzneimittelforschung*, *61*(5), 317–325.
Cross, G. A. M., Wirtz, L. E., & Navarro, M. (1998). Regulation of vsg expression site transcription and switching in Trypanosoma brucei. *Molecular and Biochemical Parasitology*, *91*(1), 77–91. http://dx.doi.org/10.1016/S0166-6851(97)00186-2.
Damper, D., & Patton, C. L. (1976a). Pentamidine transport and sensitivity in brucei group trypanosomes. *Journal of Protozoology*, *23*(2), 349–356.
Damper, D., & Patton, C. L. (1976b). Pentamidine transport in Trypanosoma brucei: Kinetics and specificity. *Biochemical Pharmacology*, *25*(3), 271–276. http://dx.doi.org/10.1016/0006-2952(76)90213-6.
De Greef, C., & Hamers, R. (1994). The serum resistance-associated (SRA) gene of Trypanosoma brucei rhodesiense encodes a variant surface glycoprotein-like protein. *Molecular and Biochemical Parasitology*, *68*(2), 277–284. http://dx.doi.org/10.1016/0166-6851(94)90172-4.
de Koning, H. P. (2001). Transporters in African trypanosomes: Role in drug action and resistance. *International Journal for Parasitology*, *31*(5–6), 512–522. http://dx.doi.org/10.1016/S0020-7519(01)00167-9.
de Koning, H. P., & Jarvis, S. M. (2001). Uptake of pentamidine in Trypanosoma brucei brucei is mediated by the P2 adenosine transporter and at least one novel, unrelated transporter. *Acta Tropica*, *80*(3), 245–250. http://dx.doi.org/10.1016/S0001-706X(01)00177-2.
Dean, M., Rzhetsky, A., & Allikmets, R. (2001). The human ATP-binding cassette (ABC) transporter superfamily. *Genome Research*, *11*(7), 1156–1166. http://dx.doi.org/10.1101/gr.GR-1649R.
Docampo, R., & Moreno, S. N. J. (2003). Current chemotherapy of human African trypanosomiasis. *Parasitology Research*, *90*(Suppl. 1), S10–S13.
Donelson, J. E., Hill, K. L., & El-Sayed, N. M. A. (1998). Multiple mechanisms of immune evasion by African trypanosomes. *Molecular and Biochemical Parasitology*, *91*, 51–66. http://dx.doi.org/10.1016/S0166-6851(97)00209-0.
Doua, F., Miezan, T. W., Sanon Singaro, J. R., Boa Yapo, F., & Baltz, T. (1996). The efficacy of pentamidine in the treatment of early-late stage Trypanosoma brucei gambiense trypanosomiasis. *American Journal of Tropical Medicine and Hygiene*, *55*(6), 586–588.
Dukes, P., Gibson, W. C., Gashumba, J. K., Hudson, K. M., Bromidge, T. J., Kaukus, A., et al. (1992). Absence of the LiTat 1.3 (CATT antigen) gene in Trypanosoma brucei gambiense stocks from Cameroon. *Acta Tropica*, *51*(2), 123–134. http://dx.doi.org/10.1016/0001-706X(92)90054-2.
Enanga, B., Keita, M., Chauvière, G., Dumas, M., & Bouteille, B. (1998). Megazol combined with suramin: A chemotherapy regimen which reversed the CNS pathology in a model of human African trypanosomiasis in mice. *Tropical Medicine and International Health*, *3*(9), 736–741.
Fairlamb, A. H., & Bowman, I. B. R. (1980). Uptake of the trypanocidal drug suramin by bloodstream forms of Trypanosoma brucei and its effect on respiration and growth rate in vivo. *Molecular and Biochemical Parasitology*, *1*(6), 315–333. http://dx.doi.org/10.1016/0166-6851(80)90050-X.

Fotiadis, D., Kanai, Y., & Palacín, M. (2013). The SLC3 and SLC7 families of amino acid transporters. *Molecular Aspects of Medicine*, *34*(2–3), 139–158. http://dx.doi.org/10.1016/j.mam.2012.10.007.

Frearson, J. A., Brand, S., McElroy, S. P., Cleghorn, L. A. T., Smid, O., Stojanovski, L., et al. (2010). N-myristoyltransferase inhibitors as new leads to treat sleeping sickness. *Nature*, *464*(7289), 728–732. http://dx.doi.org/10.1038/nature08893.

Gehrig, S., & Efferth, T. (2008). Development of drug resistance in Trypanosoma brucei rhodesiense and Trypanosoma brucei gambiense. Treatment of human africa trypanosomiasis with natural products (review). *International Journal of Molecular Medicine*, *22*(4), 411–419. http://dx.doi.org/10.3892/ijmm_00000037.

Gibson, W. (2002). Will the real Trypanosoma brucei rhodesiense please step forward? *Trends in Parasitology*, *18*(11), 486–490. http://dx.doi.org/10.1016/S1471-4922(02)02390-5.

Grab, D. J., & Kennedy, P. G. E. (2008). Traversal of human and animal trypanosomes across the blood-brain barrier. *Journal of Neurovirology*, *14*(5), 344–351. http://dx.doi.org/10.1080/13550280802282934.

Haberkorn, A., & Gönnert, R. (1972). Animal experimental investigation into the activity of nifurtimox against Trypanosoma cruzi. *Arzneimittelforschung*, *22*(9), 1570–1582.

Hackett, F., Ford, L. B., Fèvre, E., & Simarro, P. P. (2014). Incorporating scale dependence in disease burden estimates: The case of human African trypanosomiasis in Uganda. *PLoS Neglected Tropical Diseases*, *8*(2), e2704.

Huber, J. D., Egleton, R. D., & Davis, T. P. (2001). Molecular physiology and pathophysiology of tight junctions in the blood -brain barrier. *Trends in Neurosciences*, *24*(12), 719–725. http://dx.doi.org/10.1016/S0166-2236(00)02004-X.

Iten, M., Mett, H., Evans, A., Enyaru, J. C., Brun, R., & Kaminsky, R. (1997). Alterations in ornithine decarboxylase characteristics account for tolerance of Trypanosoma brucei rhodesiense to D, L-alpha-difluoromethylornithine. *Antimicrobial Agents and Chemotherapy*, *41*(9), 1922–1925.

Jamonneau, V., Ilboudo, H., Kaboré, J., Kaba, D., Koffi, M., Solano, P., et al. (2012). Untreated human infections by Trypanosoma brucei gambiense are not 100% fatal. *PLoS Neglected Tropical Diseases*, *6*(6), e1691. http://dx.doi.org/10.1371/journal.pntd.0001691.

Jeganathan, S., Sanderson, L., Dogruel, M., Rodgers, J., Croft, S., & Thomas, S. A. (2011). The distribution of nifurtimox across the healthy and trypanosome-infected murine blood-brain and blood-cerebrospinal fluid barriers. *Journal of Pharmacology and Experimental Therapeutics*, *336*(2), 506–515. http://dx.doi.org/10.1124/jpet.110.172981.

Jennings, F. W. (1993). Combination chemotherapy of CNS trypanosomiasis. *Acta Tropica*, *54*(3–4), 205–213. http://dx.doi.org/10.1016/0001-706X(93)90093-Q.

Jennings, F. W., Gichuki, C. W., Kennedy, P. G. E., Rodgers, J., Hunter, C. A., Murray, M., et al. (1997). The role of the polyamine inhibitor eflornithine in the neuropathogenesis of experimental murine African trypanosomiasis. *Neuropathology and Applied Neurobiology*, *23*(3), 225–234. http://dx.doi.org/10.1111/j.1365-2990.1997.tb01206.x.

Kageyama, T., Nakamura, M., Matsuo, A., Yamasaki, Y., Takakura, Y., Hashida, M., et al. (2000). The 4F2hc/LAT1 complex transports l-DOPA across the blood-brain barrier. *Brain Research*, *879*(1–2), 115–121. http://dx.doi.org/10.1016/S0006-8993(00)02758-X.

Kennedy, P. G. E. (2004). Human African trypanosomiasis of the CNS: Current issues and challenges. *Journal of Clinical Investigation*, *113*(4), 496–504. http://dx.doi.org/10.1172/JCI200421052.

Kennedy, P. G. E. (2013). Clinical features, diagnosis, and treatment of human African trypanosomiasis (sleeping sickness). *The Lancet Neurology*, *12*(2), 186–194. http://dx.doi.org/10.1016/S1474-4422(12)70296-X.

Koepsell, H., Lips, K., & Volk, C. (2007). Polyspecific organic cation transporters: Structure, function, physiological roles, and biopharmaceutical implications. *Pharmaceutical Research*, *24*(7), 1227–1251. http://dx.doi.org/10.1007/s11095-007-9254-z.

Kotthaus, J., Kotthaus, J., Schade, D., Schwering, U., Hungeling, H., Müller-Fielitz, H., et al. (2011). New prodrugs of the antiprotozoal drug pentamidine. *ChemMedChem, 6*(12), 2233–2242. http://dx.doi.org/10.1002/cmdc.201100422.

Kristensson, K., Nygård, M., Bertini, G., & Bentivoglio, M. (2010). African trypanosome infections of the nervous system: Parasite entry and effects on sleep and synaptic functions. *Progress in Neurobiology, 91*(2), 152–171. http://dx.doi.org/10.1016/j.pneurobio.2009.12.001.

Lambrecht, F. L. (1985). Trypanosomes and hominid evolution. *Bioscience, 35*(10), 640–646.

Lejon, V., Boelaert, M., Jannin, J., Moore, A., & Büscher, P. (2003). The challenge of Trypanosoma brucei gambiense sleeping sickness diagnosis outside Africa. *The Lancet Infectious Diseases, 3*(12), 804–808. http://dx.doi.org/10.1016/S1473-3099(03)00834-X.

Lutje, V., Seixas, J., & Kennedy, A. (2010). Chemotherapy for second-stage human African trypanosomiasis. *Cochrane Database of Systematic Reviews (Online), 8*, CD006201.

Maser, P., & Kaminsky, R. (1998). Identification of three ABC transporter genes in Trypanosoma brucei spp. *Parasitology Research, 84*(2), 106–111. http://dx.doi.org/10.1007/s004360050365.

Masocha, W., Rottenberg, M. E., & Kristensson, K. (2007). Migration of African trypanosomes across the blood-brain barrier. *Physiology and Behavior, 92*(1–2), 110–114. http://dx.doi.org/10.1016/j.physbeh.2007.05.045.

Matovu, E., Seebeck, T., Enyaru, J. C. K., & Kaminsky, R. (2001). Drug resistance in Trypanosoma brucei spp., the causative agents of sleeping sickness in man and nagana in cattle. *Microbes and Infection, 3*(9), 763–770. http://dx.doi.org/10.1016/S1286-4579(01)01432-0.

Matovu, E., Stewart, M. L., Geiser, F., Brun, R., Mäser, P., Wallace, L. J. M., et al. (2003). Mechanisms of arsenical and diamidine uptake and resistance in Trypanosoma brucei. *Eukaryotic Cell, 2*(5), 1003–1008. http://dx.doi.org/10.1128/EC.2.5.1003-1008.2003.

Ming, X., Ju, W., Wu, H., Tidwell, R. R., Hall, J. E., & Thakker, D. R. (2009). Transport of dicationic drugs pentamidine and furamidine by human organic cation transporters. *Drug Metabolism and Disposition, 37*(2), 424–430. http://dx.doi.org/10.1124/dmd.108.024083.

Mpia, B., & Pépin, J. (2002). Combination of eflornithine and melarsoprol for melarsoprol-resistant Gambian trypanosomiasis. *Tropical Medicine and International Health*, 7(9), 775–779. http://dx.doi.org/10.1046/j.1365-3156.2002.00933.x.

Mueckler, M., & Thorens, B. (2013). The SLC2 (GLUT) family of membrane transporters. *Molecular Aspects of Medicine, 34*(2–3), 121–138. http://dx.doi.org/10.1016/j.mam.2012.07.001.

Mulenga, C., Mhlanga, J. D. M., Kristensson, K., & Robertson, B. (2001). Trypanosoma brucei brucei crosses the blood-brain barrier while tight junction proteins are preserved in a rat chronic disease model. *Neuropathology and Applied Neurobiology*, 27(1), 77–85. http://dx.doi.org/10.1046/j.0305-1846.2001.00306.x.

Nare, B., Wring, S., Bacchi, C., Beaudet, B., Bowling, T., Brun, R., et al. (2010). Discovery of novel orally bioavailable oxaborole 6-carboxamides that demonstrate cure in a murine model of late-stage central nervous system African trypanosomiasis. *Antimicrobial Agents and Chemotherapy, 54*(10), 4379–4388. http://dx.doi.org/10.1128/AAC.00498-10.

Ni, Z., Bikadi, Z., Rosenberg, M. F., & Mao, Q. (2010). Structure and function of the human breast cancer resistance protein (BCRP/ABCG2). *Current Drug Metabolism, 11*(7), 603–617. http://dx.doi.org/10.2174/138920010792927325.

Nok, A. J. (2003). Arsenicals (melarsoprol), pentamidine and suramin in the treatment of human African trypanosomiasis. *Parasitology Research, 90*(1), 71–79.

Odiit, M., Kansiime, F., & Enyaru, J. C. K. (1997). Duration of symptoms and case fatality of sleeping sickness caused by Trypanosoma brucei rhodesiense in Tororo, Uganda. *East African Medical Journal*, 74(12), 792–795.

Ohtsuki, S., Ikeda, C., Uchida, Y., Sakamoto, Y., Miller, F., Glacial, F., et al. (2013). Quantitative targeted absolute proteomic analysis of transporters, receptors and junction proteins for validation of human cerebral microvascular endothelial cell line hCMEC/D3 as a human blood-brain barrier model. *Molecular Pharmaceutics*, *10*(1), 289–296. http://dx.doi.org/10.1021/mp3004308.

O'Kane, R. L., & Hawkins, R. A. (2003). Na + -dependent transport of large neutral amino acids occurs at the abluminal membrane of the blood-brain barrier. *American Journal of Physiology - Endocrinology and Metabolism*, *285*(6), E1167–E1173. http://dx.doi.org/10.1152/ajpendo.00193.2003.

O'Kane, R. L., Viña, J. R., Simpson, I., Zaragozá, R., Mokashi, A., & Hawkins, R. A. (2006). Cationic amino acid transport across the blood-brain barrier is mediated exclusively by system y +. *American Journal of Physiology Endocrinology and Metabolism*, *291*(2), E412–E419. http://dx.doi.org/10.1152/ajpendo.00007.2006.

Pal, A., Hall, B. S., & Field, M. C. (2002). Evidence for a non-LDL-mediated entry route for the trypanocidal drug suramin in Trypanosoma brucei. *Molecular and Biochemical Parasitology*, *122*(2), 217–221. http://dx.doi.org/10.1016/S0166-6851(02)00096-8.

Pardridge, W. M. (2005). The blood-brain barrier: Bottleneck in brain drug development. *NeuroRx*, *2*(1), 3–14. http://dx.doi.org/10.1602/neurorx.2.1.3.

Pepin, J., & Milord, F. (1994). The treatment of human African trypanosomiasis. *Advances in Parasitology*, *33*, 1–47.

Pépin, J., Milord, F., Khonde, A., Niyonsenga, T., Loko, L., & Mpia, B. (1994). Gambiense trypanosomiasis: Frequency of, and risk factors for, failure of melarsoprol therapy. *Transactions of the Royal Society of Tropical Medicine and Hygiene*, *88*(4), 447–452. http://dx.doi.org/10.1016/0035-9203(94)90430-8.

Pepin, J., Milord, F., Mpia, B., Meurice, F., Ethier, L., DeGroof, D., et al. (1989). An open clinical trial of nifurtimox for arseno-resistant Trypanosoma brucei gambiense sleeping sickness in central Zaire. *Transactions of the Royal Society of Tropical Medicine and Hygiene*, *83*(4), 514–517. http://dx.doi.org/10.1016/0035-9203(89)90270-8.

Philip, K. A., Dascombe, M. J., Fraser, P. A., & Pentreath, V. W. (1994). Blood-brain barrier damage in experimental African trypanosomiasis. *Annals of Tropical Medicine and Parasitology*, *88*(6), 607–616.

Picozzi, K., Carrington, M., & Welburn, S. C. (2008). A multiplex PCR that discriminates between Trypanosoma brucei brucei and zoonotic T. b. rhodesiense. *Experimental Parasitology*, *118*(1), 41–46. http://dx.doi.org/10.1016/j.exppara.2007.05.014.

Picozzi, K., Fèvre, E. M., Odiit, M., Carrington, M., Eisler, M. C., Maudlin, I., et al. (2005). Sleeping sickness in Uganda: A thin line between two fatal diseases. *British Medical Journal*, *331*(7527), 1238–1241.

Priotto, G., Kasparian, S., Mutombo, W., Ngouama, D., Ghorashian, S., Arnold, U., et al. (2009). Nifurtimox-eflornithine combination therapy for second-stage African Trypanosoma brucei gambiense trypanosomiasis: A multicentre, randomised, phase III, non-inferiority trial. *The Lancet*, *374*(9683), 56–64. http://dx.doi.org/10.1016/S0140-6736(09)61117-X.

Priotto, G., Kasparian, S., Ngouama, D., Ghorashian, S., Arnold, U., Ghabri, S., et al. (2007). Nifurtimox-eflornithine combination therapy for second-stage Trypanosoma brucei gambiense sleeping sickness: A randomized clinical trial in Congo. *Clinical Infectious Diseases*, *45*(11), 1435–1442. http://dx.doi.org/10.1086/522982.

Radwanska, M., Claes, F., Magez, S., Magnus, E., Perez-Morga, D., Pays, E., et al. (2002). Novel primer sequences for polymerase chain reaction-based detection of Trypanosoma brucei gambiense. *American Journal of Tropical Medicine and Hygiene*, *67*(3), 289–295.

Raseroka, B. H., & Ormerod, W. E. (1986). The trypanocidal effect of drugs in different parts of the brain. *Transactions of the Royal Society of Tropical Medicine and Hygiene*, *80*(4), 634–641. http://dx.doi.org/10.1016/0035-9203(86)90162-8.

Sanderson, L., Dogruel, M., Rodgers, J., Bradley, B., & Thomas, S. A. (2008). The blood-brain barrier significantly limits eflornithine entry into Trypanosoma brucei brucei infected mouse brain. *Journal of Neurochemistry*, *107*(4), 1136–1146. http://dx.doi.org/10.1111/j.1471-4159.2008.05706.x.

Sanderson, L., Dogruel, M., Rodgers, J., De Koning, H. P., & Thomas, S. A. (2009). Pentamidine movement across the murine blood-brain and blood-cerebrospinal fluid barriers: Effect of trypanosome infection, combination therapy, P-glycoprotein, and multidrug resistance-associated protein. *Journal of Pharmacology and Experimental Therapeutics*, *329*(3), 967–971. http://dx.doi.org/10.1124/jpet.108.149872.

Sanderson, L., Khan, A., & Thomas, S. (2007). Distribution of suramin, an antitrypanosomal drug, across the blood-brain and blood-cerebrospinal fluid interfaces in wild-type and P-glycoprotein transporter-deficient mice. *Antimicrobial Agents and Chemotherapy*, *51*(9), 3136–3146. http://dx.doi.org/10.1128/AAC.00372-07.

Sands, M., Kron, M. A., & Brown, R. B. (1985). Pentamidine: A review. *Reviews of Infectious Diseases*, 7(5), 625–634.

Simarro, P. P., Diarra, A., Postigo, J. A. R., Franco, J. R., & Jannin, J. G. (2011). The human African trypanosomiasis control and surveillance programme of the world health organization 2000–2009: The way forward. *PLoS Neglected Tropical Diseases*, *5*(2), e1007. http://dx.doi.org/10.1371/journal.pntd.0001007.

Steverding, D. (2008). The history of African trypanosomiasis. *Parasites and Vectors*, *1*(3). PMCID:PMC2270819 http://dx.doi.org/10.1186/1756-3305-1-3.

Sturk, L. M., Brock, J. L., Bagnell, C. R., Hall, J. E., & Tidwell, R. R. (2004). Distribution and quantitation of the anti-trypanosomal diamidine 2,5-bis(4-amidinophenyl)furan (DB75) and its N-methoxy prodrug DB289 in murine brain tissue. *Acta Tropica*, *91*(2), 131–143. http://dx.doi.org/10.1016/j.actatropica.2004.03.010.

Sun, T., & Zhang, Y. (2008). Pentamidine binds to tRNA through non-specific hydrophobic interactions and inhibits aminoacylation and translation. *Nucleic Acids Research*, *36*(5), 1654–1664. http://dx.doi.org/10.1093/nar/gkm1180.

Tatipaka, H. B., Gillespie, J. R., Chatterjee, A. K., Norcross, N. R., Hulverson, M. A., Ranade, R. M., et al. (2014). Substituted 2-phenylimidazopyridines: A new class of drug leads for human African trypanosomiasis. *Journal of Medicinal Chemistry*, *57*(3), 828–835. http://dx.doi.org/10.1021/jm401178t.

Thuita, J. K., Wolf, K. K., Murilla, G. A., Liu, Q., Mutuku, J. N., Chen, Y., et al. (2013). Safety, pharmacokinetic, and efficacy studies of oral DB868 in a first stage vervet monkey model of human African trypanosomiasis. *PLoS Neglected Tropical Diseases*, 7(6), e2230. http://dx.doi.org/10.1371/journal.pntd.0002230.

Torreele, E., Bourdin Trunz, B., Tweats, D., Kaiser, M., Brun, R., Mazué, G., et al. (2010). Fexinidazole—A new oral nitroimidazole drug candidate entering clinical development for the treatment of sleeping sickness. *PLoS Neglected Tropical Diseases*, *4*(12), e923. http://dx.doi.org/10.1371/journal.pntd.0000923.

Truc, P., Lejon, V., Magnus, E., Jamonneau, V., Nangouma, A., Verloo, D., et al. (2002). Evaluation of the micro-CATT, CATT/Trypanosoma brucei gambiense, and LATEX/T.b. gambiense methods for serodiagnosis and surveillance of human African trypanosomiasis in west and central Africa. *Bulletin of the World Health Organization*, *80*(11), 882–886.

Turner, C. M. R. (1997). The rate of antigenic variation in fly-transmitted and syringe-passaged infections of Trypanosoma brucei. *FEMS Microbiology Letters*, *153*(1), 227–231. http://dx.doi.org/10.1016/S0378-1097(97)00266-8.

Uchida, Y., Ohtsuki, S., Katsukura, Y., Ikeda, C., Suzuki, T., Kamiie, J., et al. (2011). Quantitative targeted absolute proteomics of human blood-brain barrier transporters and receptors. *Journal of Neurochemistry*, *117*(2), 333–345. http://dx.doi.org/10.1111/j.1471-4159.2011.07208.x.

Van Xong, H., Vanhamme, L., Chamekh, M., Chimfwembe, C. E., Van Den Abbeele, J., Pays, A., et al. (1998). A VSG expression site-associated gene confers resistance to human serum in Trypanosoma rhodesiense. *Cell, 95*(6), 839–846. http://dx.doi.org/10.1016/S0092-8674(00)81706-7.

Vincent, I. M., Creek, D., Watson, D. G., Kamleh, M. A., Woods, D. J., Wong, P. E., et al. (2010). A molecular mechanism for eflornithine resistance in African trypanosomes. *PLoS Pathogens, 6*(11), e1001204. http://dx.doi.org/10.1371/journal.ppat.1001204.

Wang, C. C. (1995). Molecular mechanisms and therapeutic approaches to the treatment of African trypanosomiasis. *Annual Review of Pharmacology and Toxicology, 35*, 93–127.

Watson, C. P., Dogruel, M., Mihoreanu, L., Begley, D. J., Weksler, B. B., Couraud, P. O., et al. (2012). The transport of nifurtimox, an anti-trypanosomal drug, in an in vitro model of the human blood-brain barrier: Evidence for involvement of breast cancer resistance protein. *Brain Research, 1436*, 111–121. http://dx.doi.org/10.1016/j.brainres.2011.11.053.

Wenzler, T., Yang, S., Braissant, O., Boykin, D. W., Brun, R., & Wang, M. Z. (2013). Pharmacokinetics, Trypanosoma brucei gambiense efficacy, and time of drug action of DB829, a preclinical candidate for treatment of second-stage human African trypanosomiasis. *Antimicrobial Agents and Chemotherapy, 57*(11), 5330–5343. http://dx.doi.org/10.1128/AAC.00398-13.

WHO Expert Committee on human African trypanosomiasis (2013) Control and surveillance of human African trypanosomiasis. WHO Technical Report Series, Volume 984, Geneva: World Health Organization Press. Published at http://apps.who.int/iris/bitstream/10665/95732/1/9789241209847_eng.pdf and last accessed on January 30th, 2014

Wilhelm, I., Fazakas, C., & Krizbai, I. A. (2011). In vitro models of the blood-brain barrier. *Acta Neurobiologiae Experimentalis, 71*(1), 113–128.

Wolburg, H., Mogk, S., Acker, S., Frey, C., Meinert, M., Schönfeld, C., et al. (2012). Late stage infection in sleeping sickness. *PLoS One*, 7(3), e34304. http://dx.doi.org/10.1371/journal.pone.0034304.

CHAPTER NINE

Delivery of Therapeutic Peptides and Proteins to the CNS

Therese S. Salameh*,†, William A. Banks*,†,1
*Geriatric Research Educational and Clinical Center, Veterans Affairs Puget Sound Health Care System, University of Washington, Seattle, Washington, USA
†Department of Medicine, Division of Gerontology and Geriatric Medicine, University of Washington, Seattle, Washington, USA
[1]Corresponding author: e-mail address: wabanks1@uw.edu

Contents

Abstract

Peptides and proteins have potent effects on the brain after their peripheral administration, suggesting that they may be good substrates for the development of CNS therapeutics. Major hurdles to such development include their relation to the blood–brain barrier (BBB) and poor pharmacokinetics. Some peptides cross the BBB by transendothelial diffusion and others cross in the blood-to-brain direction by saturable transporters. Some regulatory proteins are also transported across the BBB and antibodies

Advances in Pharmacology, Volume 71
ISSN 1054-3589
http://dx.doi.org/10.1016/bs.apha.2014.06.004

can enter the CNS via the extracellular pathways. Glycoproteins and some antibody fragments can be taken up and cross the BBB by mechanisms related to adsorptive endocytosis/transcytosis. Many peptides and proteins are transported out of the CNS by saturable efflux systems and enzymatic activity in the blood, CNS, or BBB are substantial barriers to others. Both influx and efflux transporters are altered by various substances and in disease states. Strategies that manipulate these interactions between the BBB and peptides and proteins provide many opportunities for the development of therapeutics. Such strategies include increasing transendothelial diffusion of small peptides, upregulation of saturable influx transporters with allosteric regulators and other posttranslational means, use of vectors and other Trojan horse strategies, inhibition of efflux transporters including with antisense molecules, and improvement in pharmacokinetic parameters to overcome short half-lives, tissue sequestration, and enzymatic degradation.

1. INTRODUCTION

Diseases of the central nervous system (CNS) are in need of effective therapeutics. However, the development of such therapeutics is hindered by the blood–brain barrier (BBB), which prevents the unregulated leakage of substances from the blood into the brain. Peptides and proteins have great potential as CNS therapeutics as they have many effects within the CNS. Many endogenous peptides and proteins can cross the BBB by a variety of mechanisms that could facilitate their development into effective CNS drugs. However, the BBB and other barriers exist to their development into effective therapeutics. This review will examine the characteristics of peptides and proteins in regards to their relations and interactions with the BBB and how those relations and interactions both facilitate and complicate their development as therapeutics.

2. OBSTACLES TO DELIVERING PROTEIN AND PEPTIDES TO THE CNS

2.1. Barriers of the CNS

Cerebrospinal fluid (CSF), which is secreted by the choroid plexuses, is contained within the cerebral ventricles and subarachnoid space. There are three barriers which limit and control molecular exchange at the interfaces between the blood and the neural tissue and its fluid spaces: (i) the vascular BBB, which is formed by cerebrovascular endothelial cells between the blood and the brain's interstitial fluid, (ii) the choroid plexus epithelium between the blood and the ventricular CSF, and (iii) the arachnoid epithelium between the blood and the subarachnoid CSF (Abbott, 2004). The distance between each of the three barriers varies, so while an individual neuron is typically found 35 μm from a brain capillary (Isaacs, Anderson, Alcantara, Black, & Greenough, 1992), it is typically millimeters or centimeters from a CSF compartment (Schlageter, Molnar, Lapin, & Groothuis, 1999). Therefore, of all the CNS barriers, the vascular BBB has the greatest control over the immediate microenvironment of brain cells.

2.2. The BBB

The BBB is the primary obstacle to overcome in the delivery of proteins and peptides to the CNS. Many peptides and regulatory proteins, for example, leptin and pituitary adenylate cyclase-activating polypeptide (PACAP), cross the BBB by saturable transport systems and affect the functions of the CNS. IL-2 does not cross the BBB and is prevented from doing so by not only the physical barrier of the capillary wall but also by an enzymatic barrier and an efflux system (Banks, Niehoff & Zalcman, 2004). To understand how and why the BBB differentiates between these peptides and regulatory proteins, we must understand the general characteristics that make up the BBB.

The BBB is a structural and functional barrier, which impedes and regulates the influx of compounds from the blood into the brain. The barrier is formed by capillary endothelial cells, surrounded by basal lamina, astrocytic perivascular endfeet, pericytes, and microglial cells (Abbott, Ronnback, & Hansson, 2006). These brain microvascular endothelial cells (BMECs) differ from endothelial cells found in other tissues both structurally and functionally. Structural differences include the absence of fenestrations and more extensive tight junctions (TJs). Functional differences include that they have sparse pinocytic vesicular transport, have increased expression of transport and carrier proteins, contain no gap junctions, and have TJs; these differences result in limited paracellular permeation and macropinocytotic transport. These characteristics of BMECs indicate that they lack the ability to produce plasma ultrafiltrate like other peripheral tissues, and thus do not leak proteins into the interstitial space of the CNS (Nag, 2011).

The structural and functional integrity of the BBB is controlled by TJs, adherens junctions, pericytes, and astrocyte end feet. TJs are present at the apical end of the interendothelial space. Review articles have stated that 98% of small molecules and ~100% of large molecules are unable to pass through the BBB as a result of TJs (Jeffrey & Summerfield, 2007; Pardridge, 2005).

TJs are comprised of a number of integral membrane proteins including claudin (isoforms 1, 3, 5 and 12), occludin, junction adhesion molecules, and cytoplasmic accessory proteins, for example, zonula occludens-1 protein, cingulin, and AF-6 (afadin) (Krause et al., 2008; Liu, Wang, Zhang, Wei, & Li, 2012; Turksen & Troy, 2004). TJ modulation at the BBB is an approach utilized to enhance delivery of proteins and peptides to the CNS. This task is completed using compounds such as calcium chelators, surfactants, cationic polymers, cyclodextrins, and hyperosmotic solutions (Deli, 2009). These compounds are not specific for TJs at the BBB, and as a result, have cytotoxic side effects. Zonula occludens toxin is a TJ modulator that is specific for the BBB. It has been shown to increase permeability selectively at the BBB (Lu et al., 2000), in a reversible and nontoxic manner (Salama, Eddington, & Fasano, 2006). Adherens junctions form adhesive contacts between the cells and are located near the basolateral side of the endothelial space. They are formed as a complex between the transmembrane glycoproteins of the cadherins family, which are linked to the cytoplasmic anchor proteins of the catenin family (Petty & Lo, 2002). Pericytes provide structural support and vasodynamic capacity to the brain microvasculature. As an example of the importance of pericytes in maintaining BBB structural integrity, it has been demonstrated that endothelial cells that are associated with pericytes are more resistant to apoptosis than isolated endothelial cells (Ramsauer, Krause, & Dermietzel, 2002). Also, the presence of pericytes improved brain endothelial cell monolayer transendothelial electrical resistance (TEER) but had no effect on albumin permeability (Dohgu & Banks, 2013). TEER is a commonly used measurement to gage the tightness of a monolayer of cells both *in vitro* and *in vivo* (Czupalla, Liebner, & Devraj, 2014). Pericytes are necessary for BBB formation during embryogenesis, given that they are recruited to the BBB prior to astrocyte generation (Daneman, Zhou, Kebede, & Barres, 2010). They regulate functional aspects of the BBB; including the formation of TJs and vesicle trafficking in CNS endothelial cells. Astrocytic end feet provide biochemical support to BMEC. They co-regulate function by the secretion of soluble cytokines such as LIF (leukemia-inhibiting factor), Ca^{2+}-dependent signals by intracellular IP-3 and gap junction-dependent pathways, and second messenger pathways involving extracellular diffusion of purinergic messengers. Astrocytes influence the formation and maintenance of the BBB *in vitro*. Physical contact, or at least close proximity, between astrocytes and endothelial cells is required for the induction of certain BBB-specific markers such as the brain-type glucose transporter

(GLUT-1) and gamma-glutamyl transpeptidase, a carboxypeptidase selectively expressed in endothelial cells of the CNS (Hurwitz, Berman, Rashbaum, & Lyman, 1993).

A unique characteristic of the BBB is that the TJs between the endothelial cells have a high TEER of 1500–2000 Ω cm^2 compared to 3–33 Ω cm^2 in other vascular tissues (Butt, Jones, & Abbott, 1990; Crone & Christensen, 1981). This high electrical resistance results in low paracellular diffusion, thus providing the brain with a highly regulated and stable microenvironment. The BBB maintains and regulates brain homeostasis, and compensates for fluctuations in the systemic circulation and increased metabolic functions; nevertheless, a number of CNS-associated diseases, including human immunodeficiency virus encephalitis (Kanmogne et al., 2006), meningitis (Barichello et al., 2012), multiple sclerosis (Zhang, Kan, Xu, Zhang, & Zhu, 2013), Alzheimer's and Parkinson's disease (Dickstein et al., 2006; Persidsky, Ramirez, Haorah, & Kanmogne, 2006), epilepsy (Arican et al., 2006), and stroke (Hu et al., 2011), have been shown or proposed to have a disrupted BBB, leading to functional breakdown.

2.3. Physicochemical characteristics of the drug

The majority of drugs that are used to treat CNS disease have a molecular weight between 150 and 500 Da and a log octanol/water partition coefficient between −0.5 and 6.0 (Bodor & Buchwald, 2003). This does not indicate that drugs with a molecular weight less than 150 or greater than 500 Da are unable to cross. Characteristics that reduce the ability of small molecules to cross the BBB include a polar surface area in excess of 80 Å, a high Lewis bond strength, and a high potential for hydrogen bond formation (Doan et al., 2002). Also, increased number of positive charges and increased flexibility contribute to BBB crossing. Lipid solubility is a clear indicator of small drugs that can pass through the BBB (Levin, 1980).

Rules for peptides have some similarities and some apparent differences from those for small drugs. Most peptides are poorly soluble in lipids and so would be expected to not penetrate the BBB very well by transendothelial diffusion. However, lipid solubility was a predictor of BBB penetration for one series of peptides that had molecular weights ranging from 486 to 6000 Da (Banks & Kastin, 1985). Delta sleep-inducing peptide and an enkephalins are examples of peptides that have a molecular weight over 600 Da and are known to cross the BBB (Banks, Kastin & Coy, 1982a; Kastin, Pearson, & Banks, 1991). The largest substance found to cross the

BBB using transmembrane diffusion thus far is cytokine-induced neutrophil chemoattractant-1, which has a molecular weight of 7800 Da (Pan & Kastin, 2001). This is thought to represent a direct correlation between BBB penetration and the ability of a drug to partition into the lipid bilayer of the cell membrane.

2.4. Pharmacokinetics of the drug

In general, peptides and regulatory proteins have very short half-lives and large volumes of distribution after their peripheral injection. This means that the opportunity for these substances to cross the BBB is reduced in terms of both the percent of the injected dose that reaches the BBB and the length of time for which that exposure lasts. Peptides are especially susceptible to enzymatic degradation (Werle, Loretz, Entstrasser, & Föger, 2007) which, along with renal and hepatic clearance, contributes to their short half-life. Regulatory proteins have smaller volumes of distribution than peptides, but can also have short half-lives in the circulation. Production of analogues with smaller volumes of distribution and longer half-lives will proportionately increase uptake by the CNS. Erythropoietin and IgG antibodies represent an example of the effects of improving the pharmacokinetics of a protein or peptide on transport into the brain (Banks, Jumbe, Farrell, Niehoff & Heatherington, 2004; Banks et al., 2002). Neither of these substances show high distribution in the brain, but they are able to gain access to the CNS through the extracellular pathways, by leaking into the brain in the same manner as albumin, and, as a result of their long residence time in blood, they are able to eventually accumulate in brain.

Enzymatic degradation is especially high when it comes to the oral delivery of therapeutic peptides and protein. Use of a chitosan–aprotinin conjugate has enhanced oral administration of therapeutic peptides and proteins that are susceptible to degradation by trypsin and chymotrypsin (Werle et al., 2007).

2.5. Binding to plasma proteins

Many peptides are known to bind to circulating proteins (Banks & Kastin, 1993). The amount of time that the unbound drug spends at the site of action mediates the intensity and duration of drug action. Since it is difficult to measure the concentration of unbound drug at the site of action, the measurement of the concentration of unbound drug in plasma is used instead (Alavijeh, Chishty, Qaiser, & Palmer, 2005). This assumes that drugs bind reversely to plasma and tissue protein and that equilibrium of unbound drug exists between plasma and tissues. So while this is an area that has been studied for over 100 years, accurate prediction of this parameter continues to be an issue. There are numerous methods for *in vitro* determination of protein binding, including equilibrium dialysis, dynamic dialysis, ultrafiltration, ultracentrifugation, and exclusion chromatography (Alavijeh et al., 2005). Protein binding is commonly determined for *in vitro* drugs during development since this is an important factor in determining their pharmacokinetics and pharmacological effects. Protein binding or uptake by circulating cells can decrease the free fraction of a substance in blood. This, in turn, can limit access to the BBB, especially for those peptides without a saturable transporter located at the BBB (Banks, Kastin & Coy, 1982a).

2.6. Enzymatic degradation at the BBB

Endothelial cells of the BBB provide a metabolic barrier for many substances by expressing a number of enzymes that modify endogenous and exogenous molecules that otherwise could bypass the physical barrier and negatively affect neuronal function (Brownson, Abbruscato, Gillespie, Hruby, & Davis, 1994; Hardebo & Owman, 1990). There are a variety of ectoenzymes, such as aminopeptidases, endopeptidases, and cholinesterases, which are expressed on the plasma membranes of the capillary endothelium, pericytes, and astrocytes (Pardridge, 2002). Patients with Parkinson's disease are treated with L-DOPA, the precursor for dopamine, because it has a higher affinity for the transporter. The ability of L-DOPA to cross the BBB is limited by the presence of the enzymes L-DOPA decarboxylase and monoamine oxidase with the capillary endothelial cells. This is evidenced by the fact that only 0.1–0.3% of a clinical dose of L-DOPA enters the brain. As a result, large amounts of L-DOPA need to be used in treatment of Parkinson's disease and sometimes, treatment is administered simultaneously with an inhibitor of L-DOPA decarboxylase (Hardebo & Owman, 1980). Brain endothelial cell enzymes are also important in peptide BBB interactions, retarding the entry of enkephalins and affecting interactions with amyloid-beta peptide (Baranczyk-Kuzma & Audus, 1987; Davies et al., 1998; Simons et al., 1998).

2.7. Brain-to-blood transporters

The BBB itself plays a role in preventing peptides and regulatory proteins from entering the brain. This includes its ability to sequester these peptides and proteins by taking them up from the blood but not transporting them into the brain. Sequestration of peptides and proteins is often harmful to the brain and results in the onset of neurodegenerative diseases. An example of this is the amyloid-beta (Aβ) peptide sequestration in Alzheimer's disease. Efflux systems transport these peptides in a brain-to-blood direction to prevent their accumulation in the brain. These efflux systems are controlled by ATP-binding cassette (ABC) transporters (Higgins, 2001). Three ABC transporters have emerged as major regulators of drug efflux: P-glycoprotein (Pgp), multidrug resistance-associated protein (MRP), and breast cancer resistance protein (BCRP). There are known inhibitors to each of these ABC transporters that prevent the expulsion of the drug from the brain.

ABC transporters are involved in clearance of some peptides from the brain, but peptides often have more specific efflux transporters as well. In the case of Aβ, the clearance not only involves Pgp (Hartz, Miller, & Bauer, 2010) but also occurs through the low-density lipoprotein receptor-related protein 1 (LRP1) (Deane et al., 2004; Pascale et al., 2011). LRP1 expression is reduced in patients with Alzheimer's disease (Kang et al., 2000). It is thought that because of this, amyloid-beta accumulates in the brains of Alzheimer's patients and is toxic to nerve cells. Efflux transporters have also been described for Tyr-MIF-1, enkephalins, arginine vasopressin, somatostatin, and a host of other peptides (Begley, 1994). Efflux can be a major regulator of brain levels of the peptide as demonstrated by Met-enkephalin or a major contributor to blood levels of the peptide as demonstrated by corticotrophin-releasing hormone (Martins, Banks, & Kastin, 1997; Plotkin, Banks, & Kastin, 1998).

3. SATURABLE MECHANISMS OF PEPTIDE AND PROTEIN PASSAGE ACROSS THE BBB

3.1. Transport proteins

Carrier-mediated transport allows substances with low lipid solubility to cross the BBB many fold faster than possible by transendothelial diffusion. Examples of transporters include the medium-chain fatty acid carrier, large neutral amino acid carrier, monocarboxylic acid carrier, cation transporter, purine carrier, nucleoside carrier, and hexose carrier (Cornford & Oldendorf, 1975; Davson & Segal, 1996; Dhopeshwarkar, 1973; Smith, Momma, Aoyagi, & Rapoport, 1987). Some of these transporters are highly selective in regards to their stereochemical requirements and as a result they will not transfer drugs with the same affinity and capacity as the endogenous substrate. An example of this is glucose, which is the primary energy substrate of the brain. It crosses the BBB by using the stereospecific, but insulin-independent, GLUT-1 transporter. The stereospecificity of the glucose-transport system allows D-glucose, but not L-glucose, to enter the brain. This transport system also allows some other hexoses, such as mannose, maltose, and fructose, to enter the brain. Low GLUT-1 expression is associated with individuals who have seizures, mental retardation, compromised brain development, and low CSF glucose concentrations (De Vivo et al., 1991).

Some small peptides cross the BBB by saturable systems as well. These include enkephalins, arginine vasopressin, a peptide-T analog, amyloid-beta peptide, and insulin (Barrera, Kastin, & Banks, 1987; Zlokovic et al., 1992, 1993; Zlokovic, Mackic, Djuricic, & Davson, 1989).

3.2. Receptor-mediated transcytosis

Larger peptides and proteins that can cross the BBB are thought to do so by binding to mobile versions of their receptors, inducing a vesicular-based transport mechanism. When a protein binds to the receptor, it is endocytosed into the endothelial cell to form a vesicle, and then released on the other side. Transport by this mechanism is unidirectional, saturable, and energy requiring. Insulin and transferrin are the classic examples usually given for blood-to-brain RMT and IgG efflux for brain-to-blood RMT. Examples exist, however, in which the transporter for a protein is not its canonical receptor. The molecular weight at which transport can no longer occur via a channel or pore is also not known.

3.3. Adsorptive-mediated endocytosis

In adsorptive-mediated endocytosis, there is thought to be a charge interaction between the protein/peptide and the luminal side of the endothelial cell. Polycationic proteins, such as histones and lectins, cross the BBB by a similar manner to receptor-mediated transcytosis (Tamai et al., 1997). However, instead of binding to a specific receptor in the membrane, these proteins absorb to the endothelial cell membrane based on charge or affinity for sugar moieties of membrane glycoproteins. The overall capacity of absorptive-mediated endocytosis is greater because the number of receptors present in the membrane does not limit it. Thus, cationization of a protein may provide a mechanism for enhancing brain uptake.

4. STRATEGIES TO ENHANCE THE DELIVERY OF PROTEINS AND PEPTIDES TO THE CNS

The BBB is lined with brain endothelial cells, sealed with paracellular protein complexes, bound by extracellular matrix, and maintained through pericyte and glial interactions (Zlokovic, 2008). Through its ability to restrict penetration of biomolecules, the BBB regulates the chemical composition of the CNS required for proper neuronal function. While vital for health and normal physiology, the BBB remains an obstacle for delivery of therapeutics into the brain. Thus, the development of noninvasive strategies to enhance macromolecule delivery across the BBB has been a long-sought objective for academic and biopharmaceutical research.

Most of the drugs currently in use for the treatment of CNS disorders have a low-molecular weight (150–500 Da) and high lipophilicity. Many potential drugs are unable to reach the brain because of enzymatic degradation, clearance by efflux mechanisms, or binding to plasma proteins. In order to enhance drug delivery to the brain, the following strategies for delivery optimization have been explored: (i) BBB modulation, which includes transient osmotic opening of the BBB; (ii) physiologically based strategies, which exploit the various transport mechanisms present at the BBB; and (iii) pharmacologically based approaches to increase the passage through the BBB by optimizing the specific biochemical attributes of a compound.

4.1. BBB modulation to increase permeability

One strategy to improve peptide and protein drug delivery to the CNS consists of combining systemic administration of the drug with transient osmotic opening of the BBB. Modulating the efficacy of the TJs between cerebral endothelial cells, so that the paracellular route of access to the brain is accessible, is an approach that has been utilized to permeabilize the BBB to drugs and enhance brain uptake. Le Fèvre and Millet, in 1926, claimed that urotropine (hexamine), given intravenously before herpes virus administration, enabled the virus to cross the BBB and initiate encephalitis in rabbits (Hurst & Davies, 1950). Although later studies involving the pathogenesis of herpetic infection of the nervous system after intravenous inoculation invalidated their findings, the interest in discovering substances that altered BBB permeability to allow the uptake of various molecules was strong. In the decades that followed, researchers discovered a number of substances that alter BBB permeability including adrenaline, theocin, urethane, histamine, coal-gas, and ether (Hurst & Davies, 1950). Currently, we are still employing this strategy of BBB modulation to deliver drugs to the CNS. Mannitol, a hypertonic solution, is administered simultaneously with drugs like methotrexate to enhance its delivery to brain tumors (Neuwelt et al., 1981). Hypertonic solutions are thought to osmotically remove water from the endothelial cells, causing the cell to shrink, which may cause cellular changes affecting the TJs. This method is transitory and the barrier closes within 10–20 min following BBB disruption. Unfortunately, this method is not selective for the drug and may allow access of other molecules, such as neurotransmitters, which could be potentially harmful. Similarly, solvents such as a high dose of ethanol or dimethylsulfide, alkylating agents like etoposide, and vasoactive agents such as bradykinin and histamine, have all been used to disrupt the BBB. Alkylglycerols have also been shown to modulate the BBB (Erdlenbruch et al., 2003; Hülper et al., 2013). The mechanism of BBB modulation has not been elucidated; however, both the normal brain and tumor BBB are opened, in contrast to osmotic opening that appears to act preferentially on the BBB of normal brain (Erdlenbruch et al., 2003). The opening of the BBB is again presumably nonselective. The use of these agents to affect BBB permeability can be highly traumatic and often results in serious side effects, such as seizures, permanent neurological disorders, and brain edema. To circumvent these problems, ultrasound and electromagnetic radiation are being employed as modulators of BBB function (Kinoshita, McDannold, Jolesz, & Hynynen, 2006; Marquet, Tung, Teichert, Ferrera, & Konofagou, 2011). An advantage of these methods is that they can be focused with some precision to a particular brain region or to a tumor, thus selectively modulating the BBB at a preferred site and not globally throughout the brain. These modifications in BBB function and integrity appear to be rapidly induced and rapidly reversed.

Few strategies have endeavored to alter the transendothelial permeation of the BBB itself. The BBB's lipid composition and permeability to lipid soluble molecules does not seem to changes during the life span (Cornford, Braun, Oldendorf, & Hill, 1982; Mooradian & Smith, 1992a), but may do so in models of diabetes mellitus and aluminum toxicity (Banks & Kastin, 1985; Mooradian & Smith, 1992b).

4.2. Physiologically based strategies

One strategy involves the exploitation of receptor-mediated and adsorptive-mediated transport systems using chimeric peptide technology. This involves coupling the peptide or protein drug to a vector, which may also be a protein/peptide, and which normally crosses the BBB either by receptor-mediated transcytosis (transferrin and insulin) or adsorptive endocytosis (cationized albumin). The following chimeric protein/peptide is endocytosed at the luminal side of the BBB following the interaction of the transport vector with its corresponding cell surface receptor. It is then carried through the membrane, released into the interstitial fluid, and the chimeric protein/peptide is cleaved to release the peptide or protein drug into the brain where it can exert a pharmacological response. The protein or peptide drug is joined to the vector using chemical linkers, polyethylene glycol linkers, or avidin–biotin technology.

Receptor-mediated vectors for brain delivery must be specific. A well-characterized transcytotic model to target drug delivery into the CNS is the transferrin receptor (TfR). It has been 30 years since Jefferies et al. discovered that brain capillaries had an abundance of TfR that delivered iron-bound transferrin into the brain (Jefferies et al., 1984). Following this discovery, they showed that TfR antibodies could cross the BBB (Dennis & Watts, 2012) and deliver therapeutic compounds such as methotrexate (Friden et al., 1991), making TfR particularly promising in brain-targeted delivery. Modifications are still being made in the use of TfR as a delivery system after studies showed that antibodies bound to the TfR were retained in the brain endothelium and not penetrating into the CNS (Couch et al., 2013). To address this problem, a "brain shuttle" approach has been developed which fuses the C-terminus of a monoclonal antibody against Aβ, the peptide that accumulates in the brain of Alzheimer's patients, to an anti-TfR F_{ab}, which facilitates the BBB transcytosis of an attached immunoglobulin (Niewoehner et al., 2014). This differs from current approaches where studies have used a TfR antibody carrying therapeutic cargo (Pardridge, 2012) or a bispecific antibody that binds TfR with low affinity and with high affinity, a disease target, for example, the enzyme β-secretase (BACE1), which processes amyloid precursor protein into Aβ peptides including those associated with Alzheimer's disease (Yu et al., 2011). Compared to the monospecific anti-BACE1 antibody, the bispecific antibody had increased accumulation in the brain and led to an increased reduction in Aβ levels (Atwal et al., 2011). Alternatively, receptor-specific monoclonal antibodies that undergo receptor-mediated endocytosis at the BBB *in vivo*, such as OX26, the mouse monoclonal antibody to the TfR, can also be used as transport vectors in this regard (Gosk, Vermehren, Storm, & Moos, 2004). Receptor-mediated transcytosis has been very useful in delivering numerous peptide and protein drugs to the CNS including VIP analogs, brain-derived neurotrophic factor, adrenocorticotrophic hormone analog, doxorubicin, dalargin, and cationized albumin.

An alternative strategy is the exploitation of carrier-mediated transport systems. The BBB contains many nutrient transporters including peptide carrier systems for small peptides such as enkephalins, thyrotropin-releasing hormone, and arginine vasopressin; amino acid carrier systems for glutamate, phenylalanine, leucine, and aspartate; nucleoside carrier systems for choline and thiamine; and hexose carrier systems for glucose and mannose. In order to utilize these transport systems, the structural properties of the drugs have to be modified to mimic those of the carried nutrient. Very few drugs are known to use BBB transport systems to enter the CNS.

This mechanism of using endogenous transporters is also often overlooked for the delivery of proteins and peptides to the CNS. Despite the growing list of peptides and proteins known to cross the BBB by saturable systems, use of transporters to deliver endogenous ligands or analogs of them has not been exploited. PACAP38 provides an example of a peptide with a saturable BBB transporter that can exert therapeutic effects in a disease model. PACAP started 24 h after four-vessel stroke and infused peripherally will prevent about 50% of CA1 hippocampal cell death (Uchida, Arimura, Somogyvari-Vigh, Shioda, & Banks, 1996).

Small molecules that are physiologic regulators of endogenous transport systems can also be used to enhance brain uptake of large proteins. Alpha adrenergics enhance the BBB uptake of both leptin and lysosomal enzymes (Banks, 2001; Urayama, Grubb, Banks, & Sly, 2007). The increase in leptin transport may explain one mechanism by which epinephrine induces weight loss.

Inhibition of efflux transporters is another method to strengthen the ability of proteins and peptides to enter the brain. Specific inhibitors to the ABC transporters have been developed as one option to allow drugs increased access to the CNS. Examples of inhibitors used to target Pgp include verapamil, cyclosporin A, LY335979, and fumitremorgin C; MRP include sulfinpyrazone and benzbromarone; BCRP include fumitremorgin C and GF120918. PACAP27 uptake by the brain is limited by the efflux system, peptide transport system-6 (PTS-6) (Dogrukol-Ak et al., 2008). Antisense targeting of PTS-6, prevented PACAP27 efflux and increased its levels in the brain. When cotreated with the antisense and PACAP27, improved cognition was observed in a mouse mode of Alzheimer's disease and infarct size was reduced after cerebral ischemia. Although the benefits of increasing the delivery of these drugs to the CNS are high, inhibition of these ABC transporters may have detrimental effects because they allow for the passage of other toxic substances through the BBB as well and require use of high concentrations to effectively block transport (Falasca & Linton, 2012).

4.3. Pharmacologically based strategies

One of the primary factors in determining whether a peptide will cross the BBB is its lipophilicity. A strategy for enhancing the ability of peptide to cross the BBB is increasing its lipophilicity. There a number of techniques to enhance a proteins lipophilicity including altering the protein structure, methylation, halogenation, or acylation (Begley, 1994; Chikhale, Ng, Burton, & Borchardt, 1994; Weber et al., 1991, 1992). Structural changes, for example covalently binding the drug to lipidic moieties, such as long-chain fatty acids, will increase the lipophilicity of a peptide (Heyl et al., 1994). Peptides with a high number of hydroxyl groups tend to promote hydrogen bonding with water, which leads to a decrease in the partition coefficient and thus, a decrease in membrane permeability. Decreasing hydrogen bonding increases membrane permeability. Ideally, there should be fewer than eight bonds when developing new drugs. Methylation is one method used to reduce hydrogen bonding. An example of how this approach has been utilized is found in the development of cyclic peptides for increased membrane permeability and oral bioavailability (White et al., 2011). In this study, they showed that on-resin N-methylation of cyclic peptides was able to increase membrane permeability and enhance oral bioavailability in rats compared to non-methylated controls. D-Penicillamine(2,5)-enkephalin (DPDPE) is a potent opioid peptide that exhibits a high selectivity for the delta-opiate receptors (Dagenais, Ducharme, & Pollack, 2001). This receptor is part of the organic anion transporting polypeptides (Oatps) family of transporters which are known to transport a wide range of amphipathic organic compounds including bile salts, steroid hormones, thyroid hormones, and organic cations; providing a potential target for therapeutic peptide delivery (Hagenbuch & Meier, 2003). Trimethylation of the Phe of DPDPE showed increased BBB transport. This study demonstrated an interesting point as four isomers of (trimethyl-Phe^{4})DPDPE were examined but only one isomer showed an effect of BBB transport (Witt et al., 2000). This illustrates an important point for peptide modifications: that the location and type of modification play a significant role in improving BBB transport of your peptide of interest.

Halogenation of peptides and proteins can also lead to increased lipophilicity and BBB permeability. The halogenation of the DPDPE peptide has been studied in great detail. The increase in BBB transport of DPDPE was dependent on which halogen was utilized; chloro and bromo additions increased BBB transport, while flouro and iodo additions had no effect (Gentry et al., 1999).

An alternative approach is acylation of the N-terminal amino acid can also increase the lipophilicity of peptides and proteins. For example, acylation of insulin improved its ability to cross the BBB while maintaining its pharmacological effects. Similarly, glycosylation has been shown to increase transport of proteins and peptides. Proteins that have been glycosylated using Amidori rearrangement have increased uptake into the CNS (Poduslo & Curran, 1994). This reaction describes the acid or base catalyzed isomerization of the N-glycoside of an aldose or the glycosylamine to the corresponding 1-amino-1-deoxy-ketose. This method has been used for deltorphin, cyclized Met-enkephalin analogues, and linear Leu-enkephalin analogues.

As an alternative to altering the chemical structure of a compound drug carriers, such as liposomes and nanoparticles, can be used to enhance the delivery of proteins and peptides to the CNS. This is referred to as the "Trojan horse" or "Universal Carrier" approach. One of the first approaches utilizing the Trojan horse strategy involved placing the cargo protein inside a liposome studded with IgG molecules to direct delivery (Weissmann, 1976).

There are many advantages to using this method for peptide and protein delivery to the brain. First, this technique allows for some control in determining where the protein and peptide are delivered to in the brain. Secondly, it is relatively easy to modify the chemical properties of the nanoparticles or liposomes to achieve a specific and selective delivery of the protein or peptide drug to the intended site of action. Since the peptides and protein drugs are carried within the nanoparticle or liposome, there is no need to change the physiochemical properties of the drugs to allow for their entry into the brain and you can deliver a large quantity of drug, as the carrier is quite large. Finally, this technique provides protection of the drug from enzymatic degradation.

Nanoparticles are solid colloidal particles, ranging in size from 1 to 1000 nm, consisting of various macromolecules in which therapeutic drugs can be absorbed, entrapped, or covalently attached. There are a variety of nanoparticles in use currently to deliver drugs across the BBB: liposomes, solid lipid nanoparticle, nonpolymeric micelles, lipoplex, dendrimers, polymeric nanoparticle, polymeric micelle, nanotubes, silica nanoparticle, quantum dots, gold nanoparticle, and magnetic nanoparticle (Gao, Pang, & Jiang, 2013). One of the most successful nanoparticles in use currently to deliver drugs to the CNS is the poly(butyl)cyanoacrylate nanoparticles (Ambruosi, Yamamoto, & Kreuter, 2005). These 250 nm nanoparticles are loaded with drugs and coated with polysorbate-80. When they are intravenously injected, their surface becomes coated with absorbed plasma proteins such as apolipoprotein E. It is thought that these nanoparticles are capable of passing the BBB because they are mistaken for low-density lipoprotein particles. A number of drugs have gained successful entrance into the brain using this method including dalargin, loperamide, and doxorubicin.

5. CONCLUSION

Diseases of the CNS are in need of effective therapeutics. A major hurdle in the development of these therapeutic agents includes their relation to the BBB and poor pharmacokinetics. This review examined the characteristics of peptides and proteins in regards to their relations and interactions with the BBB and how those relations and interactions both facilitate and complicate their development as therapeutics. Strategies that manipulate these interactions between the BBB and peptides and proteins provide many opportunities for the development of therapeutics. Such strategies include increasing transendothelial diffusion of small peptides, upregulation of saturable influx transporters with allosteric regulators and other posttranslational means, use of vectors and other Trojan horse strategies, inhibition of efflux transporters including with antisense molecules, and improvement in pharmacokinetic parameters to overcome short half-lives, tissue sequestration, and enzymatic degradation. While major advancements have been made in this area, there is still much space for improvement.

CONFLICT OF INTEREST

The authors have no conflicts of interest.

ACKNOWLEDGMENTS

This work was supported by VA merit review and NIH grant RO1 AG029839. T. S. S. is supported by NIA T32AG000258.

REFERENCES

Abbott, N. J. (2004). Evidence for bulk flow of brain interstitial fluid: Significance for physiology and pathology. *Neurochemistry International*, *45*(4), 545–552. http://dx.doi.org/10.1016/j.neuint.2003.11.006.

Abbott, N. J., Ronnback, L., & Hansson, E. (2006). Astrocyte-endothelial interactions at the blood-brain barrier. *Nature Reviews. Neuroscience*, 7(1), 41–53.

Alavijeh, M. S., Chishty, M., Qaiser, M. Z., & Palmer, A. M. (2005). Drug metabolism and pharmacokinetics, the blood-brain barrier, and central nervous system drug discovery. *NeuroRx*, *2*(4), 554–571.

Ambruosi, A., Yamamoto, H., & Kreuter, J. (2005). Body distribution of polysorbate-80 and doxorubicin-loaded [14C]poly(butyl cyanoacrylate) nanoparticles after i.v. administration in rats. *Journal of Drug Targeting*, *13*(10), 535–542. http://dx.doi.org/10.1080/10611860500411043.

Arican, N., Kaya, M., Kalayci, R., Uzun, H., Ahishali, B., Bilgic, B., et al. (2006). Effects of lipopolysaccharide on blood-brain barrier permeability during pentylenetetrazole-induced epileptic seizures in rats. *Life Sciences*, *79*(1), 1–7. http://dx.doi.org/10.1016/j.lfs.2005.12.035.

Atwal, J. K., Chen, Y., Chiu, C., Mortensen, D. L., Meilandt, W. J., Liu, Y., et al. (2011). A therapeutic antibody targeting BACE1 inhibits amyloid-β production in vivo. *Science Translational Medicine*, *3*(84), 84ra43.

Banks, W. A. (2001). Enhanced leptin transport across the blood-brain barrier by alpha1-adrenergic agents. *Brain Research*, *899*, 209–217.

Banks, W. A., Jumbe, N. L., Farrell, C. L., Niehoff, M. L., & Heatherington, A. (2004a). Passage of erythropoietic agents across the blood-brain barrier: A comparison of human and murine erythropoietin and the analog Darbopoetin alpha. *European Journal of Pharmacology*, *505*, 93–101.

Banks, W. A., & Kastin, A. J. (1985). Peptides and the blood-brain barrier: Lipophilicity as a predictor of permeability. *Brain Research Bulletin*, *15*, 287–292.

Banks, W. A., & Kastin, A. J. (1993). Peptide binding in blood and passage across the blood–brain barrier. In J. P. Tillement, H. Eckert, E. Albengres, J. Barre, P. Baumann, & F. Belpare, et al. (Eds.), *Proceedings of the international symposium on blood binding and drug transfer* (pp. 223–242). Paris: Fort and Clair (Reprinted from: IN FILE).

Banks, W. A., Kastin, A. J., & Coy, D. H. (1982a). Delta sleep-inducing peptide crosses the blood-brain-barrier in dogs: Some correlations with protein binding. *Pharmacology, Biochemistry, and Behavior*, *17*, 1009–1014.

Banks, W. A., Niehoff, M. L., & Zalcman, S. (2004b). Permeability of the mouse blood-brain barrier to murine interleukin-2: Predominance of a saturable efflux system. *Brain, Behavior, and Immunity*, *18*, 434–442.

Banks, W. A., Terrell, B., Farr, S. A., Robinson, S. M., Nonaka, N., & Morley, J. E. (2002). Transport of amyloid protein antibody across the blood-brain barrier in an animal model of Alzheimer's disease. *Peptides*, *23*, 2223–2226.

Baranczyk-Kuzma, A., & Audus, K. L. (1987). Characteristics of aminopeptidase activity from bovine brain microvessel endothelium. *Journal of Cerebral Blood Flow and Metabolism*, 7, 801–805.

Barichello, T., Fagundes, G. D., Generoso, J. S., Paula Moreira, A., Costa, C. S., Zanatta, J. R., et al. (2012). Brain-blood barrier breakdown and pro-inflammatory mediators in neonate rats submitted meningitis by Streptococcus pneumoniae. *Brain Research*, *1471*(0), 162–168. http://dx.doi.org/10.1016/j.brainres.2012.06.054.

Barrera, C. M., Kastin, A. J., & Banks, W. A. (1987). D-[Ala 1]-peptide T-amide is transported from blood to brain by a saturable system. *Brain Research Bulletin*, *19*, 629–633.

Begley, D. J. (1994). Strategies for delivery of peptide drugs to the central nervous system: Exploiting molecular structure. *Journal of Controlled Release*, *29*, 293–306.

Bodor, N., & Buchwald, P. (2003). Brain-targeted drug delivery. *American Journal of Drug Delivery*, *1*(1), 13–26. http://dx.doi.org/10.2165/00137696-200301010-00002.

Brownson, E. A., Abbruscato, T. J., Gillespie, T. J., Hruby, V. J., & Davis, T. P. (1994). Effect of peptidases at the blood brain barrier on the permeability of enkephalin. *Journal of Pharmacology and Experimental Therapeutics*, *270*, 675–680.

Butt, A. M., Jones, H. C., & Abbott, N. J. (1990). Electrical resistance across the blood-brain barrier in anaesthetized rats: A developmental study. *The Journal of Physiology*, *429*(1), 47–62.

Chikhale, E. G., Ng, K. Y., Burton, P. S., & Borchardt, R. T. (1994). Hydrogen bonding potential as a determinant of the in vitro and in situ blood-brain barrier permeability of peptides. *Pharmaceutical Research*, *11*, 412–419.

Cornford, E. M., Braun, L. D., Oldendorf, W. H., & Hill, M. A. (1982). Comparison of lipid-mediated blood-brain-barrier penetrability in neonates and adults. *American Journal of Physiology*, *243*, C161–C168.

Cornford, E. M., & Oldendorf, W. (1975). Independent blood-brain barrier transport systems for nucleic acid precursors. *Biochimica et Biophysica Acta*, *394*, 211–219.

Couch, J. A., Yu, Y. J., Zhang, Y., Tarrant, J. M., Fuji, R. N., Meilandt, W. J., et al. (2013). Addressing safety liabilities of TfR bispecific antibodies that cross the blood-brain barrier. *Science Translational Medicine*, *5*(183), 183ra157.

Crone, C., & Christensen, O. (1981). Electrical resistance of a capillary endothelium. *The Journal of General Physiology*, 77(4), 349–371. http://dx.doi.org/10.1085/jgp.77.4.349.

Czupalla, C., Liebner, S., & Devraj, K. (2014). In vitro models of the blood-brain barrier. In R. Milner (Ed.), *Vol. 1135. Cerebral angiogenesis* (pp. 415–437). New York: Springer.

Dagenais, C., Ducharme, J., & Pollack, G. M. (2001). Uptake and efflux of the peptidic delta-opioid receptor agonist [D-penicillamine2,5]-enkephalin at the murine blood-brain barrier by in situ perfusion. *Neuroscience Letters*, *301*(3), 155–158. http://dx.doi.org/10.1016/S0304-3940(01)01640-8.

Daneman, R., Zhou, L., Kebede, A. A., & Barres, B. A. (2010). Pericytes are required for blood–brain barrier integrity during embryogenesis. *Nature*, *468*(7323), 562–566. http://www.nature.com/nature/journal/v468/n7323/abs/nature09513.html#supplementary-information.

Davies, T. A., Billingslea, A., Long, H. J., Tibbles, H., Wells, J. M., Eisenhauer, P. B., et al. (1998). Brain endothelial cell enzymes cleave platelet-retained amyloid precursor protein. *Journal of Laboratory and Clinical Medicine*, *132*, 341–350.

Davson, H., & Segal, M. B. (1996). *Special aspects of the blood-brain barrier physiology of the CSF and blood-brain barriers*. (pp. 303–485). Boca Raton: CRC Press (Reprinted from: IN FILE).

De Vivo, D. C., Trifiletti, R. R., Jacobson, R. I., Ronen, G. M., Behmand, R. A., & Harik, S. I. (1991). Defective glucose transport across the blood-brain barrier as a cause of persistent hypoglycorrhachia, seizures, and developmental delay. *New England Journal of Medicine*, *325*, 703–709.

Deane, R., Wu, Z., Sagare, A., Davis, J., Du Yan, S., Hamm, K., et al. (2004). LRP/amyloid beta-peptide interaction mediates differential brain efflux of Abeta isoforms. *Neuron*, *43*(3), 333–344.

Deli, M. A. (2009). Potential use of tight junction modulators to reversibly open membranous barriers and improve drug delivery. *Biochimica et Biophysica Acta (BBA)-Biomembranes*, *1788*(4), 892–910. http://dx.doi.org/10.1016/j.bbamem.2008.09.016.

Dennis, M. S., & Watts, R. J. (2012). Transferrin antibodies into the brain. *Neuropsychopharmacology*, *37*(1), 302–303.

Dhopeshwarkar, G. A. (1973). Uptake and transport of fatty acids into the brain and the role of the blood-brain barrier system. *Advances in Lipid Research*, *11*, 109–142.

Dickstein, D. L., Biron, K. E., Ujiie, M., Pfeifer, C. G., Jeffries, A. R., & Jefferies, W. A. (2006). Aβ peptide immunization restores blood-brain barrier integrity in Alzheimer disease. *The FASEB Journal*, *20*(3), 426–433. http://dx.doi.org/10.1096/fj.05-3956com.

Doan, K. M. M., Humphreys, J. E., Webster, L. O., Wring, S. A., Shampine, L. J., Serabjit-Singh, C. J., et al. (2002). Passive permeability and P-glycoprotein-mediated efflux differentiate central nervous system (CNS) and non-CNS marketed drugs. *Journal of Pharmacology and Experimental Therapeutics*, *303*(3), 1029–1037. http://dx.doi.org/10.1124/jpet.102.039255.

Dogrukol-Ak, D., Kumar, V. B., Ryerse, J. S., Farr, S. A., Verma, S., Nonaka, N., et al. (2008). Isolation of peptide transport system-6 from brain endothelial cells: Therapeutic effects with antisense inhibition in Alzheimer and stroke models. *Journal of Cerebral Blood Flow and Metabolism*, *29*(2), 411–422.

Dohgu, S., & Banks, W. (2013). Brain pericytes increase the lipopolysaccharide-enhanced transcytosis of HIV-1 free virus across the in vitro blood-brain barrier: Evidence for cytokine-mediated pericyte-endothelial cell crosstalk. *Fluids and Barriers of the CNS*, *10*(1), 23.

Erdlenbruch, B., Alipour, M., Fricker, G., Miller, D. S., Kugler, W., Eibl, H., et al. (2003). Alkylglycerol opening of the blood-brain barrier to small and large fluorescence markers in normal and C6 glioma-bearing rats and isolated rat brain capillaries. *British Journal of Pharmacology*, *140*(7), 1201–1210. http://dx.doi.org/10.1038/sj.bjp.0705554.

Falasca, M., & Linton, K. J. (2012). Investigational ABC transporter inhibitors. *Expert Opinion on Investigational Drugs*, *21*(5), 657–666. http://dx.doi.org/10.1517/13543784.2012.679339.

Friden, P. M., Walus, L. R., Musso, G. F., Taylor, M. A., Malfroy, B., & Starzyk, R. M. (1991). Anti-transferrin receptor antibody and antibody-drug conjugates cross the blood-brain barrier. *Proceedings of the National Academy of Sciences*, *88*(11), 4771–4775.

Gao, H., Pang, Z., & Jiang, X. (2013). Targeted delivery of nano-therapeutics for major disorders of the central nervous system. *Pharmaceutical Research*, *30*(10), 2485–2498. http://dx.doi.org/10.1007/s11095-013-1122-4.

Gentry, C. L., Egleton, R. D., Gillespie, T., Abbruscato, T. J., Bechowski, H. B., Hruby, V. J., et al. (1999). The effect of halogenation on blood-brain barrier permeability of a novel peptide drug. *Peptides*, *20*(10), 1229–1238. http://dx.doi.org/10.1016/S0196-9781(99)00127-8.

Gosk, S., Vermehren, C., Storm, G., & Moos, T. (2004). Targeting anti-transferrin receptor antibody (OX26) and OX26-conjugated liposomes to brain capillary endothelial cells using in situ perfusion. *Journal of Cerebral Blood Flow and Metabolism*, *24*(11), 1193–1204.

Hagenbuch, B., & Meier, P. J. (2003). The superfamily of organic anion transporting polypeptides. *Biochimica et Biophysica Acta (BBA) - Biomembranes*, *1609*(1), 1–18. http://dx.doi.org/10.1016/S0005-2736(02)00633-8.

Hardebo, J. E., & Owman, C. (1980). Barrier mechanisms for neurotransmitter monoamines and their precursors at the blood-brain interface. *Annals of Neurology*, *8*(1), 1–11. http://dx.doi.org/10.1002/ana.410080102.

Hardebo, J. E., & Owman, C. (1990). Enzymatic barrier mechanisms for neurotransmitter monoamines and their precursors at the blood-brain barrier. In B. B. Johansson, C. Owman, & H. Widner (Eds.), *Pathophysiology of the blood-brain barrier* (pp. 41–55). Amsterdam: Elsevier (Reprinted from: NOT IN FILE).

Hartz, A. M. S., Miller, D. S., & Bauer, B. (2010). Restoring blood-brain barrier p-glycoprotein reduces brain amyloid-beta in a mouse model of Alzheimer's disease. *Molecular Pharmacology*, 77, 715–723.

Heyl, D. L., Sefler, A. M., He, J. X., Sawyer, T. K., Wustrow, D. J., Akunne, H. C., et al. (1994). Structure-activity and conformational studies of a series of modified C-terminal hexapeptide neurotensin analogues. *International Journal of Peptide and Protein Research, 44*, 233–238.

Higgins, C. F. (2001). ABC transporters: Physiology, structure and mechanism—An overview. *Research in Microbiology, 152*(3–4), 205–210. http://dx.doi.org/10.1016/S0923-2508(01)01193-7.

Hu, Q., Chen, C., Khatibi, N. H., Li, L., Yang, L., Wang, K., et al. (2011). Lentivirus-mediated transfer of MMP-9 shRNA provides neuroprotection following focal ischemic brain injury in rats. *Brain Research, 1367*(0), 347–359. http://dx.doi.org/10.1016/j.brainres.2010.10.002.

Hülper, P., Veszelka, S., Walter, F. R., Wolburg, H., Fallier-Becker, P., Piontek, J., et al. (2013). Acute effects of short-chain alkylglycerols on blood-brain barrier properties of cultured brain endothelial cells. *British Journal of Pharmacology, 169*(7), 1561–1573. http://dx.doi.org/10.1111/bph.12218.

Hurst, E. W., & Davies, O. L. (1950). Studies on the blood-brain barrier. II. Attempts to influence the passage of substances into the brain. *British Journal of Pharmacology, 5*, 147–164.

Hurwitz, A. A., Berman, J. W., Rashbaum, W. K., & Lyman, W. D. (1993). Human fetal astrocytes induce the expression of blood-brain barrier specific proteins by autologous endothelial cells. *Brain Research, 625*(2), 238–243. http://dx.doi.org/10.1016/0006-8993(93)91064-Y.

Isaacs, K. R., Anderson, B. J., Alcantara, A. A., Black, J. E., & Greenough, W. T. (1992). Exercise and the brain: Angiogenesis in the adult rat cerebellum after vigorous physical activity and motor skill learning. *Journal of Cerebral Blood Flow and Metabolism, 12*, 110–119.

Jefferies, W. A., Brandon, M. R., Hunt, S. V., Williams, A. F., Gatter, K. C., & Mason, D. Y. (1984). Transferrin receptor on endothelium of brain capillaries. *Nature, 312*(5990), 162–163.

Jeffrey, P., & Summerfield, S. G. (2007). Challenges for blood-brain barrier (BBB) screening. *Xenobiotica, 37*(10–11), 1135–1151. http://dx.doi.org/10.1080/00498250701570285.

Kang, D. E., Pietrzik, C. U., Baum, L., Chevallier, N., Merriam, D. E., Kounnas, M. Z., et al. (2000). Modulation of amyloid β-protein clearance and Alzheimer's disease susceptibility by the LDL receptor-related protein pathway. *The Journal of Clinical Investigation, 106*(9), 1159–1166. http://dx.doi.org/10.1172/JCI11013.

Kanmogne, G. D., Schall, K., Leibhart, J., Knipe, B., Gendelman, H. E., & Persidsky, Y. (2006). HIV-1 gp120 compromises blood-brain barrier integrity and enhance monocyte migration across blood-brain barrier: Implication for viral neuropathogenesis. *Journal of Cerebral Blood Flow and Metabolism, 27*(1), 123–134.

Kastin, A. J., Pearson, M. A., & Banks, W. A. (1991). EEG evidence that morphine and an enkephalin analog cross the blood-brain barrier. *Pharmacology, Biochemistry, and Behavior, 40*(4), 771–774. http://dx.doi.org/10.1016/0091-3057(91)90084-F.

Kinoshita, M., McDannold, N., Jolesz, F. A., & Hynynen, K. (2006). Noninvasive localized delivery of Herceptin to the mouse brain by MRI-guided focused ultrasound-induced blood-brain barrier disruption. *Proceedings of the National Academy of Sciences, 103*(31), 11719–11723.

Krause, G., Winkler, L., Mueller, S. L., Haseloff, R. F., Piontek, J., & Blasig, I. E. (2008). Structure and function of claudins. *Biochimica et Biophysica Acta (BBA) - Biomembranes, 1778*(3), 631–645. http://dx.doi.org/10.1016/j.bbamem.2007.10.018.

Levin, V. A. (1980). Relationship of octanol/water partition coefficient and molecular weight to rat brain capillary permeability. *Journal of Medicinal Chemistry, 23*(6), 682–684. http://dx.doi.org/10.1021/jm00180a022.

Liu, W.-Y., Wang, Z.-B., Zhang, L.-C., Wei, X., & Li, L. (2012). Tight junction in blood-brain barrier: An overview of structure, regulation, and regulator substances. *CNS Neuroscience & Therapeutics*, *18*(8), 609–615. http://dx.doi.org/10.1111/j.1755-5949.2012.00340.

Lu, R., Wang, W., Uzzau, S., Vigorito, R., Zielke, H. R., & Fasano, A. (2000). Affinity purification and partial characterization of the zonulin/zonula occludens toxin (Zot) receptor from human brain. *Journal of Neurochemistry*, *74*(1), 320–326. http://dx.doi.org/10.1046/j.1471-4159.2000.0740320.

Marquet, F., Tung, Y.-S., Teichert, T., Ferrera, V. P., & Konofagou, E. E. (2011). Noninvasive, transient and selective blood-brain barrier opening in non-human primates in vivo. *PLoS One*, *6*(7), e22598. http://dx.doi.org/10.1371/journal.pone.0022598.

Martins, J. M., Banks, W. A., & Kastin, A. J. (1997). Transport of CRH from mouse brain directly affects peripheral production of· beta-endorphin by the spleen. *American Journal of Physiology*, *273*, E1083–E1089.

Mooradian, A. D., & Smith, T. L. (1992a). The effect of age on lipid composition and order of rat cerebral microvessels. *Neurochemical Research*, *17*, 233–237.

Mooradian, A. D., & Smith, T. L. (1992b). The effect of experimentally induced diabetes mellitus on the lipid order and composition of rat cerebral microvessels. *Neuroscience Letters*, *145*, 145–148.

Nag, S. (2011). Morphology and properties of brain endothelial cells. In S. Nag (Ed.), *Vol. 686. The blood-brain and other neural barriers* (pp. 3–47). New Jersey: Humana Press.

Neuwelt, E. A., Diehl, J. T., Vu, L. H., Hill, S. A., Michael, A. J., & Frenkel, E. P. (1981). Monitoring of methotrexate delivery in patients with malignant brain tumors after osmotic blood-brain barrier disruption. *Annals of Internal Medicine*, *94*(4_Part_1), 449–454. http://dx.doi.org/10.7326/0003-4819-94-4-449.

Niewoehner, J., Bohrmann, B., Collin, L., Urich, E., Sade, H., Maier, P., et al. (2014). Increased brain penetration and potency of a therapeutic antibody using a monovalent molecular shuttle. *Neuron*, *81*(1), 49–60. http://dx.doi.org/10.1016/j.neuron.2013.10.061.

Pan, W., & Kastin, A. J. (2001). Changing the chemokine gradient: CINC1 crosses the blood-brain barrier. *Journal of Neuroimmunology*, *115*(1–2), 64–70. http://dx.doi.org/10.1016/S0165-5728(01)00256-9.

Pardridge, W. M. (2002). Drug and gene delivery to the brain: The vascular route. *Neuron*, *36*(4), 555–558. http://dx.doi.org/10.1016/S0896-6273(02)01054-1.

Pardridge, W. M. (2005). The blood-brain barrier: Bottleneck in brain drug development. *NeuroRx*, *2*(1), 3–14.

Pardridge, W. M. (2012). Drug transport across the blood-brain barrier. *Journal of Cerebral Blood Flow and Metabolism*, *32*(11), 1959–1972.

Pascale, C., Miller, M., Chiu, C., Boylan, M., Caralopoulos, I., Gonzalez, L., et al. (2011). Amyloid-beta transporter expression at the blood-CSF barrier is age-dependent. *Fluids and Barriers of the CNS*, *8*(1), 21.

Persidsky, Y., Ramirez, S., Haorah, J., & Kanmogne, G. (2006). Blood-brain barrier: Structural components and function under physiologic and pathologic conditions. *Journal of Neuroimmune Pharmacology*, *1*(3), 223–236. http://dx.doi.org/10.1007/s11481-006-9025-3.

Petty, M. A., & Lo, E. H. (2002). Junctional complexes of the blood-brain barrier: Permeability changes in neuroinflammation. *Progress in Neurobiology*, *68*(5), 311–323. http://dx.doi.org/10.1016/S0301-0082(02)00128-4.

Plotkin, S. R., Banks, W. A., & Kastin, A. J. (1998). Enkephalin, PPE, mRNA, and PTS-1 in alcohol withdrawal seizure-prone and -resistant mice. *Alcohol*, *15*, 25–31.

Poduslo, J. F., & Curran, G. L. (1994). Glycation increases the permeability of proteins across the blood-nerve and blood-brain barriers. *Brain Research. Molecular Brain Research*, *1*(2), 157–162.

Ramsauer, M., Krause, D., & Dermietzel, R. (2002). Angiogenesis of the blood-brain barrier in vitro and the function of cerebral pericytes. *The FASEB Journal*, *16*(10), 1274–1276. http://dx.doi.org/10.1096/fj.01-0814fje.

Salama, N. N., Eddington, N. D., & Fasano, A. (2006). Tight junction modulation and its relationship to drug delivery. *Advanced Drug Delivery Reviews*, *58*(1), 15–28. http://dx.doi.org/10.1016/j.addr.2006.01.003.

Schlageter, K. E., Molnar, P., Lapin, G. D., & Groothuis, D. R. (1999). Microvessel organization and structure in experimental brain tumors: Microvessel populations with distinctive structural and functional properties. *Microvascular Research*, *58*(3), 312–328. http://dx.doi.org/10.1006/mvre.1999.2188.

Simons, E. R., Marshall, D. C., Long, H. J., Otto, K., Billingslea, A., Tibbles, H., et al. (1998). Blood brain barrier endothelial cells express candidate amyloid precursor protein-cleaving secretases. *Amyloid*, *5*, 153–162.

Smith, Q. R., Momma, S., Aoyagi, M., & Rapoport, S. I. (1987). Kinetics of neutral amino acid transport across the blood-brain barrier. *Journal of Neurochemistry*, *49*, 1651–1658.

Tamai, I., Sai, Y., Kobayashi, H., Kamata, M., Wakamiya, T., & Tsuji, A. (1997). Structure-internalization relationship for adsorptive-mediated endocytosis of basic peptides at the blood-brain barrier. *Journal of Pharmacology and Experimental Therapeutics*, *280*(1), 410–415.

Turksen, K., & Troy, T.-C. (2004). Barriers built on claudins. *Journal of Cell Science*, *117*(12), 2435–2447. http://dx.doi.org/10.1242/jcs.01235.

Uchida, D., Arimura, A., Somogyvari-Vigh, A., Shioda, S., & Banks, W. A. (1996). Prevention of ischemia-induced death of hippocampal neurons by pituitary adenylate cyclase activating polypeptide. *Brain Research*, *736*, 280–286.

Urayama, A., Grubb, J. H., Banks, W. A., & Sly, W. S. (2007). Epinephrine enhances lysosomal enzyme delivery across the blood-brain barrier by up-regulation of the mannose 6-phosphate receptor. *Proceedings of the National Academy of Sciences United States of America*, *31*, 12873–12878.

Weber, S. J., Greene, D. L., Hruby, V. J., Yamamura, H. I., Porreca, F., & Davis, T. P. (1992). Whole body and brain distribution of [3H]cyclic[D-Pen 2, D-Pen 5] enkephalin after intraperitoneal, intravenous, oral and subcutaneous administration. *Journal of Pharmacology and Experimental Therapeutics*, *263*, 1308–1316.

Weber, S. J., Greene, D. L., Sharma, S. D., Yamamura, H. I., Kramer, T. H., Burks, T. F., et al. (1991). Distribution and analgesia of [3 H][D-Pen 2, D-Pen 5]enkephalin and two halogenated analogs after intravenous administration. *Journal of Pharmacology and Experimental Therapeutics*, *259*, 1109–1117.

Weissmann, G. (1976). Experimental enzyme replacement in genetic and other disorders. *Hospital Practice*, *11*, 49–58.

Werle, M., Loretz, B., Entstrasser, D., & Föger, F. (2007). Design and evaluation of a chitosan–aprotinin conjugate for the perioral delivery of therapeutic peptides and proteins susceptible to enzymatic degradation. *Journal of Drug Targeting*, *15*(5), 327–333. http://dx.doi.org/10.1080/10611860701349141.

White, T. R., Renzelman, C. M., Rand, A. C., Rezai, T., McEwen, C. M., Gelev, V. M., et al. (2011). On-resin N-methylation of cyclic peptides for discovery of orally bioavailable scaffolds. *Nature Chemical Biology*, 7(11), 810–817. http://www.nature.com/nchembio/journal/v7/n11/abs/nchembio.664.html#supplementary-information.

Witt, K. A., Slate, C. A., Egleton, R. D., Huber, J. D., Yamamura, H. I., Hruby, V. J., et al. (2000). Assessment of stereoselectivity of trimethylphenylalanine analogues of δ-opioid [D-Pen2, D-Pen5]-enkephalin. *Journal of Neurochemistry*, *75*(1), 424–435. http://dx.doi.org/10.1046/j.1471-4159.20000750424.

Yu, Y. J., Zhang, Y., Kenrick, M., Hoyte, K., Luk, W., Lu, Y., et al. (2011). Boosting brain uptake of a therapeutic antibody by reducing its affinity for a transcytosis target. *Science Translational Medicine*, *3*(84), 84ra44.

Zhang, S., Kan, Q.-C., Xu, Y., Zhang, G.-X., & Zhu, L. (2013). Inhibitory effect of matrine on blood-brain barrier disruption for the treatment of experimental autoimmune encephalomyelitis. *Mediators of Inflammation*, *2013*, 10. http://dx.doi.org/10.1155/2013/736085.

Zlokovic, B. V. (2008). The blood-brain barrier in health and chronic neurodegenerative disorders. *Neuron*, *57*(2), 178–201. http://dx.doi.org/10.1016/j.neuron.2008.01.003.

Zlokovic, B. V., Banks, W. A., El Kadi, H., Erchegyi, J., Mackic, J. B., McComb, J. G., et al. (1992). Transport, uptake, and metabolism of blood-borne vasopressin by the blood-brain barrier. *Brain Research*, *590*, 213–218.

Zlokovic, B. V., Ghiso, J., Mackic, J. B., McComb, J. G., Weiss, M. H., & Frangione, B. (1993). Blood-brain barrier transport of circulating Alzheimer's amyloid. *Biochemical and Biophysical Research Communications*, *197*, 1034–1040.

Zlokovic, B. V., Mackic, J. B., Djuricic, B. M., & Davson, H. (1989). Kinetic analysis of leucine-enkephalin cellular uptake at the luminal side of the blood-brain barrier of an in situ perfused guinea pig brain. *Journal of Neurochemistry*, *53*, 1333–1340.

CHAPTER TEN

Engineering and Pharmacology of Blood–Brain Barrier-Permeable Bispecific Antibodies

Danica Stanimirovic*[,1], Kristin Kemmerich*, Arsalan S. Haqqani*, Graham K. Farrington[†]

*Human Health Therapeutics Portfolio, National Research Council of Canada, Ottawa, Ontario, Canada
[†]Biogen Idec Inc., 12 Cambridge Center, Cambridge, Massachusetts, USA
[1]Corresponding author: e-mail address: danica.stanimirovic@nrc-cnrc.gc.ca

Contents

Abstract

The development and approval of antibody-based therapeutics have progressed rapidly over the past decade. However, poor blood–brain barrier (BBB) permeability hinders the progress of antibody therapies for conditions in which the target is located in the central nervous system (CNS). Increased brain penetration of therapeutic antibodies can be achieved by engineering bispecific antibodies in which one antibody binding specificity recognizes a BBB receptor that undergoes receptor-mediated transcytosis (RMT) from the circulatory compartment into brain parenchyma, and the second binding specificity recognizes a therapeutic target within the CNS. These bispecific antibodies can be built using various antibody fragments as "building blocks," including monomeric

Advances in Pharmacology, Volume 71
ISSN 1054-3589
http://dx.doi.org/10.1016/bs.apha.2014.06.005

single-domain antibodies, the smallest antigen-binding fragments of immunoglobulins. The development of BBB-crossing bispecific antibodies requires targeted antibody engineering to optimize multiple characteristics of "BBB carrier" and therapeutic arms, as well as other antibody properties impacting pharmacokinetics and effector function. Whereas several BBB-crossing bispecific antibodies have been developed using transferrin receptor antibodies as BBB carriers, the principal obstacle for capitalizing on the future promise of CNS-active antibodies remains the scarcity of known, characterized RMT receptors which could be exploited for the development of BBB carriers. This chapter reviews the recent advances and guiding principles for designing, engineering, and evaluating BBB-crossing bispecific antibodies and discusses approaches to identify and characterize novel BBB-crossing antibodies and RMT receptors.

ABBREVIATIONS

AD Alzheimer's disease
AUC area under the curve
BBB blood–brain barrier
BEC brain endothelial cells
bsAb bispecific antibody
CSF cerebrospinal fluid
Da Daltons
IgG immunoglobulin G
ILIS isotopically labeled internal standard
IR insulin receptor
ISF interstitial fluid
LDL low-density lipoprotein
LRP low-density lipoprotein receptor-related protein
NPY neuropeptide Y
PK/PD pharmacokinetics/pharmacodynamics
RMT receptor-mediated transcytosis
TfR transferrin receptor
V_HH camelid single-domain antibody

1. INTRODUCTION

The invention of methods for producing monoclonal antibodies (mAbs) revolutionized biomedical research giving rise to a whole new class of therapeutics, more complex yet more "precise" than synthetic small molecule drugs. Initially isolated from mice to study the immune system, mAbs began to unfold their broad therapeutic potential with the development of chimeric antibodies and the "humanization" of rodent mAbs (Güssow & Seemann, 1991; Jolliffe, 1993; Jones, Dear, Foote, Neuberger, & Winter, 1986) the generation of phage-display libraries of fully human mAbs (Marks et al., 1991; McCafferty, Griffiths, Winter, & Chiswell, 1990; Persson, 1993) as well as the development of transgenic mice, carrying human immunoglobulin genes (Brüggemann et al., 1989; Lee et al., 2014). Antibody-based treatments make up a third of the current biologics market (La Merie Publishing, 2013) and include approved therapeutic products for various types of cancers, immune- and infectious diseases, and many more in late-stage clinical trials.

Antibodies differ substantially from small molecule pharmaceuticals in the way they are produced, and in their physicochemical and functional properties. Salient differences between antibodies and small molecule drugs that guide and impact their preclinical and clinical development as therapeutics are summarized in Table 1. Antibodies are large, complex and inherently multifunctional molecules that can be selected to exhibit exquisite target and epitope selectivity and binding affinity (subpicomolar). Unlike small molecule drugs, antibodies persist in peripheral circulation for several days to

Table 1 Essential differences between antibodies and small molecule drugs that influence their preclinical and clinical development as therapeutics

mAb	Small molecule drug
150,000 Da	200–500 Da
Biological production process—*heterogeneous* (posttranslational modifications; glycosylation)	Chemical production process—homogeneous
High *species selectivity*	Generally less selective
Multifunctional—target binding, Fc effector function, FcRn binding	Single target
Long plasma pharmacokinetics—FcRn-mediated recycling	Shorter pharmacokinetics
Target can affect PK behavior (target-mediated drug disposition)	Mostly linear PK; nonlinearity from saturation of metabolic pathways
Toxicity—largely "*on-target*"-mediated exaggerated pharmacology	Toxicity—often "off-target" mediated
Poor extravasation and limited tissue diffusion	Easy extravasation and wide tissue distribution
Drug–drug interaction (DDI)—few examples; mostly PD related	DDI—many examples; metabolic and/or PD related
Immunogenicity sometimes observed	Immunogenicity rarely observed

weeks. However, due to size (~150 kDa) and complexity, antibodies can have poor extravasation and limited tissue penetration, even in organs supplied with fenestrated vessels. In contrast to small molecule drugs which exhibit "off-target" toxicity, antibodies can trigger exaggerated "on-target" pharmacology and may be immunogenic triggering production of autoantibodies. However, antibodies can nowadays be engineered to enhance their therapeutic properties (such as target affinity or specificity), to eliminate unwanted effects (e.g., characteristics which can cause immunogenicity and on-target toxicity), to add additional functionalities (multispecificity), or to reduce size and complexity. The recent advances in antibody engineering, combined with industrialization of mAb manufacturing and high approval rates by regulatory agencies (in comparison to small molecule drugs), have fueled the development of therapeutic antibodies as a "new wave" of targeted therapeutics.

2. MAKING THE CASE FOR ANTIBODIES AS CENTRAL NERVOUS SYSTEM THERAPEUTICS

Antibodies have been enjoying success as potent and efficacious therapeutics meeting multiple therapeutic needs in specific instances where small molecules have not been successful. Examples include the "blockbuster" antibody Humira that binds and blocks TNFα (e.g., for treatment of rheumatoid arthritis) and the anti-CD20 antibody Rituxan (e.g., for treatment of B-cell lymphoma) (La Merie Publishing, 2013). Tysabri is an effective antibody for the treatment of the neuroimmune disease multiple sclerosis that suppresses activation of the majority of T-cell subtypes and most monocytes (Deloire et al., 2004) of the immune system peripherally and therefore does not need to penetrate the brain parenchyma for therapeutic efficacy.

Despite the successes of antibodies in treating "peripheral" diseases, the overwhelming majority (99%) of all central nervous system (CNS) therapeutics remain small molecules (PharmaBiotech, 2010) and there are currently no approved therapeutic antibodies for treatment of brain diseases such as Alzheimer's or Parkinson's disease, amyotrophic lateral sclerosis, and brain tumors (e.g., glioblastoma), all of which currently have no disease-modifying treatments. The principal hurdle in developing biologics that target the CNS is their insufficient penetration across the blood–brain barrier (BBB). The tight junctions of endothelial cells that make up the BBB prevent the free diffusion of hydrophilic molecules larger than 500 Da (Daltons) (Abbott, Patabendige, Dolman, Yusof, & Begley, 2010; Pardridge, 2002).

Transport of macromolecules, including antibodies, is severely restricted, essentially preventing therapeutically efficacious antibody concentrations to reach the brain parenchyma (Pardridge, 2002). In addition, the physical size of an antibody, its molecular charge, and binding to heparan-sulfate proteoglycans in combination with the tortuosity of the brain extracellular space, severely limit antibody diffusion to their targets within the brain parenchyma (Wolak & Thorne, 2013).

Several examples from clinical development and therapeutic applications of antibodies demonstrate how the peripheral restriction of antibodies by the BBB negatively impacts their efficacy within the CNS. The humanized, recombinant mAb trastuzumab (Herceptin) that binds specifically to the human epidermal growth factor receptor 2 protein (HER2) was developed for the treatment of HER2-positive breast cancer (25–30% of all breast cancer patients). Interestingly, due to good control of the peripheral disease with this antibody and extended life span of HER2-positive cancer patients, the incidence of brain metastases in patients treated with trastuzumab has increased over the last decade. This exemplified how the BBB and blood-cerebrospinal fluid barrier (BCSFB) prevent trastuzumab from reaching efficacious concentrations in the brain after standard intravenous administration (Braen et al., 2010).

The development of an immunotherapy to treat Alzheimer's disease (AD) has generated intense interest and led to several clinical trials with antibodies against amyloid beta (Aβ) that accumulates and deposits excessively in the brain parenchyma of AD patients causing neuronal toxicity. The hypothesis driving the immunotherapy development for AD, the "peripheral sink hypothesis" (DeMattos et al., 2001; Zlokovic, 2011), contends that Aβ-binding antibodies disturb the equilibrium between central and peripheral Aβ pools by accelerating the removal of the circulating Aβ pool and mobilizing efflux of brain parenchymal amyloid into the circulation by reverse transport across the BBB, presumed to be mediated by the low-density lipoprotein receptor-related protein 1 (LRP) transporter (Sagare, Deane, & Zlokovic, 2012; Stanimirovic & Friedman, 2012). Despite enormous investment (e.g., $1B trial cost for Pfizer, J&J, and Elan's antibody bapineuzumab) in the development, engineering, and clinical testing of several Aβ-binding antibodies, anti-Aβ immunotherapy failed to produce benefit in several phase III clinical trials, questioning the importance of Aβ as therapeutic target for AD. Rather than dismissing Aβ as a potential therapeutic target, a recent study (Henderson et al., 2014) disputed the "sink hypothesis" by demonstrating that the peripherally restricted, engineered Aβ-degrading enzyme neprilysin, did not alter brain or cerebrospinal fluid (CSF) Aβ levels after a chronic (up to 4 months) administration in mice, rats, and non-human primates, despite severe depletion of circulating Aβ. The study showed that the rate of "reverse transport" of brain Aβ across the BBB triggered by the peripheral depletion was too slow to affect the brain Aβ pool. This study reconfirmed that predominantly peripherally restricted actions of Aβ antibody therapy were not sufficient to produce a central therapeutic effect. In contrast, Levites et al. (2006) demonstrated that centrally delivered Aβ-binding antibody fragments are highly effective in preventing Aβ deposition in CRND8-transgenic mice, which normally develop plaques at an early age.

With hurdles such as overcoming the restricted brain penetration and diffusion, one might question whether therapeutic antibodies are feasible therapeutics for CNS targets hidden beyond brain barriers. Many experimental studies and some clinical syndromes demonstrate the strong therapeutic impact that CNS-acting antibodies can have when they are injected directly or produced within the brain. Two paraneoplastic syndromes (Darnell & Posner, 2003) provide examples where target-specific autoantibodies against extracellular epitopes of the *N*-methyl-D-aspartate (NMDA) or gamma-aminobutyric acid-A (GABA) receptors are produced by brain infiltrating neoplastic B cells and cause central symptoms of these diseases (Bien et al., 2012; Petit-Pedrol et al., 2014). Antibodies generated against the cell surface expressed N-terminal domain of the NR1 subunit of the NMDA receptor, for example, drive receptor internalization by cross-linking, resulting in a decrease of synaptic NMDAR-mediated currents and in severe forms of the syndrome in increasing NMDAR clustering and loss of function (Dalmau, Lancaster, Martinez-Hernandez, Rosenfeld, & Balice-Gordon, 2011; Hughes et al., 2010). Similarly, $GABA_A$ receptor autoantibodies have been implicated in symptoms of encephalitis, seizures, and refractory status epilepticus (Petit-Pedrol et al., 2014). These examples demonstrate the potent pharmacological effects, though undesirable in these cases, that antibodies targeting brain parenchymal targets can achieve when available in sufficient concentrations beyond the BBB.

Potential advantages of antibodies for CNS indications include their strong selectivity against specific epitopes, such as those expressed in ion channels and G-protein-coupled receptors, that small molecule drugs cannot achieve. This subtype and epitope selectivity of antibodies should ameliorate the "off-target" side effects often seen with small molecule CNS drugs. Antibodies can also expand the CNS target space by addressing numerous targets not suitable for small molecules, including immunomodulators and growth factors secreted into the extracellular microenvironment. To capitalize on the promise of therapeutic antibodies for CNS indications, it is critical to *integrate the development of BBB-delivery technologies into the development of therapeutic antibodies for CNS indications.*

3. BBB SHUTTLES FOR MACROMOLECULES

The development of successful antibody therapies targeting parenchymal CNS molecules will largely be tied to the development of innovative BBB-delivery methods since the concentration of antibodies in the brain and CSF following peripheral administration is generally less than 0.1% of the circulating concentration (Pepinsky, Shao, Ji, & Wang, 2011). The current methods for improving CNS delivery of antibodies and biologics, including osmotic or focussed ultrasound BBB disruption, convection-enhanced diffusion, intrathecal infusion, intracerebral implantation of genetically engineered viruses or cells, require neurosurgical intervention, hospitalization, use of expensive equipment and can only be applied to a small subset of patients due to side effects and limited clinical benefit (Gabathuler, 2009).

In contrast, transvascular delivery of macromolecules across the BBB after systemic administration is noninvasive and is amenable to chronic diseases and repetitive dosing regimens (Pardridge, 2002). Delivery of nutrients required for brain function and elimination of unwanted molecules is accomplished by carrier-mediated transporters, present at both the apical (blood) and basolateral (brain) side of the BBB, respectively (Neuwelt et al., 2011). These carriers are usually highly stereospecific and transport small molecules such as ions, energy sources, and amino acids. Delivery of macromolecules, important for brain physiology, relies on vesicular transport via nonspecific macropinocytosis, adsorptive-mediated endocytosis/transcytosis (AME), and receptor-mediated transcytosis (RMT) (Jones & Shusta, 2007; Pardridge & Boado, 2012; Spencer & Verma, 2007). Whereas AME is mediated by nonspecific and nonselective charge-based interactions of polycationic molecules with the highly negatively charged glycocalyx of brain endothelial cells (BEC), brain influx of nutrients such as iron, insulin, and leptin occurs by energy-dependent RMT (Abbott et al., 2010). Ligand binding to the receptor presented on the luminal (blood) side of the BEC initiates RMT and triggers subsequent receptor clustering, membrane invagination and the formation of intracellular transport vesicles. The transport vesicles are subject to sorting within the cellular endocytic compartments that result in ligand release on the abluminal surface of the endothelial cell and receptor recycling back to the luminal membrane (Jones & Shusta, 2007; Smith & Gumbleton, 2006). The RMT pathway is selective for BBB-expressed receptors and can be initiated by antibodies which bind RMT receptors. The presently known RMT receptors can be grouped broadly into one of three types: (1) iron transporters (e.g., transferrin receptor (TfR)), (2) insulin transporters (e.g., insulin receptor (IR)), and (3) lipid transporters (e.g., low-density lipoprotein (LDL) and LRP1), all of which have different capacities to channel ligands into the brain.

3.1. Antibodies targeting RMT receptors

"Carriers" for therapeutic delivery into the brain have been developed against all three "types" of RMT receptors. Antibodies have been developed against TfR and IR as BBB-delivery carriers for macromolecules, whereas the LRP-1 system has so far been targeted only by various peptide ligands.

The presently best studied RMT receptor is the TfR, enriched in the BBB endothelial cells (Jefferies et al., 1984; Pardridge, Eisenberg, & Yang, 1987) and important for maintaining brain iron homeostasis. However, TfR is also expressed in most other organs and cell types, including hepatocytes, a major iron storage site, reticulocytes, and enterocytes of the crypts and villi, localized in the portions of the gastrointestinal tract involved in iron absorption (Anderson, Powell, & Halliday, 1990).

The murine antibody OX26 developed against rat TfR (Jefferies et al., 1984) demonstrated the ability to cross the BBB (Friden et al., 1991; Pardridge, Buciak, & Friden, 1991) and became the foundation molecule for the "Trojan horse" hypothesis, the brain delivery of biologics across the BBB by hitching a ride on a protein that transcytoses the BBB as part of its normal function. Multiple proteins have been fused to OX26 and evaluated *in vivo* including, among others, brain-derived neurotrophic factor, epidermal growth factor, and beta-galactosidase (Pardridge, 2007a). The antibody exhibited high affinity against rat TfR, but had no cross-reactivity against mouse or human TfR, limiting its use to selected preclinical models. The original findings of efficient brain delivery of OX26-attached therapeutics became a matter of controversy, as some groups reported antibody "trapping" in brain microvessels and its limited brain penetration (Alata, Paris-Robidas, Emond, Bourasset, & Calon, 2014; Moos & Morgan,

2001). However, OX26-conjugated therapeutics demonstrated pharmacological efficacy in several animal models despite limited transcytosis (Pardridge, 2007a).

A mouse mAb against the IR which is highly expressed by BBB endothelial cells (Pardridge, Eisenberg, & Yang, 1985) was generated and characterized (Pardridge, Kang, Buciak, & Yang, 1995) showing rapid transport across an *in vitro* BBB model. This antibody was subsequently humanized (HIRMAb), shown to enter the brain of a rhesus monkey (Pardridge, 2007b) and used to create a multitude of C-terminal fusion proteins including neuroptrophins, enzymes, type II tumor necrosis factor receptor, and bispecific anti-amyloid antibodies that are summarized in Pardridge and Boadoo (2012). The species restrictive nature of this antibody (i.e., cross-reactivity with human and monkey) is unfortunate, preventing its use for screening fusion proteins in various animal models of disease. Boado, Hui, Lu, and Pardridge (2012) did not observe significant toxicity of HIRMAb fused to glial-derived growth factor in rhesus monkeys; however, the same molecule was found to produce focal pancreatic metaplasia (ADM) and cardiotoxicity without evidence of neuroprotection in Parkinsonian monkeys (Ohshima-Hosoyama et al., 2012). Nevertheless, HIRMAb conjugated to the enzyme idunorate 2-sulfatase has proceeded to clinical trials for the orphan lysosomal storage disease, mucopolysaccharoidosis Type II (Hunter's syndrome) characterized by the severe central involvement due to genetic deficiency of the enzyme.

Lipid transporters described as potential RMT receptors include the LDL (Dehouck et al., 1997) and the low-density lipoprotein receptor-related protein (LRP) family (Gabathuler, 2009). LRP-1 consists of an 85 kDa membrane bound carboxyl fragment, the β chain, and a non-covalently associated amino terminal fragment, the 515 kDa α chain (Harris-White & Frautschy, 2005). The molecule functions as a cell surface endocytic receptor that binds and internalizes molecules bound for degradation in the lysosomal system. LRP-1 interacts with more than 40 different ligands, including receptor-associated protein and aprotinin. Specific Kunitz domain peptides that have high rates of transcytosis across the BBB (Demeule, Currie, et al., 2008; Demeule, Régina, et al., 2008) were synthesized from aprotinin and are currently being evaluated in phase II clinical trials as peptide-paclitaxel conjugates for treatment of primary and metastatic brain tumors (Kurzrock et al., 2012; Régina et al., 2008; Thomas et al., 2009).

3.2. Workflows to identify new BBB-transmigrating antibodies and RMT receptors

Most RMT targets currently exploited for the delivery of large molecules across the BBB are highly and broadly expressed in tissues and are implicated in metabolically critical cellular functions creating safety risks (Couch et al., 2013; Ohshima-Hosoyama et al., 2012). To overcome these limitations, new approaches have been developed to identify and validate novel receptor–antibody pairs that undergo BBB shuttling. These approaches, in principle, utilize two intersecting workflows: (1) the first approach is a "top-down" identification of new RMT receptors from databases generated by molecular profiling of the BBB using "omics" (proteomics, genomics, etc.) approaches (Badhwar, Stanimirovic, Hamel, & Haqqani, 2014; Calabria & Shusta, 2006, 2008; Enerson & Drewes, 2006; Haqqani, Hill, Mullen, & Stanimirovic, 2011; Stutz, Zhang, & Shusta, 2014) combined with functional characterization of selected targets. Antibodies are then raised against identified targets and further characterized for their "Trojan horse" potential; (2) the second approach utilizes phenotypic *in vitro* or *in vivo* screening (panning) of antibody (and in some cases peptide) libraries, displayed in various formats including phage and yeast (Muruganandam, Tanha, Narang, & Stanimirovic, 2002; Stutz et al., 2014; Tanha, Muruganandam, & Stanimirovic, 2003; Wang, Cho, & Shusta, 2007), to select BBB transmigrating antibodies. Once the BBB-transmigrating antibodies are selected, their antigens—RMT receptors—are identified by various biochemical approaches including immunoprecipitation or cross-linking coupled with mass spectrometry-based sequencing (Wang et al., 2007). The phenotypic screening approaches have so far yielded several published single-chain variable fragments (scFv) with selective BBB binding (Jones, Stutz, Zhou, Marks, & Shusta, 2014) as well as two novel BBB-crossing single-domain antibodies that can be optimized as BBB carriers for macromolecules (Muruganandam et al., 2002).

In the latter example, a phage-displayed library of single-domain antibodies from a non-immunized (naïve) llama (camelid single-domain antibody (V_HHs)) was panned for antibody fragments that bind and internalize into primary human BBB forming BEC but do not interact with primary human lung endothelial cells. Human BEC internalizing and binding V_HHs were selected and tested for their ability to transmigrate a human BEC monolayer *in vitro* (Fig. 1; Muruganandam et al., 2002). This selection protocol (Tanha et al., 2003) yielded two candidate single-domain antibodies, FC5 (GenBank No. AF441486) and FC44 (GenBank No. AF441487) that were

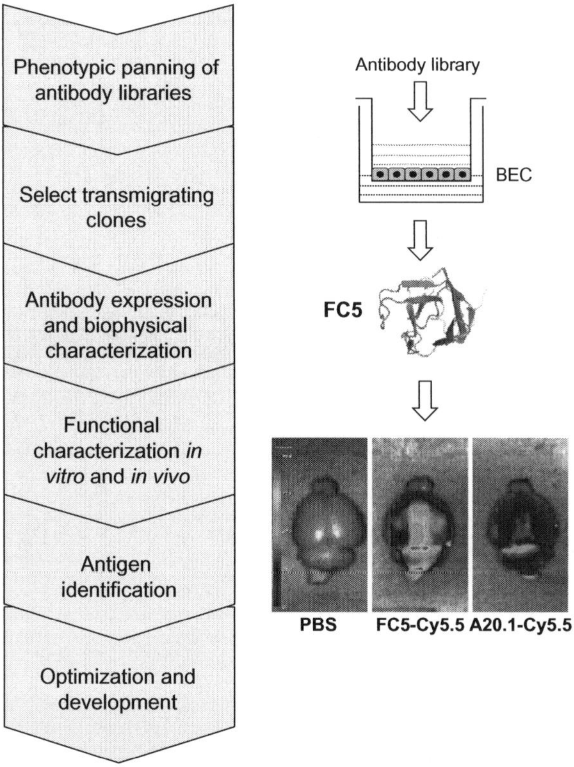

Figure 1 A generic workflow for phenotypic selection and characterization of blood–brain barrier (BBB) crossing antibodies from a phage-display library (left). A similar workflow as depicted on the right was used to isolate the blood–brain barrier-crossing single-domain antibody FC5 from a high diversity library of single-domain antibodies from a non-immunized (naïve) llama (V_HHs) (Muruganandam et al., 2002). FC5 V_HH (NMR structure shown) was characterized *in vitro* and *in vivo*, showing improved brain targeting compared to other V_HHs from the same library, as shown by optical imaging of perfused brains *ex vivo* 30 min after systemic injection of 6 mg/kg of FC5 or control V_HH A20.1 conjugated with fluorescent contrast agent Cy5.5.

subsequently expressed, characterized, and compared to other single-domain antibodies. FC5 and FC44, compared to control V_HHs A20.1 (anti-*Clostridium difficile* toxin A) and EG2 (anti-epidermal growth factor receptor) (Haqqani, Caram-Salas, et al., 2013), demonstrated a 5–100-fold enhanced rate of transport across a rat *in vitro* BBB model. FC5 and FC44 both showed elevated CSF levels in rats, compared to co-dosed control V_HHs despite their similar serum pharmacokinetics. Moreover, both FC5 and FC44 were detected in brain vessels and in brain parenchyma by immunofluorescence and mass spectrometry finger printing, respectively (Haqqani, Caram-Salas, et al., 2013). FC5 was subsequently shown to bind a glycosylated luminal BEC protein, tentatively identified as Cdc50A, that undergoes energy-dependent endocytosis via clathrin-coated vesicles (Abulrob, Sprong, Van Bergen en Henegouwen, & Stanimirovic, 2005). It is worth noting that, while both FC5 and FC44 were selected using human BEC, they showed a broad species cross-reactivity, including mouse, rat, and primate BECs, beneficial for their preclinical development.

This example demonstrates that workflows based on *phenotypic selection* of BBB-crossing molecules, using naïve or immune antibody libraries, have a potential to yield novel BBB "Trojan horses" that can subsequently be optimized through antibody engineering to generate a platform for delivery of brain-targeting biologics.

4. ENGINEERING BBB-PERMEABLE BISPECIFIC ANTIBODIES

4.1. Bispecific antibodies

A bispecific antibody (bsAb) is designed to possess two binding specificities against two different antigens in one antibody molecule. The antigenic epitopes may be on the same target molecule (biparatopic), on two different molecules on the same cell, or on different cells. The desired therapeutic effects are either potentiated or cannot be achieved by a combination of two monospecific antibodies. bsAbs have been developed primarily for oncology indications. For example, enhanced therapeutic effects can be achieved by effector-cell-recruitment using a bsAb with one binding specificity directed against a target on tumor cells and the other against antigens expressed on immune effector cells (Wickramasinghe, 2013). The prototypic example of such a bsAb is the bispecific T-cell engager antibody, consisting of two linked scFvs, one targeting CD3, found on T cells, and the other targeting a tumor-specific antigen (Aigner et al., 2013).

BBB delivery of therapeutic antibodies has recently emerged as a novel application for bsAbs (Niewoehner et al., 2014; Sumbria, Hui, Lu, Boado, & Pardridge, 2013; Yu et al., 2011). BBB-crossing bsAbs have been engineered to incorporate one specificity against a BBB RMT receptor, which drives their transmigration across the BBB, and the second specificity against a CNS therapeutic target to produce a pharmacological effect. Because brain penetration of therapeutic antibodies is minimal, their *central therapeutic effect can only be achieved in a bispecific format* (Fig. 2).

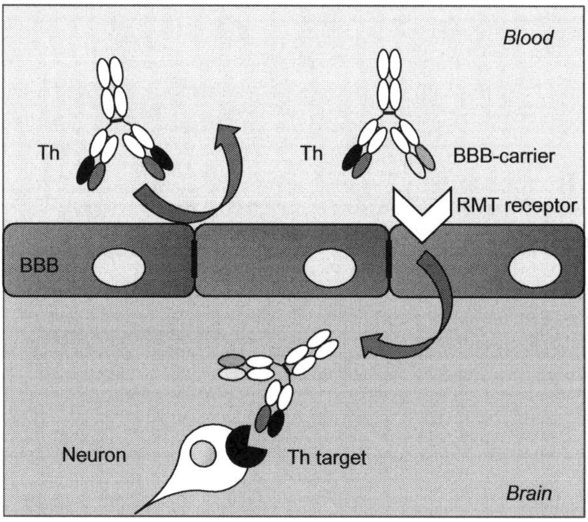

Figure 2 The concept of bispecific blood–brain barrier (BBB)-crossing antibodies. Therapeutic antibodies are unable to cross the blood–brain barrier and cannot reach their targets within the brain parenchyma. Bispecific antibodies (bsAbs) are engineered to contain two antigen specificities in the same molecule: specificity against the CNS therapeutic target (black in print version) and specificity against a BBB receptor (grey in print version) that undergoes receptor-mediated transcytosis (RMT). This BBB "shuttling" arm of the antibody facilitates brain penetration of the antibody thus enabling the therapeutic "arm" of the antibody to engage its CNS target.

Dual specificities in antibodies have been achieved by combining various antigen-recognizing domains (schematically shown in Fig. 3A) including Fabs, single-chain variable fragments (scFv) and single-domain antibodies (sdAb) as "building blocks" in various ingenious formats (Chames & Baty, 2009; Wickramasinghe, 2013). bsAbs can be "built" using different strategies and designs, including the fusion of antibody fragments to the N- or C-terminus of an immunoglobulin, or the heterodimerization of two "half-antibodies," allowing each targeting antibody fragment to be present in a mono-, bi-, or other multivalent format, with some examples being shown in Fig. 3. One such heterodimerization strategy is the "Knobs-into-holes" technology, in which knobs were created by replacing small amino side chains at the interface between CH3 domains with larger ones, whereas holes were constructed by replacing large side chains with smaller ones (Ridgway, Presta, & Carter, 1996; Shatz et al., 2013). This and other heterodimerization approaches, which use different engineered proprietary amino acid changes or point mutations in the CH3 region, result in bsAbs

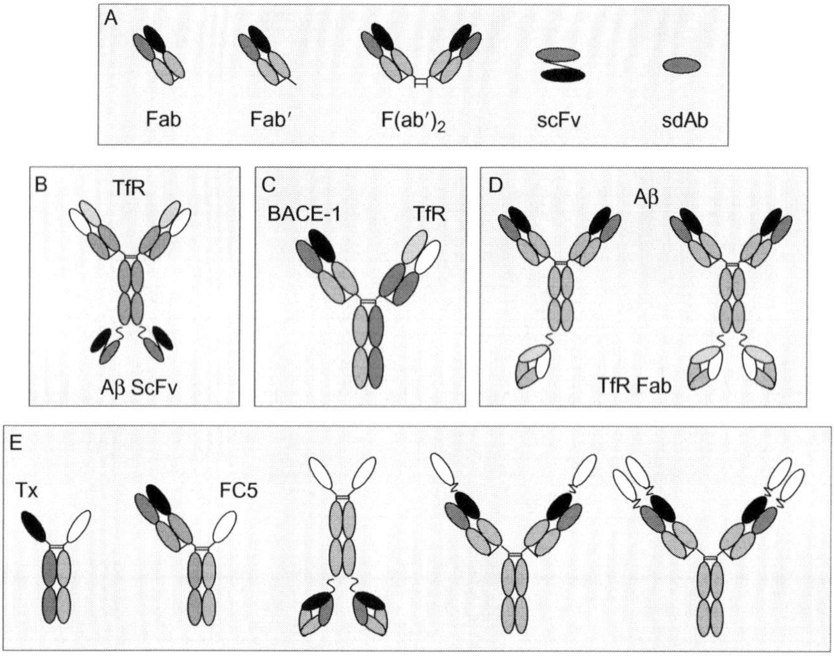

Figure 3 Building blocks and designs of blood–brain barrier (BBB)-crossing bispecific antibodies. Bispecific antibodies (bsAbs) are created using antibody fragments (A), including mono- or bivalent Fabs, single-chain fragment variable (scFv), and single-domain antibodies (sdAbs), combined in various ways. The principal strategies to generate bsAbs include heterodimerization of "half-antibodies," and fusion of various antibody fragments with IgG molecules. Different BBB-crossing antibodies have been built using these strategies. BBB-crossing bsAbs using the transferrin receptor (TfR) antibody as the BBB carrier are shown in the middle panel: (B) Aβ-recognizing scFv fused to the C-terminus of an anti-TfR antibody; (C) bsAb created by heterodimerization of a TfR antibody- and anti-BACE1 antibody-heavy chain using the knobs-into-holes strategy that allows to display each antigen-specific antibody in a monovalent format; (D) bsAb generated by fusing a TfR Fab to the C-terminus of an anti-Aβ-antibody (IgG) to have either mono- or bivalent display. The bottom panel (E) shows BBB-crossing bsAb designs using the single-domain antibody FC5 as a modular BBB carrier. FC5 is active in either mono- or bivalent display and can be used in both heterodimeric- and fusion-derived bispecific antibodies. FC5 is active only when linked to the N-terminus of the therapeutic antibody.

similar in structure to natural immunoglobulin G (IgGs), where each specificity "arm" binds the antigen in a monovalent manner; however, they are often difficult to produce effectively to homogeneity, not only because of the inherent problem of improper light-chain pairing (Spiess et al., 2013; Spreter Von Kreudenstein, Lario, & Dixit, 2014; Von Kreudenstein et al., 2013). In contrast, the fusion approach can produce easily scalable bsAbs which bind antigens in either bivalent or multivalent fashion; however, their complex designs often departs from the "natural" structure of IgGs and could carry a risk of immunogenicity.

4.2. BBB-crossing bsAbs

The principles that govern engineering of brain-targeting bsAbs are different from those typically used for building bsAbs for oncology targets. For the selection of the BBB, RMT receptor and the targeting antibody several factors should be taken into consideration, which are summarized in Table 2. The RMT target selection should be guided by the following: (a) the RMT receptor should have high expression levels in BBB endothelial cells versus other endothelial cells and peripheral tissues; (b) the RMT

Table 2 Key characteristics of RMT receptor influencing design of RMT receptor-targeting antibodies, and other key antibody engineering considerations important for the development of BBB-crossing bispecific antibodies

RMT receptor	BBB carrier arm
• Selectivity of expression in BBB endothelium versus peripheral tissues	• Specific for RMT receptor
• Transport capacity	• Affinity-optimized to facilitate transcytosis
• Receptor downregulation by cross-linking	• Antibody formats that do not trigger receptor cross-linking
• Physiological function of the receptor	• Antibody binding to receptor must not interfere with the binding of natural ligand
• Receptor abundance in peripheral tissues	• Optimization of pharmacokinetics
• Modulation of receptor in disease	• Dosing strategies
Key antibody design considerations	
Fc engineering	• Effector function
	• Circulatory pharmacokinetics versus brain clearance
Bispecific format	• Heterodimeric or fusion; mono- or multivalent "arms"
Therapeutic "arm"	• Binding affinity, epitope selectivity, etc.

receptor should have high transport capacity; (c) antibodies raised against the RMT receptor should not interfere with the biological function of the receptor; ideally, the receptor should not be involved in essential physiological processes; (d) the RMT receptor might be modulated in disease states, which would likely affect the efficiency of transport; (e) the RMT receptor might be removed from the surface and targeted for degradation upon cross-linking of the receptor; this might require engineering of antibodies that do not cause receptor cross-linking. TfR antibodies developed as BBB-carrier arms in bsAbs are illustrative of the importance of these principles.

Several bsAb formats incorporating anti-TfR antibodies have been developed and evaluated. In one example (Sumbria et al., 2013), a scFv against amyloid beta was fused to the carboxyl terminus of each heavy chain of a high-affinity chimeric mAbs against the mouse TfR, yielding a tetravalent bsAb designated cTfRMAb–scFv fusion protein (Fig. 3B). This antibody had a short circulation half-life of only 3 h, due to high-affinity binding to peripheral targets. The antibody was therefore administered by daily subcutaneous injections of 5 mg/kg for 12 consecutive weeks to presenilin-1/amyloid precursor protein (APP) double transgenic PSAPP mice resulting in ~60% reduction of amyloid plaques. Although affinities and binding properties of each antigen-specific component of this bsAb have not been described, the study suggested that this bsAb engaged central deposits of Aβ and facilitated its elimination, allegedly via FcRn-mediated efflux of the antibody–amyloid β complex.

Another bsAb-targeting TfR and BACE1, an enzyme that cleaves the pathogenic form of Aβ from the APP (Atwal et al., 2011; Ghosh, Brindisi, & Tang, 2012), was produced by Genentech using the "knobs-into-holes" heterodimerization method (Fig. 3C; Atwal et al., 2011; Yu et al., 2011). The BBB-carrier "arm" was engineered to bind TfR remote from the transferrin-binding site to minimize interference with the physiological function of the receptor, and variants having a range of monovalent binding affinities (20–600 nM) were generated. Lower affinity TfR binding variants demonstrated higher brain penetration of TfR-BACE1 bsAb, improved BACE1 inhibition and reduced Aβ accumulation which was attributed to facilitated abluminal release of the bsAb (Yu et al., 2011). In contrast, high-affinity TfR binding bsAb remained trapped within vascular compartments and did not reach the parenchymal BACE1 target. Follow-on studies revealed that high-affinity TfR binding TfR-BACE1 bispecific variants were targeted to lysosomal degradation, resulting in downregulation of TfR in BEC, while low-affinity TfR binding variants were sorted to early endosomes and directed towards abluminal externalization (Bien-Ly et al., 2014). Importantly, TfR engaged by low-affinity binding was able to effectively recycle to the membrane and was not downregulated in either BBB endothelium or neurons. Several other recently published studies (Alata et al., 2014; Moos & Morgan, 2001) using high-affinity TfR antibodies in conventional IgG formats confirmed their "trapping" within cerebral vasculature and minimal transcytosis into brain parenchyma. In addition to favoring transendothelial crossing, low-affinity TfR variants exhibited improved circulating pharmacokinetics and were not subject to the rapid "target-mediated" depletion seen with high-affinity anti-TfR antibodies (Yu et al., 2011). Improved exposure of the bsAb with a low-affinity TfR arm to the target within the brain was likely the combined result of improved circulatory pharmacokinetics, reduced TfR and TfR–bsAb complex removal and lysosomal degradation within the BEC, and facilitated abluminal antibody release from recycling endosomes.

An alternative design of TfR-targeting bsAb was developed recently by Roche (Niewoehner et al., 2014), where anti-TfR Fab fragments were fused to the C-terminus of an amyloid-β-binding IgG to obtain either mono- or bivalent formats (Fig. 3D). Despite having relatively high affinity (~20 nM), the monovalent TfR Fab fusion exhibited transcytosis across the BBB *in vitro* and *in vivo*, whereas the cross-linking of TfR by bivalent TfR Fab resulted in preferential lysosomal targeting and degradation (Bell & Ehlers, 2014; Niewoehner et al., 2014). While this study argued that it was the binding valency as opposed to the binding affinity that determined TfR–Aβ complex sorting (i.e., bivalent binding targets the receptor–antibody complex for degradation, whereas monovalent binding regardless of affinity facilitates transmigration), it is important to note that the TfR antibodies used in the two bsAb designs by Genentech (heterodimeric) and by Roche (fusion) are different antibodies that may not bind the same receptor epitope. A recent study (Sade et al., 2014) also suggested that the fate of TfR antibodies is determined not only by their affinities at extracellular pH but also correlates with their relative affinities at endosomal pH. An antibody with reduced affinity at pH 5.5 showed significant transcytosis, while an antibody with comparable affinity that did not change at pH 5.5, remained trapped within the endosomal compartments and was ultimately degraded. A schematic of intracellular trafficking and transcytosis pathways triggered by various TfR antibody formats is shown in Fig. 4.

Although the above-mentioned examples demonstrated that the TfR antibody "arm" in a bsAb can be optimized to deliver pharmacologically

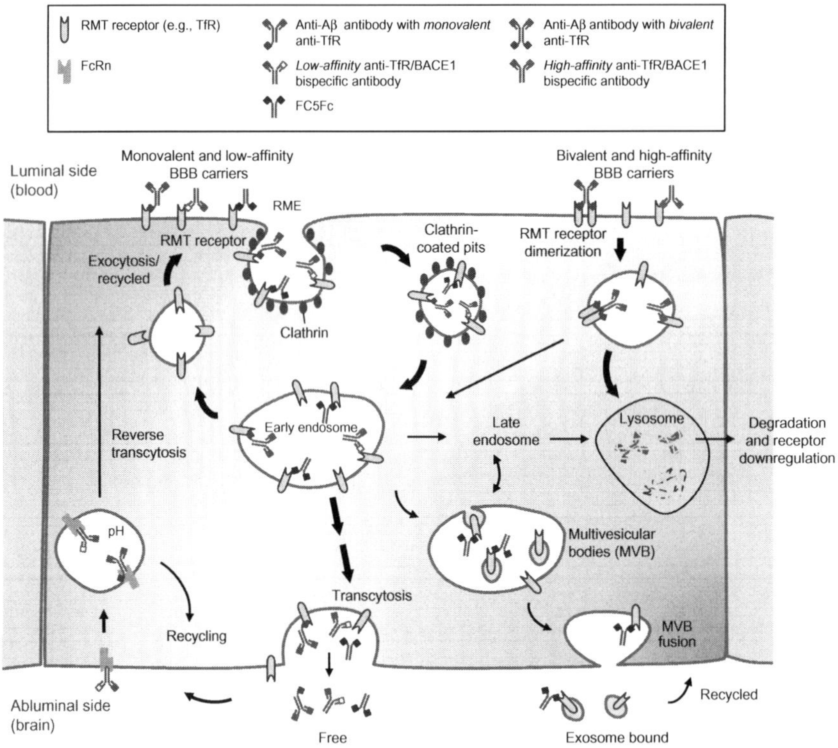

Figure 4 A schematic depiction of intracellular trafficking pathways triggered by the blood–brain barrier-crossing bispecific antibodies. Low-affinity or monovalent antibodies against transferrin receptor (TfR) as well as the single-domain antibody FC5 trigger internalization of the antibody–RMT receptor complex via clathrin-coated vesicles; shown is their preferential trafficking into early endosomes and their transcytosis/exocytosis at the abluminal endothelial membrane. The RMT receptor is then recycled back to the luminal membrane via recycling endosomes. The receptor–antibody complex can also be trafficked between early and late endosomes as well as into multivesicular bodies (MVBs); the BBB-crossing single-domain antibody FC5 externalizes as both "free" antibody and as a part of shed exosomes, likely originating from MVBs. In contrast, high-affinity and bivalent anti-TfR antibodies preferentially direct the receptor–antibody complex to the lysosomal compartment where both undergo degradation resulting in TfR downregulation. Some evidence suggests that antibodies released on the abluminal side of the BBB undergo recycling and reverse transcytosis via abluminally expressed neonatal FcRn receptor.

relevant levels of the antibody into the brain, they also underscored potential drawbacks of TfR as BBB shuttle receptor—its high expression in peripheral organs and cells affects the pharmacokinetics of targeting antibodies and creates a potential safety liability. Whereas low-affinity TfR binding of the

BBB-crossing arm ameliorated some PK and target toxicity issues (Couch et al., 2013; Yu et al., 2011) and increased the brain penetration, it also necessitated very high systemic dosing of this bsAb.

4.3. BBB-crossing bsAbs engineered with single-domain antibodies

sdAbs are small (15 kDa), monomeric antigen-binding fragments of antibodies which provide various advantages over other antibody fragments as "building blocks" for bsAbs. They occur in nature as the antigen-binding portion of heavy chain antibodies in camelid species (called V_HH) and cartilaginous fish (called V_{NAR}) or can be generated from conventional IgGs by obtaining or engineering monomeric, stable VH or VL domains (Hamers-Casterman et al., 1993; Hussack et al., 2012; Kim et al., 2014; Nuttall, 2012; Ward, Güssow, Griffiths, Jones, & Winter, 1989). sdAbs are highly stable and compact and they can access recessed epitopes in proteins, such as receptor cavities or the active sites of enzymes, which are often "hidden" from conventional IgGs and can achieve target binding affinities comparable to those of conventional antibodies (Lauwereys et al., 1998; Staus et al., 2014). These monomeric antigen-binding units do not pair with light chains, which make them excellent building blocks for heterodimerized bsAbs as they avoid difficulties of improper light-chain pairing (Hamers-Casterman et al., 1993; Saerens, Ghassabeh, & Muyldermans, 2008). Heterodimeric bsAbs can be created with one or both "arms" being sdAb, the latter being similar in structure to camelid heavy-chain antibodies (Fig. 3E). sdAbs can also be used in various mono-, bi-, or tetravalent fusions with conventional therapeutic antibodies or Fabs (Fig. 3E), generally resulting in smaller, less complex molecules, compared to those generated with scFvs or Fabs as building blocks, which tend to be biophysically well behaved and easy to produce (Holliger & Hudson, 2005). Humanization of V_HHs as well as engineering of sdAbs is well described, allowing to readily generate human(ized) sdAbs with optimal target affinity and exceptional biophysical properties (Vincke et al., 2009).

To evaluate the potential use of the camelid V_HH FC5 as a BBB carrier within bispecific CNS-targeting antibodies, monovalent and bivalent fusions (N- and C-terminus) of FC5 with human Fc were designed and evaluated *in vitro* and *in vivo* (Farrington et al., 2014). Apparent binding affinity (Kd_{app}) to rat BEC of the bivalent FC5Fc fusion was 75 nM, whereas monovalent FC5Fc binding was in the micromolar range. The analyses of apparent transmigration rates (P_{app}) across an *in vitro* BBB model, apparent CNS exposure derived from serum/CSF pharmacokinetics of systemically administered antibody constructs, and pharmacological responses elicited by chemically conjugated BBB-impermeable neuroactive peptides in Hargreaves pain model, provided the evidence of enhanced BBB transport of these large (75 kDa) antibody molecules mediated by FC5: (1) *in vitro* P_{app} values were ~200 cm/min for both mono- and bivalent N-terminal Fc fusion molecules (FC5Fc) compared to 4–8 cm/min for control V_HH A20.1Fc or EG2Fc fusions; (2) the apparent CNS exposure of the FC5Fc fusion was 30-fold higher compared to control domain antibody–Fc fusions; (3) systemic pharmacological potency of FC5Fc conjugates with neuropeptides dalargin or galanin in Hargreaves inflammatory pain model were up to 60-fold higher compared to monomeric FC5–neuropeptide conjugates. This result was attributed to the long circulatory half-life (~96 h) of FC5Fc– compared to FC5–neuropeptide conjugates; (4) various control V_HH–Fc neuropeptide conjugates showed no systemic efficacy; (5) fusion of FC5 to the C-terminus of Fc resulted in attenuated BBB-crossing capacity. In contrast to TfR-targeting BBB-carrier antibodies, both mono- and bivalent FC5Fc fusion proteins showed a similar rate of transcytosis *in vitro*, similar plasma/CSF pharmacokinetic profiles, and similar systemic potency in the pharmacodynamics model *in vivo*, despite differences in apparent binding affinity and valency (Farrington et al., 2014). These studies demonstrated that the BBB-crossing single-domain antibody FC5 can be used as a platform BBB carrier in both, heterodimerized "half-antibodies" and as the more readily scalable bi- or tetravalent fusion to conventional IgGs (Farrington et al., 2014).

Another potential advantage of V_HHs as BBB carriers is their natural resistance to extreme biophysical challenges, such as temperature and pH, as well as to protease degradation (Kim et al., 2014), often encountered in various endocytic compartments during transcytosis. Both FC5 and FC5Fc fusions are internalized into BEC via clathrin-coated vesicles, and are sorted to early endosomes. Interestingly, FC5 was also found to stimulate shedding of extracellular microvesicles (exosomes) from BEC (Haqqani, Caram-Salas, et al., 2013; Haqqani, Delaney, et al., 2013) in which both FC5 and increased levels of its putative receptor Cdc50A were detected by Western blot and targeted mass spectrometry. This study suggested that shed exosomes may be the final vesicle of the RMT pathway released from the abluminal surface carrying the receptor-antibody complex (schematically shown in Fig. 4). The RMT pathway and exosome formation share some notable similarities. As outlined in the first discovery of exosomes, an anti-TfR antibody was tracked by electron microscopy in reticulocytes

(Théry, 2011) from the surface of the cells, into clathrin-coated pits, inside early endosomes, on the surface of internal vesicles of multivesicular endosomes and finally on the released exosomes after fusion of the multivesicular endosomes with the plasma membrane (Fig. 4). RMT appears to unfold in a similar fashion and the BEC extracellular microvesicles have been shown to contain several receptors known to carry macromolecules across the BBB via RMT, including TfR, LRPs, LDLR, and IR (Haqqani, Delaney, et al., 2013).

From the described studies, it should be evident that the BBB carrier arm of CNS-targeting bsAb requires careful optimization for each RMT receptor. Important considerations in designing CNS-targeting bsAbs are discussed below in view of "lessons-learned" from TfR-BACE1 bsAb development and from our own work with FC5 as a BBB-carrier antibody.

4.4. Engineering the Fc domain of CNS-targeting antibodies

The Fc domain of an IgG, essential for the dimerization of the two antibody heavy chains into one immunoglobulin molecule, plays also an important role in conferring the long circulatory half-life to the antibody through interactions with the neonatal Fc receptor (FcRn) and can upon binding to various other Fc receptors activate immune responses, collectively referred to as "effector function."

FcRn binding: The improvement of circulatory half-life of FC5 by its fusion to an FcRn-binding Fc domain (from 20 min to 96 h) has been shown to dramatically improve brain exposure and pharmacological potency (>60-fold) of biconjugated centrally active peptides (Farrington et al., 2014; Haqqani, Caram-Salas, et al., 2013). The Fc domain of antibodies can be engineered to increase binding affinity to the endothelial FcRn at pH 6.0, but not at neutral pH, to obtain a very long (weeks) circulatory half-life (Chen & Balthasar, 2012; Olafsen, 2012). This is desirable for treating chronic conditions since it increases target exposure, reduces frequency of antibody dosing and improves patient compliance.

However, FcRn has been proposed to also actively remove antibodies from the CNS via polarized reverse transcytosis across BEC (Cooper et al., 2013; Schlachetzki, Zhu, & Pardridge, 2002; Fig. 4). This creates an important dilemma for developers of CNS-targeting antibodies since increasing antibody half-life by reengineering high-affinity FcRn binding to improve target exposure could lead to undesired faster elimination of antibodies delivered across the BBB.

In an early study by Pardridge and colleagues (Schlachetzki et al., 2002), the estimated kinetics of the FcRn-mediated radioactively labeled antibody efflux from the brain was fast, resulting in a brain residence half-life of ~45 min. In a more recent study, investigating brain elimination of antibodies with different FcRn affinities after intracranial injection, a high-affinity-FcRn binding variant cleared faster compared to the low-affinity FcRn-binding variant (Cooper et al., 2013). The significance of this FcRn-mediated antibody efflux in overall brain exposure of antibodies has been challenged recently by studies comparing blood/brain area under the curve (AUC) of IgGs in various FcRn knock-out strains (Abuqayyas & Balthasar, 2013; Cao, Balthasar, & Jusko, 2013). The disposition of 8C2, a murine monoclonal IgG1 antibody, showed no difference in brain–plasma AUC ratios after intravenous administration in FcRn α-chain knock-out mice, FcγRIIb knock-out mice, FcγRI/RIII knock-out mice, and C57BL/6 control mice (Abuqayyas & Balthasar, 2013). The predicted 8C2 brain efflux clearance in these experiments was ~135-fold faster than the brain uptake, which correlated with the low ratio of brain–blood exposure, indicating that neither FcRn nor FcγR are limiting factors for mAb uptake into the brain (Abuqayyas & Balthasar, 2013). It is important to note that this study used antibodies that were not "enabled" with the BBB-carrier arm and therefore have very low blood-to-brain transport rates. Although definitive studies using BBB-enabled antibodies are needed, the current literature evidence suggests that the shorter circulatory half-life of antibodies engineered to have reduced binding to FcRn would override any advantage in brain exposure gained by extending their brain residence time.

Effector function: Binding of the antibody's Fc domain to Fcγ receptors on immune cells activates these cells and can trigger antibody-dependent cell-mediated cytotoxicity and complement-dependent cytotoxicity. As the activation of the immune system is highly desired for treatment of most cancers, the effector function is often engineered in antibodies for oncology indications to enhance their therapeutic efficacy (Strohl, 2009; Withoff, Helfrich, de Leij, & Molema, 2001). In contrast, Fc domain engineering of CNS-targeting antibodies aims to reduce immune system recruitment and adverse reactions to often abundant and broadly distributed RMT targets. Therefore, introducing specific mutations in the Fc region of the antibody that either remove or attenuate its effector function is an essential safety consideration (Vafa et al., 2014).

The importance of reengineering the Fc effector function has been convincingly demonstrated for the TfR-BACE1 bsAb (Couch et al., 2013).

Acute clinical side effects have been observed in mice when treated with the effector-competent high-affinity, bivalent TfR antibody. The most prominent sign of "on-target" toxicity was acute lysis of TfR-rich reticulocytes. This immunotoxicity was subsequently ameliorated by reengineering the Fc region to reduce effector function and by creating monovalent and low-affinity TfR binding bsAbs (Couch et al., 2013).

4.5. The therapeutic arm of brain-targeting bsAbs

Detailed discussion on engineering desired properties of the therapeutic "arm" in a CNS-targeting bsAb is beyond the scope of this chapter since this is highly target-specific. The CNS is a vast source of therapeutic targets, including a myriad of neuronal and glial receptors, voltage- and ligand-gated ion channels, neurotransmitter transporters, secreted neuromodulators, misfolded proteins and enzymes involved in their production or degradation, among many others, that are amenable for antibody targeting. It is important to emphasize that both the nature of the therapeutic target and characteristics of the targeting antibody (e.g., neutralizing, receptor modulating, agonist or antagonist, etc.) developed against that target determine the optimal "on-target" levels required to produce a desired pharmacological response. Given that small amounts of antibodies, estimated at $\sim$ 0.01% of an injected dose (St-Amour et al., 2013), penetrate the BBB via a non-specific mechanisms, the argument has also been made that a very high-affinity antibody against CNS target may exert pharmacological effect even without specific engineering to enhance BBB-crossing. This would require a very high systemic dosing, as well as a careful choice of targets that are highly selective for CNS and virtually absent in the periphery. Besides such targets being very rare, clinical experience so far argues for the necessity to augment brain delivery of biologics. Preclinically evaluated antibody Trojan horses, including various engineered TfR antibodies, the IR antibody and FC5, increase brain delivery of antibodies to roughly 1–2.5% of the injected dose, levels close to those achieved in the brain by several efficacious small molecule CNS drugs (Garberg et al., 2005). Although a clinical proof of mechanism for BBB Trojan horse antibodies is still lacking, it is reasonable to argue that the progress in understanding mechanisms of RMT, as well as the sophistication achieved in selection and fine tuning of various carrier and therapeutic antibody properties will accelerate the translation of BBB-enabled bsAbs into clinical realm. Improved cross-BBB transport would also significantly lower the dosing of therapeutic antibodies with neurospecific targets, since the efficiency of parenchymal delivery would be much higher.

5. ANALYTICAL CHALLENGES AND PHARMACOKINETICS/PHARMACODYNAMICS MODELS

The development of systemically effective biologics targeting the CNS is an emerging field and requires reevaluation of widely accepted pharmacological principles and models developed for small molecules. The primary challenge posed by the unique nature of biologics is their accurate quantification in various systemic and CNS compartments. A typical approach used in the field is radioactive labeling of antibodies followed by "trace dosing" and quantitation of the radioactivity partition in systemic and CNS compartments. This often involves the removal of the brain vasculature-"trapped" antibodies by microvessel depletion (Iqbal, Abulrob, & Stanimirovic, 2011). The differences in estimated BBB transport rates using trace versus therapeutic dosing of antibodies have been clearly demonstrated with the TfR-BACE1 antibody (Yu et al., 2011). To avoid drawbacks of antibody labeling with tracers, highly sensitive ELISAs and targeted mass spectrometry methods have been developed to quantify non-labeled antibodies in body fluids and tissues. For example, the recently described nanoLC–MS/MS single reaction monitoring coupled with isotopically labeled internal standards (ILIS) (Haqqani, Caram-Salas, et al., 2013; Haqqani, Kelly, & Stanimirovic, 2008) achieves exquisite sensitivity (limit of detection at attomolar levels) of antibody quantification in miniscule (less than 5 μl) samples from complex body fluids including blood, CSF, and ECF, as well as small tissue samples procured by the laser-capture microdissection microscopy. This analytical technique can be multiplexed to allow quantification of several antibodies in the same sample and is exceptionally suited for PK analyses of coinjected antibodies (internal positive and negative controls) as well as for simultaneous quantification of the therapeutic antibody and its target engagement biomarkers (Haqqani, Caram-Salas, et al., 2013). With the development of highly sensitive analytical techniques and availability of BBB-enabled bsAbs, the field of therapeutic CNS-targeted antibodies is now in a position to begin building appropriate pharmacokinetics/pharmacodynamics (PK/PD) models to guide predictive translation to clinical studies. Basic elements of such a model depicting various CNS compartments and exchange routes as well as rate-limiting "fluxes" for macromolecules among these compartments are shown in Fig. 5.

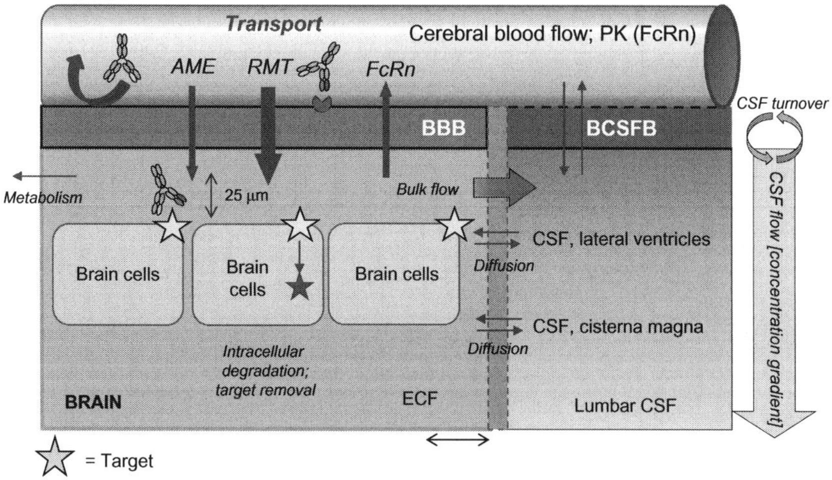

Figure 5 Principles that govern PK/PD models for systemically administered blood–brain barrier (BBB)-enabled antibodies. Antibodies can engage brain targets if engineered with BBB carriers that utilize an RMT receptor (e.g., bispecific antibodies or antibody-carrier conjugates). The abundance, capacity, and rate of recycling of the RMT receptor are rate-limiting parameters in modeling antibody influx. The BBB efflux pumps, typically a major component of brain distribution models for synthetic molecules, are not involved in antibody trafficking across the BBB; however, a potential role of reverse transcytosis via FcRn in antibody efflux from the brain should be considered, although rates and significance of this elimination route have been disputed. The following additional considerations should be built into PK/PD models for CNS-targeting antibodies: (1) very limited diffusion distances due to their size and interactions with the extracellular matrix; (2) target-mediated disposition through interaction with parenchymal receptors; (3) the role of bulk flow in antibody elimination into perivascular spaces and ventricular cerebrospinal fluid. It is important to note that the blood-cerebrospinal fluid (BCSF) barrier, though often permissive to small molecules, is highly restrictive for antibodies.

5.1. Surrogate measures of brain delivery of antibodies

Ideally, evaluation of brain target exposure by BBB-enabled antibodies *in vivo* should be based on their quantitation in the CNS interstitial space (Fig. 5) sampled by intracerebral microdialysis. However, neither microdialysis nor target occupancy studies using position emission tomography (PET) or single-photon emission tomography are well suited for antibodies due to their size and long half-life, respectively.

CSF levels of drugs are often used to extrapolate brain interstitial fluid (at target) levels (De Lange & Danhof, 2002; Lin, 2008; Pepinsky et al., 2011; Shen, Artru, & Adkison, 2004). Approximately, two-thirds of the CSF is produced by the choroid plexus as an ultrafiltrate with low concentrations of most blood-derived proteins and drugs (Johanson, Stopa, & McMillan, 2011), while only one-third of the CSF originates from the extracellular space of the brain and spinal cord (Johanson et al., 2011). The BCSFB (i.e., apical tight junctions of the choroid plexus epithelium) is highly restrictive for macromolecules. The steady state serum/CSF albumin ratio is about 0.005 and the serum/CSF IgG ratio is about 0.0027 (Johanson et al., 2011; Strazielle & Ghersi-Egea, 2013). No diffusional barrier exists between the interstitial space of the nervous tissue and the CSF due to the fenestrated nature of the lining ependima and even large molecules can exchange between the interstitial space of the nervous tissue and CSF by diffusion. It is important to note that the diffusion of antibodies within neuropil is highly restricted due to the tortuosity of the extracellular space, and antibody binding to both target and extracellular matrix heparin sulfate proteoglycans (Wolak & Thorne, 2013). A continuous flow within the extracellular space of the brain and spinal cord toward the CSF space (Abbott, 2004; Iliff et al., 2012; Szentistványi, Patlak, Ellis, & Cserr, 1984) prevents the establishment of equal drug concentrations in the CSF space and extracellular fluid of the brain by diffusion (CSF sink). The elimination of free antibody from the ECS into CSF occurs mostly via a bulk flow of interstitial fluid (ISF). One of the hallmarks of bulk flow, compared to simple diffusion, is the independence of solute movement from molecular size (Wolak & Thorne, 2013). ISF drainage rates for albumin estimated for various brain regions range between 0.18 and 0.29 μl g brain^{-1} min^{-1} and flow of ISF into bulk CSF sampled from the cisterna magna accounted for 60–75% of efflux from midbrain but only 10–15% of efflux from caudate nucleus or internal capsule (Cserr, Cooper, Suri, & Patlak, 1981; Szentistványi et al., 1984). The other potential drainage routes of macromolecules delivered across the BBB into ISF are perivascular spaces (Iliff et al., 2012) and deep cervical lymph nodes (Szentistványi et al., 1984).

With these elimination rates in mind, it is possible to design a predictive model that estimates ISF ("at target") levels of BBB-delivered antibodies from serial blood and CSF sampling from a cannulated cisterna magna. Using this approach, we have recently described the AUC_{CSF}/AUC_{serum} ratio as a surrogate measure of apparent CNS exposure of coinjected BBB-crossing FC5Fc and control A20.1Fc using MRM-ILIS analytical quantification (Farrington et al., 2014). This paired analysis of coinjected molecules with essentially the same serum PK and molecular weight, allowed us to control for choroid plexus filtration rates contributing to CSF levels of antibodies in the same animal and to demonstrate up to

40-fold increases in apparent CNS exposure achieved with the BBB-enabled FC5Fc compared to the control A20.1Fc.

5.2. Surrogate measures of CNS target engagement

To complement true or surrogate measures of "at-target" levels of CNS therapeutic antibodies, PK–PD models require quantitative and correlative dose–response measures of desired target engagement. The excellent example of incorporating PK–PD evaluation in bsAb development is the TfR-BACE1 antibody, where brain BACE1 enzyme inhibition was used as a direct "target engagement" correlate for various bsAb designs (Yu et al., 2011). However, the therapeutic antibody does not always have an obvious "target engagement" read-out. "Typical" CNS targets that have well validated and measurable electrophysiological or behavioral consequences, such as ion channels or GPCRs are "difficult" targets for antibody development. The majority of CNS targets currently pursued for antibody development are either misfolded proteins, such are β-amyloid or α-synuclein or proteins secreted into the brain extracellular milieu that are implicated in chronic pathophysiology or long-term regenerative processes. Evaluation of improved efficacy of such molecules when engineered for increased BBB delivery requires preclinical "disease models," often transgenic in nature, lengthy treatments, and complex outcome measures that are difficult to interpret and translate. Due to species selectivity of antibodies, the use of humanized models (Proetzel & Roopenian, 2014) or "surrogate" murine-specific antibodies is often required. In these cases, the use of surrogate PD read outs that enable direct dose–response correlation with at-target therapeutic antibody levels are important for building predictive scale-up models. Typically, such read outs for small molecules can be achieved by PET imaging studies of CNS receptor occupancy. Given difficulties in applying PET imaging in evaluation of CNS-targeting antibodies, an alternative approach is the coupling of the BBB-enabled bsAb to a surrogate molecule that acts on a central target and triggers a quantifiable response which can be benchmarked against a standard. This read-out molecule could be either fused or chemically conjugated to a bsAb creating a trispecific molecule (i.e., BBB carrier, therapeutic, and secondary read-out target specificity). Examples of such read-out molecules are various BBB impenetrable neuropeptides, notably analgesic peptides acting on well-characterized opioid receptors. We have used this surrogate PD read-out approach (Farrington et al., 2014) to establish a correlation between serum/CSF pharmacokinetics with the central mu receptor engagement using the opioid peptide Dalargin chemically conjugated to FC5Fc- or FC5-therapeutic IgG bsAbs. The receptor engagement after various dosing paradigms could only be achieved with FC5-enabled bsAbs and was measured by suppression of thermal hyperalgesia in an inflammatory pain model (Farrington et al., 2014). These surrogate PD approaches enabled evaluation of BBB delivery and the establishment of a PK–PD relationship of variously designed bsAbs, without lengthy efficacy studies in animal disease models that have poor predictive value.

6. CONCLUSION

Despite setbacks, clinical trial failures and many barriers, not the least of which is the BBB, the development of antibody therapeutics for CNS indications is forging forward. The appetite to break into CNS markets with more efficacious therapeutics that have better success rates and safety profiles is high, despite the risks. The excitement generated from initial preclinical successes of BBB-enabled bsAbs is aided by rapid advancements in antibody engineering. For the first time, the field has on its disposal a pipeline of improved BBB carriers that can be used as building blocks for designing novel CNS-targeting biologics. The focus on understanding mechanistic aspects of RMT will provide further foundation for optimizing BBB carriers and BBB-enabled bsAbs. With accompanying advances in analytical techniques and PD assessment, novel, predictive, and scalable PK–PD models for CNS-targeting antibodies can be developed to ensure clinical translation. Many challenges remain—the most important being to demonstrate that BBB Trojan horses work in humans. BBB-enabled bsAbs carry a double risk of failure in clinical development—that of BBB carrier failure and that of therapeutic failure. Therefore, it will be important to design clinical studies and surrogate biomarker assays that dissociate two proofs of concepts. Early demonstration of successful delivery (i.e., that the BBB carrier works) in phase I would catalyze further development of improved CNS-targeting antibodies increasing chances of their eventual success.

CONFLICT OF INTEREST

The authors have no conflict of interest to declare.

REFERENCES

Abbott, N. J. (2004). Evidence for bulk flow of brain interstitial fluid: Significance for physiology and pathology. *Neurochemistry International*, *45*, 545–552.

Abbott, N. J., Patabendige, A. A. K., Dolman, D. E. M., Yusof, S. R., & Begley, D. J. (2010). Structure and function of the blood-brain barrier. *Neurobiology of Disease*, *37*, 13–25.

Abulrob, A., Sprong, H., Van Bergen en Henegouwen, P., & Stanimirovic, D. (2005). The blood-brain barrier transmigrating single domain antibody: Mechanisms of transport and antigenic epitopes in human brain endothelial cells. *Journal of Neurochemistry*, *95*, 1201–1214.

Abuqayyas, L., & Balthasar, J. P. (2013). Investigation of the role of FcγR and FcRn in mAb distribution to the brain. *Molecular Pharmaceutics*, *10*, 1505–1513.

Aigner, M., Feulner, J., Schaffer, S., Kischel, R., Kufer, P., Schneider, K., et al. (2013). T lymphocytes can be effectively recruited for ex vivo and in vivo lysis of AML blasts by a novel CD33/CD3-bispecific BiTE antibody construct. *Leukemia*, *27*, 1107–1115.

Alata, W., Paris-Robidas, S., Emond, V., Bourasset, F., & Calon, F. (2014). Brain uptake of a fluorescent vector targeting the transferrin receptor: A novel application of in situ brain perfusion. *Molecular Pharmaceutics*, *11*, 243–253.

Anderson, G. J., Powell, L. W., & Halliday, J. W. (1990). Transferrin receptor distribution and regulation in the rat small intestine. Effect of iron stores and erythropoiesis. *Gastroenterology*, *98*, 576–585.

Atwal, J. K., Chen, Y., Chiu, C., Mortensen, D. L., Meilandt, W. J., Liu, Y., et al. (2011). A therapeutic antibody targeting BACE1 inhibits amyloid-B production in vivo. *Science Translational Medicine*, *3*, 84ra43.

Badhwar, A., Stanimirovic, D. B., Hamel, E., & Haqqani, A. S. (2014). The proteome of mouse cerebral arteries. *Journal of Cerebral Blood Flow & Metabolism*, *34*, 1033–1046.

Bell, R. D., & Ehlers, M. D. (2014). Breaching the blood-brain barrier for drug delivery. *Neuron*, *81*, 1–3.

Bien, C. G., Vincent, A., Barnett, M. H., Becker, A. J., Blümcke, I., Graus, F., et al. (2012). Immunopathology of autoantibody-associated encephalitides: Clues for pathogenesis. *Brain*, *135*, 1622–1638.

Bien-Ly, N., Yu, Y. J., Bumbaca, D., Elstrott, J., Boswell, C. A., Zhang, Y., et al. (2014). Transferrin receptor (TfR) trafficking determines brain uptake of TfR antibody affinity variants. *The Journal of Experimental Medicine*, *211*, 233–244.

Boado, R., Hui, E., Lu, J., & Pardridge, W. (2012). IgG-enzyme fusion protein: Pharmacokinetics and anti-drug antibody response in rhesus monkeys. *Bioconjugate Chemistry*, *1*, 97–104.

Braen, A. P. J. M., Perron, J., Tellier, P., Catala, A. R., Kolaitis, G., & Geng, W. (2010). A 4-week intrathecal toxicity and pharmacokinetic study with Trastuzumab in cynomolgus monkeys. *International Journal of Toxicology*, *29*, 259–267.

Brüggemann, M., Caskey, H. M., Teale, C., Waldmann, H., Williams, G. T., Surani, M. A., et al. (1989). A repertoire of monoclonal antibodies with human heavy chains from transgenic mice. *Proceedings of the National Academy of Sciences of the United States of America*, *86*, 6709–6713.

Calabria, A. R., & Shusta, E. V. (2006). Blood-brain barrier genomics and proteomics: Elucidating phenotype, identifying disease targets and enabling brain drug delivery. *Drug Discovery Today*, *11*, 792–799.

Calabria, A. R., & Shusta, E. V. (2008). A genomic comparison of in vivo and in vitro brain microvascular endothelial cells. *Journal of Cerebral Blood Flow & Metabolism*, *28*, 135–148.

Cao, Y., Balthasar, J. P., & Jusko, W. J. (2013). Second-generation minimal physiologically-based pharmacokinetic model for monoclonal antibodies. *Journal of Pharmacokinetics and Pharmacodynamics*, *40*, 597–607.

Chames, P., & Baty, D. (2009). Bispecific antibodies for cancer therapy: The light at the end of the tunnel? *MAbs*, *1*, 539–547.
Chen, Y., & Balthasar, J. P. (2012). Evaluation of a catenary PBPK model for predicting the in vivo disposition of mAbs engineered for high-affinity binding to FcRn. *The AAPS Journal*, *14*, 850–859.
Cooper, P. R., Ciambrone, G. J., Kliwinski, C. M., Maze, E., Johnson, L., Li, Q., et al. (2013). Efflux of monoclonal antibodies from rat brain by neonatal Fc receptor, FcRn. *Brain Research*, *1534*, 13–21.
Couch, J. A., Yu, Y. J., Zhang, Y., Tarrant, J. M., Fuji, R. N., Meilandt, W. J., et al. (2013). Addressing safety liabilities of TfR bispecific antibodies that cross the blood-brain barrier. *Science Translational Medicine*, *5*, 1–12, 183ra57.
Cserr, H. F., Cooper, D. N., Suri, P. K., & Patlak, C. S. (1981). Efflux of radiolabeled polyethylene glycols and albumin from rat brain. *The American Journal of Physiology*, *240*, F319–F328.
Dalmau, J., Lancaster, E., Martinez-Hernandez, E., Rosenfeld, M. R., & Balice-Gordon, R. (2011). Clinical experience and laboratory investigations in patients with anti-NMDAR encephalitis. *The Lancet Neurology*, *10*, 63–74.
Darnell, R. B., & Posner, J. B. (2003). Paraneoplastic syndromes involving the nervous system. *The New England Journal of Medicine*, *349*, 1543–1554.
De Lange, E. C. M., & Danhof, M. (2002). Considerations in the use of cerebrospinal fluid pharmacokinetics to predict brain target concentrations in the clinical setting: Implications of the barriers between blood and brain. *Clinical Pharmacokinetics*, *41*, 691–703.
Dehouck, B., Fenart, L., Dehouck, M. P., Pierce, A,., Torpier, G., & Cecchelli, R. (1997). A new function for the LDL receptor: Transcytosis of LDL across the blood-brain barrier. *The Journal of Cell Biology*, *138*, 877–889.
Deloire, M. S. A., Touil, T., Brochet, B., Dousset, V., Caillé, J.-M., & Petry, K. G. (2004). Macrophage brain infiltration in experimental autoimmune encephalomyelitis is not completely compromised by suppressed T-cell invasion: In vivo magnetic resonance imaging illustration in effective anti-VLA-4 antibody treatment. *Multiple Sclerosis*, *10*, 540–548.
DeMattos, R. B., Bales, K. R., Cummins, D. J., Dodart, J. C., Paul, S. M., & Holtzman, D. M. (2001). Peripheral anti-A beta antibody alters CNS and plasma A beta clearance and decreases brain A beta burden in a mouse model of Alzheimer's disease. *Proceedings of the National Academy of Sciences of the United States of America*, *98*, 8850–8855.
Demeule, M., Currie, J.-C., Bertrand, Y., Ché, C., Nguyen, T., Régina, A., et al. (2008). Involvement of the low-density lipoprotein receptor-related protein in the transcytosis of the brain delivery vector angiopep-2. *Journal of Neurochemistry*, *106*, 1534–1544.
Demeule, M., Régina, A., Ché, C., Poirier, J., Nguyen, T., Gabathuler, R., et al. (2008). Identification and design of peptides as a new drug delivery system for the brain. *The Journal of Pharmacology and Experimental Therapeutics*, *324*, 1064–1072.
Enerson, B. E., & Drewes, L. R. (2006). The rat blood-brain barrier transcriptome. *Journal of Cerebral Blood Flow & Metabolism*, *26*, 959–973.
Farrington, G. K., Caram-Salas, N., Haqqani, A. S., Brunette, E., Eldredge, J., Pepinsky, R. B., et al. (2014). A novel platform for engineering blood-brain barrier crossing bispecific biologics. *FASEB Journal*, in press.
Friden, P. M., Walus, L. R., Musso, G. F., Taylor, M. a, Malfroy, B., & Starzyk, R. M. (1991). Anti-transferrin receptor antibody and antibody-drug conjugates cross the blood-brain barrier. *Proceedings of the National Academy of Sciences of the United States of America*, *88*, 4771–4775.
Gabathuler, R. (2009). Blood-brain barrier transport of drugs for the treatment of brain diseases. *CNS & Neurological Disorders: Drug Targets*, *8*, 195–204.

Garberg, P., Ball, M., Borg, N., Cecchelli, R., Fenart, L., Hurst, R. D., et al. (2005). In vitro models for the blood-brain barrier. *Toxicology in Vitro, 19*, 299–334.

Ghosh, A. K., Brindisi, M., & Tang, J. (2012). Developing B-secretase inhibitors for treatment of Alzheimer's disease. *Journal of Neurochemistry, 120*(Suppl.), 71–83.

Güssow, D., & Seemann, G. (1991). Humanization of monoclonal antibodies. *Methods in Enzymology, 203*, 99–121.

Hamers-Casterman, C., Atarhouch, T., Muyldermans, S., Robinson, G., Hamers, C., Songa, E. B., et al. (1993). Naturally occurring antibodies devoid of light chains. *Nature, 363*, 446–448.

Haqqani, A. S., Caram-Salas, N., Ding, W., Brunette, E., Delaney, C. E., Baumann, E., et al. (2013). Multiplexed evaluation of serum and CSF pharmacokinetics of brain-targeting single-domain antibodies using a nanoLC-SRM-ILIS method. *Molecular Pharmaceutics, 10*, 1542–1556.

Haqqani, A. S., Delaney, C. E., Tremblay, T.-L., Sodja, C., Sandhu, J. K., & Stanimirovic, D. B. (2013). Method for isolation and molecular characterization of extracellular microvesicles released from brain endothelial cells. *Fluids and Barriers of the CNS, 10*, 4.

Haqqani, A. S., Hill, J. J., Mullen, J., & Stanimirovic, D. B. (2011). Methods to study glycoproteins at the blood-brain barrier using mass spectrometry. *Methods in Molecular Biology, 686*, 337–353.

Haqqani, A. S., Kelly, J. F., & Stanimirovic, D. B. (2008). Quantitative protein profiling by mass spectrometry using label-free proteomics. *Methods in Molecular Biology, 439*, 241–256.

Harris-White, M. E., & Frautschy, S. A. (2005). Low density lipoprotein receptor-related proteins (LRPs), Alzheimer's and cognition. *Current Drug Targets CNS and Neurological Disorders, 4*, 469–480.

Henderson, S. J., Andersson, C., Narwal, R., Janson, J., Goldschmidt, T. J., Appelkvist, P., et al. (2014). Sustained peripheral depletion of amyloid-B with a novel form of neprilysin does not affect central levels of amyloid-B. *Brain, 137*, 553–564.

Holliger, P., & Hudson, P. J. (2005). Engineered antibody fragments and the rise of single domains. *Nature Biotechnology, 23*, 1126–1136.

Hughes, E. G., Peng, X., Gleichman, A. J., Lai, M., Zhou, L., Tsou, R., et al. (2010). Cellular and synaptic mechanisms of anti-NMDA receptor encephalitis. *The Journal of Neuroscience, 30*, 5866–5875.

Hussack, G., Keklikian, A., Alsughayyir, J., Hanifi-Moghaddam, P., Arbabi-Ghahroudi, M., van Faassen, H., et al. (2012). A V(L) single-domain antibody library shows a high-propensity to yield non-aggregating binders. *Protein Engineering, Design & Selection, 25*, 313–318.

Iliff, J. J., Wang, M., Liao, Y., Plogg, B. A., Peng, W., Gundersen, G. A., et al. (2012). A paravascular pathway facilitates CSF flow through the brain parenchyma and the clearance of interstitial solutes, including amyloid B. *Science Translational Medicine, 4*, 147ra111.

Iqbal, U., Abulrob, A., & Stanimirovic, D. B. (2011). Integrated platform for brain imaging and drug delivery across the blood-brain barrier. *Methods in Molecular Biology, 686*, 465–481.

Jain PharmaBiotech. (2010). *Drug delivery in central nervous system disorders: Technologies, companies and markets.*

Jefferies, W. A., Brandon, M. R., Hunt, S. V., Williams, A. F., Gatter, K. C., & Mason, D. Y. (1984). Transferrin receptor on endothelium of brain capillaries. *Nature, 312*, 162–163.

Johanson, C. E., Stopa, E. G., & McMillan, P. N. (2011). The blood-cerebrospinal fluid barrier: Structure and functional significance. *Methods in Molecular Biology, 686*, 101–131.

Jolliffe, L. K. (1993). Humanized antibodies: Enhancing therapeutic utility through antibody engineering. *International Reviews of Immunology, 10*, 241–250.

Jones, P. T., Dear, P. H., Foote, J., Neuberger, M. S., & Winter, G. (1986). Replacing the complementarity-determining regions in a human antibody with those from a mouse. *Nature*, *321*, 522–525.

Jones, A. R., & Shusta, E. V. (2007). Blood-brain barrier transport of therapeutics via receptor-mediation. *Pharmaceutical Research*, *24*, 1759–1771.

Jones, A. R., Stutz, C. C., Zhou, Y., Marks, J. D., & Shusta, E. V. (2014). Identifying blood-brain-barrier selective single-chain antibody fragments. *Biotechnology Journal*, *9*, 664–674.

Kim, D. Y., To, R., Kandalaft, H., Ding, W., van Faassen, H., Luo, Y., et al. (2014). Antibody light chain variable domains and their biophysically improved versions for human immunotherapy. *MAbs*, *6*, 219–235.

Kurzrock, R., Gabrail, N., Chandhasin, C., Moulder, S., Smith, C., Brenner, A., et al. (2012). Safety, pharmacokinetics, and activity of GRN1005, a novel conjugate of angiopep-2, a peptide facilitating brain penetration, and paclitaxel, in patients with advanced solid tumors. *Molecular Cancer Therapeutics*, *11*, 308–316.

La Merie Publishing. (2013). *Antibody technologies and attrition rates: An industry analysis*.

Lauwereys, M., Arbabi Ghahroudi, M., Desmyter, A., Kinne, J., Hölzer, W., De Genst, E., et al. (1998). Potent enzyme inhibitors derived from dromedary heavy-chain antibodies. *The EMBO Journal*, *17*, 3512–3520.

Lee, E.-C., Liang, Q., Ali, H., Bayliss, L., Beasley, A., Bloomfield-Gerdes, T., et al. (2014). Complete humanization of the mouse immunoglobulin loci enables efficient therapeutic antibody discovery. *Nature Biotechnology*, *32*, 356–363.

Levites, Y., Smithson, L. A., Price, R. W., Dakin, R. S., Yuan, B., Sierks, M. R., et al. (2006). Insights into the mechanisms of action of anti-abeta antibodies in Alzheimer's disease mouse models. *FASEB Journal*, *20*, 2576–2578.

Lin, J. H. (2008). CSF as a surrogate for assessing CNS exposure: An industrial perspective. *Current Drug Metabolism*, *9*, 46–59.

Marks, J. D., Hoogenboom, H. R., Bonnert, T. P., McCafferty, J., Griffiths, A. D., & Winter, G. (1991). By-passing immunization. Human antibodies from V-gene libraries displayed on phage. *Journal of Molecular Biology*, *222*, 581–597.

McCafferty, J., Griffiths, A. D., Winter, G., & Chiswell, D. J. (1990). Phage antibodies: Filamentous phage displaying antibody variable domains. *Nature*, *348*, 552–554.

Moos, T., & Morgan, E. H. (2001). Restricted transport of anti-transferrin receptor antibody (OX26) through the blood-brain barrier in the rat. *Journal of Neurochemistry*, *79*, 119–129.

Muruganandam, A., Tanha, J., Narang, S., & Stanimirovic, D. (2002). Selection of phage-displayed llama single-domain antibodies that transmigrate across human blood-brain barrier endothelium. *FASEB Journal*, *16*, 240–242.

Neuwelt, E. A., Bauer, B., Fahlke, C., Fricker, G., Iadecola, C., Janigro, D., et al. (2011). Engaging neuroscience to advance translational research in brain barrier biology. *Nature Reviews Neuroscience*, *12*, 169–182.

Niewoehner, J., Bohrmann, B., Collin, L., Urich, E., Sade, H., Maier, P., et al. (2014). Increased brain penetration and potency of a therapeutic antibody using a monovalent molecular shuttle. *Neuron*, *81*, 49–60.

Nuttall, S. D. (2012). Overview and discovery of IgNARs and generation of VNARs. *Methods in Molecular Biology (Clifton, N.J.)*, *911*, 27–36.

Ohshima-Hosoyama, S., Simmons, H. A., Goecks, N., Joers, V., Swanson, C. R., Bondarenko, V., et al. (2012). A monoclonal antibody-GDNF fusion protein is not neuroprotective and is associated with proliferative pancreatic lesions in Parkinsonian monkeys. *PLoS One*, 7, e39036.

Olafsen, T. (2012). Fc engineering: Serum half-life modulation through FcRn binding. *Methods in Molecular Biology*, *907*, 537–556.

Pardridge, W. M. (2002). Drug and gene delivery to the brain: The vascular route. *Neuron*, *36*, 555–558.

Pardridge, W. M. (2007a). Drug targeting to the brain. *Pharmaceutical Research, 24*, 1733–1744.
Pardridge, W. M. (2007b). Blood-brain barrier delivery. *Drug Discovery Today, 12*, 54–61.
Pardridge, W. M., & Boado, R. J. (2012). Reengineering biopharmaceuticals for targeted delivery across the blood-brain barrier. *Methods in Enzymology, 503*, 269–292.
Pardridge, W., Buciak, L., & Friden, P. M. (1991). Selective transport of an anti-transferrin through the blood-brain barrier in Vivo1 receptor antibody. *Journal of Pharmacology and Experimental Therapeutics, 259*, 66–70.
Pardridge, W. M., Eisenberg, J., & Yang, J. (1985). Human blood-brain barrier insulin receptor. *Journal of Neurochemistry, 44*, 1771–1778.
Pardridge, W. M., Eisenberg, J., & Yang, J. (1987). Human blood-brain barrier transferrin receptor. *Metabolism, 36*, 892–895.
Pardridge, W. M., Kang, Y. S., Buciak, J. L., & Yang, J. (1995). Human insulin receptor monoclonal antibody undergoes high affinity binding to human brain capillaries in vitro and rapid transcytosis through the blood-brain barrier in vivo in the primate. *Pharmaceutical Research, 12*, 807–816.
Pepinsky, R., Shao, Z., Ji, B., & Wang, Q. (2011). Exposure levels of anti-LINGO-1 Li81 antibody in the central nervous system and dose-efficacy relationships in rat spinal cord remyelination models after systemic administration. *Journal of Pharmacology and Experimental Therapeutics, 339*, 519–529.
Persson, M. A. (1993). Combinatorial libraries. *International Reviews of Immunology, 10*, 153–163.
Petit-Pedrol, M., Armangue, T., Peng, X., Bataller, L., Cellucci, T., Davis, R., et al. (2014). Encephalitis with refractory seizures, status epilepticus, and antibodies to the GABAA receptor: A case series, characterisation of the antigen, and analysis of the effects of antibodies. *Lancet Neurology, 13*, 14–16.
Proetzel, G., & Roopenian, D. C. (2014). Humanized FcRn mouse models for evaluating pharmacokinetics of human IgG antibodies. *Methods, 65*, 148–153.
Régina, A., Demeule, M., Ché, C., Lavallée, I., Poirier, J., Gabathuler, R., et al. (2008). Antitumour activity of ANG1005, a conjugate between paclitaxel and the new brain delivery vector angiopep-2. *British Journal of Pharmacology, 155*, 185–197.
Ridgway, J. B., Presta, L. G., & Carter, P. (1996). "Knobs-into-holes" engineering of antibody CH3 domains for heavy chain heterodimerization. *Protein Engineering, 9*, 617–621.
Sade, H., Baumgartner, C., Hugenmatter, A., Moessner, E., Freskgård, P.-O., & Niewoehner, J. (2014). A human blood-brain barrier transcytosis assay reveals antibody transcytosis influenced by pH-dependent receptor binding. *PLoS One, 9*, e96340.
Saerens, D., Ghassabeh, G. H., & Muyldermans, S. (2008). Single-domain antibodies as building blocks for novel therapeutics. *Current Opinion in Pharmacology, 8*, 600–608.
Sagare, A. P., Deane, R., & Zlokovic, B. V. (2012). Low-density lipoprotein receptor-related protein 1: A physiological Aβ homeostatic mechanism with multiple therapeutic opportunities. *Pharmacology & Therapeutics, 136*, 94–105.
Schlachetzki, F., Zhu, C., & Pardridge, W. M. (2002). Expression of the neonatal Fc receptor (FcRn) at the blood-brain barrier. *Journal of Neurochemistry, 81*, 203–206.
Shatz, W., Chung, S., Li, B., Marshall, B., Tejada, M., Phung, W., et al. (2013). Knobs-into-holes antibody production in mammalian cell lines reveals that asymmetric afucosylation is sufficient for full antibody-dependent cellular cytotoxicity. *MAbs, 5*, 872–881.
Shen, D. D., Artru, A. A., & Adkison, K. K. (2004). Principles and applicability of CSF sampling for the assessment of CNS drug delivery and pharmacodynamics. *Advanced Drug Delivery Reviews, 56*, 1825–1857.
Smith, M. W., & Gumbleton, M. (2006). Endocytosis at the blood-brain barrier: From basic understanding to drug delivery strategies. *Journal of Drug Targeting, 14*, 191–214.
Spencer, B. J., & Verma, I. M. (2007). Targeted delivery of proteins across the blood-brain barrier. *Proceedings of the National Academy of Sciences of the United States of America, 104*, 7594–7599.

Spiess, C., Merchant, M., Huang, A., Zheng, Z., Yang, N.-Y., Peng, J., et al. (2013). Bispecific antibodies with natural architecture produced by co-culture of bacteria expressing two distinct half-antibodies. *Nature Biotechnology, 31*, 753–758.

Spreter Von Kreudenstein, T., Lario, P. I., & Dixit, S. B. (2014). Protein engineering and the use of molecular modeling and simulation: The case of heterodimeric Fc engineering. *Methods, 65*, 77–94.

St-Amour, I., Paré, I., Alata, W., Coulombe, K., Ringuette-Goulet, C., Drouin-Ouellet, J., et al. (2013). Brain bioavailability of human intravenous immunoglobulin and its transport through the murine blood-brain barrier. *Journal of Cerebral Blood Flow & Metabolism, 33*, 1983–1992.

Stanimirovic, D. B., & Friedman, A. (2012). Pathophysiology of the neurovascular unit: Disease cause or consequence? *Journal of Cerebral Blood Flow & Metabolism, 32*, 1207–1221.

Staus, D. P., Wingler, L. M., Strachan, R. T., Rasmussen, S. G. F., Pardon, E., Ahn, S., et al. (2014). Regulation of β2-adrenergic receptor function by conformationally selective single-domain intrabodies. *Molecular Pharmacology, 85*, 472–481.

Strazielle, N., & Ghersi-Egea, J. F. (2013). Physiology of blood-brain interfaces in relation to brain disposition of small compounds and macromolecules. *Molecular Pharmaceutics, 10*, 1473–1491.

Strohl, W. R. (2009). Optimization of Fc-mediated effector functions of monoclonal antibodies. *Current Opinion in Biotechnology, 20*, 685–691.

Stutz, C. C., Zhang, X., & Shusta, E. V. (2014). Combinatorial approaches for the identification of brain drug delivery targets. *Current Pharmaceutical Design, 20*, 1564–1576.

Sumbria, R. K., Hui, E. K.-W., Lu, J. Z., Boado, R. J., & Pardridge, W. M. (2013). Disaggregation of amyloid plaque in brain of Alzheimer's disease transgenic mice with daily subcutaneous administration of a tetravalent bispecific antibody that targets the transferrin receptor and the abeta amyloid peptide. *Molecular Pharmaceutics, 10*, 3507–3513.

Szentistványi, I., Patlak, C. S., Ellis, R. A., & Cserr, H. F. (1984). Drainage of interstitial fluid from different regions of rat brain. *The American Journal of Physiology, 246*, F835–F844.

Tanha, J., Muruganandam, A., & Stanimirovic, D. (2003). Phage display technology for identifying specific antigens on brain endothelial cells. *Methods in Molecular Medicine, 89*, 435–449.

Théry, C. (2011). Exosomes: Secreted vesicles and intercellular communications. *F1000 Biology Reports, 3*, 15.

Thomas, F. C., Taskar, K., Rudraraju, V., Goda, S., Thorsheim, H. R., Gaasch, J. A., et al. (2009). Uptake of ANG1005, a novel paclitaxel derivative, through the blood-brain barrier into brain and experimental brain metastases of breast cancer. *Pharmaceutical Research, 26*, 2486–2494.

Vafa, O., Gilliland, G. L., Brezski, R. J., Strake, B., Wilkinson, T., Lacy, E. R., et al. (2014). An engineered Fc variant of an IgG eliminates all immune effector functions via structural perturbations. *Methods, 65*, 114–126.

Vincke, C., Loris, R., Saerens, D., Martinez-Rodriguez, S., Muyldermans, S., & Conrath, K. (2009). General strategy to humanize a camelid single-domain antibody and identification of a universal humanized nanobody scaffold. *The Journal of Biological Chemistry, 284*, 3273–3284.

Von Kreudenstein, T. S., Escobar-Carbrera, E., Lario, P. I., D'Angelo, I., Brault, K., Kelly, J., et al. (2013). Improving biophysical properties of a bispecific antibody scaffold to aid developability: Quality by molecular design. *MAbs, 5*, 646–654.

Wang, X. X., Cho, Y. K., & Shusta, E. V. (2007). Mining a yeast library for brain endothelial cell-binding antibodies. *Nature Methods, 4*, 143–145.

Ward, E. S., Güssow, D., Griffiths, A. D., Jones, P. T., & Winter, G. (1989). Binding activities of a repertoire of single immunoglobulin variable domains secreted from Escherichia coli. *Nature, 341*, 544–546.

Wickramasinghe, D. (2013). Tumor and T cell engagement by BiTE. *Discovery Medicine, 16*, 149–152.
Withoff, S., Helfrich, W., de Leij, L. F., & Molema, G. (2001). Bi-specific antibody therapy for the treatment of cancer. *Current Opinion in Molecular Therapeutics, 3*, 53–62.
Wolak, D. J., & Thorne, R. G. (2013). Diffusion of macromolecules in the brain: Implications for drug delivery. *Molecular Pharmaceutics, 10*, 1492–1504.
Yu, Y. J., Zhang, Y., Kenrick, M., Hoyte, K., Luk, W., Lu, Y., et al. (2011). Boosting brain uptake of a therapeutic antibody by reducing its affinity for a transcytosis target. *Science Translational Medicine, 3*, 84ra44.
Zlokovic, B. V. (2011). Neurovascular pathways to neurodegeneration in Alzheimer's disease and other disorders. *Nature Reviews. Neuroscience, 12*, 723–738.

CHAPTER ELEVEN

Pharmacological Significance of Prostaglandin E_2 and D_2 Transport at the Brain Barriers

Masanori Tachikawa*, Ken-ichi Hosoya†, Tetsuya Terasaki*,[1]
*Division of Membrane Transport and Drug Targeting, Graduate School of Pharmaceutical Sciences, Tohoku University, Sendai, Japan
†Department of Pharmaceutics, Graduate School of Pharmaceutical Sciences, University of Toyama, Toyama, Japan
[1]Corresponding author: e-mail address: terasaki.tetsuya@m.tohoku.ac.jp

Contents

Abstract

Prostaglandin (PG) E_2 and PGD_2, which are biosynthesized from arachidonic acid generated by enzymatic cleavage of membrane phospholipid in response to various stimuli, play key roles in multiple brain pathophysiological processes, including modulation of synaptic plasticity, neuroinflammation, and sleep promotion. Concentrations of PGE_2 and PGD_2 in brain interstitial fluid (ISF) and cerebrospinal fluid (CSF) are maintained at appropriate levels for normal brain function by regulatory systems. The blood–brain barrier (BBB) and the blood–CSF barrier (BCSFB) possess ISF/CSF-to-blood efflux transport systems that are the primary cerebral clearance pathways for PGE_2 and PGD_2. However, regulatory dysfunction at the brain barriers may seriously affect brain function. In a mouse inflammation model, significant reduction of PGE_2 efflux transport at the BBB has been observed. Several kinds of cephalosporin antibiotics and nonsteroidal anti-inflammatory drugs inhibit the BBB- and BCSFB-mediated efflux transport of PGE_2

Advances in Pharmacology, Volume 71
ISSN 1054-3589
http://dx.doi.org/10.1016/bs.apha.2014.06.006

and PGD_2. Especially, drugs that inhibit multidrug resistance-associated protein 4 (MRP4)-mediated PGE_2 transport are capable of reducing PGE_2 efflux at the BBB. Thus, it might be important in the treatment of inflammatory and infectious diseases to use drugs that do not inhibit clearance of PGE_2 at the brain barriers, in order to avoid unexpected adverse CNS effects. Further, considering that PGD_2 in CSF is a natural sleep-promoting factor, changes in the activity of the PGD_2 efflux transport system at the BCSFB may modify the PGD_2 level in CSF, thus affecting physiological sleep. These findings indicate that the efflux transport systems at the brain barriers play key roles in the pathophysiology and pharmacology of PGE_2 and PGD_2.

ABBREVIATIONS

ABC ATP-binding cassette
BBB blood–brain barrier
BEI brain efflux index
CNS central nervous system
COX cyclooxygenase
BCSFB blood–CSF barrier
CSF cerebrospinal fluid
DP D-type prostanoid
EP E-type prostanoid
IL-1 interleukin-1
ISF interstitial fluid
LPS lipopolysaccharide
MRP/Mrp multidrug resistance-associated protein
NSAIDs nonsteroidal anti-inflammatory drugs
NVU neurovascular unit
OAT/Oat organic anion transporter
OATP/Oatp organic anion transporting polypeptide
OCT organic cation transporter
PG prostaglandin
PGE_2 prostaglandin E_2
Pgt prostaglandin transporter
mPGES microsomal prostaglandin E synthase
SLC/Slc solute carrier

1. INTRODUCTION

Prostaglandins (PGs), which are biosynthesized from arachidonic acid generated by enzymatic cleavage of membrane phospholipid in response to various stimuli (Fig. 1), have multiple pharmacological impacts in the body. In the central nervous system (CNS), prostaglandin E_2 (PGE_2) and PGD_2 play key roles in modulating the functional activities of neurons

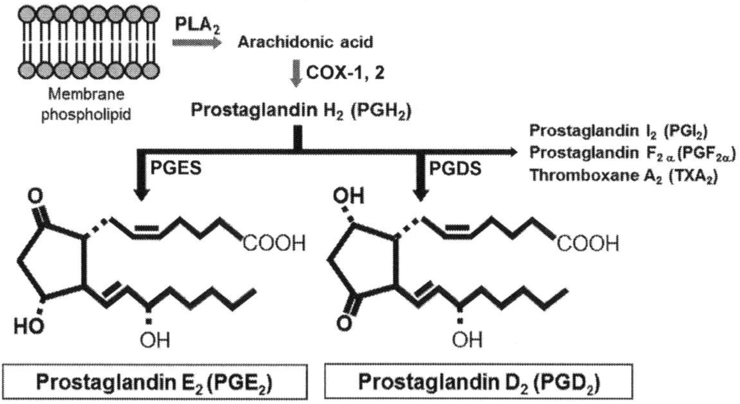

Figure 1 Biosynthetic pathway and structures of PGE_2 and PGD_2. PLA_2, phospholipase A_2; COX, cyclooxygenase; PGES, prostaglandin E synthase; PGDS, prostaglandin D synthase.

and the neurovascular unit (NVU) under normal and pathological conditions (Fig. 2). Therefore, regulatory systems for PGE_2 and PGD_2 levels in brain interstitial fluid (ISF) and cerebrospinal fluid (CSF) are considered essential for normal CNS function.

The rates of production and clearance of PGE_2 and PGD_2 need to be well balanced to precisely regulate PGs levels in the brain under normal conditions. However, regulatory dysfunction, e.g., increased production and/or reduced elimination, under pathological conditions would change the levels and biological activities of PGE_2 and PGD_2 in the brain and may seriously affect CNS function. Indeed, it has been reported that the brain concentration of PGE_2 increases in an animal model of inflammation, using lipopolysaccharide (LPS) endotoxin administration (Inoue et al., 2002). Montine et al. (1999) reported increased levels of PGE_2 in CSF of patients with Alzheimer's disease (Montine et al., 1999).

The production–clearance rate balance may also be affected by drug administration. β-Lactam cephalosporin antibiotics are often prescribed to treat a variety of infectious diseases. However, there have been reports of CNS adverse effects, such as encephalitis (Schliamser, Cars, & Norrby, 1991). PGE_2 is at least partly involved in the CNS symptoms (Phillis, Horrocks, & Farooqui, 2006), and therefore we considered that PGE_2 production and/or clearance might be altered by these drugs, and this in turn might result in an increase of PGE_2 brain levels.

Regarding the elimination of PGs from adult brain, PGs are not extensively inactivated because the adult brain shows little expression or activity of

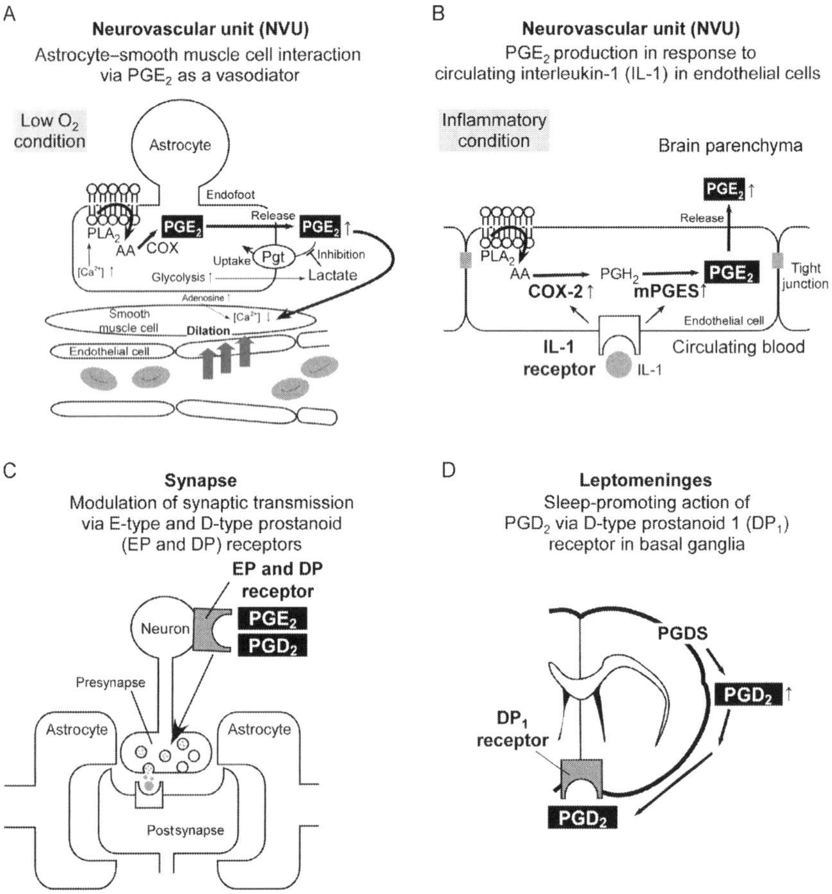

Figure 2 Sites of action of PGE_2 and PGD_2 in the brain.

15-hydroxyprostaglandin dehydrogenase, the rate-limiting enzyme for PGs catabolism (Alix, Schmitt, Strazielle, & Ghersi-Egea, 2008). It is thus likely that the primary clearance pathway for PGs from the brain is brain parenchyma/ISF-to-blood and/or the CSF-to-blood vectorial efflux transport across the blood–brain barrier (BBB) and blood–CSF barrier (BCSFB), respectively. Furthermore, since PGs (pK_a ~5) are anionic at physiological pH, simple diffusion would not be a major biological membrane permeation process at the brain barriers. This strongly suggests that carrier-mediated efflux transport processes across the brain barriers serve as the major components of the PGs clearance system.

In this review, we cover the role of efflux transport systems at the BBB and BCSFB as a regulatory system of PGE_2 and PGD_2 levels in the brain ISF and CSF and discuss their pharmacological relevance to drug therapeutics in inflammation.

2. ROLES AND KINETICS OF PGE_2 AND PGD_2 IN THE CNS

PGE_2 and PGD_2 have multiple pharmacological effects at multiple sites of action in the brain. The action sites of PGE_2 and PGD_2 in the CNS are summarized in Fig. 2. At the NVU, PGE_2 acts as a vasodilator at low oxygen levels, inducing increased local blood flow (Fig. 2A) (Gordon, Choi, Rungta, Ellis-Davies, & MacVicar, 2008). The mechanism is considered to be as follows (Gordon, Howarth, & MacVicar, 2011): (i) PGE_2 is extensively produced in astrocytes and released from the cells. (ii) Increasing levels of extracellular lactate due to enhanced glycolysis attenuate prostaglandin transporter (Pgt/Slco2a1)-mediated PGE_2 uptake from the extracellular space, causing accumulation of extracellular PGE_2 and relaxation of smooth muscle cells.

Under inflammatory conditions, PGE_2 is extensively produced at the BBB and serves as a messenger to activate E-type prostanoid (EP) receptors in the brain parenchyma. Brain endothelial cells induce PGE_2 synthesis by increasing the expression of cyclooxygenase (COX) and microsomal prostaglandin E synthase-1 (mPGES-1) in response to circulating interleukin-1 (IL-1) and release PGE_2 into the brain ISF (Ek et al., 2001; Engblom et al., 2002). This idea is supported by the observation that IL-1-evoked PGE_2 release in cultured brain endothelial cells is four times greater on the basal side than on the apical side (Moore, Spector, & Hart, 1988). Inoue et al. (2002) proposed that mPGES-1-mediated production of PGE_2 in blood vessels causes fever, an acute neuroinflammatory response. Thus, it appears that increased production of PGE_2 in the endothelial cells triggers CNS immune responses, such as fever, fatigue, and appetite loss (Fig. 2B). Furthermore, Nishijima et al. reported that PGE_2 released during neuronal excitation acts as a trigger for serum-derived IGF-I entry across the BBB (Nishijima et al., 2010). This indicates that PGE_2 is also involved in neuronal activity-dependent BBB transport.

In the brain parenchyma, both PGE_2 and PGD_2 modulate synaptic signaling, excitability, and neuroinflammatory responses via specific EP and D-type prostanoid (DP) receptors (Andreasson, 2010) (Fig. 2C). PGD_2 is an endogenous sleep-promoting factor that regulates physiological sleep, both nonrapid eye movement sleep and rapid eye movement sleep, through the DP_1 receptor (Huang, Urade, & Hayaishi, 2007). Because the DP_1 receptor is localized predominantly in CSF-facing arachnoid trabecular cells (Tachikawa, Tsuji, et al., 2012), the CSF concentration of PGD_2 will be a key determinant of the action of DP_1 receptors (Fig. 2D). Considering that the CSF levels of PGD_2 exhibit a significant circadian fluctuation (Pandey, Ram, Matsumura, & Hayaishi, 1995), regulatory systems for the generation and/or elimination of PGD_2 in the CSF may generate circadian rhythm.

3. TRANSPORTERS FOR PGs AND INTERSPECIES DIFFERENCES

Table 1 summarizes the characteristics of various transporters that accept PGs as substrates. Polarized brain capillary endothelial cells and choroid plexus epithelial cells with complex tight junctions engage in transporter(s)-mediated brain ISF/CSF-to-blood vectorial transport. There are two types of transporters most likely involved in the brain ISF/CSF-to-blood efflux transport of PGE_2 and PGD_2 at the BBB and BCSFB (Fig. 3): at the BBB (1) influx transporter across the abluminal membrane of endothelial cells from the brain ISF into the cells and (2) efflux transporter across the luminal membrane from the cells into the circulating blood, and at the BCSFB (1) influx transporter across brush-border membrane of choroid plexus epithelial cells from the CSF into the cells and (2) efflux transporter across the basolateral membrane from the cells into the blood.

At the BBB, studies using quantitative targeted absolute proteomics (QTAP) indicated that organic anion transporter 3 (Oat3/Slc22a8) and multidrug resistance-associated protein 4 (Mrp4/ABCC4) were expressed in mouse isolated brain capillaries in amounts of 1.97 and 1.59 (fmol/μg protein), respectively (Kamiie et al., 2008; Uchida et al., 2013). Mrp4 is localized at the luminal membrane of brain capillary endothelial cells (Leggas et al., 2004), whereas Oat3 is localized at the abluminal membrane of endothelial cells (Mori et al., 2003). As shown in Fig. 3, interplay of Oat3 and Mrp4 at the BBB could enable vectorial transport of PGs across the endothelial cells from the brain ISF to the circulating blood. It should be noted that OAT3 (SLC22A8), a potent homolog of rodent Oat3, is under the limit of quantification in human (<0.348 fmol/μg protein) and monkey (<0.404 fmol/μg protein) isolated brain capillaries, although MRP4 (ABCC4) was detected in human and monkey isolated brain capillaries in amounts of 0.195 and 0.286 fmol/μg protein, respectively (Ito et al., 2011; Uchida et al., 2011). Luminal membrane localization of MRP4 has

Table 1 Characteristics of transporters for PGs

Transporter	Species	Affinity (K_m) (expression system)	PG substrates	References
SLCO3A1 (OATP-D/ PGT-2)	Human	E_1: 48.5 nM E_2: 55 nM (oocyte)	D_2, E_1, E_2, $F_{2\alpha}$	Adachi et al. (2003)
SLC22A6 (OAT1)	Human	E_2: 970 nM $F_{2\alpha}$: 575 nM (S_2 cell)	E_2, $F_{2\alpha}$	Kimura et al. (2002)
SLC22A7 (OAT2)	Human	E_2: 713 nM (S_2 cell)	E_2, $F_{2\alpha}$	Kimura et al. (2002)
SLC22A8 (OAT3)	Human	E_2: 345 nM $F_{2\alpha}$: 1092 nM (S_2 cell)	E_2, $F_{2\alpha}$	Kimura et al. (2002)
SLC22A11 (OAT4)	Human	E_2: 154 nM $F_{2\alpha}$: 692 nM (S_2 cell)	E_2, $F_{2\alpha}$	Kimura et al. (2002)
SLC22A1 (OCT1)	Human	E_2: 657 nM $F_{2\alpha}$: 477 nM (S_2 cell)	E_2, $F_{2\alpha}$	Kimura et al. (2002)
SLC22A3 (OCT2)	Human	E_2: 28.9 nM $F_{2\alpha}$: 334 nM (S_2 cell)	E_2, $F_{2\alpha}$	Kimura et al. (2002)
ABCC4 (MRP4)	Human	E_1: 2.1 μM E_2: 3.4 μM (Sf9 vesicle)	E_1, E_2	Reid et al. (2003)
ABCC4 (MRP4)	Human	E_2: 3.5 μM $F_{2\alpha}$: 12.6 μM (V79 vesicle)	E_2, $F_{2\alpha}$	Rius, Thon, Keppler, and Nies (2005)
Slco2b1 (Oatp2b1/ moat1)	Rat	D_2: 35.5 nM (oocyte)	D_2, E_1, E_2	Nishio et al. (2000)
Slco1a5 (Oatp3/ oatp1a2)	Rat	E_2: 35 μM (oocyte)	E_2	Cattori et al. (2001)
Slco1a3 (OAT-K2)	Rat	ND	E_2	Masuda et al. (1999)
Slco1b2 (Oatp4/ oatp1b2)	Rat	E_2: 13 μM (oocyte)	E_2	Cattori et al. (2001)
Slco3a1 (OATP-D/ PGT-2)	Rat	ND	E_1, E_2, $F_{2\alpha}$	Adachi et al. (2003)

Continued

Table 1 Characteristics of transporters for PGs—cont'd

Transporter	Species	Affinity (K_m) (expression system)	PG substrates	References
Slco2a1 (PGT)	Rat	E_1: 70 nM E_2: 94 nM $F_{2\alpha}$: 104 nM (HeLa cell)	E_1, E_2, $F_{2\alpha}$	Kanai et al. (1995)
Slc22a22 (OAT-PG)	Rat	E_2: 143 nM (S_2 cells)	E_2	Hatano et al. (2012)
Slc22a8 (Oat3)	Mouse	ND	E_2, $F_{2\alpha}$	Kobayashi et al. (2004)
Slc22a22 (OAT-PG)	Mouse	E_1: 156.8 nM E_2: 118.3 nM $F_{2\alpha}$: 158.2 nM D_2: 371.6 nM (S_2 cells)	E_1, E_2, $F_{2\alpha}$, D_2	Shiraya et al. (2010)

ND, not determined. S_2 cells, second portion of proximal tubule cells.

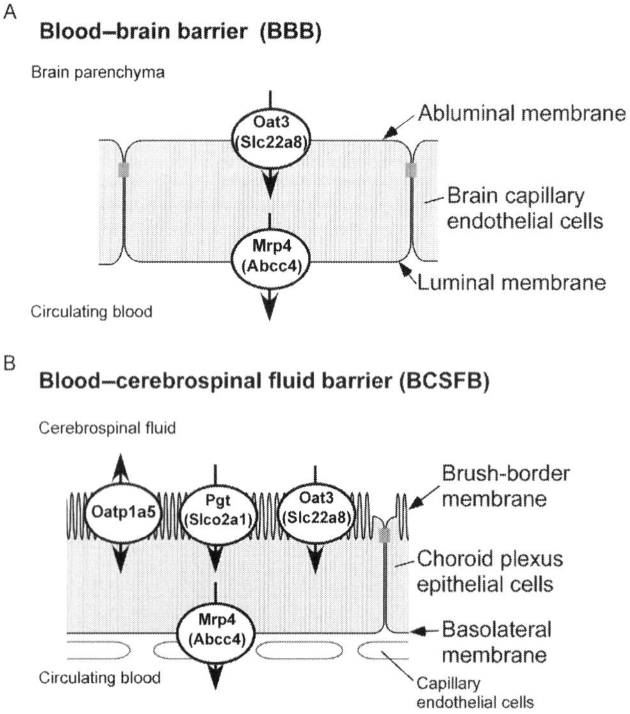

Figure 3 PGs transporters localized at the BBB and BCSFB.

also been demonstrated in human brain capillary endothelial cells (Nies et al., 2004). One possible explanation of the interspecies differences is that even small amounts of OAT3 are sufficient to play a functional role at the BBB. Another possibility is that human BBB and monkey BBB possess an alternative organic anion transporter(s). This remains a key issue relating to mechanisms of PGs transport at the human BBB.

At the BCSFB, transcellular transport activities for PGE_2 in the apical-to-basolateral direction exist in polarized choroid plexus epithelial cells, without inactivation of PGE_2 in the cells (Khuth, Strazielle, Giraudon, Belin, & Ghersi-Egea, 2005). It has also been reported that the choroid plexus takes up $PGF_{2\alpha}$ via a saturable transport process (DiBenedetto & Bito, 1986). Although QTAP analysis of rodent and human BCSFB transporters has not yet been reported, there is accumulating evidence of the expression of organic anion transporters at the rodent BCSFB. Oat3 (Nagata, Kusuhara, Endou, & Sugiyama, 2002), Pgt/Slco2a1 (Adachi et al., 2003; Kis et al., 2006), organic anion transporting polypeptide 1a5 (oatp1a5/oatp3/Slco1a5) (Kusuhara et al., 2003; Ohtsuki et al., 2004), and Mrp4 (Leggas et al., 2004) are expressed in the rodent choroid plexus. Oat3, Pgt, and Oatp1a5 are localized on the brush-border membrane of choroid plexus epithelial cells, whereas Mrp4 is localized on the basolateral membrane of epithelial cells (Nagata et al., 2002; Ohtsuki et al., 2004; Tachikawa, Tsuji, et al., 2012). These lines of evidence suggest that interplay of Oat3, Pgt, and Oatp1a5 at the brush-border membrane and Mrp4 at the basolateral membrane may regulate transcellular transport of PGs in the CSF-to-circulating blood direction, although the contribution of each transporter remains to be clarified.

It is further intriguing to pursue the possibility that the other PG transporters (Table 1), for which there is no information on BBB and BCSFB localization, are involved in the BBB and BCSFB transport, especially under pathological conditions.

4. PGE_2 EFFLUX TRANSPORT SYSTEM AT THE BBB

4.1. Effect of cephalosporin antibiotics on PGE_2 efflux transport at the BBB

Brain efflux index (BEI) analysis revealed that $[^3H]PGE_2$ microinjected into the secondary somatosensory cortex region undergoes carrier-mediated efflux transport from the brain parenchyma to the circulating blood with a half-life of 16.3 min in normal mice (Fig. 4) (Akanuma et al., 2010). As

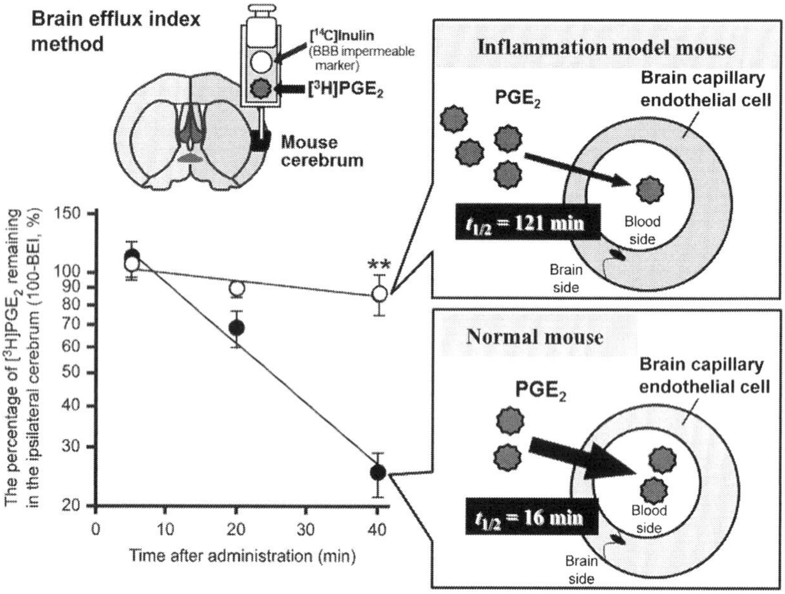

Figure 4 Reduction of PGE_2 efflux transport across the mouse blood–brain barrier (BBB) under inflammatory conditions. Time-course of $[^3H]PGE_2$ in the ipsilateral cerebrum after intracerebral microinjection in LPS-treated mice (open circles) and saline-treated mice (closed circles). Each point represents the mean $\pm$ SEM ($n=4$–5). $^{**}p<0.01$, significantly different from the saline-treated mice. *The figure is adapted from Akanuma, Uchida, Ohtsuki, Tachikawa, et al. (2011).*

much as 48% of the total ^3H radioactivity in jugular venous plasma collected 5 min after $[^3H]PGE_2$ intracerebral microinjection was detected in the form of intact PGE_2 (Akanuma et al., 2010). Considering that (i) the adult brain exhibits little activity of the rate-limiting enzyme for PGs catabolism (Alix et al., 2008) and (ii) $[^3H]PGE_2$ is extensively metabolized within 5 min after systemic administration in rats (Eguchi, Kaneko, Urade, Hayashi, & Hayaishi, 1992), it is likely that $[^3H]PGE_2$ microinjected into the brain undergoes brain-to-blood efflux transport as the intact form, and is metabolized rapidly in the peripheral tissues. These findings suggest that brain ISF-to-blood efflux transport functions as a clearance system for intact PGE_2 produced in the brain. In this regard, the interplay of mPGES-1-mediated PGE_2 production in perivascular sheets of astrocytes and PGE_2 clearance across the BBB (Fig. 2A) appears to be an efficient way of terminating the vasodilation reaction in an NVU.

The cephalosporin antibiotic cefmetazole is a high-affinity substrate for MRP4 with a K_m value of 28.5 μM (Uchida, Kamiie, Ohtsuki, & Terasaki,

2007) and an intrinsic transport activity per human MRP4 protein of 1.31 nL/(min·fmol MRP4) (Table 2). When cefmetazole is administered intravenously prior to $[^3H]PGE_2$ microinjection into secondary somatosensory cortex region, $[^3H]PGE_2$ elimination from the brain was significantly reduced with an ID_{50} value of 120 mg/kg in mice (Akanuma et al., 2010). *In vitro* uptake study showed that cefmetazole inhibited $[^3H]PGE_2$ uptake by human MRP4-expressing membrane vesicles with an IC_{50} value of 10.2 μM (Akanuma et al., 2010). Because this IC_{50} value is similar to the K_m value of human MRP4-mediated cefmetazole transport, MRP4 is likely to be involved in $[^3H]PGE_2$ efflux transport across the BBB. Intravenous administration of cefazoline, which causes significant inhibition of MRP4-mediated $[^3H]PGE_2$ uptake, also reduced the *in vivo* $[^3H]PGE_2$ efflux transport (Table 2). In contrast, intravenous administration of cefotaxime and ceftriaxone had no inhibitory effect on *in vivo* $[^3H]PGE_2$ efflux transport, even although both drugs can significantly inhibit MRP4-mediated $[^3H]PGE_2$ uptake (Table 2) (Akanuma et al., 2010). One possible explanation of these apparent discrepancies is that cefmetazole and cefazoline are substrates of oatp1a4, which is localized at both the luminal and abluminal membranes of brain capillary endothelial cells, at least in rodents (Gao, Stieger, Noe, Fritschy, & Meier, 1999), but cefotaxime and ceftriaxone are not substrates (Nakakariya et al., 2008). To produce a *cis*-inhibitory effect on MRP4-mediated PGE_2 transport at the luminal membrane of capillary endothelial cells, drugs needs to be transported into the cells at sufficient concentrations. In support of this notion, the inhibitory effect of cefmetazole was diminished when oatp1a4 was inhibited by intravenous administration of amiodarone (Akanuma, Uchida, Ohtsuki, Tachikawa, et al., 2011).

A similar situation is seen in the case of the nonsteroidal anti-inflammatory drug (NSAID) ketoprofen: intravenously administered ketoprofen showed no inhibitory effect on *in vivo* brain-to-blood efflux transport of $[^3H]PGE_2$, although ketoprofen had a significant inhibitory effect on human MRP4-mediated $[^3H]PGE_2$ uptake (Table 2). This discrepancy could be explained by the lack of an influx transport system for ketoprofen at the luminal membrane of capillary endothelial cells. These lines of evidence strongly suggest that intravenous administration of some cephalosporin antibiotics and NSAIDs reduces MRP4-mediated PGE_2 clearance from the brain.

As shown in Fig. 5, it appears that the inhibitory effect of cephalosporin antibiotics and NSAIDs on human MRP4-mediated $[^3H]PGE_2$ transport is

Table 2 Effect of cephalosporin antibiotics and other compounds on [^{3}H]PGE_2 transport

Compounds	Inhibitory effect on *in vivo* brain-to-blood efflux transport of [^{3}H]PGE_2 in mice (Akanuma et al., 2010) (% of control)	Inhibitory effect (20 μM) on [^{3}H]PGE_2 uptake in human MRP4-expressing vesicles (Akanuma et al., 2010) (% of control)	Transport activity per human MRP4 protein (Akanuma, Uchida, Ohtsuki, Kamiie, et al., 2011) (nL/(min·fmol MRP4))	Substrate of rat oatp1a4 (Nakakariya et al., 2008) (Yes: substrate, No: not substrate)
Control	100 ± 3	100 ± 4		
Cephem antibiotics				
Cefmetazole	75.4 ± 8.2**	–	1.31	Yes
Cefazolin	80.6 ± 8.4*	63.2 ± 3.3**	–	Yes
Cefotaxime	115 ± 4	34.5 ± 6.4**	–	No
Ceftriaxone	98.9 ± 1.8	6.62 ± 5.05**	1.15	No
Cephalexin	105 ± 3	109 ± 3	0.0939	Yes
Cefaclor	106 ± 4	100 ± 4	–	–
Cefsulodin	100 ± 3	106 ± 2	–	Yes
Organic anion transporter inhibitors and NSAIDs				
Dipyridamole	71.6 ± 18.6*	42.7 ± 4.2**	–	–
Taurocholate	90.3 ± 8.5	101 ± 2	–	–
Ketoprofen	99.7 ± 7.9	49.1 ± 2.4**	–	–
Diclofenac	111 ± 7.1	94.8 ± 0.7	–	

Each % of control value represents the mean ± SEM ($n = 3$–15). In *in vivo* brain-to-blood efflux transport of [^{3}H]PGE_2, inhibitory effect of intravenous administration of cephalosporin antibiotics (200 mg/kg) and other compounds (10–40 mg/kg) are investigated in mice. Transport activities of cephalosporin antibiotics and other compounds per human MRP4 protein are estimated by using human MRP4-expressing vesicles and quantitative targeted absolute proteomics.

*$p < 0.05$, **$p < 0.01$, significantly different from control.

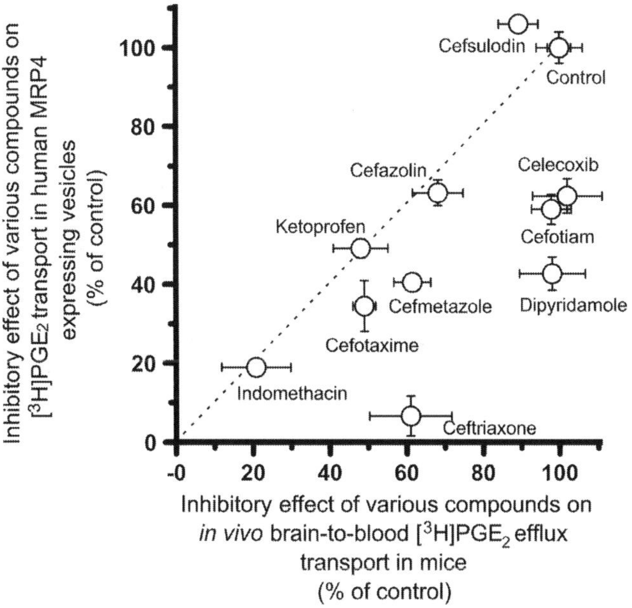

Figure 5 Correlation between inhibition of human MRP4-mediated [^{3}H]PGE$_2$ transport and *in vivo* [^{3}H]PGE$_2$ efflux transport in mice. In *in vivo* brain-to-blood efflux transport of [^{3}H]PGE$_2$, inhibitory effect of intracerebral administration of cephalosporin antibiotics and other compounds is investigated. *Data are cited from Akanuma et al. (2010).*

in good agreement with that of the intracerebrally administered drugs on *in vivo* [^{3}H]PGE$_2$ efflux transport in mice. However, an exception can be found in the case of ceftriaxone: although ceftriaxone at a concentration of 20 μM produces more than 90% inhibition of human MRP4-mediated [^{3}H]PGE$_2$ transport, its inhibition ratio of *in vivo* [^{3}H]PGE$_2$ efflux transport is only around 60%. This is presumably due to the lack of an efficient influx transport system for ceftriaxone at the abluminal membrane of capillary endothelial cells. Taking the example of cefotaxime, its intracerebral administration showed an inhibitory effect of 50% on *in vivo* brain-to-blood [^{3}H]PGE$_2$ efflux transport (Fig. 5), whereas its intravenous administration had no effect (Table 2). These apparently contradictory results could be explained by the fact that cefotaxime potentially inhibits [^{3}H]PGE$_2$ transport at the abluminal membrane of capillary endothelial cells. Hence, drugs that do not inhibit PGE$_2$ clearance may be preferable for the treatment of inflammatory and infectious diseases. Assessment of inhibitory activity toward

MRP4-mediated PGE_2 transport and uptake by endothelial cells could be useful to predict adverse effects in the CNS.

4.2. Changes in PGE_2 efflux transport at the BBB under inflammatory conditions

We have found that the PGE_2 elimination rate across the BBB in an LPS-induced mouse model of inflammation is decreased to 13.0% of that in saline-treated normal mice (Fig. 4) (Akanuma, Uchida, Ohtsuki, Tachikawa, et al., 2011), although there was no significant difference in the percentage of the BBB-impermeable [^{14}C]inulin recovery between LPS-treated mice and saline-treated mice. These results strongly suggest that increasing levels of PGE_2 in inflammation reflects a significant reduction of PGE_2 efflux transport capacity at the BBB, as well as the induction of PGE_2-synthesizing enzymes, such as COX-2 and microsomal PGES-1, in the brain (Inoue et al., 2002; Tachikawa, Ozeki, et al., 2012).

QTAP analysis revealed that the Mrp4 protein level was not changed in LPS-treated mouse brain capillaries, whereas the levels of Oat3 and Oatp1a4 were significantly decreased by 25.7% and 39.0%, respectively, in LPS-treated mice (Akanuma, Uchida, Ohtsuki, Tachikawa, et al., 2011). Because the reduction of Oat3 and Oatp1a4 expression is insufficient to fully account for the 87.0% decrease in the PGE_2 elimination rate, Oat3 and Oatp1a4 may not play substantial roles in PGE_2 elimination in mice. One possible mechanism is a reduction of the intrinsic transport activity due to protein modification, such as phosphorylation. Indeed, LPS treatment decreased P-glycoprotein intrinsic activity, without changing its protein expression level, via protein kinase C activation (Bauer, Hartz, & Miller, 2007; Fattori et al., 2007; Hartz, Bauer, Fricker, & Miller, 2006). Another possibility is that increasing levels of endogenous PGE_2 inhibited MRP4-mediated [^{3}H]PGE_2 efflux transport from the brain. In support of this notion, the expression levels of COX-2 and microsomal PGES-1 in mouse brain capillaries were increased by LPS administration (Chung et al., 2010; Yamagata et al., 2001)

Intracerebral and intravenous preadministration of cefmetazole inhibited PGE_2 efflux transport across the BBB in LPS-treated mice (Akanuma, Uchida, Ohtsuki, Tachikawa, et al., 2011). These results suggest that cefmetazole administration has the potential to further inhibit PGE_2 elimination from the brain under inflammatory conditions. Considering that cefmetazole induces adverse effects such as fever (Jones, 1989), it appears to reduce PGE_2 efflux transport in inflammation. This is expected to result in increased cerebral accumulation of PGE_2, presumably leading to fever. In humans, cefmetazole is intravenously administered at the dosage of 2 g per person, and the maximum serum unbound concentration of cefmetazole was reported to be 80.0 μM at this dose (Ko, Cathcart, Griffith, Peters, & Adams, 1989; Komiya, Kikuchi, Tachibana, & Yano, 1981). Since the unbound concentration of cefmetazole in human circulating blood is greater than its IC_{50} value for Mrp4-mediated PGE_2 transport, inhibition of PGE_2 elimination across the BBB following intravenous administration of cefmetazole may occur in humans. However, it should be noted that we need to consider the intracellular unbound concentration of cefmetazole in endothelial cells to precisely estimate the *in vivo* inhibition at the human BBB.

5. PGE_2 AND PGD_2 EFFLUX TRANSPORT SYSTEMS AT THE BCSFB

5.1. Drug–PGE_2 efflux transport interaction at the BCSFB

PGE_2 is the crucial mediator of propagating neuroinflammation induced by ischemia and bacterial infection. Because there is a positive correlation between the PGE_2 level in the CSF and the severity and clinical outcome of stroke (Carasso, Vardi, Rabay, Zor, & Streifler, 1977), the CSF levels of PGE_2 appears to be a key determinant of neuroinflammation progression. The rapid $[^3H]PGE_2$ elimination clearance from CSF in rats *in vivo* (half-life = 3.4 min) was eightfold greater than that of D-mannitol, which is considered to reflect CSF bulk flow (Tachikawa, Ozeki, et al., 2012). The *in vivo* PGE_2 elimination process was inhibited by the simultaneous injection of unlabeled PGE_2 and β-lactam antibiotics, such as benzylpenicillin, cefazolin, and ceftriaxone (Tachikawa, Ozeki, et al., 2012). Thus, several kinds of cephalosporins may attenuate PGE_2 efflux transport at the BCSFB as well as the BBB. As summarized in Table 3, PGE_2 uptake by freshly isolated choroid plexus was inhibited by unlabeled PGE_2, PGB_1, diclofenac, an NSAID, and β-lactam antibiotics, such as benzylpenicillin, cefazolin, and ceftriaxone, which are substrates and/or inhibitors of Oat3 (Tachikawa, Ozeki, et al., 2012). The K_m value (23.0 μM) of PGE_2 uptake by the choroid plexus is similar to that of Oat3-mediated PGE_2 transport (4 μM) (Table 3). Since the K_m value of PGE_2 uptake by the choroid plexus is almost four orders of magnitude greater than the PGE_2 concentrations in rat CSF under normal (1.2 nM) and inflammatory (~3.4 nM) conditions (Gao et al., 2009), it is likely that PGE_2 uptake without saturation results

Table 3 Characteristics of PGE_2 transport in isolated rat choroid plexus and rat Oat3-expressing oocytes

	Isolated rat choroid plexus		**Rat Oat3-expressing oocytes**	
Affinity (K_m, μM)	**23.0 ± 8.0**		**4.24 ± 0.79**	
Inhibitory effect	**Concentration (mM)**	**% of control**	**Concentration (mM)**	**% of control**
Control		100 ± 5		100 ± 5
PGE_2	0.16	38.8 ± 2.5*	0.01	28.2 ± 2.4*
PGB_1	1	17.0 ± 1.0*	0.1	12.8 ± 0.6*
Diclofenac	1	16.0 ± 0.4*	0.1	15.1 ± 0.6*
Bromocresolgreen	1	16.5 ± 0.2*	1	28.4 ± 1.0*
Benzylpenicillin	1	49.9 ± 2.2*	1	15.6 ± 0.5*
p-Aminohippuric acid (PAH)	1	82.5 ± 3.8*	1	86.0 ± 8.3
Cefazolin	1	53.2 ± 3.3*		ND
Cefmetazole	1	41.4 ± 1.8*		ND

Rat freshly isolated choroid plexus and rat Oat3-expressing *Xenopus* oocytes were incubated with $[^3H]PGE_2$ in the absence (control) or presence of inhibitors at 37 °C and 20 °C for 1 min and 1 h, respectively. Each K_m value represents the mean ± SD (n = 6–10). Each % of control value represents the mean ± SEM (n = 3–5).
*$p < 0.01$, significantly different from control.
Data are cited from Tachikawa, Ozeki, et al. (2012).

in continuous removal of PGE_2 from the CSF. These results suggest that the system regulating the PGE_2 level in CSF involves at least partially Oat3-mediated PGE_2 uptake by choroid plexus epithelial cells, acting as a cerebral clearance pathway via the BCSFB, although contributions by oatp1a5 and Pgt cannot be ruled out (Tachikawa, Ozeki, et al., 2012).

In rats that received intracisternal LPS, an experimental model of bacterial meningitis, reduced uptake of benzylpenicillin by the choroid plexus has been reported (Han, Kim, Lee, Shim, & Chung, 2002). Since Oat3 is responsible for the uptake of PGE_2 as well as benzylpenicillin (Table 3), it appears that PGE_2 clearance from CSF is reduced under inflammatory conditions. As described in Section 4.1, cefmetazole, cefazolin, ceftriaxone, and cefotaxime, administered intravenously to mice, significantly inhibit brain-to-blood $[^3H]PGE_2$ efflux transport across the BBB most likely because of the inhibition of MRP4 (Akanuma et al., 2010). This might explain the risk of adverse effects, such as encephalitis, induced by some cephalosporins (Schliamser et al., 1991). Similarly, it has been reported that Mrp4, which is localized at the basolateral membrane of choroid plexus epithelial cells (Fig. 3), mediates active efflux transport of PGE_2 from the cells (Reid et al., 2003). From this viewpoint, the interaction between the drugs, which potentially inhibit Oat3 and Mrp4, and PGE_2 efflux transport at the BCSFB may cause the accumulation of PGE_2 in the CSF, thus exacerbating neuroinflammation in the brain.

For instance, intravenous administration of ceftriaxone is clinically useful for the treatment of bacterial meningitis (Scheld, 1984). Since the K_i value of ceftriaxone for human OAT3-mediated [^{3}H]estrone-3-sulfate transport is estimated to be 4.39 μM (Takeda, Babu, Narikawa, & Endou, 2002), ceftriaxone does not inhibit PGE_2 uptake by the choroid plexus at a clinically relevant concentration. On the other hand, ceftriaxone strongly inhibits human MRP4-mediated PGE_2 transport (Table 2). Although it needs to be considered whether the uptake transporter like oatp1a4 at the BBB can achieve a sufficient concentration of ceftriaxone in the cells, the possibility of chorionic inhibition should be taken into consideration when selecting therapeutic drugs, as well as in the development of new drugs.

5.2. PGD_2 efflux transport at the BCSFB as a regulatory system for sleep promotion

According to the National Institutes of Health in United States, roughly 30% of the general population complains of sleep disruption (http://sleepfoundation.org/). Although various insomnia medications are available, including over-the-counter and prescription drugs, major classes of insomnia medication are benzodiazepine and nonbenzodiazepine hypnotics, the sleep-promoting mechanism of which differs from that of endogenous sleep. Considering that PGD_2 in the CSF is an endogenous sleep-promoting factor (Huang et al., 2007), a natural sleep-promoting drug that targets PGD_2 kinetics in the CSF may be desirable.

[^{3}H]PGD_2, after intracerebroventricular administration in rats, is rapidly eliminated from the CSF with a half-life of 1.1 min, most likely as the intact form (Tachikawa, Tsuji, et al., 2012). This result supports the idea that the circadian fluctuation in CSF PGD_2 levels ranging from 1 to 3 nM (Pandey et al., 1995) is due to PGD2 generation via lipocalin-type prostaglandin D synthetase (L-PGDS), which is predominantly localized in leptomeninges facing the CSF (Tachikawa, Tsuji, et al., 2012). As summarized in Table 4, the inhibition profiles on [^{3}H]PGD_2 uptake by the isolated choroid plexus are almost identical to those of Pgt- and/or Oat3-mediated

Table 4 Characteristics of PGD_2 transport in isolated rat choroid plexus, mouse Pgt-expressing oocytes, and rat Oat3-expressing oocytes

		Isolated rat choroid plexus	**Mouse Pgt-expressing oocytes**	**Rat Oat3-expressing oocytes**
Affinity (K_m, μM)		–	**1.07 ± 0.32**	**7.32 ± 1.27**
Inhibition	**Concentration (mM)**	**% of control**		
Control		100 ± 2	100 ± 5	100 ± 5
PGD_2	0.1	43.2 ± 2.8*	5.43 ± 0.34*	ND
PGB_1	0.1	28.6 ± 0.6*	12.1 ± 0.6*	41.8 ± 3.2*
Bromocresolgreen	1	20.8 ± 0.4*	8.13 ± 0.37*	48.9 ± 1.4*
Dehydroepiandrosterone-3-sulfate (DHEAS)	1 (choroid plexus) 0.1 (oocyte)	24.9 ± 1.0*	68.8 ± 6.9*	65.5 ± 8.0*
Benzylpenicillin	1	46.2 ± 5.1*	99.1 ± 6.2	38.1 ± 3.2*
Indomethacin	0.1	73.6 ± 0.9*	ND	53.1 ± 2.9*
Diclofenac	0.1	ND	ND	38.6 ± 1.8*

Rat freshly isolated choroid plexus and mouse Pgt/rat Oat3-expressing *Xenopus* oocytes were incubated with $[^3H]PGD_2$ in the absence (control) or presence of inhibitors at 37 °C and 20 °C for 1 min and 1 h, respectively. Each K_m value represents the mean ± SD (n = 6–15). Each % of control value represents the mean ± SEM (n = 3–15).
ND, not determined.
ND, not determined.
*$p < 0.01$, significantly different from control.
Data are cited from Tachikawa, Tsuji, et al. (2012).

PGD_2 uptake. These results support the belief that the regulatory system of the PGD_2 level in CSF involves Pgt- and Oat3-mediated PGD_2 uptake at the brush-border membrane of choroid plexus epithelial cells, acting as a clearance pathway for continuous PGD_2 elimination from the CSF. Because PGE_2 and indomethacin are transportable substrates (Cattori et al., 2001) and/or inhibitors (Kusuhara et al., 2003) of oatp1a5 (Slco1a5), the involvement of oatp1a5 cannot be ruled out. The K_m values of PGD_2 transport mediated by Pgt (1.07 μM) and Oat3 (7.32 μM) are almost three orders of magnitude greater than the CSF levels of PGD_2 (1–3 nM; Pandey et al., 1995) and PGE_2 (1.2 nM; Gao et al., 2009). This suggests that at least Pgt and Oat3 mediate PGD_2 clearance without saturation, thus enabling continuous removal of PGD_2 from the CSF. The inhibition of Pgt- and Oat3-mediated PGD_2 clearance at the BCSFB may modify the PGD_2 level in the CSF, thus affecting physiological sleep. This idea provide a new insight, i.e., that inhibition of PGD_2 transport in the choroid plexus might be useful as a new target for treatment of insomnia. Indeed, the commonly used NSAIDs indomethacin and diclofenac inhibit Oat3-mediated [^{3}H]PGD_2 transport and/or [^{3}H]PGD_2 uptake by isolated choroid plexus (Table 3; Tachikawa, Tsuji, et al., 2012). However, it should be noted here that the BCSFB clearance system for PGE_2 shares the same transporters, such as Oat3 and Mrp4 (Tachikawa, Ozeki, et al., 2012). Since PGE_2 is a factor in neuroinflammation progression, the inhibition of PGD_2 clearance would need to be controlled in a time-dependent manner.

6. CONCLUSION

The BBB and BCSFB possess ISF/CSF-to-blood efflux transport systems that are the primary cerebral clearance pathways for PGE_2 and PGD_2. These efflux transport systems at the brain barriers represent a new therapeutic target for the treatment of neuroinflammation and insomnia. The efflux transport activities at the BBB and BCSFB are reduced by administration of several kinds of cephalosporin antibiotics and NSAIDs, which inhibit Mrp4 and/or Oat3-mediated PGE_2 transport. A mouse model of inflammation showed a significant reduction of PGE_2 efflux transport at the BBB. Therefore, drugs that do not inhibit clearance of PGE_2 may be preferable for the treatment of inflammatory and infectious diseases. Also, PGD_2 in CSF is a natural sleep-promoting factor, and so the PGD_2 efflux transport system at the BCSFB may modify the PGD_2 level in CSF, thus affecting physiological sleep. These findings indicate that the PGE_2 and PGD_2 efflux transport systems at the brain barriers play key roles in the pathophysiology and pharmacology of the PGs in the CNS.

CONFLICT OF INTEREST

The authors declare no conflicts of interest.

ACKNOWLEDGMENTS

We would like to acknowledge the collaboration of Dr. S. Akanuma (University of Toyama). This work was supported, in part, by a Grant-in-Aid for Scientific Research from the Japan Society for the Promotion of Science.

REFERENCES

Adachi, H., Suzuki, T., Abe, M., Asano, N., Mizutamari, H., Tanemoto, M., et al. (2003). Molecular characterization of human and rat organic anion transporter OATP-D. *American Journal of Physiology Renal Physiology. 285*, F1188–F1197.

Akanuma, S., Hosoya, K., Ito, S., Tachikawa, M., Terasaki, T., & Ohtsuki, S. (2010). Involvement of multidrug resistance-associated protein 4 in efflux transport of prostaglandin E2 across mouse blood-brain barrier and its inhibition by intravenous administration of cephalosporins. *The Journal of Pharmacology and Experimental Therapeutics, 333*, 912–919.

Akanuma, S., Uchida, Y., Ohtsuki, S., Kamiie, J., Tachikawa, M., Terasaki, T., et al. (2011). Molecular-weight-dependent, anionic-substrate-preferential transport of beta-lactam antibiotics via multidrug resistance-associated protein 4. *Drug Metabolism and Pharmacokinetics, 26*, 602–611.

Akanuma, S., Uchida, Y., Ohtsuki, S., Tachikawa, M., Terasaki, T., & Hosoya, K. (2011). Attenuation of prostaglandin E2 elimination across the mouse blood-brain barrier in lipopolysaccharide-induced inflammation and additive inhibitory effect of cefmetazole. *Fluids and Barriers of the CNS, 8*, 24.

Alix, E., Schmitt, C., Strazielle, N., & Ghersi-Egea, J. F. (2008). Prostaglandin E2 metabolism in rat brain: Role of the blood-brain interfaces. *Cerebrospinal Fluid Research, 5*, 5.

Andreasson, K. (2010). Emerging roles of PGE_2 receptors in models of neurological disease. *Prostaglandins & Other Lipid Mediators, 91*, 104–112.

Bauer, B., Hartz, A. M., & Miller, D. S. (2007). Tumor necrosis factor alpha and endothelin-1 increase P-glycoprotein expression and transport activity at the blood-brain barrier. *Molecular Pharmacology, 71*, 667–675.

Carasso, R. L., Vardi, J., Rabay, J. M., Zor, U., & Streifler, M. (1977). Measurement of prostaglandin E_2 in cerebrospinal fluid in patients suffering from stroke. *Journal of Neurology, Neurosurgery, and Psychiatry, 40*, 967–969.

Cattori, V., van Montfoort, J. E., Stieger, B., Landmann, L., Meijer, D. K., Winterhalter, K. H., et al. (2001). Localization of organic anion transporting polypeptide 4 (Oatp4) in rat liver and comparison of its substrate specificity with Oatp1, Oatp2 and Oatp3. *Pflügers Archiv, 443*, 188–195.

Chung, D. W., Yoo, K. Y., Hwang, I. K., Kim, D. W., Chung, J. Y., Lee, C. H., et al. (2010). Systemic administration of lipopolysaccharide induces cyclooxygenase-2 immunoreactivity in endothelium and increases microglia in the mouse hippocampus. *Cellular and Molecular Neurobiology, 30*, 531–541.

DiBenedetto, F. E., & Bito, L. Z. (1986). Transport of prostaglandins and other eicosanoids by the choroid plexus: Its characterization and physiological significance. *Journal of Neurochemistry*, *46*, 1725–1731.

Eguchi, N., Kaneko, T., Urade, Y., Hayashi, H., & Hayaishi, O. (1992). Permeability of brain structures and other peripheral tissues to prostaglandins D_2, E_2 and F_2 alpha in rats. *The Journal of Pharmacology and Experimental Therapeutics*, *262*, 1110–1120.

Ek, M., Engblom, D., Saha, S., Blomqvist, A., Jakobsson, P. J., & Ericsson-Dahlstrand, A. (2001). Inflammatory response: Pathway across the blood-brain barrier. *Nature*, *410*, 430–431.

Engblom, D., Ek, M., Saha, S., Ericsson-Dahlstrand, A., Jakobsson, P. J., & Blomqvist, A. (2002). Prostaglandins as inflammatory messengers across the blood-brain barrier. *Journal of Molecular Medicine*, *80*, 5–15.

Fattori, S., Becherini, F., Cianfriglia, M., Parenti, G., Romanini, A., & Castagna, M. (2007). Human brain tumors: Multidrug-resistance P-glycoprotein expression in tumor cells and intratumoral capillary endothelial cells. *Virchows Archiv*, *451*, 81–87.

Gao, W., Schmidtko, A., Wobst, I., Lu, R., Angioni, C., & Geisslinger, G. (2009). Prostaglandin D_2 produced by hematopoietic prostaglandin D synthase contributes to LPS-induced fever. *Journal of Physiology and Pharmacology*, *60*, 145–150.

Gao, B., Stieger, B., Noe, B., Fritschy, J. M., & Meier, P. J. (1999). Localization of the organic anion transporting polypeptide 2 (Oatp2) in capillary endothelium and choroid plexus epithelium of rat brain. *The Journal of Histochemistry and Cytochemistry*, *47*, 1255–1264.

Gordon, G. R., Choi, H. B., Rungta, R. L., Ellis-Davies, G. C., & MacVicar, B. A. (2008). Brain metabolism dictates the polarity of astrocyte control over arterioles. *Nature*, *456*, 745–749.

Gordon, G. R., Howarth, C., & MacVicar, B. A. (2011). Bidirectional control of arteriole diameter by astrocytes. *Experimental Physiology*, *96*, 393–399.

Han, H., Kim, S. G., Lee, M. G., Shim, C. K., & Chung, S. J. (2002). Mechanism of the reduced elimination clearance of benzylpenicillin from cerebrospinal fluid in rats with intracisternal administration of lipopolysaccharide. *Drug Metabolism and Disposition*, *30*, 1214–1220.

Hartz, A. M., Bauer, B., Fricker, G., & Miller, D. S. (2006). Rapid modulation of P-glycoprotein-mediated transport at the blood-brain barrier by tumor necrosis factor-alpha and lipopolysaccharide. *Molecular Pharmacology*, *69*, 462–470.

Hatano, R., Onoe, K., Obara, M., Matsubara, M., Kanai, Y., Muto, S., et al. (2012). Sex hormones induce a gender-related difference in renal expression of a novel prostaglandin transporter, OAT-PG, influencing basal PGE_2 concentration. *American Journal of Physiology. Renal Physiology*, *302*, F342–F3496.

Huang, Z. L., Urade, Y., & Hayaishi, O. (2007). Prostaglandins and adenosine in the regulation of sleep and wakefulness. *Current Opinion in Pharmacology*, *7*, 33–38.

Inoue, W., Matsumura, K., Yamagata, K., Takemiya, T., Shiraki, T., & Kobayashi, S. (2002). Brain-specific endothelial induction of prostaglandin E_2 synthesis enzymes and its temporal relation to fever. *Neuroscience Research*, *44*, 51–61.

Ito, K., Uchida, Y., Ohtsuki, S., Aizawa, S., Kawakami, H., Katsukura, Y., et al. (2011). Quantitative membrane protein expression at the blood-brain barrier of adult and younger cynomolgus monkeys. *Journal of Pharmaceutical Sciences*, *100*, 3939–3950.

Jones, R. N. (1989). Cefmetazole (CS-1170), a "new" cephamycin with a decade of clinical experience. *Diagnostic Microbiology and Infectious Disease*, *12*, 367–379.

Kamiie, J., Ohtsuki, S., Iwase, R., Ohmine, K., Katsukura, Y., Yanai, K., et al. (2008). Quantitative atlas of membrane transporter proteins: Development and application of a highly sensitive simultaneous LC/MS/MS method combined with novel in-silico peptide selection criteria. *Pharmaceutical Research*, *25*, 1469–1483.

Kanai, N., Lu, R., Satriano, J. A., Bao, Y., Wolkoff, A. W., & Schuster, V. L. (1995). Identification and characterization of a prostaglandin transporter. *Science*, *268*, 866–869.

Khuth, S. T., Strazielle, N., Giraudon, P., Belin, M. F., & Ghersi-Egea, J. F. (2005). Impairment of blood-cerebrospinal fluid barrier properties by retrovirus-activated T lymphocytes: Reduction in cerebrospinal fluid-to-blood efflux of prostaglandin E_2. *Journal of Neurochemistry*, *94*, 1580–1593.

Kimura, H., Takeda, M., Narikawa, S., Enomoto, A., Ichida, K., & Endou, H. (2002). Human organic anion transporters and human organic cation transporters mediate renal transport of prostaglandins. *The Journal of Pharmacology and Experimental Therapeutics*, *301*, 293–298.

Kis, B., Isse, T., Snipes, J. A., Chen, L., Yamashita, H., Ueta, Y., et al. (2006). Effects of LPS stimulation on the expression of prostaglandin carriers in the cells of the blood-brain and blood-cerebrospinal fluid barriers. *Journal of Applied Physiology*, *100*, 1392–1399.

Ko, H., Cathcart, K. S., Griffith, D. L., Peters, G. R., & Adams, W. J. (1989). Pharmacokinetics of intravenously administered cefmetazole and cefoxitin and effects of probenecid on cefmetazole elimination. *Antimicrobial Agents and Chemotherapy*, *33*, 356–361.

Kobayashi, Y., Ohshiro, N., Tsuchiya, A., Kohyama, N., Ohbayashi, M., & Yamamoto, T. (2004). Renal transport of organic compounds mediated by mouse organic anion transporter 3 (mOat3): Further substrate specificity of mOat3. *Drug Metabolism and Disposition*, *32*, 479–483.

Komiya, M., Kikuchi, Y., Tachibana, A., & Yano, K. (1981). Pharmacokinetics of new broad-spectrum cephamycin, YM09330, parenterally administered to various experimental animals. *Antimicrobial Agents and Chemotherapy*, *20*, 176–183.

Kusuhara, H., He, Z., Nagata, Y., Nozaki, Y., Ito, T., Masuda, H., et al. (2003). Expression and functional involvement of organic anion transporting polypeptide subtype 3 (Slc21a7) in rat choroid plexus. *Pharmaceutical Research*, *20*, 720–727.

Leggas, M., Adachi, M., Scheffer, G. L., Sun, D., Wielinga, P., Du, G., et al. (2004). Mrp4 confers resistance to topotecan and protects the brain from chemotherapy. *Molecular and Cellular Biology*, *24*, 7612–7621.

Masuda, S., Ibaramoto, K., Takeuchi, A., Saito, H., Hashimoto, Y., & Inui, K. I. (1999). Cloning and functional characterization of a new multispecific organic anion transporter, OAT-K2, in rat kidney. *Molecular Pharmacology*, *55*, 743–752.

Montine, T. J., Sidell, K. R., Crews, B. C., Markesbery, W. R., Marnett, L. J., Roberts, L. J., et al. (1999). Elevated CSF prostaglandin E_2 levels in patients with probable AD. *Neurology*, *53*, 1495–1498.

Moore, S. A., Spector, A. A., & Hart, M. N. (1988). Eicosanoid metabolism in cerebromicrovascular endothelium. *The American Journal of Physiology*, *254*, C37–C44.

Mori, S., Takanaga, H., Ohtsuki, S., Deguchi, T., Kang, Y. S., Hosoya, K., et al. (2003). Rat organic anion transporter 3 (rOAT3) is responsible for brain-to-blood efflux of homovanillic acid at the abluminal membrane of brain capillary endothelial cells. *Journal of Cerebral Blood Flow and Metabolism*, *23*, 432–440.

Nagata, Y., Kusuhara, H., Endou, H., & Sugiyama, Y. (2002). Expression and functional characterization of rat organic anion transporter 3 (rOat3) in the choroid plexus. *Molecular Pharmacology*, *61*, 982–988.

Nakakariya, M., Shimada, T., Irokawa, M., Koibuchi, H., Iwanaga, T., Yabuuchi, H., et al. (2008). Predominant contribution of rat organic anion transporting polypeptide-2 (Oatp2) to hepatic uptake of beta-lactam antibiotics. *Pharmaceutical Research*, *25*, 578–585.

Nies, A. T., Jedlitschky, G., Konig, J., Herold-Mende, C., Steiner, H. H., Schmitt, H. P., et al. (2004). Expression and immunolocalization of the multidrug resistance proteins, MRP1-MRP6 (ABCC1-ABCC6), in human brain. *Neuroscience*, *129*, 349–360.

Nishijima, T., Piriz, J., Duflot, S., Fernandez, A. M., Gaitan, G., Gomez-Pinedo, U., et al. (2010). Neuronal activity drives localized blood-brain-barrier transport of serum insulin-like growth factor-I into the CNS. *Neuron, 67*, 834–846.

Nishio, T., Adachi, H., Nakagomi, R., Tokui, T., Sato, E., Tanemoto, M., et al. (2000). Molecular identification of a rat novel organic anion transporter moat1, which transports prostaglandin D_2, leukotriene C_4, and taurocholate. *Biochemical and Biophysical Research Communications, 275*, 831–838.

Ohtsuki, S., Takizawa, T., Takanaga, H., Hori, S., Hosoya, K., & Terasaki, T. (2004). Localization of organic anion transporting polypeptide 3 (oatp3) in mouse brain parenchymal and capillary endothelial cells. *Journal of Neurochemistry, 90*, 743–749.

Pandey, H. P., Ram, A., Matsumura, H., & Hayaishi, O. (1995). Concentration of prostaglandin D_2 in cerebrospinal fluid exhibits a circadian alteration in conscious rats. *Biochemistry and Molecular Biology International, 37*, 431–437.

Phillis, J. W., Horrocks, L. A., & Farooqui, A. A. (2006). Cyclooxygenases, lipoxygenases, and epoxygenases in CNS: Their role and involvement in neurological disorders. *Brain Research Reviews, 52*, 201–243.

Reid, G., Wielinga, P., Zelcer, N., van der Heijden, I., Kuil, A., de Haas, M., et al. (2003). The human multidrug resistance protein MRP4 functions as a prostaglandin efflux transporter and is inhibited by nonsteroidal antiinflammatory drugs. *Proceedings of the National Academy of Sciences of the United States of America, 100*, 9244–9249.

Rius, M., Thon, W. F., Keppler, D., & Nies, A. T. (2005). Prostanoid transport by multidrug resistance protein 4 (MRP4/ABCC4) localized in tissues of the human urogenital tract. *The Journal of Urology, 174*, 2409–2414.

Scheld, W. M. (1984). Rationale for optimal dosing of beta-lactam antibiotics in therapy for bacterial meningitis. *European Journal of Clinical Microbiology, 3*, 579–591.

Schliamser, S. E., Cars, O., & Norrby, S. R. (1991). Neurotoxicity of beta-lactam antibiotics: Predisposing factors and pathogenesis. *The Journal of Antimicrobial Chemotherapy, 27*, 405–425.

Shiraya, K., Hirata, T., Hatano, R., Nagamori, S., Wiriyasermkul, P., Jutabha, P., et al. (2010). A novel transporter of SLC22 family specifically transports prostaglandins and co-localizes with 15-hydroxyprostaglandin dehydrogenase in renal proximal tubules. *The Journal of Biological Chemistry, 285*, 22141–22151.

Tachikawa, M., Ozeki, G., Higuchi, T., Akanuma, S., Tsuji, K., & Hosoya, K. (2012). Role of the blood-cerebrospinal fluid barrier transporter as a cerebral clearance system for prostaglandin E_2 produced in the brain. *Journal of Neurochemistry, 123*, 750–760.

Tachikawa, M., Tsuji, K., Yokoyama, R., Higuchi, T., Ozeki, G., Yashiki, A., et al. (2012). A clearance system for prostaglandin D2, a sleep-promoting factor, in cerebrospinal fluid: Role of the blood-cerebrospinal barrier transporters. *The Journal of Pharmacology and Experimental Therapeutics, 343*, 608–616.

Takeda, M., Babu, E., Narikawa, S., & Endou, H. (2002). Interaction of human organic anion transporters with various cephalosporin antibiotics. *European Journal of Pharmacology, 438*, 137–142.

Uchida, Y., Kamiie, J., Ohtsuki, S., & Terasaki, T. (2007). Multichannel liquid chromatography-tandem mass spectrometry cocktail method for comprehensive substrate characterization of multidrug resistance-associated protein 4 transporter. *Pharmaceutical Research, 24*, 2281–2296.

Uchida, Y., Ohtsuki, S., Katsukura, Y., Ikeda, C., Suzuki, T., Kamiie, J., et al. (2011). Quantitative targeted absolute proteomics of human blood-brain barrier transporters and receptors. *Journal of Neurochemistry, 117*, 333–345.

Uchida, Y., Tachikawa, M., Obuchi, W., Hoshi, Y., Tomioka, Y., Ohtsuki, S., et al. (2013). A study protocol for quantitative targeted absolute proteomics (QTAP) by LC-MS/MS: Application for inter-strain differences in protein expression levels of transporters, receptors, claudin-5, and marker proteins at the blood–brain barrier in ddY, FVB, and C57BL/6 J mice. *Fluids and Barriers of the CNS*, *10*, 21.

Yamagata, K., Matsumura, K., Inoue, W., Shiraki, T., Suzuki, K., Yasuda, S., et al. (2001). Coexpression of microsomal-type prostaglandin E synthase with cyclooxygenase-2 in brain endothelial cells of rats during endotoxin-induced fever. *The Journal of Neuroscience*, *21*, 2669–2677.

CHAPTER TWELVE

Steroids and the Blood–Brain Barrier: Therapeutic Implications

Ken A. Witt[1], Karin E. Sandoval
Pharmaceutical Sciences, School of Pharmacy, Southern Illinois University, Edwardsville, Illinois, USA
[1]Corresponding author: e-mail address: kwitt@siue.edu

Contents

Abstract

Steroids have a wide spectrum of impact, serving as fundamental regulators of nearly every physiological process within the human body. Therapeutic applications of steroids are equally broad, with a diverse range of medications and targets. Within the central nervous system (CNS), steroids influence development, memory, behavior, and disease outcomes. Moreover, steroids are well recognized as to their impact on the vascular endothelium. The blood–brain barrier (BBB) at the level of the brain microvascular endothelium serves as the principle interface between the peripheral circulation and the brain. Steroids have been identified to impact several critical properties of the BBB, including cellular efflux mechanisms, nutrient uptake, and tight junction integrity. Such actions not only influence brain homeostasis but also the delivery of CNS-targeted therapeutics. A greater understanding of the respective steroid–BBB interactions may shed further light on the differential treatment outcomes observed across CNS pathologies. In this chapter, we examine the current therapeutic implications of steroids respective to BBB structure and function, with emphasis on glucocorticoids and estrogens.

Advances in Pharmacology, Volume 71
ISSN 1054-3589
http://dx.doi.org/10.1016/bs.apha.2014.06.018

ABBREVIATIONS

ABC adenosine triphosphate (ATP)-binding cassette
AR androgen receptor
BBB blood–brain barrier
BCRP breast cancer-related protein
CAMs cellular adhesion molecules
CNS central nervous system
CRASH Corticosteroid Randomization After Significant Head-Injury
DHEAS dehydroepiandrosterone sulfate
ER estrogen receptor
GLUT1 glucose transporter-1
GPER1 G-protein-coupled estrogen receptor
GR glucocorticoid receptor
ICAM-1 intercellular adhesion molecule-1
IL-1β interleukin-1β
JAM-A junctional adhesion molecule-A
MCP1 monocyte-chemoattractant protein-1
MDR1 multidrug resistance protein-1
MMPs matrix metalloproteinases
MR mineralocorticoid receptor
NFκB nuclear factor kappa-light-chain-enhancer of activated B cells
NVU neurovascular unit
OAT organic anion transporter
PR progesterone receptor
PXR pregnane X Receptor
TEER transendothelial electrical resistance
TIMPs tissue inhibitors of matrix metalloproteinases
TJ tight junction
TNF tumor necrosis factor
TNFα tumor necrosis factor α
VCAM-1 vascular cell adhesion protein-1
VE vascular endothelial
VEGF vascular endothelial growth factor
WEST Women's Estrogen for Stroke Trial
WHI Women's Health Initiative
WHIMS Women's Health Initiative Memory Study
ZO zonula occluden

1. INTRODUCTION

There is an ever increasing focus on disorders of the central nervous system (CNS) and the search for new treatments. Yet, it should also be understood that "new" treatments are not solely restricted to the development of novel therapeutics. Ultimately, the objective is to effectively meet the unmet medical needs of the patient, which includes the further understanding of current therapeutics and their alternate applications. In this regard, steroids have been proposed as an additional treatment option for a number of CNS conditions, as: (1) steroids play a primary role in general brain function, (2) certain steroids have neuroprotective effects, (3) steroid level decline with advancing age correlates to altered CNS function, (4) CNS disorders associated with inflammation can be mitigated via select steroids, and (5) much is already known respective to steroid side effects and pharmacokinetic properties (Joels, Sarabdjitsingh, & Karst, 2012; Schumacher et al., 2003). Nevertheless, when targeting the CNS with any therapeutic, the blood–brain barrier (BBB) becomes a central focus. The BBB represents the principle interface between the periphery and CNS. This highly dynamic structure is not only involved in the protection of sensitive neuronal tissues but also in nutrient uptake, waste removal, and enzymatic processes. Furthermore, the BBB mediates drug transport into the CNS, greatly limiting the vast proportion of drug molecules currently on the market from entering the brain. Beyond the critical aspects of drug transport, understanding how steroid therapeutics impact the BBB itself, in coordination with both CNS and peripheral influences, must also be considered. Indeed, the significant implications of BBB dysregulation contributing to and potentially preceding disorders of the CNS make it a prime therapeutic target. Given the broad use of steroids and the distinctions of each respective steroid class, there is further need to understand and delineate their effects at the BBB and corresponding ramifications.

2. BLOOD–BRAIN BARRIER

The BBB is composed of specialized cerebrovascular endothelial cells (i.e., brain microvessels) that work in concert with neighboring cells (pericytes, astrocytes, neurons), which are collectively defined as the neurovascular unit (NVU). The NVU in turn interacts with circulatory components and inflammatory cells capable of altering microvascular integrity/function and thereby brain homeostasis. BBB endothelial cells are differentiated from peripheral endothelial cells by the general lack of fenestrations, limited pinocytosis, and the presence of tight junctions (TJs) (Abbott, Patabendige, Dolman, Yusof, & Begley, 2010). Moreover, BBB endothelial cells have an elevated mitochondrial content (Oldendorf, Cornford, & Brown, 1977), required for numerous energy-dependent processes necessary for its normal functioning. Lastly, BBB endothelial cells express many enzymes capable of degrading various molecules, as well as highly efficacious efflux transporters. These features are the basis for the BBB endothelium being the primary cellular obstacle to drug transport into the brain, as well as the reason the brain is preserved as an immune-privileged site.

2.1. Tight junctions

One of the essential functions of the BBB is the restriction of paracellular permeability via the TJs. The TJs, along with the adherens junctions, exist between adjacent endothelial cells, separating the luminal from the abluminal side of the plasma membrane and imparting a high trans-endothelial electrical resistance (TEER) (Butt, Jones, & Abbott, 1990). Under normal physiological conditions, polar substances do not readily transverse the BBB TJs. Nevertheless, the TJs are not necessarily uniform over the length of a microvessel and may vary in TEER dependent on brain region, relative localization to arterioles and venules, and extracellular interactions (Sandoval & Witt, 2008). The essential transmembrane proteins of the BBB TJs include occludin, claudins (-3, -5, and -12), and junctional adhesion molecule-A (JAM-A). Although, occludin is not required for the formation of TJs (Saitou et al., 1998), evidence consistently identifies occludin as a critical regulatory protein, capable of mediating paracellular permeability during conditions of pathology and inflammatory stress (Feldman, Mullin, & Ryan, 2005; Sandoval & Witt, 2008). Moreover, it has been hypothesized that occludin acts as a primary "shock absorber," respective to TJ responses to acute changes in vascular dynamics (Sandoval & Witt, 2008). The claudins have also been identified in the formation of the TJ seal (Piontek et al., 2008). Specifically, claudin-5 has shown to mediate small molecule paracellular permeability at the BBB. Increased claudin-5 expression has shown to increase TEER and decrease BBB permeability (Burek, Arias-Loza, Roewer, & Forster, 2010; Burek, Steinberg, & Forster, 2014; Honda et al., 2006). JAMs are a family of immunoglobulin superfamily proteins that localize within the intercellular cleft and are associated with leukocyte diapedesis (Weber, Fraemohs, & Dejana, 2007). Additionally, homophilic JAM-A interactions have been shown to stabilize cellular junctions and decrease paracellular permeability (Liu et al., 2000; Mandell, McCall, & Parkos, 2004). Principle cytoplasmic scaffolding proteins that link the transmembrane TJ proteins to the actin cytoskeleton include the zonula occludens (ZO-1, -2, -3), cingulin, 7H6, and AF-6 (Abbott et al., 2010). While the traditionally defined TJ proteins are most often identified as the primary mediators of the fully formed junctional seal, the adherens junction proteins are also critical for the stabilization and development of the intercellular junction. The cadherins family of transmembrane proteins maintain the adherens junction in a calcium-dependent manner, with vascular endothelial (VE)-cadherin also playing a significant role in gene transcription and regulation of the TJ proteins (Giannotta, Trani, & Dejana, 2013; Sajja, Prasad, & Cucullo, 2014). Holistically, the cellular localization, protein–protein interaction, and posttranslational modification of these transmembrane and cytoplasmic proteins all contribute to the regulation of the TJ seal. Yet, perhaps more critical respective to drug delivery and pathological influences are the numerous signaling pathways which govern the end functional response. Evidence supports steroidal interaction and mediation of these pathways, as well as direct regulation of BBB TJ proteins under physiological and pathological conditions (Forster et al., 2005; Kang, Ahn, Kang, & Gye, 2006; Salvador, Shityakov, & Forster, 2013; Sandoval & Witt, 2011; Ye et al., 2003).

2.2. Transport

Given the restricted paracellular flux across the BBB, transport of substances into the brain is predominated by passive diffusion, solute carriers, and transcytotic mechanisms (Abbott et al., 2010). Effective passive diffusion favors relatively lipophilic compounds of neutral charge and relatively low-molecular weight (<500 Da). Molecules with high polar surface areas (>80 A^2) and an increased number of rotatable bonds within a molecule further reduce diffusion rates (Pajouhesh & Lenz, 2005). While enhanced lipophilicity is generally identified to increase passive diffusion, lipophilic molecules lend themselves to enhanced affinity for efflux mechanisms, reducing their entry into the brain (Miller & Cannon, 2013). Beyond diffusional transport, many polar nutrients (e.g., glucose, amino acids) use widely expressed solute carriers that are distributed between the luminal and abluminal membranes (e.g., glucose transporter-1 (GLUT1), large neutral amino acid transporter) (Abbott et al., 2010). Specific transcytotic mechanisms also exist for key large molecular weight molecules (e.g., transferrin, insulin), and include receptor-mediated and adsorptive-mediated transcytosis (Abbott et al., 2010). While molecules can be designed to target these mechanisms for enhanced brain uptake, any alteration in BBB function has the potential to significantly alter the actual brain bioavailability of such substances. Thus, drug delivery strategies need to take into account not only the targeted mode of transport and efflux potential but also any health-related conditions or therapeutics that may impact BBB function. This is highlighted by the use of certain steroids (e.g., dexamethasone) in the media of *in vitro* BBB models, which not only enhances TEER but also induces efflux transporter expression (Bauer, Hartz, Fricker, & Miller, 2004; Chan et al., 2013). In this regard, such effects may significantly decrease the permeability of other molecules, and potentially reduce the ability to accurately extrapolate drug uptake data between various models. It should be emphasized that the broad reaching impact of each steroid class throughout the CNS, as well as periphery, have compounding/interactive effects on the transport of nutrients and therapeutics that may further alter drug pharmacokinetics and brain bioavailability.

2.3. Pathology

Dysregulation of BBB function has been shown in a number of CNS pathologies (e.g., Alzheimer's disease, Parkinson's disease, multiple sclerosis, stroke), with corresponding alterations in drug/nutrient transport, enzyme induction/inhibition, and TJ integrity (Abbott et al., 2010). Such changes may also precede a given pathology, and hence the BBB is frequently the cause of significant debate respective to pathological initiation, outcomes, and treatment approaches. While the mechanisms of BBB dysregulation are multifactorial, inflammation often plays a predominant role. This is further supported by studies showing peripheral inflammatory conditions (e.g., inflammatory pain, systemic infections, metabolic syndrome) are capable of altering BBB integrity and function (Banks & Erickson, 2010; Giannotta et al., 2013; Ouyang et al., 2014). Additionally, the BBB itself secretes many inflammatory mediators, including prostaglandins, nitric oxide, and various cytokines, which may subsequently impact surrounding tissues (Banks & Erickson, 2010). Thus, the nature of the BBB lends itself to being a key component and contributor to the inflammatory response. In this regard, various steroid therapeutics have been proposed for the treatment of CNS pathologies associated with BBB inflammatory dysregulation (Joels et al., 2012; Schumacher et al., 2003). Conversely, loss or depletion of endogenous steroids with age and/or disease may contribute to BBB dysregulation, promoting CNS pathology and altering drug delivery to the brain.

3. STEROIDS AND THE BRAIN

Steroids are vital substances that mediate a wide variety of physiological functions, including water regulation, metabolism, general immune functions, sexual differentiation, events during pregnancy, and brain function. Steroids are formally defined by their chemical structure, having three cyclohexane rings and one cyclopentane ring that vary by the functional groups attached to the ring structures and by the oxidation state. There are five classes of steroid hormones: androgens, estrogens, progestogens, glucocorticoids, and mineralocorticoids, each with distinctive receptors. Endogenous steroids are synthesized from cholesterol as needed, primarily by the adrenal glands or gonads, and secreted into the blood stream in a highly regulated manner. Synthetically derived steroids encompass a wide spectrum of therapeutics capable of interacting with endogenous receptors, although there are many nonsteroids also capable of interacting with steroid receptors (Proteau, 2011). Steroids as a whole are relatively small and lipophilic, allowing entry into cells via passive diffusion. Thus, unconjugated steroids within the systemic circulation can readily cross the BBB and impact CNS function. Some steroids that regulate neural function (i.e., "neuroactive steroids") may also be synthesized locally by neurons and glia, and as such have been further delineated as neurosteroids (Baulieu, 1997). Neurosteroids are not structurally unique from peripherally generated steroids and/or their metabolites, albeit they consist of relative subsets (i.e., pregnane, androstane, and sulfated forms) and have been strongly affiliated with nongenomic actions through modulation of specific ion channels and membrane receptors (e.g., *N*-methyl-D-aspartate (NMDA), GABA-A, Sigma) (Reddy, 2010). Classic genomic theory of action dictates steroids, bound to their receptors, exert positive (transactivation) or negative (transrepression) effects on the expression of target genes. Nevertheless, over the past two decades, a great deal of attention has been focused on the more rapid acting nongenomic actions of steroids, relative to membrane and cytoplasmic signaling pathways. Ultimately, steroids have a means of signaling and modulation of cellular action that may include both genomic and nongenomic pathways, which are dependent on the target receptor.

3.1. Neuroactive steroids

Steroids, whether originating from endogenous or exogenous sources, have been identified to have a significant, multifaceted, and many yet to be fully defined effects within the CNS (Giatti, Boraso, Melcangi, & Viviani, 2012; Melcangi & Panzica, 2013; Schumacher et al., 2003). The concentration and form of respective steroids in the body depends on an individual's age, gender, current health, diet, and originating source of the steroid. Moreover, as steroids have variable plasma–protein binding rates, blood levels may not accurately reflect brain bioavailability (Kancheva et al., 2011; Melcangi & Panzica, 2013). The complexity grows as steroids undergo highly dynamic interconversions. Metabolic conversion of a steroid may produce other active forms (e.g., aromatase converts testosterone to estradiol), as well as inactive metabolites (Melcangi & Panzica, 2013). Nevertheless, there appears to be few, if any, brain regions not affected by steroidal action. Neuroactive steroids have long since been identified with development, impacting synaptic connectivity and neuronal differentiation in the limbic system, hypothalamic areas, pituitary, cerebellum, cerebral cortex, and hippocampus (Melcangi, Panzica, & Garcia-Segura, 2011). Yet, it has also become increasingly clear that steroidal actions within the CNS reach well beyond development, influencing memory, behavior, pathology, and general brain health.

Not surprisingly, each of the five classes of steroid hormones has receptors within the CNS. The traditionally defined "gonadal" steroids (i.e., androgens, estrogens, progestogens) are strongly affiliated with sexual differentiation and control of normal reproductive function. Androgens are classically known as "male" steroid hormones, given their impact on skeletal muscle and male sexual differentiation. Estrogens and progestogens are in turn known as "female" steroid hormones, given their involvement in pregnancy and enhancement of female sexual differentiation. Nevertheless, such gender classification is relative to abundance and not absolute presence or absence given these steroids are indeed present in both genders with associated interconversions. The androgen receptor (AR) has two isoforms (AR-A, AR-B), as does the progesterone receptor (PR) with two isoforms (PR-A, PR-B) (Schumacher et al., 2014). Additionally, the progesterone receptor membrane component 1 (PGRMC1) is regulated by progesterone, although its role in signaling remains unclear (Su et al., 2012). There are two distinct estrogen receptors (ERα, ERβ) encoded by different genes, yet with multiple splice variants. Additionally, the G-protein-coupled estrogen receptor (GPER1, formerly GPR30) has been identified to bind estrogen and mediate rapid nongenomic signaling events (Rettberg, Yao, & Brinton, 2014). Although the gonadal steroids have similar regional distributions in the brain, actual concentrations are highly gender dependent (Vest & Pike, 2013; Wierman, 2007). Such gender dependency has implications in neuronal viability and conductivity, glial cell responses, and overall brain tissue activity, giving rise to gender-related differences in behavior and brain functioning (Schumacher et al., 2003). Alternately, glucocorticoids and mineralocorticoids are derived from the adrenal cortex, each having specific genes encoding their receptors. Even though only two genes encode for these receptors, respectively, there are associated isoforms that give rise to variable expression levels and transcriptional activity within the brain (Joels et al., 2012). The glucocorticoid receptor (GR) is quite ubiquitous in its expression and distribution in glial and neurons (Joels et al., 2012), while the mineralocorticoid receptor (MR) has a more restricted brain distribution, with various degrees of expression in the hippocampus, hypothalamus, cortex, and choroid plexus (Birmingham, Sar, & Stumpf, 1984; Nakano, Hirooka, Matsukawa, Ito, & Sunagawa, 2013; Oki, Gomez-Sanchez, & Gomez-Sanchez, 2012). Additionally, GR and MR isoforms have different affinities for many of the same endogenous and synthetic steroids, so changes in steroid concentrations in the brain can lead to variable shifts between MR and GR activity (Joels et al., 2012). Also of note is that certain endogenous glucocorticoids (i.e., corticosterone) have a pulsatile release pattern which is maintained across the BBB to target regions in the brain (Droste et al., 2008), implicating changes in brain tissue concentrations are dependent on a circadian cycle. The compounding factors of variable steroid levels, receptor isoforms, receptor density/localization, tissue function/health, endogenous versus synthetic ligands, enzymatic contributions, and ligand–receptor affinities each plays a role in determining steroidal action in the brain.

3.2. Therapeutic targeting of the CNS

Beyond what has been identified as traditional "housekeeping" roles, it is recognized that certain steroids (e.g., 17β-estradiol, progesterone) have a degree of neuroprotective action. Neuroprotection has been attributed to reducing edema, alleviating inflammatory processes, activating antiapoptotic pathways, counteracting excitotoxicity and oxidative stress, stimulating survival-promoting factors, myelin repair, and stabilizing the BBB

(Johann & Beyer, 2013; Reddy, 2010). As such, the list of specific CNS diseases/conditions proposed to be mitigated through steroidal-based treatments has grown almost exponentially over the last decade, often linked with gender-dependent variables (e.g., Parkinson's disease, Alzheimer's disease, Huntington's disease, stroke, schizophrenia, depression, epilepsy, drug dependence) (Giatti et al., 2012; Luchetti, Huitinga, & Swaab, 2011; Melcangi & Panzica, 2013; Melcangi et al., 2011; Reddy, 2010). Yet such proposals must be balanced by the wide array of side effects. For instance, while it has been demonstrated that some estrogens and progesterone are neuroprotective in various experimental models of acute neuronal injury (Johann & Beyer, 2013; Melcangi et al., 2011), chronic use may well contribute to cardiovascular disease and exacerbation of CNS pathology (Howard & Rossouw, 2013). Similarly, with the recent surge in marketing of testosterone to men, concerns have arisen regarding the detrimental contributions of androgens respective to stroke and neuroinflammation (Gonzales, 2013; Quillinan, Deng, Grewal, & Herson, 2014).

Glucocorticoid and mineralocorticoid use have a long therapeutic history, with glucocorticoids well noted for their immunosuppressive, antiinflammatory, and antiallergic activities. In this regard, glucocorticoids are utilized for numerous CNS conditions, in both direct treatment and prophylactically, as highlighted by their significant use in neurooncology. More than 50 years ago, it was shown that the glucocorticoid dexamethasone could alleviate cerebral edema due to tumors (Galicich, French, & Melby, 1961), via reducing BBB TJ permeability (Heiss et al., 1996; Papadopoulos et al., 2004). Glucocorticoids are not only beneficial in reducing brain tumor edema and intracranial pressure but also diminish chemotherapy-associated emesis, help control tumor-associated pain, and improve patient appetite (Dietrich, Rao, Pastorino, & Kesari, 2011). Nevertheless, while the use of glucocorticoids in the treatment of CNS diseases is well founded, there remain significant repercussions respective to side effects, both peripherally (e.g., infection, diabetes, glaucoma, osteoporosis) and centrally (e.g., psychosis, depression, memory decline, seizures) (Ciriaco et al., 2013; Poetker & Reh, 2010).

4. STEROID:BBB INTERACTION

Steroids have been identified to impact BBB transport processes and barrier integrity through various interdependent mechanisms. To date, much of what is known regarding such interactions has focused on estrogenic and glucocorticoid effects, for pragmatic reasons. First, both estrogens and glucocorticoids have many clinical uses, with various synthetic derivatives. Second, their impact on vascular endothelium has established clinical implications. Third, estrogen and GRs have been identified at the level of the cerebral microvasculature and shown to directly impact BBB regulation. A qualifying note respective to BBB–steroid interactions is that much of what is currently understood at the molecular level is derived from animal studies and/or various endothelial and epithelial cell studies, with numerous model variables and interpretation of results. Nevertheless, such data have shown to be invaluable in the understanding of clinical outcomes, as well as providing critical insight into CNS drug delivery irregularities.

4.1. Efflux transport

Many lipophilic molecules are effectively prevented from entering the brain via BBB efflux transporters. Such efflux is largely due to the expression of the adenosine triphosphate ATP-binding cassette (ABC) super family of transporters. The ABC efflux transporters at the BBB include P-glycoprotein (multidrug resistance protein-1 (MDR1); ABCB1), multidrug resistance-associated protein (multidrug resistance-associated protein (MRP); ABCC1,2,4,5), and breast cancer-related protein (BCRP; ABCG2) (Miller & Cannon, 2013). While evolutionarily ABC transporters help limit brain exposure to potentially toxic substances, they remain a substantial impediment to CNS-directed therapeutics. Many cellular processes contribute to the regulation of ABC efflux transporter activity, including transcriptional regulation that can be augmented via steroidal action.

Evidence shows certain endogenous (e.g., cortisol) and synthetic (e.g., dexamethasone) glucocorticoids are P-glycoprotein transporter substrates, limiting their access to the brain (Chan et al., 2013; Karssen et al., 2001; Meijer et al., 1998). Furthermore, in murine evaluations such glucocorticoids have been shown to be effective inducers of P-glycoprotein expression at the BBB (Bauer et al., 2004, 2006; Narang et al., 2008). Such induction has been identified to occur through the activation of both the GR and nuclear pregnane X receptor (PXR) pathways. Upon activation, PXR can promote the transcription of MDR1 and mdr1a/1b genes, which encode P-glycoprotein in humans and rodents, respectively (Cui,

Gunewardena, Rockwell, & Klaassen, 2010; Geick, Eichelbaum, & Burk, 2001). Given the significant structural diversity of agents that serve as ligands to PXR, including steroids, bile acids, dietary constituents, and various therapeutics (Chang & Waxman, 2006), multiple interactions and outcomes exist. Dexamethasone highlights such potential issues. Dexamethasone, a common use drug for numerous conditions including cancer chemotherapy, is a potent agonist of PXR/GR and an inducer of P-glycoprotein expression at the BBB (Bauer et al., 2004, 2006; Chan, Hoque, Cummins, & Bendayan, 2011). As many cancer chemotherapeutics are well-established substrates for P-glycoprotein (Nobili, Landini, Mazzei, & Mini, 2012), dexamethasone administration may lead to altered pharmacokinetics and diminished brain uptake of such therapeutics. Another corresponding implication of such effects is the impact of glucocorticoids on the developing brain. P-glycoprotein protection of the fetal brain has been shown to increase progressively with gestational age, with enhanced functioning also shown with dexamethasone administration (Iqbal, Gibb, & Matthews, 2011; Petropoulos, Gibb, & Matthews, 2010). In this regard, use of glucocorticoids may prove protective to the developing CNS under certain conditions of maternal exposure to toxicants.

Estrogenic actions have been particularly noted with respect to BCRP, as evaluated *ex vivo* via rodent brain capillaries. The use of 17β-estradiol has shown to modulate BCRP activity through both ERα and ERβ, reducing BBB BCRP transport activity at nanomolar concentrations (Hartz, Mahringer, Miller, & Bauer, 2010). Yet interestingly, extended 17β-estradiol exposure (6 h) has shown to reduce both activity and expression strictly via ERβ-mediated processes (Hartz, Madole, Miller, & Bauer, 2010; Mahringer & Fricker, 2010). The ERβ signaling pathways have been shown to increase the ubiquitination of the BCRP protein, leading to its degradation by the proteasome (Hartz, Madole, et al., 2010). These findings have broad reaching implications, especially when placed in context of hormone-replacement therapies and enhanced cerebrovascular complications with age, or even within the context of exposure to environmental xenoestrogens (e.g., pesticides, dichlorodiphenyltrichloroethane (DDT), bisphenol). Effectively reducing BCRP efflux activity may not only enhance brain exposure to toxins but may also alter the normal brain levels of endogenous estrogens. Given the observed decrease in cognitive function in postmenopausal women on estrogen therapy (Espeland et al., 2004; Resnick et al., 2004), the questions must be asked as to whether the impact on the BBB may in part play some role. Alternatively, it may be viable to use targeted estrogens to reduce BCRP transport activity as a means to enhance brain uptake of other known BCRP substrates (e.g., cancer chemotherapeutics) (Noguchi, Katayama, & Sugimoto, 2014).

Another category often overlooked respective to efflux at the BBB is the organic anion transporters (OATs), which form a superfamily of Na-independent transport systems that mediate the transmembrane transport of a wide range of amphipathic endogenous and exogenous organic anions. Certain OATs have been identified in the efflux of amphipathic and hydrophilic organic acidic substances, Oatp1a4 (Slco1a4) and Oat-3 (Slc22a8), respectively, at the BBB (Emami Riedmaier, Nies, Schaeffeler, & Schwab, 2012). Oatp1a4 and Oat-3 appear to mediate the efflux of dehydroepiandrosterone sulfate (DHEAS) from the murine brain (Asaba et al., 2000; Miyajima, Kusuhara, Fujishima, Adachi, & Sugiyama, 2011). DHEAS is the sulfate ester of DHEA, which is produced in the CNS and periphery with wide-reaching impact. Moreover, AR-mediated regulation of Oat-3 function at the *in vitro* BBB has also been shown through induction of dihydrotestosterone, which lies downstream of DHEAS (Ohtsuki et al., 2005). Actions of Oat-3 also extend to transport regulation of cortisol and estradiol-17β-glucuronide (Emami Riedmaier et al., 2012). Given the number of other therapeutics and endogenous molecules impacted by OATs, there remains limited understanding as to how these transporters may impact the direct function of the BBB or contribute to CNS pathology.

4.2. Nutrient transport

Nutrient transporters at the BBB are relatively well defined, yet species differences have been reported, along with variations in expression and function dependent on model used. Additionally, gene expression has been shown for many transporters without full functional characterization to date (Dahlin, Royall, Hohmann, & Wang, 2009). Currently, evaluations of nutrient transport at the BBB have identified estrogenic interactions with the Na–K–Cl cotransporter- and sodium-independent GLUT1.

Recent studies have been geared toward identifying whether neuroprotective/anti-edema effects of estrogens corresponding with ischemic stroke may be derived through the BBB Na–K–Cl cotransporter. The impact of 17β-estradiol was assessed respective to the lumenal Na–K–Cl cotransporter at the BBB in ischemic stroke modeling (rodent), as well as in extracted cerebral microvascular endothelial cells (bovine) with hypoxia (Chang, O'Donnell, & Barakat, 2008; O'Donnell, Lam, Tran, Foroutan, & Anderson, 2006). These evaluations showed an estrogen-dependent regulation of the Na–K–Cl cotransporter, corresponding with the ability to mitigate brain swelling and lesion volume. Interestingly, 17β-estradiol also played a role in shear-stress-related regulation of the Na–K–Cl cotransporter (Chang et al., 2008), as well as reducing the aquaporin-4 abundance on the astrocytic end feet (Rutkowsky, Wallace, Wise, & O'Donnell, 2011). Such interactions highlight steroidal impact across the various components of the NVU, and in this case helping to reduce ischemia-induced brain edema.

Arguably, the most critical moment-to-moment transporter at the BBB is the GLUT1, which ensures adequate glucose uptake to the brain (Cornford, Nguyen, & Landaw, 2000; Leybaert, 2005). While GLUT1 is a low-affinity transporter, it is extremely sensitive to alterations in glucose levels. 17β-Estradiol has been shown to enhance GLUT1 expression, inducing rapid response changes in glucose uptake into the brain (Cheng, Cohen, Wang, & Bondy, 2001; Shi & Simpkins, 1997; Shi, Zhang, & Simpkins, 1997). Additionally, reduced estrogen concentrations via ovariectomization of female rats corresponded to reduced GLUT1 mRNA, which was reversible with 17β-estradiol treatment (Shi et al., 1997). Such effects correlate to neurodegenerative disease incidence. For example, the increased incidence of Alzheimer's disease in postmenopausal females corresponds with declining GLUT1 transporter levels (Liu, Liu, Iqbal, Grundke-Iqbal, & Gong, 2008; Simpson & Davies, 1994; Vest & Pike, 2013). Thus, it is plausible that the neuroprotective effects identified with estrogens may in part be related to the enhanced nutrient transport across the BBB.

4.3. Barrier integrity

Alterations in BBB interendothelial integrity may be brought about by mechanical (e.g., shear stress), biochemical (e.g., enzymes, inflammatory mediators), and/or molecular (e.g., transactivation/transrepression) pathways. Such mechanisms directly or indirectly impact the TJ proteins, with corresponding changes in paracellular permeability. Steroidal contributions to the BBB TJ response are complex and often condition specific. For instance, shortly after glucocorticoids were introduced for the treatment of brain tumor edema (Galicich et al., 1961), high-dose glucocorticoids became commonplace in the treatment of traumatic brain injury owing to the assumed benefits. However, multiple clinical trials in the 1980s and 1990s found no clear benefit in this regard. In fact, the large-scale Corticosteroid Randomization After Significant Head-Injury (CRASH) trial had to be terminated early due to unexpected increased mortality associated with glucocorticoids (Roberts et al., 2004). It has been proposed that the high-dose use of glucocorticoids (methylprednisolone) may have had too broad of an impact on the inflammatory response (Beauchamp, Mutlak, Smith, Shohami, & Stahel, 2008), with little consideration as to the time frame of initiation, dose, and BBB effects.

It has been established for quite some time that glucocorticoids directly influence BBB integrity through the TJ proteins. Evaluations of BBB integrity against dexamethasone in rodent models showed regional reductions in TJ permeability under standard conditions, with a corresponding rebound in permeability subsequent to discontinuation (Ziylan, LeFauconnier, Bernard, & Bourre, 1988; Ziylan, Lefauconnier, Bernard, & Bourre, 1989). Glucocorticoids have been shown to restore and/or preserve the TJs via upregulation of both occludin and claudin-5 to the TJ cleft, with associated two- to threefold increases in TEER (mouse and human endothelial cells) (Forster et al., 2008, 2005; Kashiwamura et al., 2011). This response is conferred via the occludin-enhancer element, demonstrated to have homology to elements in other steroid-responsive junctional genes including claudin-5 (retinal endothelial cells) (Felinski, Cox, Phillips, & Antonetti, 2008; Keil, Liu, & Antonetti, 2013). Glucocorticoid treatment has also shown to increase VE-cadherin protein levels at the adherens junction in murine brain endothelial cEND cells (Blecharz, Drenckhahn, & Forster, 2008). Interestingly, VE-cadherin has shown to upregulate the gene encoding for claudin-5 in peripheral endothelial cells (Taddei et al., 2008), identifying overlapping pathways in which glucocorticoids may effect TJ integrity. Whether such interactions hold true at the level of the BBB endothelium have yet to be elucidated.

Glucocorticoid repression of inflammatory mechanisms has also been identified to mitigate BBB TJ permeability and leukocyte diapedesis with corresponding benefits. At the level of the endothelium, glucocorticoids affect many inflammatory response genes and cellular response signals. Glucocorticoids inhibit nuclear factor kappa-light-chain-enhancer of activated B cells (NFκB) signaling, counteracting the inflammatory expression of cellular adhesion molecules (CAMs) (Dietrich, 2006). CAMs provide for leukocyte–endothelial cell interactions necessary for diapedesis. Various

CNS pathologies are associated with enhanced leukocyte transmigration (e.g., multiple sclerosis, bacterial meningitis), with corresponding enhancement of BBB TJ permeability (Abbott et al., 2010). Glucocorticoids have also shown to reduce tumor necrosis factor α (TNFα)-induced intercellular adhesion molecule-1 (ICAM-1) and vascular cell adhesion protein-1 (VCAM-1) expression in human brain endothelial cells (Gelati et al., 2000). Moreover, the loss of TJ integrity with administration of TNFα has been shown to be reversed via glucocorticoid treatment in human brain endothelial cells (hCMEC/D3), associated with the relative stabilization of occludin protein expression levels (Forster et al., 2008). The corresponding impact on circulating inflammatory activators is also critical. For instance, monocyte-chemoattractant protein-1 (MCP1/CCL2) is a key chemokine that regulates migration and infiltration of monocytes/macrophages, demonstrated to be involved in various CNS conditions, including human immunodeficiency virus (HIV) dementia, Alzheimer's disease, stroke, and multiple sclerosis (Yao & Tsirka, 2014). MCP1 has shown to increase BBB permeability, via redistribution of TJ proteins affiliated with actin-myosin contraction (Song & Pachter, 2004; Stamatovic et al., 2005; Yao & Tsirka, 2014), as well as disruption of the adherens junctions (Roberts et al., 2012). Glucocorticoid treatment has shown to reduce the upregulation of secreted MCP1 after activation by TNFα, interleukin-1β (IL-1β), and interferon-γ (IFNγ) (Harkness, Sussman, Davies-Jones, Greenwood, & Woodroofe, 2003). Another key aspect involves glucocorticoid impact on the enzymatic degradation of the BBB extracellular matrix. Inflammatory induction of matrix metalloproteinases (MMPs) contributes to the degradation of the extracellular matrix, affiliated with BBB TJ disruption in conditions such as multiple sclerosis and ischemic stroke (Mirshafiey, Asghari, Ghalamfarsa, Jadidi-Niaragh, & Azizi, 2014; Sandoval & Witt, 2008; Yang & Rosenberg, 2011). In murine microvessel, endothelial cells exposed to serum from multiple sclerosis patients, the enhancement of MMP-9 expression corresponded with the downregulation of occludin and claudin-5 mRNA and protein levels (Blecharz et al., 2010). Active MMPs can be blocked via endogenous MMP inhibitors (tissue inhibitors of MMPs; tissue inhibitors of matrix metalloproteinases (TIMPs)). In this regard, glucocorticoids have been identified to upregulate TIMP-1 and TIMP-3 (Forster, Kahles, Kietz, & Drenckhahn, 2007; Hartmann et al., 2009), thus inhibiting the MMP-mediated breakdown of the extracellular matrix.

Neovascularization also contributes to altered BBB integrity, which may occur in tandem with inflammatory and neurodegenerative processes.

Endothelial growth factors are well identified with neovascularization under such conditions (Sandoval & Witt, 2008). In this context, the majority of BBB evaluations to date have focused on vascular endothelial growth factor (VEGF), a key regulator of angiogenesis. VEGF has been identified to increase TJ permeability via VEGF receptor-2 activation, corresponding with decreased ZO-1 and occludin expression in brain microvessel endothelial cells (Harhaj & Antonetti, 2004; Wang, Dentler, & Borchardt, 2001). In turn, another growth factor, angiopoietin-1 has shown to block VEGF-induced BBB TJ permeability, as well as decrease MMP-9 activity (Valable et al., 2005). Glucocorticoids have shown to increase angiopoietin-1 mRNA and protein in the brain, with corresponding stabilization of the BBB and reduced paracellular permeability (Kim et al., 2008). In animal modeling of acute ischemic stroke, angiopoietin-1 actions have been shown to prevent ischemic lesion volume and plasma leakage into the brain (Thurston et al., 2000; Zhang & Chopp, 2002). Nevertheless, actual clinical applications are not straight forward along these lines, as glucocorticoid treatment applied to acute ischemic stroke in humans appears either ineffective or actually harmful (Poungvarin, 2004). Nevertheless, controversy and conflicting opinions as to glucocorticoid use in ischemic stroke remain (Norris, 2004). The implication being that time frame of initiation, dose, comorbidities, and the peripheral impact of glucocorticoids must also be factored in and appropriately evaluated against short- and long-term recovery measures.

While not as robust as glucocorticoids, estrogens have been shown to reduce endothelial inflammatory activation. Estrogens inhibit cytokine-mediated endothelial CAM transcriptional activation. In brain endothelial cells, 17β-estradiol inhibited the IL-1β-mediated activation of NFκB and expression of the ICAM-1 (Galea et al., 2002). Similarly, 17β-estradiol has shown to inhibit TNFα-induced NFκB activation of VCAM-1 through ERα-mediated mechanisms (Mori, Tsukahara, Yoshioka, Irie, & Ohta, 2004). As addressed previously, NFκB activation at the BBB enhances TJ permeability (Dietrich, 2006; Huber, Campos, Mark, & Davis, 2005). Moreover, 17β-estradiol has been shown to attenuate astrocyte-derived release of NFκB, IL-1β, TNFα, and MMP-9 in models of inflammatory injury (Dodel, Du, Bales, Gao, & Paul, 1999; Lewis, Johnson, Stohlgren, Harms, & Sohrabji, 2008), as well as increase angiotensin-1 and microvessel density in experimental stroke (Ardelt et al., 2005). Thus, neuroprotective actions of estrogens may in part be from the mitigation of BBB permeability respective to a reduction of inflammatory mediators. In animal models of stroke, estrogen has been shown to be protective of the brain when given as a pretreatment (Dubal et al., 1998) as well as subsequent to the ischemic injury (Liu et al., 2005; Yang, Liu, Wu, & Simpkins, 2003), respective to reduced infarct volumes. Correspondingly, estrogen treatment in women has shown to enhance recovery subsequent to cerebral ischemia (Paganini-Hill, Ross, & Henderson, 1988; Schmidt et al., 1996). Yet once again controversies arise, as estrogen's effects are not only dependent on dose and time of exposure but also highly dependent on reproductive/postmenopausal age (Rettberg et al., 2014; Sohrabji, Bake, & Lewis, 2013). Case-in-point, chronic 17β-estradiol treatment given to postmenopausal women (Women's Estrogen for Stroke Trial; WEST) was identified with an increased risk of fatal stroke and a worsening of neurological outcomes (Viscoli et al., 2001). Similar increased stroke risk has been shown with estrogen and estrogen-progestin treatment (Women's Health Initiative; WHI) (Wassertheil-Smoller et al., 2003). In this regard, age of treatment initiation appears a critical factor, as the aforementioned studies incorporated women of an age that was well beyond normal menopause onset (age averages: WEST, 71 years; WHI, 63 years). These studies parallel the Women's Health Initiative Memory Study (WHIMS), which identified chronic estrogen use was detrimental if initiated well after menopause, giving rise to the "critical window" theory of hormone replacement (Brinton, 2005; Rettberg et al., 2014). Subsequent investigations in animal models of ischemic stroke corroborate this theory, as chronic estrogen treatment in ovariectomized senescent female rats was shown to increase infarct volumes compared to younger treatment-matched females (Leon, Li, Huber, & Rosen, 2012; Selvamani & Sohrabji, 2010). The idea that the aging brain is refractory to the neuroprotective attributes of estrogens, or at least as it corresponds to long-term administration, underscores the importance of treatment time frame respective to age/menopausal onset. As to the contributions of altered BBB integrity to such disparities, age-dependent inflammatory responses may provide some insight. Estrogen replacement in young ovariectomized animals has been shown to decrease brain IL-1β levels, whereas estrogen treatment enhanced IL-1β expression in ovariectomized aged females (Nordell, Scarborough, Buchanan, & Sohrabji, 2003). Similar effects have also been noted with MMP-9 and TNFα (Johnson & Sohrabji, 2005). As such, the altered inflammatory responses/mediators with increasing age may result in a comparatively proinflammatory state, corresponding to a BBB with a reduced resilience to injury.

Factors beyond overt inflammation have also been identified respective to estrogen effects on BBB integrity. Nevertheless, age remains a primary element. Compounded aging effects associated with reduced cerebral-blood flow (Schultz et al., 1999), altered NVU interactions and angiogenic responses (Sohrabji et al., 2013), and general declines in endogenous hormones are all likely contributors. While the pathways by which estrogens mediate brain responses and neuroprotection have been strongly linked to ERα activation, ERβ and the ERα/ERβ ratios have also been strongly implicated respective to the cerebrovasculature (Spence & Voskuhl, 2012). In rat brain microvessels, expression of ERα and ERβ has been shown to decrease with age and ovariectomization, which was reversible with 17β-estradiol treatment (Jesmin et al., 2003; Sandoval & Witt, 2011; Stirone, Duckles, & Krause, 2003). Correspondingly, in ovariectomized aged rats, paracellular permeability (hippocampus and olfactory bulb) was shown to be significantly higher than in matched younger animals (Bake & Sohrabji, 2004). Furthermore, young animals treated with 17β-estradiol showed a greater reversal of paracellular permeability than aged animals, with the aged rats actually showing an exacerbation of hippocampal permeability (Bake & Sohrabji, 2004). In a similar evaluation, occludin expression levels where shown to effectively rebound in young ovariectomized animals when treated with 17β-estradiol; whereas aged animals showed no changes in occludin expression with 17β-estradiol treatment (Sandoval & Witt, 2011). Yet interestingly, both young and aged animals showed increased claudin-5 and ERα expression with 17β-estradiol treatment (Sandoval & Witt, 2011). 17β-Estradiol has been shown to increase claudin-5 promoter activity, mRNA, and protein levels corresponding to enhancement of TEER readings in murine microvascular endothelial cells (Burek et al., 2010; Burek et al., 2014). Taken together, this would implicate occludin as an estrogen-responsive and age-dependent component of the TJ protein; whereas claudin-5 appears to be estrogen-responsive regardless of the age component. Also of recent note are the GPER1-mediated actions of estrogens. GPER1 has been identified in human and mouse cerebral endothelial cells, capable of modulating the nitric oxide (NO) pathway corresponding to ischemic/hypoxic responsive actions and antiproliferative mechanisms (Holm, Baldetorp, Olde, Leeb-Lundberg, & Nilsson, 2011; Murata, Dietrich, Xiang, & Dacey, 2013; Tu & Jufri, 2013). To date, age-associated effects of GPER1 on the cerebrovasculature have yet to be investigated. In the end, estrogen regulation of BBB integrity appears to be dependent on a complex interaction of age, inflammatory mediation, and estrogen receptor activity, as well as form of estrogen-replacement therapy used.

4.4. Other considerations

As our knowledge of BBB structure and function progresses, the impact of the NVU as a whole becomes more apparent. Neuronal-endothelial communications are thought to be principally routed through astrocytes (Koehler, Gebremedhin, & Harder, 2006), and may well incorporate nongenomic pathways. While the understanding of nongenomic steroid action is still in its infancy, such pathways would fit the criteria for rapid signaling responses to the BBB endothelium necessary to meet the moment-to-moment needs of the brain. In this regard, differences in localization of respective steroid receptors within the brain may account for certain regional variations in BBB integrity. Additionally, astrocytes have come to the forefront as mediators of cerebral-blood flow, brain edema, and inflammation (Johann & Beyer, 2013; Sohrabji et al., 2013). Though not unexpected given the highly supportive nature of astrocytes, astrocyte–steroid interactions respective to BBB function is only beginning to be addressed. Lastly, steroid impact on pericytes has been almost entirely overlooked to date.

Another critical aspect is the effect of steroids at the level of the mitochondria within the BBB endothelium. With the numerous energy-dependent processes required of the BBB, mitochondrial alterations and associated shifts in bioenergetics may underlie changes in function and integrity. A substantial number of signal pathways regulated by estrogens converge upon the mitochondria, linking cerebrovascular disease, inflammation, and aging (Rettberg et al., 2014). Studies have shown ERα and ERβ directly bind mitochondrial DNA (mtDNA) through mitochondrial estrogen-response elements, with 17β-estradiol increasing the associated binding response (Chen, Eshete, Alworth, & Yager, 2004). Furthermore, 17β-estradiol increases mitochondrial biogenesis and suppresses mitochondrial production of reactive oxygen species in human brain microvascular endothelial cells via ERα (Guo et al., 2010; Razmara et al., 2008). Given the potential of mtDNA damage with age and pathology, the mitochondrial protective effects of estrogens may be essential to the preservation of BBB function.

Though the direct effects of progestogens, androgens, and mineralocorticoids have not been extensively investigated in regards to BBB effects, the actions of their respective receptors do impact overall brain function, inflammation, and blood flow with corresponding implications. Neuroprotective actions of progestogens have been noted for many conditions, through genomic and nongenomic pathways similar to estrogen. Progesterone has shown to attenuate cerebral edema by inhibiting MMP-9 levels and reducing astrocyte aquaporin-4 expression (Wang et al., 2013). Treatment with progesterone plus tissue plasminogen activator (tPA) has shown to ameliorate hemorrhage, edema, BBB permeability, MMP-9 induction, and VEGF levels compared with controls (Won, Lee, Wali, Stein, & Sayeed, 2014). Androgens have a more dubious reputation, affiliated with proinflammatory actions and detrimental outcomes mediated through ARs at the cerebrovasculature (Gonzales, 2013; Gonzales, Duckles, & Krause, 2009). Yet, some condition dependent antiinflammatory activities for androgens have also been noted, subject to the time frame of use (Gonzales, 2013). Mineralocorticoid impact on the BBB is primary related to blood pressure (Joels et al., 2012). However, aldosterone has also been identified to interact with GPER1. While controversy remains over aldosterone–GPER1 interactions, a functional cross talk between MR and GPER1 does appear to exist, capable of impacting acute vascular responses within the body (Evans, Bayliss, & Reale, 2014; Prossnitz & Barton, 2014). Nevertheless, the greatest impact of progestogens, androgens, and mineralocorticoids on BBB function may actually be through their subsequent metabolism and/or impact on other steroid receptors. For instance, progesterone has well-established antiandrogen and antimineralocorticoid effects (Schumacher et al., 2014), and testosterone can be readily converted to 17β-estradiol, thus impact ERs (Gonzales, 2013).

5. CONCLUSION

Therapeutics targeted to the steroid receptors continue to serve as primary medications for various acute and chronic conditions. Moreover, the significant potential of such medications to mitigate CNS pathology and age-dependent cognitive dysfunctions put them at the forefront of medical research. It is well recognized that the BBB is a primary focus of CNS-targeted therapies, not simply as the impediment to brain delivery but as a potential contributor to pathological outcomes and as a therapeutic target itself. Yet while our understanding of steroid–BBB interactions has grown, much remains to be elucidated. What is the impact of continuous synthetic steroid use versus the regulated release of endogenous steroids on BBB function? Does the BBB play a role in glucocorticoid/estrogen resistance? Perhaps foremost, how may steroid-based therapeutics, agonists and antagonists, be optimized with consideration to BBB dynamics? Further investigations of the genomic and nongenomic steroid pathways and their impact on BBB regulation are clearly required. Given the added complexity respective the other components of the NVU and the associated steroidal interactions therein, it is safe to say we have only touch the surface.

CONFLICT OF INTEREST

The authors have no conflicts of interest.

REFERENCES

Abbott, N. J., Patabendige, A. A., Dolman, D. E., Yusof, S. R., & Begley, D. J. (2010). Structure and function of the blood-brain barrier. *Neurobiology of Disease*, *37*, 13–25.

Ardelt, A. A., McCullough, L. D., Korach, K. S., Wang, M. M., Munzenmaier, D. H., & Hurn, P. D. (2005). Estradiol regulates angiopoietin-1 mRNA expression through estrogen receptor-alpha in a rodent experimental stroke model. *Stroke*, *36*, 337–341.

Asaba, H., Hosoya, K., Takanaga, H., Ohtsuki, S., Tamura, E., Takizawa, T., et al. (2000). Blood-brain barrier is involved in the efflux transport of a neuroactive steroid, dehydroepiandrosterone sulfate, via organic anion transporting polypeptide 2. *Journal of Neurochemistry*, *75*, 1907–1916.

Bake, S., & Sohrabji, F. (2004). 17beta-Estradiol differentially regulates blood-brain barrier permeability in young and aging female rats. *Endocrinology*, *145*, 5471–5475.

Banks, W. A., & Erickson, M. A. (2010). The blood-brain barrier and immune function and dysfunction. *Neurobiology of Disease*, *37*, 26–32.

Bauer, B., Hartz, A. M., Fricker, G., & Miller, D. S. (2004). Pregnane X receptor up-regulation of P-glycoprotein expression and transport function at the blood-brain barrier. *Molecular Pharmacology*, *66*, 413–419.

Bauer, B., Yang, X., Hartz, A. M., Olson, E. R., Zhao, R., Kalvass, J. C., et al. (2006). In vivo activation of human pregnane X receptor tightens the blood-brain barrier to methadone through P-glycoprotein up-regulation. *Molecular Pharmacology*, *70*, 1212–1219.

Baulieu, E. E. (1997). Neurosteroids: Of the nervous system, by the nervous system, for the nervous system. *Recent Progress in Hormone Research*, *52*, 1–32.

Beauchamp, K., Mutlak, H., Smith, W. R., Shohami, E., & Stahel, P. F. (2008). Pharmacology of traumatic brain injury: Where is the "golden bullet"? *Molecular Medicine*, *14*, 731–740.

Birmingham, M. K., Sar, M., & Stumpf, W. E. (1984). Localization of aldosterone and corticosterone in the central nervous system, assessed by quantitative autoradiography. *Neurochemical Research*, *9*, 333–350.

Blecharz, K. G., Drenckhahn, D., & Forster, C. Y. (2008). Glucocorticoids increase VE-cadherin expression and cause cytoskeletal rearrangements in murine brain endothelial cEND cells. *Journal of Cerebral Blood Flow and Metabolism*, *28*, 1139–1149.

Blecharz, K. G., Haghikia, A., Stasiolek, M., Kruse, N., Drenckhahn, D., Gold, R., et al. (2010). Glucocorticoid effects on endothelial barrier function in the murine brain endothelial cell line cEND incubated with sera from patients with multiple sclerosis. *Multiple Sclerosis*, *16*, 293–302.

Brinton, R. D. (2005). Investigative models for determining hormone therapy-Induced outcomes in brain: Evidence in support of a healthy cell bias of estrogen action. *Annals of the New York Academy of Sciences*, *1052*, 57–74.

Burek, M., Arias-Loza, P. A., Roewer, N., & Forster, C. Y. (2010). Claudin-5 as a novel estrogen target in vascular endothelium. *Arteriosclerosis, Thrombosis, and Vascular Biology*, *30*, 298–304.

Burek, M., Steinberg, K., & Forster, C. Y. (2014). Mechanisms of transcriptional activation of the mouse claudin-5 promoter by estrogen receptor alpha and beta. *Molecular and Cellular Endocrinology*, *392*(1–2), 144–151.

Butt, A. M., Jones, H. C., & Abbott, N. J. (1990). Electrical resistance across the blood-brain barrier in anaesthetized rats: A developmental study. *The Journal of Physiology*, *429*, 47–62.

Chan, G. N., Hoque, M. T., Cummins, C. L., & Bendayan, R. (2011). Regulation of P-glycoprotein by orphan nuclear receptors in human brain microvessel endothelial cells. *Journal of Neurochemistry*, *118*, 163–175.

Chan, G. N., Saldivia, V., Yang, Y., Pang, H., de Lannoy, I., & Bendayan, R. (2013). In vivo induction of P-glycoprotein expression at the mouse blood-brain barrier: An intracerebral microdialysis study. *Journal of Neurochemistry*, *127*, 342–352.

Chang, E., O'Donnell, M. E., & Barakat, A. I. (2008). Shear stress and 17beta-estradiol modulate cerebral microvascular endothelial Na-K-Cl cotransporter and Na/H exchanger protein levels. *American Journal of Physiology. Cell Physiology*, *294*, C363–C371.

Chang, T. K., & Waxman, D. J. (2006). Synthetic drugs and natural products as modulators of constitutive androstane receptor (CAR) and pregnane X receptor (PXR). *Drug Metabolism Reviews*, *38*, 51–73.

Chen, J. Q., Eshete, M., Alworth, W. L., & Yager, J. D. (2004). Binding of MCF-7 cell mitochondrial proteins and recombinant human estrogen receptors alpha and beta to human mitochondrial DNA estrogen response elements. *Journal of Cellular Biochemistry*, *93*, 358–373.

Cheng, C. M., Cohen, M., Wang, J., & Bondy, C. A. (2001). Estrogen augments glucose transporter and IGF1 expression in primate cerebral cortex. *Faseb Journal*, *15*, 907–915.

Ciriaco, M., Ventrice, P., Russo, G., Scicchitano, M., Mazzitello, G., Scicchitano, F., et al. (2013). Corticosteroid-related central nervous system side effects. *Journal of Pharmacology and Pharmacotherapeutics*, *4*, S94–S98.

Cornford, E. M., Nguyen, E. V., & Landaw, E. M. (2000). Acute upregulation of blood-brain barrier glucose transporter activity in seizures. *American Journal of Physiology. Heart and Circulatory Physiology*, *279*, H1346–H1354.

Cui, J. Y., Gunewardena, S. S., Rockwell, C. E., & Klaassen, C. D. (2010). ChIPing the cistrome of PXR in mouse liver. *Nucleic Acids Research*, *38*, 7943–7963.

Dahlin, A., Royall, J., Hohmann, J. G., & Wang, J. (2009). Expression profiling of the solute carrier gene family in the mouse brain. *The Journal of Pharmacology and Experimental Therapeutics*, *329*, 558–570.

Dietrich, J. (2006). Glucocorticoid hormones and estrogens: Their interaction with the endothelial cells of the blood-brain barrier. In R. Dermietzel, D. C. Spray, & M. Nedergaard (Eds.), *Blood-brain interfaces: From ontogeny to artificial barriers: Vol. 1.* (pp. 287–312): Weinheim, Germany: Wiley.

Dietrich, J., Rao, K., Pastorino, S., & Kesari, S. (2011). Corticosteroids in brain cancer patients: Benefits and pitfalls. *Expert Review of Clinical Pharmacology*, *4*, 233–242.

Dodel, R. C., Du, Y., Bales, K. R., Gao, F., & Paul, S. M. (1999). Sodium salicylate and 17beta-estradiol attenuate nuclear transcription factor NF-kappaB translocation in cultured rat astroglial cultures following exposure to amyloid A beta(1–40) and lipopolysaccharides. *Journal of Neurochemistry*, *73*, 1453–1460.

Droste, S. K., de Groote, L., Atkinson, H. C., Lightman, S. L., Reul, J. M., & Linthorst, A. C. (2008). Corticosterone levels in the brain show a distinct ultradian rhythm but a delayed response to forced swim stress. *Endocrinology, 149*, 3244–3253.

Dubal, D. B., Kashon, M. L., Pettigrew, L. C., Ren, J. M., Finklestein, S. P., Rau, S. W., et al. (1998). Estradiol protects against ischemic injury. *Journal of Cerebral Blood Flow and Metabolism, 18*, 1253–1258.

Emami Riedmaier, A., Nies, A. T., Schaeffeler, E., & Schwab, M. (2012). Organic anion transporters and their implications in pharmacotherapy. *Pharmacological Reviews, 64*, 421–449.

Espeland, M. A., Rapp, S. R., Shumaker, S. A., Brunner, R., Manson, J. E., Sherwin, B. B., et al. (2004). Conjugated equine estrogens and global cognitive function in postmenopausal women: Women's Health Initiative Memory Study. *JAMA, 291*, 2959–2968.

Evans, P. D., Bayliss, A., & Reale, V. (2014). GPCR-mediated rapid, non-genomic actions of steroids: Comparisons between DmDopEcR and GPER1 (GPR30). *General and Comparative Endocrinology, 195*, 157–163.

Feldman, G. J., Mullin, J. M., & Ryan, M. P. (2005). Occludin: Structure, function and regulation. *Advanced Drug Delivery Reviews, 57*, 883–917.

Felinski, E. A., Cox, A. E., Phillips, B. E., & Antonetti, D. A. (2008). Glucocorticoids induce transactivation of tight junction genes occludin and claudin-5 in retinal endothelial cells via a novel cis-element. *Experimental Eye Research, 86*, 867–878.

Forster, C., Burek, M., Romero, I. A., Weksler, B., Couraud, P. O., & Drenckhahn, D. (2008). Differential effects of hydrocortisone and TNFalpha on tight junction proteins in an in vitro model of the human blood-brain barrier. *The Journal of Physiology, 586*, 1937–1949.

Forster, C., Kahles, T., Kietz, S., & Drenckhahn, D. (2007). Dexamethasone induces the expression of metalloproteinase inhibitor TIMP-1 in the murine cerebral vascular endothelial cell line cEND. *The Journal of Physiology, 580*, 937–949.

Forster, C., Silwedel, C., Golenhofen, N., Burek, M., Kietz, S., Mankertz, J., et al. (2005). Occludin as direct target for glucocorticoid-induced improvement of blood-brain barrier properties in a murine in vitro system. *The Journal of Physiology, 565*, 475–486.

Galea, E., Santizo, R., Feinstein, D. L., Adamsom, P., Greenwood, J., Koenig, H. M., et al. (2002). Estrogen inhibits NF kappa B-dependent inflammation in brain endothelium without interfering with I kappa B degradation. *Neuroreport, 13*, 1469–1472.

Galicich, J. H., French, L. A., & Melby, J. C. (1961). Use of dexamethasone in treatment of cerebral edema associated with brain tumors. *The Journal-Lancet, 81*, 46–53.

Geick, A., Eichelbaum, M., & Burk, O. (2001). Nuclear receptor response elements mediate induction of intestinal MDR1 by rifampin. *The Journal of Biological Chemistry, 276*, 14581–14587.

Gelati, M., Corsini, E., Dufour, A., Massa, G., Giombini, S., Solero, C. L., et al. (2000). High-dose methylprednisolone reduces cytokine-induced adhesion molecules on human brain endothelium. *The Canadian Journal of Neurological Sciences, 27*, 241–244.

Giannotta, M., Trani, M., & Dejana, E. (2013). VE-cadherin and endothelial adherens junctions: Active guardians of vascular integrity. *Developmental Cell, 26*, 441–454.

Giatti, S., Boraso, M., Melcangi, R. C., & Viviani, B. (2012). Neuroactive steroids, their metabolites, and neuroinflammation. *Journal of Molecular Endocrinology, 49*, R125–R134.

Gonzales, R. J. (2013). Androgens and the cerebrovasculature: Modulation of vascular function during normal and pathophysiological conditions. *Pflügers Archiv, 465*, 627–642.

Gonzales, R. J., Duckles, S. P., & Krause, D. N. (2009). Dihydrotestosterone stimulates cerebrovascular inflammation through NFkappaB, modulating contractile function. *Journal of Cerebral Blood Flow and Metabolism, 29*, 244–253.

Guo, J., Krause, D. N., Horne, J., Weiss, J. H., Li, X., & Duckles, S. P. (2010). Estrogen-receptor-mediated protection of cerebral endothelial cell viability and mitochondrial function after ischemic insult in vitro. *Journal of Cerebral Blood Flow and Metabolism*, *30*, 545–554.

Harhaj, N. S., & Antonetti, D. A. (2004). Regulation of tight junctions and loss of barrier function in pathophysiology. *The International Journal of Biochemistry & Cell Biology*, *36*, 1206–1237.

Harkness, K. A., Sussman, J. D., Davies-Jones, G. A., Greenwood, J., & Woodroofe, M. N. (2003). Cytokine regulation of MCP-1 expression in brain and retinal microvascular endothelial cells. *Journal of Neuroimmunology*, *142*, 1–9.

Hartmann, C., El-Gindi, J., Lohmann, C., Lischper, M., Zeni, P., & Galla, H. J. (2009). TIMP-3: A novel target for glucocorticoid signaling at the blood-brain barrier. *Biochemical and Biophysical Research Communications*, *390*, 182–186.

Hartz, A. M., Madole, E. K., Miller, D. S., & Bauer, B. (2010). Estrogen receptor beta signaling through phosphatase and tensin homolog/phosphoinositide 3-kinase/Akt/glycogen synthase kinase 3 down-regulates blood-brain barrier breast cancer resistance protein. *The Journal of Pharmacology and Experimental Therapeutics*, *334*, 467–476.

Hartz, A. M., Mahringer, A., Miller, D. S., & Bauer, B. (2010). 17-beta-Estradiol: A powerful modulator of blood-brain barrier BCRP activity. *Journal of Cerebral Blood Flow and Metabolism*, *30*, 1742–1755.

Heiss, J. D., Papavassiliou, E., Merrill, M. J., Nieman, L., Knightly, J. J., Walbridge, S., et al. (1996). Mechanism of dexamethasone suppression of brain tumor-associated vascular permeability in rats. Involvement of the glucocorticoid receptor and vascular permeability factor. *The Journal of Clinical Investigation*, *98*, 1400–1408.

Holm, A., Baldetorp, B., Olde, B., Leeb-Lundberg, L. M., & Nilsson, B. O. (2011). The GPER1 agonist G-1 attenuates endothelial cell proliferation by inhibiting DNA synthesis and accumulating cells in the S and G2 phases of the cell cycle. *Journal of Vascular Research*, *48*, 327–335.

Honda, M., Nakagawa, S., Hayashi, K., Kitagawa, N., Tsutsumi, K., Nagata, I., et al. (2006). Adrenomedullin improves the blood-brain barrier function through the expression of claudin-5. *Cellular and Molecular Neurobiology*, *26*, 108–118.

Howard, B. V., & Rossouw, J. E. (2013). Estrogens and cardiovascular disease risk revisited: The Women's Health Initiative. *Current Opinion in Lipidology*, *24*, 493–499.

Huber, J. D., Campos, C. R., Mark, K. S., & Davis, T. P. (2005). Alterations in blood-Brain barrier ICAM-1 expression and brain microglial activation following {lambda}-carrageenan induced inflammatory pain. *American Journal of Physiology. Heart and Circulatory Physiology*, *290*(2), H732–H740.

Iqbal, M., Gibb, W., & Matthews, S. G. (2011). Corticosteroid regulation of P-glycoprotein in the developing blood-brain barrier. *Endocrinology*, *152*, 1067–1079.

Jesmin, S., Hattori, Y., Sakuma, I., Liu, M. Y., Mowa, C. N., & Kitabatake, A. (2003). Estrogen deprivation and replacement modulate cerebral capillary density with vascular expression of angiogenic molecules in middle-aged female rats. *Journal of Cerebral Blood Flow and Metabolism*, *23*, 181–189.

Joels, M., Sarabdjitsingh, R. A., & Karst, H. (2012). Unraveling the time domains of corticosteroid hormone influences on brain activity: Rapid, slow, and chronic modes. *Pharmacological Reviews*, *64*, 901–938.

Johann, S., & Beyer, C. (2013). Neuroprotection by gonadal steroid hormones in acute brain damage requires cooperation with astroglia and microglia. *The Journal of Steroid Biochemistry and Molecular Biology*, *137*, 71–81.

Johnson, A. B., & Sohrabji, F. (2005). Estrogen's effects on central and circulating immune cells vary with reproductive age. *Neurobiology of Aging*, *26*, 1365–1374.

Kancheva, R., Hill, M., Novak, Z., Chrastina, J., Kancheva, L., & Starka, L. (2011). Neuroactive steroids in periphery and cerebrospinal fluid. *Neuroscience*, *191*, 22–27.
Kang, H. S., Ahn, H. S., Kang, H. J., & Gye, M. C. (2006). Effect of estrogen on the expression of occludin in ovariectomized mouse brain. *Neuroscience Letters*, *402*, 30–34.
Karssen, A. M., Meijer, O. C., van der Sandt, I. C., Lucassen, P. J., de Lange, E. C., de Boer, A. G., et al. (2001). Multidrug resistance P-glycoprotein hampers the access of cortisol but not of corticosterone to mouse and human brain. *Endocrinology*, *142*, 2686–2694.
Kashiwamura, Y., Sano, Y., Abe, M., Shimizu, F., Haruki, H., Maeda, T., et al. (2011). Hydrocortisone enhances the function of the blood-nerve barrier through the up-regulation of claudin-5. *Neurochemical Research*, *36*, 849–855.
Keil, J. M., Liu, X., & Antonetti, D. A. (2013). Glucocorticoid induction of occludin expression and endothelial barrier requires transcription factor p54 NONO. *Investigative Ophthalmology & Visual Science*, *54*, 4007–4015.
Kim, H., Lee, J. M., Park, J. S., Jo, S. A., Kim, Y. O., Kim, C. W., et al. (2008). Dexamethasone coordinately regulates angiopoietin-1 and VEGF: A mechanism of glucocorticoid-Induced stabilization of blood-Brain barrier. *Biochemical and Biophysical Research Communications*, *372*, 243–248.
Koehler, R. C., Gebremedhin, D., & Harder, D. R. (2006). Role of astrocytes in cerebrovascular regulation. *Journal of Applied Physiology*, *100*, 307–317.
Leon, R. L., Li, X., Huber, J. D., & Rosen, C. L. (2012). Worsened outcome from middle cerebral artery occlusion in aged rats receiving 17beta-estradiol. *Endocrinology*, *153*, 3386–3393.
Lewis, D. K., Johnson, A. B., Stohlgren, S., Harms, A., & Sohrabji, F. (2008). Effects of estrogen receptor agonists on regulation of the inflammatory response in astrocytes from young adult and middle-aged female rats. *Journal of Neuroimmunology*, *195*, 47–59.
Leybaert, L. (2005). Neurobarrier coupling in the brain: A partner of neurovascular and neurometabolic coupling? *Journal of Cerebral Blood Flow and Metabolism*, *25*, 2–16.
Liu, Y., Liu, F., Iqbal, K., Grundke-Iqbal, I., & Gong, C. X. (2008). Decreased glucose transporters correlate to abnormal hyperphosphorylation of tau in Alzheimer disease. *FEBS Letters*, *582*, 359–364.
Liu, Y., Nusrat, A., Schnell, F. J., Reaves, T. A., Walsh, S., Pochet, M., et al. (2000). Human junction adhesion molecule regulates tight junction resealing in epithelia. *Journal of Cell Science*, *113*(Pt 13), 2363–2374.
Liu, R., Wen, Y., Perez, E., Wang, X., Day, A. L., Simpkins, J. W., et al. (2005). 17beta-Estradiol attenuates blood-brain barrier disruption induced by cerebral ischemia-Reperfusion injury in female rats. *Brain Research*, *1060*, 55–61.
Luchetti, S., Huitinga, I., & Swaab, D. F. (2011). Neurosteroid and GABA-A receptor alterations in Alzheimer's disease, Parkinson's disease and multiple sclerosis. *Neuroscience*, *191*, 6–21.
Mahringer, A., & Fricker, G. (2010). BCRP at the blood-brain barrier: Genomic regulation by 17beta-estradiol. *Molecular Pharmaceutics*, 7, 1835–1847.
Mandell, K. J., McCall, I. C., & Parkos, C. A. (2004). Involvement of the junctional adhesion molecule-1 (JAM1) homodimer interface in regulation of epithelial barrier function. *The Journal of Biological Chemistry*, *279*, 16254–16262.
Meijer, O. C., de Lange, E. C., Breimer, D. D., de Boer, A. G., Workel, J. O., & de Kloet, E. R. (1998). Penetration of dexamethasone into brain glucocorticoid targets is enhanced in mdr1A P-glycoprotein knockout mice. *Endocrinology*, *139*, 1789–1793.
Melcangi, R. C., & Panzica, G. C. (2013). Neuroactive steroids and the nervous system: Further observations on an incomplete tricky puzzle. *Journal of Neuroendocrinology*, *25*, 957–963.

Melcangi, R. C., Panzica, G., & Garcia-Segura, L. M. (2011). Neuroactive steroids: Focus on human brain. *Neuroscience*, *191*, 1–5.

Miller, D. S., & Cannon, R. E. (2013). Signaling pathways that regulate basal ABC transporter activity at the blood-Brain barrier. *Current Pharmaceutical Design*, *20*(10), 1463–1471.

Mirshafiey, A., Asghari, B., Ghalamfarsa, G., Jadidi-Niaragh, F., & Azizi, G. (2014). The significance of matrix metalloproteinases in the immunopathogenesis and treatment of multiple sclerosis. *Sultan Qaboos University Medical Journal*, *14*, e13–e25.

Miyajima, M., Kusuhara, H., Fujishima, M., Adachi, Y., & Sugiyama, Y. (2011). Organic anion transporter 3 mediates the efflux transport of an amphipathic organic anion, dehydroepiandrosterone sulfate, across the blood-brain barrier in mice. *Drug Metabolism and Disposition*, *39*, 814–819.

Mori, M., Tsukahara, F., Yoshioka, T., Irie, K., & Ohta, H. (2004). Suppression by 17beta-estradiol of monocyte adhesion to vascular endothelial cells is mediated by estrogen receptors. *Life Sciences*, *75*, 599–609.

Murata, T., Dietrich, H. H., Xiang, C., & Dacey, R. G., Jr. (2013). G protein-coupled estrogen receptor agonist improves cerebral microvascular function after hypoxia/reoxygenation injury in male and female rats. *Stroke*, *44*, 779–785.

Nakano, M., Hirooka, Y., Matsukawa, R., Ito, K., & Sunagawa, K. (2013). Mineralocorticoid receptors/epithelial Na(+) channels in the choroid plexus are involved in hypertensive mechanisms in stroke-prone spontaneously hypertensive rats. *Hypertension Research*, *36*, 277–284.

Narang, V. S., Fraga, C., Kumar, N., Shen, J., Throm, S., Stewart, C. F., et al. (2008). Dexamethasone increases expression and activity of multidrug resistance transporters at the rat blood-brain barrier. *American Journal of Physiology Cell Physiology*, *295*, C440–C450.

Nobili, S., Landini, I., Mazzei, T., & Mini, E. (2012). Overcoming tumor multidrug resistance using drugs able to evade P-glycoprotein or to exploit its expression. *Medicinal Research Reviews*, *32*, 1220–1262.

Noguchi, K., Katayama, K., & Sugimoto, Y. (2014). Human ABC transporter ABCG2/BCRP expression in chemoresistance: Basic and clinical perspectives for molecular cancer therapeutics. *Pharmacogenomics and Personalised Medicine*, 7, 53–64.

Nordell, V. L., Scarborough, M. M., Buchanan, A. K., & Sohrabji, F. (2003). Differential effects of estrogen in the injured forebrain of young adult and reproductive senescent animals. *Neurobiology of Aging*, *24*, 733–743.

Norris, J. W. (2004). Steroids may have a role in stroke therapy. *Stroke*, *35*, 228–229.

O'Donnell, M. E., Lam, T. I., Tran, L. Q., Foroutan, S., & Anderson, S. E. (2006). Estradiol reduces activity of the blood-brain barrier Na-K-Cl cotransporter and decreases edema formation in permanent middle cerebral artery occlusion. *Journal of Cerebral Blood Flow and Metabolism*, *26*(10), 1234–1249.

Ohtsuki, S., Tomi, M., Hata, T., Nagai, Y., Hori, S., Mori, S., et al. (2005). Dominant expression of androgen receptors and their functional regulation of organic anion transporter 3 in rat brain capillary endothelial cells; comparison of gene expression between the blood-brain and -retinal barriers. *Journal of Cellular Physiology*, *204*, 896–900.

Oki, K., Gomez-Sanchez, E. P., & Gomez-Sanchez, C. E. (2012). Role of mineralocorticoid action in the brain in salt-sensitive hypertension. *Clinical and Experimental Pharmacology & Physiology*, *39*, 90–95.

Oldendorf, W. H., Cornford, M. E., & Brown, W. J. (1977). The large apparent work capability of the blood-brain barrier: A study of the mitochondrial content of capillary endothelial cells in brain and other tissues of the rat. *Annals of Neurology*, *1*, 409–417.

Ouyang, S., Hsuchou, H., Kastin, A. J., Wang, Y., Yu, C., & Pan, W. (2014). Diet-induced obesity suppresses expression of many proteins at the blood-brain barrier. *Journal of Cerebral Blood Flow and Metabolism, 34*, 43–51.
Paganini-Hill, A., Ross, R. K., & Henderson, B. E. (1988). Postmenopausal oestrogen treatment and stroke: A prospective study. *BMJ, 297*, 519–522.
Pajouhesh, H., & Lenz, G. R. (2005). Medicinal chemical properties of successful central nervous system drugs. *NeuroRx, 2*, 541–553.
Papadopoulos, M. C., Saadoun, S., Binder, D. K., Manley, G. T., Krishna, S., & Verkman, A. S. (2004). Molecular mechanisms of brain tumor edema. *Neuroscience, 129*, 1011–1020.
Petropoulos, S., Gibb, W., & Matthews, S. G. (2010). Developmental expression of multidrug resistance phosphoglycoprotein (P-gp) in the mouse fetal brain and glucocorticoid regulation. *Brain Research, 1357*, 9–18.
Piontek, J., Winkler, L., Wolburg, H., Muller, S. L., Zuleger, N., Piehl, C., et al. (2008). Formation of tight junction: Determinants of homophilic interaction between classic claudins. *Faseb Journal, 22*, 146–158.
Poetker, D. M., & Reh, D. D. (2010). A comprehensive review of the adverse effects of systemic corticosteroids. *Otolaryngologic Clinics of North America, 43*, 753–768.
Poungvarin, N. (2004). Steroids have no role in stroke therapy. *Stroke, 35*, 229–230.
Prossnitz, E. R., & Barton, M. (2014). Estrogen biology: New insights into GPER function and clinical opportunities. *Molecular and Cellular Endocrinology, 389*(1–2), 71–83.
Proteau, P. J. (2011). Steroid hormones and therapeutically related compounds. In J. M. Beale, & J. H. Block (Eds.), *Wilson and Gisvold's textbook of organic medicinal and pharmaceutical chemistry*. 12th ed. (pp. 819–867). Baltimore, MD: Wolters Kluwer, Lippincott Williams.
Quillinan, N., Deng, G., Grewal, H., & Herson, P. S. (2014). Androgens and stroke: Good, bad or indifferent? *Experimental Neurology, S0014–4886*(14), 00039–00049.
Razmara, A., Sunday, L., Stirone, C., Wang, X. B., Krause, D. N., Duckles, S. P., et al. (2008). Mitochondrial effects of estrogen are mediated by estrogen receptor alpha in brain endothelial cells. *The Journal of Pharmacology and Experimental Therapeutics, 325*, 782–790.
Reddy, D. S. (2010). Neurosteroids: Endogenous role in the human brain and therapeutic potentials. *Progress in Brain Research, 186*, 113–137.
Resnick, S. M., Coker, L. H., Maki, P. M., Rapp, S. R., Espeland, M. A., & Shumaker, S. A. (2004). The Women's Health Initiative Study of Cognitive Aging (WHISCA): A randomized clinical trial of the effects of hormone therapy on age-associated cognitive decline. *Clinical Trials, 1*, 440–450.
Rettberg, J. R., Yao, J., & Brinton, R. D. (2014). Estrogen: A master regulator of bioenergetic systems in the brain and body. *Frontiers in Neuroendocrinology, 35*, 8–30.
Roberts, T. K., Eugenin, E. A., Lopez, L., Romero, I. A., Weksler, B. B., Couraud, P. O., et al. (2012). CCL2 disrupts the adherens junction: Implications for neuroinflammation. *Laboratory Investigation, 92*, 1213–1233.
Roberts, I., Yates, D., Sandercock, P., Farrell, B., Wasserberg, J., Lomas, G., et al. (2004). Effect of intravenous corticosteroids on death within 14 days in 10008 adults with clinically significant head injury (MRC CRASH trial): Randomised placebo-controlled trial. *Lancet, 364*, 1321–1328.
Rutkowsky, J. M., Wallace, B. K., Wise, P. M., & O'Donnell, M. E. (2011). Effects of estradiol on ischemic factor-induced astrocyte swelling and AQP4 protein abundance. *American Journal of Physiology Cell Physiology, 301*, C204–C212.
Saitou, M., Fujimoto, K., Doi, Y., Itoh, M., Fujimoto, T., Furuse, M., et al. (1998). Occludin-deficient embryonic stem cells can differentiate into polarized epithelial cells bearing tight junctions. *The Journal of Cell Biology, 141*, 397–408.

Sajja, R. K., Prasad, S., & Cucullo, L. (2014). Impact of altered glycaemia on blood-Brain barrier endothelium: An in vitro study using the hCMEC/D3 cell line. *Fluids and Barriers of the CNS*, *11*, 8.

Salvador, E., Shityakov, S., & Forster, C. (2013). Glucocorticoids and endothelial cell barrier function. *Cell and Tissue Research*, *355*(3), 597–605.

Sandoval, K. E., & Witt, K. A. (2008). Blood-brain barrier tight junction permeability and ischemic stroke. *Neurobiology of Disease*, *32*, 200–219.

Sandoval, K. E., & Witt, K. A. (2011). Age and 17beta-estradiol effects on blood-brain barrier tight junction and estrogen receptor proteins in ovariectomized rats. *Microvascular Research*, *81*, 198–205.

Schmidt, R., Fazekas, F., Reinhart, B., Kapeller, P., Fazekas, G., Offenbacher, H., et al. (1996). Estrogen replacement therapy in older women: A neuropsychological and brain MRI study. *Journal of the American Geriatrics Society*, *44*, 1307–1313.

Schultz, S. K., O'Leary, D. S., Boles Ponto, L. L., Watkins, G. L., Hichwa, R. D., & Andreasen, N. C. (1999). Age-related changes in regional cerebral blood flow among young to mid-life adults. *Neuroreport*, *10*, 2493–2496.

Schumacher, M., Mattern, C., Ghoumari, A., Oudinet, J. P., Liere, P., Labombarda, F., et al. (2014). Revisiting the roles of progesterone and allopregnanolone in the nervous system: Resurgence of the progesterone receptors. *Progress in Neurobiology*, *113*, 6–39.

Schumacher, M., Weill-Engerer, S., Liere, P., Robert, F., Franklin, R. J., Garcia-Segura, L. M., et al. (2003). Steroid hormones and neurosteroids in normal and pathological aging of the nervous system. *Progress in Neurobiology*, *71*, 3–29.

Selvamani, A., & Sohrabji, F. (2010). Reproductive age modulates the impact of focal ischemia on the forebrain as well as the effects of estrogen treatment in female rats. *Neurobiology of Aging*, *31*, 1618–1628.

Shi, J., & Simpkins, J. W. (1997). 17 beta-Estradiol modulation of glucose transporter 1 expression in blood-brain barrier. *The American Journal of Physiology*, *272*, E1016–E1022.

Shi, J., Zhang, Y. Q., & Simpkins, J. W. (1997). Effects of 17beta-estradiol on glucose transporter 1 expression and endothelial cell survival following focal ischemia in the rats. *Experimental Brain Research*, *117*, 200–206.

Simpson, I. A., & Davies, P. (1994). Reduced glucose transporter concentrations in brains of patients with Alzheimer's disease. *Annals of Neurology*, *36*, 800–801.

Sohrabji, F., Bake, S., & Lewis, D. K. (2013). Age-related changes in brain support cells: Implications for stroke severity. *Neurochemistry International*, *63*, 291–301.

Song, L., & Pachter, J. S. (2004). Monocyte chemoattractant protein-1 alters expression of tight junction-associated proteins in brain microvascular endothelial cells. *Microvascular Research*, *67*, 78–89.

Spence, R. D., & Voskuhl, R. R. (2012). Neuroprotective effects of estrogens and androgens in CNS inflammation and neurodegeneration. *Frontiers in Neuroendocrinology*, *33*, 105–115.

Stamatovic, S. M., Shakui, P., Keep, R. F., Moore, B. B., Kunkel, S. L., Van Rooijen, N., et al. (2005). Monocyte chemoattractant protein-1 regulation of blood-brain barrier permeability. *Journal of Cerebral Blood Flow and Metabolism*, *25*, 593–606.

Stirone, C., Duckles, S. P., & Krause, D. N. (2003). Multiple forms of estrogen receptor-alpha in cerebral blood vessels: Regulation by estrogen. *American Journal of Physiology Endocrinology and Metabolism*, *284*, E184–E192.

Su, C., Rybalchenko, N., Schreihofer, D. A., Singh, M., Abbassi, B., & Cunningham, R. L. (2012). Cell models for the study of sex steroid hormone neurobiology. *Journal of Steroids & Hormonal Science*, Suppl 2: 003.

Taddei, A., Giampietro, C., Conti, A., Orsenigo, F., Breviario, F., Pirazzoli, V., et al. (2008). Endothelial adherens junctions control tight junctions by VE-cadherin-mediated upregulation of claudin-5. *Nature Cell Biology*, *10*, 923–934.

Thurston, G., Rudge, J. S., Ioffe, E., Zhou, H., Ross, L., Croll, S. D., et al. (2000). Angiopoietin-1 protects the adult vasculature against plasma leakage. *Nature Medicine*, *6*, 460–463.
Tu, J., & Jufri, N. F. (2013). Estrogen signaling through estrogen receptor beta and G-protein-coupled estrogen receptor 1 in human cerebral vascular endothelial cells: Implications for cerebral aneurysms. *BioMed Research International*, *2013*, 524324.
Valable, S., Montaner, J., Bellail, A., Berezowski, V., Brillault, J., Cecchelli, R., et al. (2005). VEGF-induced BBB permeability is associated with an MMP-9 activity increase in cerebral ischemia: Both effects decreased by Ang-1. *Journal of Cerebral Blood Flow and Metabolism*, *25*, 1491–1504.
Vest, R. S., & Pike, C. J. (2013). Gender, sex steroid hormones, and Alzheimer's disease. *Hormones and Behavior*, *63*, 301–307.
Viscoli, C. M., Brass, L. M., Kernan, W. N., Sarrel, P. M., Suissa, S.; & Horwitz, R. I. (2001). A clinical trial of estrogen-replacement therapy after ischemic stroke. *The New England Journal of Medicine*, *345*, 1243–1249.
Wang, W., Dentler, W. L., & Borchardt, R. T. (2001). VEGF increases BMEC monolayer permeability by affecting occludin expression and tight junction assembly. *American Journal of Physiology Heart and Circulatory Physiology*, *280*, H434–H440.
Wang, X., Zhang, J., Yang, Y., Dong, W., Wang, F., Wang, L., et al. (2013). Progesterone attenuates cerebral edema in neonatal rats with hypoxic-Ischemic brain damage by inhibiting the expression of matrix metalloproteinase-9 and aquaporin-4. *Experimental and Therapeutic Medicine*, *6*, 263–267.
Wassertheil-Smoller, S., Hendrix, S. L., Limacher, M., Heiss, G., Kooperberg, C., Baird, A., et al. (2003). Effect of estrogen plus progestin on stroke in postmenopausal women: The Women's Health Initiative: A randomized trial. *JAMA*, *289*, 2673–2684.
Weber, C., Fraemohs, L., & Dejana, E. (2007). The role of junctional adhesion molecules in vascular inflammation. *Nature Reviews Immunology*, 7, 467–477.
Wierman, M. E. (2007). Sex steroid effects at target tissues: Mechanisms of action. *Advances in Physiology Education*, *31*, 26–33.
Won, S., Lee, J. H., Wali, B., Stein, D. G., & Sayeed, I. (2014). Progesterone attenuates hemorrhagic transformation after delayed tPA treatment in an experimental model of stroke in rats: Involvement of the VEGF-MMP pathway. *Journal of Cerebral Blood Flow and Metabolism*, *34*, 72–80.
Yang, S. H., Liu, R., Wu, S. S., & Simpkins, J. W. (2003). The use of estrogens and related compounds in the treatment of damage from cerebral ischemia. *Annals of the New York Academy of Sciences*, *1007*, 101–107.
Yang, Y., & Rosenberg, G. A. (2011). MMP-mediated disruption of claudin-5 in the blood-brain barrier of rat brain after cerebral ischemia. *Methods in Molecular Biology*, *762*, 333–345.
Yao, Y., & Tsirka, S. E. (2014). Monocyte chemoattractant protein-1 and the blood-Brain barrier. *Cellular and Molecular Life Sciences*, *71*, 683–697.
Ye, L., Martin, T. A., Parr, C., Harrison, G. M., Mansel, R. E., & Jiang, W. G. (2003). Biphasic effects of 17-beta-estradiol on expression of occludin and transendothelial resistance and paracellular permeability in human vascular endothelial cells. *Journal of Cellular Physiology*, *196*, 362–369.
Zhang, Z., & Chopp, M. (2002). Vascular endothelial growth factor and angiopoietins in focal cerebral ischemia. *Trends in Cardiovascular Medicine*, *12*, 62–66.
Ziylan, Y. Z., LeFauconnier, J. M., Bernard, G., & Bourre, J. M. (1988). Effect of dexamethasone on transport of alpha-Aminoisobutyric acid and sucrose across the blood-Brain barrier. *Journal of Neurochemistry*, *51*, 1338–1342.
Ziylan, Y. Z., Lefauconnier, J. M., Bernard, G., & Bourre, J. M. (1989). Regional alterations in blood-to-brain transfer of alpha-aminoisobutyric acid and sucrose, after chronic administration and withdrawal of dexamethasone. *Journal of Neurochemistry*, *52*, 684–689.

CHAPTER THIRTEEN

Combination Approaches to Attenuate Hemorrhagic Transformation After tPA Thrombolytic Therapy in Patients with Poststroke Hyperglycemia/Diabetes

Xiang Fan*, Yinghua Jiang*,†, Zhanyang Yu*, Jing Yuan*,‡, Xiaochuan Sun*,†, Shuanglin Xiang*,‡, Eng H. Lo*, Xiaoying Wang*,[1]

*Neuroprotection Research Laboratory, Department of Neurology and Radiology, Massachusetts General Hospital, Neuroscience Program, Harvard Medical School, Boston, Massachusetts, USA

†Department of Neurosurgery, The First Affiliated Hospital, Chongqing Medical University, Chongqing, PR China

‡Key Laboratory of Protein Chemistry and Developmental Biology of State Education Ministry of China, College of Life Sciences, Hunan Normal University, Changsha, Hunan, PR China

[1]Corresponding author: e-mail address: wangxi@helix.mgh.harvard.edu

Contents

Abstract

To date, tissue type plasminogen activator (tPA)-based thrombolytic stroke therapy is the only FDA-approved treatment for achieving vascular reperfusion and clinical benefit, but this agent is given to only about 5% of stroke patients in the USA. This may be related, in part, to the elevated risk of symptomatic intracranial hemorrhage, and consequently limited therapeutic time window. Clinical investigations demonstrate that

Advances in Pharmacology, Volume 71
ISSN 1054-3589
http://dx.doi.org/10.1016/bs.apha.2014.06.007

poststroke hyperglycemia is one of the most important risk factors that cause intracerebral hemorrhage and worsen neurological outcomes. There is a knowledge gap in understanding the underlying molecular mechanisms, and lack of effective therapeutics targeting the severe complication. This short review summarizes clinical observations and experimental investigations in preclinical stroke models of the field. The data strongly suggest that interactions of multiple pathogenic factors including hyperglycemia-mediated vascular oxidative stress and inflammation, ischemic insult, and tPA neurovascular toxicity in concert contribute to the BBB damage–intracerebral hemorrhagic transformation process. Development of combination approaches targeting the multiple pathological cascades may help to attenuate the hemorrhagic complication.

1. INTRODUCTION

Ischemic stroke is a cerebrovascular event, tissue type plasminogen activator (tPA) thrombolytic stroke therapy is based on the "re-canalization hypothesis," i.e., that reopening of occluded vessels by lyses of the clot improves clinical outcome in acute ischemic stroke through regional reperfusion and salvage of threatened tissues (Whiteley et al., 2014). Recanalization is an important predictor of stroke outcome in all the modalities of thrombolysis. Despite enormous research efforts including many clinical trials, intravenous administration of recombinant tPA remains the only FDA-approved and the most beneficial proven intervention for emergency treatment of stroke (Chapman et al., 2014; Whiteley et al., 2014). However, risk of hemorrhagic transformation, short treatment time window, poor thrombolytic perfusion rate, and tPA neurotoxicity comprise the major limitations to the application (Alexandrov & Grotta, 2002; Bambauer, Johnston, Bambauer, & Zivin, 2006; Weintraub, 2006). Although other thrombolytic agents are being tested, none has been established as effective or as a replacement for tPA (Adams et al., 2007). Importantly, exogenous tPA may worsen ischemia-induced blood–brain barrier disruption, elevate risks of symptomatic intracranial hemorrhage, and in part consequently reduce therapeutic time window (Chapman et al., 2014). Recent clinical investigations have indicated the potential and opportunity to improve tPA therapy. For instance, PWI (Perfusion-weighted magnetic resonance imaging)-DWI (Diffusion-weighted magnetic resonance imaging) mismatch MRI studies suggest that some individual patients may benefit from treatment beyond 3-h time window, if there is low bleeding risk and salvageable mismatch (Thomalla, Kohrmann, Rother, & Schellinger, 2007; Thomalla et al., 2006). European ECASS III trial showed that intravenous tPA given up to

4.5 h after symptom onset benefited clinical outcomes. However, tPA is still associated with increased intracranial transformation and remains the most threaten complication for thrombolytic stroke therapy (Hacke et al., 2008).

2. INCREASED HEMORRHAGIC TRANSFORMATION AFTER tPA THROMBOLYTIC THERAPY

There are a number of risk factors in association with tPA stroke therapy-mediated hemorrhagic transformation, including poststroke hyperglycemia, older age, larger infarct, and high blood pressure (Faigle, Sharrief, Marsh, Llinas, & Urrutia, 2014; Miller, Simpson, & Silver, 2011). Poststroke hyperglycemia is presented in all preexisting diabetes (about 37% of stroke patients) and 50% of nondiabetic stroke patients (Allport et al., 2006; Kruyt, Biessels, Devries, & Roos, 2010), and the severity of the poststroke hyperglycemia and history of diabetes mellitus (DM) are associated with poor clinical outcome after stroke and thrombolysis (Ahmed et al., 2010; Bruno et al., 2008; Desilles et al., 2013; Poppe et al., 2009; Ribo et al., 2005). For example, in the NINDS rt-PA Stroke Trial treated with tPA within 3 h of onset, only serum glucose was an independent predictor of symptomatic hemorrhagic transformation (Bruno et al., 2002). This was replicated in the PROACT II trial, where symptomatic hemorrhagic transformation occurred in 35% of patients with serum glucose values greater than 200 mg/dL (Kase et al., 2001). In another study using data from the prospective, multicenter Canadian Alteplase for Stroke Effectiveness Study (CASES), the cohort of IV-tPA-treated stroke patients, admission hyperglycemia was independently associated with increased risk of death, hemorrhagic transformation, and poor functional status at 90 days (Poppe et al., 2009). Although the evidence supports an increased risk of hemorrhage due to tPA in patients with hyperglycemia, the mechanisms of this effect remain poorly known. Thus, better understanding the underlying mechanism and developing therapeutic approaches targeting this complication to improve tPA thrombolytic therapy is considered one of the highest clinical priorities (Ishrat, Soliman, Guan, Saler, & Fagan, 2012; Whiteley et al., 2014).

3. UNDERLYING MECHANISMS: MULTIPLE PATHOLOGICAL PATHWAYS

A large knowledge gap remains in the understanding of insight molecular mechanisms to the BBB disruption-mediated hemorrhagic transformation after tPA stroke therapy in patients with hyperglycemia/diabetes (Arnold et al., 2012; Desilles et al., 2013). These mechanisms are likely to be complex, with a strong correlation between deleterious pathways. Among a variety of pathological factors and cascades, experimental investigations strongly suggest that interactions of multiple pathogenic factors including hyperglycemia-mediated vascular oxidative stress and inflammation, ischemic insult, and tPA neurovascular toxicity in concert contribute to the extracellular proteolysis dysfunction–BBB damage–intracerebral hemorrhagic transformation process (Hafez, Coucha, Bruno, Fagan, & Ergul, 2014; Lo, Wang, & Cuzner, 2002; Wang & Lo, 2003; Wang et al., 2004; Won, Tang, Suh, Yenari, & Swanson, 2011).

4. DM AND HYPERGLYCEMIA-MEDIATED VASCULAR PATHOLOGY

DM is one of the risk factors to cardiovascular and cerebrovascular diseases (Peters, Huxley, & Woodward, 2014). It has been suggested that many complex pathways contribute to the pathobiology of diabetic vascular injuries and elevated vascular permeability, including hyperglycemia itself, overproduction of ROS derived from NAD(P)H oxidases (Nox), matrix metalloproteinase (MMP) activation, production of advanced glycation end products and interaction with its receptor (RAGE), vascular inflammation, and the activation of vasoactive systems (Allen & Bayraktutan, 2009; Gray & Jandeleit-Dahm, 2014; Hamilton & Watts, 2013; Kamada, Yu, Nito, & Chan, 2007; Won et al., 2011).

Experimental evidence have demonstrated that hyperglycemia may cause endothelial dysfunction by oxidative stress, inflammation, elevated protease activity-mediated BBB and extracellular matrix degradation, resulting in BBB permeability increase (Ceriello et al., 2013). In streptozotocin-induced type 1 diabetes rats, permeability to [(14)C] sucrose increased concurrently with decreased production of BBB tight junction proteins occludin and zona occludens 1 (ZO-1), at early 14 days after streptozotocin injection(Hawkins, Lundeen, Norwood, Brooks, & Egleton, 2007). Plasma MMP activity increase was also detected (Hawkins et al., 2007). Another study reported that after 60 days of streptozotocin injection, BBB disruption was observed by monitoring leakages of fluorescent dyes differing in molecular weight: fluorescein, fluorescein isothiocyanate (FITC)-dextran, and Evans blue (Karolczak, Rozalska, Wieczorek, Labieniec-Watala, & Watala, 2012).

In cultured human brain microvascular endothelial cell cultures, hyperglycemia promotes cerebral barrier dysfunction through the activation of PKC-β and consequent stimulations of oxidative stress, MMP-2 activation, and tight junction dissolution (Shao & Bayraktutan, 2013). Using an *in vitro* model of human BBB comprising human brain microvascular endothelial cells and astrocytes, hyperglycemia evoked *in vitro* barrier dysfunction with markedly increased RhoA/Rho-kinase protein expressions and RhoA activities while concurrently reducing the expression of tight junction protein occludin. Normalization of glucose levels and silencing PKC-β activity neutralized the effects of hyperglycemia on occludin and RhoA/Rho-kinase/MLC2 expression, localization, and activity and consequently improved *in vitro* barrier integrity and function (Srivastava, Shao, & Bayraktutan, 2013). Furthermore, hyperglycemia can induce endothelial cell expression and activity of the collagenase, MMP-1 and MMP-2; interestingly, hyperglycemia also induces expression and activity of MMP-9 from monocyte-derived macrophages (Death, Fisher, McGrath, & Yue, 2003). Taken together, experimental investigations suggested crucial roles of hyperglycemia itself in mediating cerebrovascular oxidative stress and inflammation. All above can be amplified by stroke-mediated pathological factors that lead to the BBB disruption and increased hemorrhagic transformation after stroke and tPA reperfusion treatment (Alves, Oliveira, Socorro, & Moreira, 2012; Hafez et al., 2014; Hawkins et al., 2007; Wang & Lo, 2003; Wang, Rosell, & Lo, 2008; Wang et al., 2004). In a clinical investigation, pretreatment baseline of blood MMP-9 level predicts intracranial hemorrhagic complications after thrombolysis in human stroke (Montaner et al., 2003).

5. ISCHEMIC STROKE AND BBB DISRUPTION

It has been well known that ischemic stroke insult weakens BBB integrity, which may result in reperfusion injury and hemorrhagic transformation (Jickling et al., 2014; Kamada et al., 2007; Sussman & Connolly, 2013). BBB disruption can be visualized by both head CT and MRI in both stroke patients and experimental stroke animals (Dankbaar et al., 2011; Jiang, Ewing, & Chopp, 2012). Loss of integrity of the BBB resulting from ischemia and reperfusion may cause hemorrhagic transformation and worse clinical outcome from the beneficial effects of tPA reperfusion. In a study using brain MRI, the BBB disruption was evidenced by delayed gadolinium enhancement of cerebrospinal fluid space in fluid-attenuated inversion recovery images that was observed in 47 (33%) of 144 patients with ischemic stroke (Warach & Latour, 2004).

Hemorrhagic transformation of acute ischemic stroke is a complex and multifactorial phenomenon (Rosell, Foerch, Murata, & Lo, 2008; Sussman & Connolly, 2013; Wang & Lo, 2003). Endothelial swelling may occur within minutes to hours of ischemic onset mainly due to a sudden energy failure, leading to narrowing of the internal diameter of the blood vessel. The decreased cerebral embolism also causes decreases of occludin and ZO-1 at the level of the tight junctions and loses contact with the astrocyte feet, contributing to increases in paracellular permeability (Kaur & Ling, 2008; Rossi, Brady, & Mohr, 2007; Sandoval & Witt, 2008). Most importantly, emerging experimental evidence suggested that all the above pathological cascades together with oxidative stress and inflammation may lead to increase in secretion and activity of proteases and photolytic dysfunction that ultimately contributes to BBB and extracellular matrix degradation-mediated hemorrhagic transformation (Lo et al., 2002; Sussman & Connolly, 2013; Wang et al., 2008).

6. tPA AND EXTRACELLULAR PROTEOLYSIS DYSFUNCTION-MEDIATED BBB DISRUPTION

Besides clot lysis, tPA may have pleiotropic actions in the brain. It has been discovered that tPA has the ability to cross both leaky and intact BBB (Benchenane et al., 2005; Wang et al., 2003; Yepes et al., 2003). At the level of the neurovascular unit, tPA can cause direct vasoactivity (Nassar et al., 2004) and bind to the NR1 subunit of the *N*-methyl-D-aspartate receptor, resulting in cleavage of the NR1 subunit and amplification of intracellular Ca^{2+} conductance (Fernandez-Monreal et al., 2004; Kaur, Zhao, Klein, Lo, & Buchan, 2004; Nicole et al., 2001). Importantly, tPA may also target nonfibrin substrates of brain extracellular matrix by activating other extracellular proteases (Lo et al., 2002). Although extracellular proteases comprise many important biological functions through extracellular proteolysis, the most important one is in promoting weakness and rupture of cerebral vasculatures, leading to cerebral hemorrhage in ischemic stroke and tPA thrombolysis (Wang et al., 2008).

In stroke, disturbed extracellular proteolysis targets multiple brain cells, cell–cell communications, and matrix degradations within the neurovascular unit (Lee, Wang, Tsuji, & Lo, 2004). The neurovascular unit is assembled from endothelial cells of the capillary wall, the extracellular matrix of the basal lamina, the end-feet of astrocytes that surround the microvessel, and the adjacent neurons (Jullienne & Badaut, 2013; Lee et al., 2004). Cell–cell and matrix–cell interactions between these various components thus provide the anatomical and functional neurovascular barrier components of the BBB (Lee et al., 2004; Lo, Broderick, & Moskowitz, 2004; Seo et al., 2012). Our previous study suggests that tPA-triggered MMP-9 upregulation is partially through binding endothelial cell-surface receptor low-density lipoprotein receptor-related protein LRP (Wang et al., 2003). Furthermore, tPA may also mediate neuroinflammation and dysregulate extracellular matrix proteolysis, leading to BBB leakage and hemorrhagic transformation after tPA stroke treatment (Jin, Yang, & Li, 2010). Although the main effect of tPA in stroke certainly occurs within the targeted vessel, these findings suggest that extravascular actions of tPA may complicate its intended role in clot lysis. Emerging experimental evidence suggested that extracellular proteolysis dysregulation represents a key pathological cascade attributable to BBB disruption and hemorrhagic transformation after ischemic stroke and tPA thrombolysis (Lee et al., 2004; Lo et al., 2004; Wang & Lo, 2003; Wang et al., 2004).

7. MULTIPLE PATHOLOGICAL FACTORS AND INTERACTIONS

There is a knowledge gap in understanding the increased damage of BBB integrity-associated hemorrhagic transformation in patients with diabetes/poststroke hyperglycemia after receiving tPA, and lack of effective therapeutics targeting the severe complication (Hafez et al., 2014; Jickling et al., 2014; Peters et al., 2014; Whiteley et al., 2014). Accumulating experimental evidence demonstrates the crucial roles of extracellular matrix proteolysis in stroke pathology and tPA thrombolytic complications (Lo et al., 2002; Wang & Lo, 2003; Wang et al., 2004). These are likely to be complex, with a strong correlation between deleterious pathways caused by hyperglycemia, energy deficits, and most importantly reperfusion injury. Among a variety of pathological factors and cascades, hyperglycemia, oxidative stress, neuroinflammation, and leukocyte recruitment are believed to be major triggers for dysregulating protease expression, secretion, and activation, and there are many points of interaction and feedback between these various pathways in this stimulation process (Adibhatla & Hatcher, 2008; Jin et al., 2010; Wang et al., 2008).

Hyperglycemia may cause vascular oxidative stress, while oxidative stress occurs very early after the onset of ischemia/reperfusion injury via overproduction of ROS. Oxidative stress generated during stroke is a critical event leading to BBB disruption with secondary vasogenic edema and hemorrhagic transformation of infarcted brain tissue, restricting the benefit of thrombolytic reperfusion (Kaur et al., 2004; Wang et al., 2004). ROS can directly oxidize and damage tissue BBB structures. Furthermore, ROS is the primary upstream of pathophysiological mechanisms during reperfusion injury, linking protease activation to vascular leakage (Gasche, Copin, Sugawara, Fujimura, & Chan, 2001; Jian Liu & Rosenberg, 2005). The importance of oxidative stress in stroke and tPA thrombolytic-related vasculature disruption has been well documented from several animal studies of antioxidant plus tPA combination treatments in embolic stroke models (Asahi, Asahi, Wang, & Lo, 2000; Lapchak et al., 2002; Lapchak, Chapman, & Zivin, 2001). In early human stroke, there was evidence of increased oxidative stress and a relationship with MMP-9 expression, supporting findings from experimental studies (Kelly et al., 2008).

Postischemic neuroinflammation-mediated BBB leakage after stroke is a progressive and interactive process, and largely depends on the activation, expression, and secretion of proinflammatory mediators (e.g., cytokines) from both cerebral and peripheral cells (Amantea et al., 2014; Gidday et al., 2005; Rosenberg, 2002). Oxidative stress is a major stimulator of inflammatory cytokine production and protease secretion by microglia, leukocytes, and brain resident cells of the neurovascular unit (Lee et al., 2004; Pun, Lu, & Moochhala, 2009; Wang & Lo, 2003). Experimental investigations have suggested that neuroinflammation-mediated extracellular matrix proteolysis dysfunction is the key pathological mechanism attributed to BBB disruption after stroke, mainly by means of early elevated cytokines, release of leukocytes into circulation, leukocyte adhesion to injured cerebrovasculature and brain infiltration, and release and activation of proteases (Najjar, Pearlman, Devinsky, Najjar, & Zagzag, 2013; Simi, Tsakiri, Wang, & Rothwell, 2007). Leukocyte–microvessel interactions, and thus infiltration of leukocytes into the ischemic brain play dominant roles (Amantea et al., 2014). This leukocyte–microvessel interaction contributes to the development of secondary damage resulting in edema, microvascular permeabilization, and hemorrhage via secreted free radicals, cytokines/chemokines, lipid-derived mediators, and proteases (Borlongan, Glover, Sanberg, & Hess, 2012; Fagan, Hess, Hohnadel, Pollock, & Ergul, 2004;

Wang & Lo, 2003). It has been clearly recognized that proteases secreted by activated leukocytes is one of the key pathogenic factors contributing to BBB leakage and hemorrhagic transformation in ischemic stroke (Bao Dang et al., 2013; Lee et al., 2004; Lo et al., 2002; Wang & Lo, 2003). Importantly, activated extracellular proteases such as MMP act as inflammatory mediators as well, for example, by triggering cytokine expression (Amantea et al., 2007; Bao Dang et al., 2013; Radisky et al., 2005).

Again, there are many points of interaction and feedback between above various pathways and cascades, with interactions also occurring between protease–protease and protease-stimulating triggers. In general, proteases in the extracellular space can be activated by other extracellular proteases, thus linking these enzymes. In the context of extracellular proteolytic dysregulation in tPA stroke thrombolysis-related hemorrhagic complication, the key representative is the tPA–MMP interactions (Adibhatla & Hatcher, 2008; Jin et al., 2010; Lakhan, Kirchgessner, Tepper, & Leonard, 2013; Wang et al., 2008). tPA amplifies MMP-9 in part, it may be nonspecifically related to oxidative stress, and additionally by stimulating neuroinflammation (Lo et al., 2004; Wang et al., 2004), or via tPA binding to LRP (Wang et al., 2003; Zhang, Polavarapu, She, Mao, & Yepes, 2007). Experimental data suggest that extracellular matrix proteolysis may target multiple cell types at the neurovascular interface, and underlie multiple cascades of BBB disruption after tPA reperfusion treatment (Lee et al., 2004; Lo et al., 2004; Seo et al., 2012).

Fundamentally, the precise pathological molecular mechanisms involved remain poorly characterized (Desilles et al., 2013; Hafez et al., 2014). One of difficulties is that assessing dynamic multiple factors and interactions is technically difficult, particularly in *in vivo* animal models. As discussed earlier, there are multiple upstream regulators of neurovascular proteolysis–BBB disruption comprising mediators of hyperglycemia, oxidative stress, and inflammation. Exogenous tPA may potentiate this pathological process (Adibhatla & Hatcher, 2008; Jin et al., 2010; Kaur et al., 2004; Lo et al., 2004; Wang et al., 2008). Therefore, in combination with tPA in patients with diabetes/poststroke hyperglycemia, targeting these upstream mechanisms or even multiple combinations may ultimately improve stroke thrombolytic therapy in both safety and efficacy (Adibhatla & Hatcher, 2008; Jin et al., 2010; Wang et al., 2008). Figure 1 presents a schematic outline to link multiple interactions between pathogenic factors and consequently mediated BBB breakdown and hemorrhagic transformation after tPA thrombolytic therapy to stroke with poststroke hyperglycemia/diabetes.

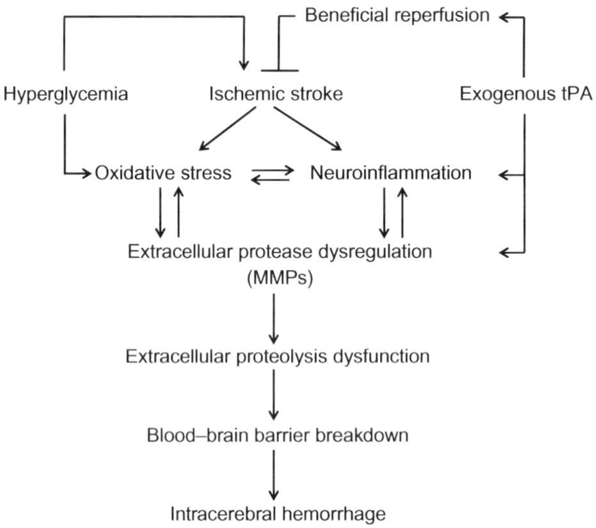

Figure 1 A schematic outline to link multiple interactions between pathogenic factors and consequently mediated BBB breakdown and hemorrhagic transformation after tPA thrombolytic therapy to stroke with poststroke hyperglycemia/diabetes. Hyperglycemia accelerates ischemic brain infarct formation, directly mediates cerebrovascular oxidative stress, and inflammation. Ischemic stroke initiates early elevation in oxidative stress and neuroinflammation and underlies extracellular matrix proteolytic dysfunction at the neurovascular interface, resulting in BBB breakdown and hemorrhagic transformation. Properly titrated use of exogenous tPA is beneficial to reperfuse ischemic brain and rescue compromised tissue. Exogenous tPA may also activate extracellular protease and neuroinflammation to potentiate extracellular proteolysis dysfunction. Targeting upstream components of hyperglycemia, vascular oxidative stress, inflammation, and extracellular proteolytic activity may improve extracellular proteolytic homeostasis and maintain BBB integrity, and thus reduce the hemorrhagic complications of tPA thrombolytic stroke therapy to patients with hyperglycemia/diabetes.

8. COMBINATION APPROACHES IN FOCAL EMBOLIC STROKE MODEL OF HYPERGLYCEMIA/DIABETIC RATS

Combination approaches targeting tPA reperfusion-mediated hemorrhagic transformation have been tested in experimental stroke animal models by targeting different signaling pathways, many of them showed beneficial effects in infarction reduction, hemorrhagic transformation reduction, and/or therapeutic time window extension in focal filament or embolic stroke rodent models(Ishrat et al., 2012; Wang et al., 2008). However, one translational limitation of above experiments is that all investigations of tPA thrombolysis performed in either nondiabetes/hyperglycemia animals or non-clot stroke models (MacDougall & Muir, 2011). Preclinical studies in experimental animal models that closely reflect human diseases ("bedside to bench" research) may potentially better understand pathophysiological mechanisms and develop new translational therapeutic approaches (Fisher et al., 2009). Thus for the first time in a commonly used embolic focal stroke rat model (Zhang, Chopp, Zhang, Jiang, & Ewing, 1997; Zhu et al., 2010), we tested neurological outcomes after tPA thrombolysis in type 1 diabetic rats and estimated the translational relevance of this animal model for future investigations (Fan et al., 2012). These rats exhibit hyperglycemia, cerebrovascular inflammation, and coagulation dysfunction (Zhang et al., 2003; Okazaki et al., 1997) that contribute to an increased risk for stroke (Hagiwara et al., 2003; Manna & Sil, 2012). In the focal embolic stroke model of type 1 diabetic rats, our results closely mimic the clinical situation (Hafez, Coucha, Bruno, Fagan, & Ergul, 2014; Capes SE et al., 2001) with increased brain infarction and hemorrhagic transformation observed after tPA thrombolysis in diabetic rats (Fan et al., 2012). A recent study reported similar findings of increased hemorrhage, inflammation and ineffective neuroprotection in focal embolic model of type 1 diabetic rats after tPA thrombolysis (Ning et al., 2012). By using this focal embolic stroke model of diabetic rats, we further investigated two translational combination approaches with tPA thrombolysis (Fan, Lo, & Wang, 2013; Fan, Ning, Lo, & Wang, 2013).

For the first combination, we tested early insulin glycemic control combined with tPA thrombolysis (Fan, Ning, et al., 2013). Clinical and experimental findings provide a rationale for attempting glycemic control in hyperglycemic stroke patients in combination with tPA administration (Poppe et al., 2009; Won et al., 2011). However, hyperglycemic correct with insulin in the acute phase of stroke did not show beneficial effects (Bellolio, Gilmore, & Stead, 2011; Rosso et al., 2012). It is possible that the lack of efficacy in these past efforts is related to the delayed institution of insulin treatments, i.e., early correction of hyperglycemia is required for therapeutic benefit, in particular to tPA reperfusion therapy (Alvarez-Sabin et al., 2004). Our experimental result showed that early insulin glycemic control at 1 h followed by tPA or saline at 1.5 h after stroke, the insulin glycemic control alone or tPA thrombolysis alone had no significant effects on ischemic infarction. However, early insulin glycemic control combined with tPA significantly reduced brain infarction, hemispheric swelling and tPA-mediated hemorrhagic transformation, and improved plasma perfusion at 24 h after stroke. We also found the combination significantly decreased plasma plasminogen activator inhibitor-1 (PAI-1) antigen level at 6 h, and PAI-1 activity at 1.5 h and 6 h after stroke. Although the underlying mechanisms need to be further investigated, this study suggests that early insulin glycemic control may be beneficial in combination with tPA thrombolysis for ischemic stroke with DM or poststroke hyperglycemia (Fan, Ning, et al., 2013).

For the second combination, we tested minocycline with tPA thrombolysis (Fan, Lo, et al., 2013). Although the pathophysiology of stroke patients with diabetic or posthyperglycemia is complex, experimental animal studies have suggested that ischemic brain tissue damage and vascular inflammation-mediated BBB disruption may be two major contributors to increased hemorrhagic transformation and worse neurological outcomes after stroke and tPA thrombolytic therapy (De Silva et al., 2010; Poppe et al., 2009; Won et al., 2011). Combination of neuroprotective and anti-inflammatory agents with tPA thrombolysis would be a reasonable approach to overcome above shortcomings(Wang et al., 2008). Minocycline might be a compelling candidate (Fagan, Cronic, & Hess, 2011; Hess & Fagan, 2010; Yong et al., 2004). Minocycline is a semisynthetic tetracycline, which has been clinically used as an antibiotic and anti-inflammatory drug. Accumulating experimental evidence has demonstrated that minocycline is neuroprotective in multiple neurological disorders including ischemic and hemorrhagic stroke (Fagan et al., 2011; Yong et al., 2004; Zhao, Hua, He, Keep, & Xi, 2011). Although its underlying molecular mechanisms remain to be fully defined, minocycline possess a wide array of anti-inflammatory, anti-apoptotic, antioxidative, and vascular protective properties (Plane, Shen, Pleasure, & Deng, 2010; Yong et al., 2004). These effects may be especially important in the context of stroke patients with vascular comorbidities. Our experimental results showed that compared to saline or tPA alone treatments, minocycline plus tPA combination therapy significantly reduced brain infarction, intracerebral hemorrhage, and hemispheric swelling at 24 h after stroke. The combination also significantly suppressed the elevated plasma levels of MMP-9 and interlukin-1. In the peri-infarct brain tissues, the combination also significantly decreased neutrophil infiltration, microglia activation, MMP-9 activity, and tight junction protein claudin-5 degradation, suggesting that these beneficial effects of tPA-minocycline combination therapy may be mediated in part by the suppression of MMP-9 activity, decrease in brain tissue inflammation, and protection against cerebrovascular damage (Fan, Lo, et al., 2013).

For future study, in addition to the acute brain infarction and hemorrhagic translation measurements, clinically relevant outcomes such as reperfusion effects and long-term neurological function also need to be assessed. Since about 30% stroke patients are diabetes and 90% of them represent type 2 diabetes (Furie et al., 2011), it would be more translational in preclinical investigations also to use type 2 diabetic animals with/without metabolic syndrome (Lucke-Wold, Turner, Lucke-Wold, Rosen, & Huber, 2012). Finally, to develop more effective and safe tPA combination therapy, we need to deeply dissect the molecular pathophysiology mechanisms of tPA-mediated increase of BBB disruption and hemorrhagic transformation. Although further translation preclinical studies to evaluate more combination therapeutic approaches are warranted, experimental results from combination of early insulin glycemic control or minocyclin with tPA in type 1 diabetic rats suggested that targeting early hyperglycemia and blocking multiple pathological pathways of oxidative stress, MMP activity, and inflammation might improve safety and efficacy of tPA thrombolysis in patients with diabetes/poststroke hyperglycemia (Fan, Lo, et al., 2013; Fan, Ning, et al., 2013).

9. CONCLUSION

There is a knowledge gap in understanding the increased damage of BBB integrity-associated hemorrhagic transformation in patients with diabetes/poststroke hyperglycemia after receiving tPA, and lack of effective therapeutics targeting the severe complication (Desilles et al., 2013; Hafez et al., 2014; Whiteley et al., 2014). Although clinical evidence is lacking, accumulating experimental findings suggest that there are interactions of multiple pathogenic factors including hyperglycemia-mediated vascular oxidative stress and inflammation, ischemic insult, and tPA neurovascular toxicity in concert contribute to the BBB disruption–intracerebral hemorrhagic transformation process (Adibhatla & Hatcher, 2008; Ishrat et al., 2012; Wang et al., 2008). Further research efforts need to deeply dissect the underlying mechanisms in clinically relevant clot stroke models of diabetes/hyperglycemia animals, and develop combination approaches targeting the multiple pathological cascades to attenuate the severe hemorrhagic complication.

CONFLICT OF INTEREST

The authors have no conflict of interest to declare.

REFERENCES

Adams, H. P., Jr., del Zoppo, G., Alberts, M. J., Bhatt, D. L., Brass, L., Furlan, A., et al. (2007). Guidelines for the early management of adults with ischemic stroke: a guideline from the American Heart Association/American Stroke Association Stroke Council, Clinical Cardiology Council, Cardiovascular Radiology and Intervention Council, and the Atherosclerotic Peripheral Vascular Disease and Quality of Care Outcomes in Research Interdisciplinary Working Groups: The American Academy of Neurology affirms the value of this guideline as an educational tool for neurologists. *Circulation, 115*, e478–e534.

Adibhatla, R. M., & Hatcher, J. F. (2008). Tissue plasminogen activator (tPA) and matrix metalloproteinases in the pathogenesis of stroke: Therapeutic strategies. *CNS & Neurological Disorders Drug Targets*, 7, 243–253.

Ahmed, N., Davalos, A., Eriksson, N., Ford, G. A., Glahn, J., Hennerici, M., et al. (2010). Association of admission blood glucose and outcome in patients treated with intravenous thrombolysis: Results from the Safe Implementation of Treatments in Stroke International Stroke Thrombolysis Register (SITS-ISTR). *Archives of Neurology, 67*, 1123–1130.

Alexandrov, A. V., & Grotta, J. C. (2002). Arterial reocclusion in stroke patients treated with intravenous tissue plasminogen activator. *Neurology, 59*, 862–867.

Allen, C. L., & Bayraktutan, U. (2009). Antioxidants attenuate hyperglycaemia-mediated brain endothelial cell dysfunction and blood-brain barrier hyperpermeability. *Diabetes, Obesity & Metabolism, 11*, 480–490.

Allport, L., Baird, T., Butcher, K., Macgregor, L., Prosser, J., Colman, P., et al. (2006). Frequency and temporal profile of poststroke hyperglycemia using continuous glucose monitoring. *Diabetes Care, 29*, 1839–1844.

Alvarez-Sabin, J., Molina, C. A., Ribo, M., Arenillas, J. F., Montaner, J., Huertas, R., et al. (2004). Impact of admission hyperglycemia on stroke outcome after thrombolysis: Risk stratification in relation to time to reperfusion. *Stroke: A Journal of Cerebral Circulation, 35*, 2493–2498.

Alves, M. G., Oliveira, P. F., Socorro, S., & Moreira, P. I. (2012). Impact of diabetes in blood-testis and blood-brain barriers: Resemblances and differences. *Current Diabetes Reviews, 8*, 401–412.

Amantea, D., Russo, R., Gliozzi, M., Fratto, V., Berliocchi, L., Bagetta, G., et al. (2007). Early upregulation of matrix metalloproteinases following reperfusion triggers neuroinflammatory mediators in brain ischemia in rat. *International Review of Neurobiology, 82*, 149–169.

Amantea, D., Tassorelli, C., Petrelli, F., Certo, M., Bezzi, P., Micieli, G., et al. (2014). Understanding the multifaceted role of inflammatory mediators in ischemic stroke. *Current Medicinal Chemistry, 21*(18), 2098–2117.

Arnold, M., Mattle, S., Galimanis, A., Kappeler, L., Fischer, U., Jung, S., et al. (2012). Impact of admission glucose and diabetes on recanalization and outcome after intra-arterial thrombolysis for ischaemic stroke. *International Journal of Stroke: Official Journal of the International Stroke Society*. http://dx.doi.org/10.1111/j.1747-4949.2012.00879.x.

Asahi, M., Asahi, K., Wang, X., & Lo, E. H. (2000). Reduction of tissue plasminogen activator-induced hemorrhage and brain injury by free radical spin trapping after embolic focal cerebral ischemia in rats. *Journal of Cerebral Blood Flow and Metabolism: Official Journal of the International Society of Cerebral Blood Flow and Metabolism, 20*, 452–457.

Bambauer, K. Z., Johnston, S. C., Bambauer, D. E., & Zivin, J. A. (2006). Reasons why few patients with acute stroke receive tissue plasminogen activator. *Archives of Neurology, 63*, 661–664.

Bao Dang, Q., Lapergue, B., Tran-Dinh, A., Diallo, D., Moreno, J. A., Mazighi, M., et al. (2013). High-density lipoproteins limit neutrophil-induced damage to the blood-brain barrier in vitro. *Journal of Cerebral Blood Flow and Metabolism: Official Journal of the International Society of Cerebral Blood Flow and Metabolism*, *33*, 575–582.

Bellolio, M. F., Gilmore, R. M., & Stead, L. G. (2011). Insulin for glycaemic control in acute ischaemic stroke. *Cochrane Database of Systematic Reviews*, (9), CD005346.

Benchenane, K., Berezowski, V., Fernandez-Monreal, M., Brillault, J., Valable, S., Dehouck, M. P., et al. (2005). Oxygen glucose deprivation switches the transport of tPA across the blood-brain barrier from an LRP-dependent to an increased LRP-independent process. *Stroke*, *36*, 1065–1070.

Borlongan, C. V., Glover, L. E., Sanberg, P. R., & Hess, D. C. (2012). Permeating the blood brain barrier and abrogating the inflammation in stroke: Implications for stroke therapy. *Current Pharmaceutical Design*, *18*, 3670–3676.

Bruno, A., Kent, T. A., Coull, B. M., Shankar, R. R., Saha, C., Becker, K. J., et al. (2008). Treatment of hyperglycemia in ischemic stroke (THIS): A randomized pilot trial. *Stroke: A Journal of Cerebral Circulation*, *39*, 384–389.

Bruno, A., Levine, S. R., Frankel, M. R., Brott, T. G., Lin, Y., Tilley, B. C., et al. (2002). Admission glucose level and clinical outcomes in the NINDS rt-PA Stroke Trial. *Neurology*, *59*, 669–674.

Capes, S. E., Hunt, D., Malmberg, K., Pathak, P., & Gerstein, H. C. (2001). Stress hyperglycemia and prognosis of stroke in nondiabetic and diabetic patients: A systematic overview. *Stroke*, *32*(10), 2426–2432.

Ceriello, A., Novials, A., Ortega, E., Canivell, S., La Sala, L., Pujadas, G., et al. (2013). Glucagon-like peptide 1 reduces endothelial dysfunction, inflammation, and oxidative stress induced by both hyperglycemia and hypoglycemia in type 1 diabetes. *Diabetes Care*, *36*, 2346–2350.

Chapman, S. N., Mehndiratta, P., Johansen, M. C., McMurry, T. L., Johnston, K. C., & Southerland, A. M. (2014). Current perspectives on the use of intravenous recombinant tissue plasminogen activator (tPA) for treatment of acute ischemic stroke. *Vascular Health and Risk Management*, *10*, 75–87.

Dankbaar, J. W., Hom, J., Schneider, T., Cheng, S. C., Bredno, J., Lau, B. C., et al. (2011). Dynamic perfusion-CT assessment of early changes in blood brain barrier permeability of acute ischaemic stroke patients. *Journal of Neuroradiology*, *38*, 161–166.

De Silva, D. A., Ebinger, M., Christensen, S., Parsons, M. W., Levi, C., Butcher, K., et al. (2010). Baseline diabetic status and admission blood glucose were poor prognostic factors in the EPITHET trial. *Cerebrovascular Diseases*, *29*, 14–21.

Death, A. K., Fisher, E. J., McGrath, K. C., & Yue, D. K. (2003). High glucose alters matrix metalloproteinase expression in two key vascular cells: Potential impact on atherosclerosis in diabetes. *Atherosclerosis*, *168*, 263–269.

Desilles, J. P., Meseguer, E., Labreuche, J., Lapergue, B., Sirimarco, G., Gonzalez-Valcarcel, J., et al. (2013). Diabetes mellitus, admission glucose, and outcomes after stroke thrombolysis: A registry and systematic review. *Stroke: A Journal of Cerebral Circulation*, *44*, 1915–1923.

Fagan, S. C., Cronic, L. E., & Hess, D. C. (2011). Minocycline development for acute ischemic stroke. *Translational Stroke Research*, *2*, 202–208.

Fagan, S. C., Hess, D. C., Hohnadel, E. J., Pollock, D. M., & Ergul, A. (2004). Targets for vascular protection after acute ischemic stroke. *Stroke*, *35*, 2220–2225.

Faigle, R., Sharrief, A., Marsh, E. B., Llinas, R. H., & Urrutia, V. C. (2014). Predictors of critical care needs after IV thrombolysis for acute ischemic stroke. *PLoS One*, *9*, e88652.

Fan, X., Lo, E. H., & Wang, X. (2013). Effects of minocycline plus tissue plasminogen activator combination therapy after focal embolic stroke in type 1 diabetic rats. *Stroke: A Journal of Cerebral Circulation*, *44*, 745–752.

Fan, X., Ning, M., Lo, E. H., & Wang, X. (2013). Early insulin glycemic control combined with tPA thrombolysis reduces acute brain tissue damages in a focal embolic stroke model of diabetic rats. *Stroke: A Journal of Cerebral Circulation*, *44*, 255–259.

Fan, X., Qiu, J., Yu, Z., Dai, H., Singhal, A. B., Lo, E. H., et al. (2012). A rat model of studying tissue-type plasminogen activator thrombolysis in ischemic stroke with diabetes. *Stroke: A Journal of Cerebral Circulation*, *43*, 567–570.

Fernandez-Monreal, M., Lopez-Atalaya, J. P., Benchenane, K., Cacquevel, M., Dulin, F., Le Caer, J. P., et al. (2004). Arginine 260 of the amino-terminal domain of NR1 subunit is critical for tissue-type plasminogen activator-mediated enhancement of N-methyl-D-aspartate receptor signaling. *Journal of Biological Chemistry*, *279*, 50850–50856.

Fisher, M., Feuerstein, G., Howells, D. W., Hurn, P. D., Kent, T. A., Savitz, S. I., et al. (2009). Update of the stroke therapy academic industry roundtable preclinical recommendations. *Stroke: A Journal of Cerebral Circulation*, *40*, 2244–2250.

Furie, K. L., Kasner, S. E., Adams, R. J., Albers, G. W., Bush, R. L., Fagan, S. C., et al. (2011). Guidelines for the prevention of stroke in patients with stroke or transient ischemic attack: A guideline for healthcare professionals from the American Heart Association/American Stroke Association. *Stroke: A Journal of Cerebral Circulation*, *42*, 227–276.

Gasche, Y., Copin, J. C., Sugawara, T., Fujimura, M., & Chan, P. H. (2001). Matrix metalloproteinase inhibition prevents oxidative stress-associated blood-brain barrier disruption after transient focal cerebral ischemia. *Journal of Cerebral Blood Flow and Metabolism*, *21*, 1393–1400.

Gidday, J. M., Gasche, Y. G., Copin, J. C., Shah, A. R., Perez, R. S., Shapiro, S. D., et al. (2005). Leukocyte-derived matrix metalloproteinase-9 mediates blood-brain barrier breakdown and is proinflammatory after transient focal cerebral ischemia. *American Journal of Physiology Heart and Circulatory Physiology*. *289*, H558–H568.

Gray, S. P., & Jandeleit-Dahm, K. (2014). The pathobiology of diabetic vascular complications—Cardiovascular and kidney disease. *Journal of Molecular Medicine*, *92*(5), 441–452.

Hacke, W., Kaste, M., Bluhmki, E., Brozman, M., Davalos, A., Guidetti, D., et al. (2008). Thrombolysis with alteplase 3 to 4.5 hours after acute ischemic stroke. *New England Journal of Medicine*, *359*, 1317–1329.

Hafez, S., Coucha, M., Bruno, A., Fagan, S. C., & Ergul, A. (2014). Hyperglycemia, acute ischemic stroke, and thrombolytic therapy. *Translational Stroke Research*, *5*(4), 442–453.

Hagiwara, H., Kaizu, K., Uriu, K., Noguchi, T., Takagi, I., Qie, Y. L., et al. (2003). Expression of type-1 plasminogen activator inhibitor in the kidney of diabetic rat models. *Thrombosis Research*, *111*, 301–309.

Hamilton, S. J., & Watts, G. F. (2013). Endothelial dysfunction in diabetes: Pathogenesis, significance, and treatment. *The Review of Diabetic Studies: RDS*, *10*, 133–156.

Hawkins, B. T., Lundeen, T. F., Norwood, K. M., Brooks, H. L., & Egleton, R. D. (2007). Increased blood-brain barrier permeability and altered tight junctions in experimental diabetes in the rat: Contribution of hyperglycaemia and matrix metalloproteinases. *Diabetologia*, *50*, 202–211.

Hess, D. C., & Fagan, S. C. (2010). Repurposing an old drug to improve the use and safety of tissue plasminogen activator for acute ischemic stroke: Minocycline. *Pharmacotherapy*, *30*, 55S–61S.

Ishrat, T., Soliman, S., Guan, W., Saler, M., & Fagan, S. C. (2012). Vascular protection to increase the safety of tissue plasminogen activator for stroke. *Current Pharmaceutical Design*, *18*, 3677–3684.

Jian Liu, K., & Rosenberg, G. A. (2005). Matrix metalloproteinases and free radicals in cerebral ischemia. *Free Radical Biology and Medicine*, *39*, 71–80.

Jiang, Q., Ewing, J. R., & Chopp, M. (2012). MRI of blood-brain barrier permeability in cerebral ischemia. *Translational Stroke Research*, *3*, 56–64.

Jickling, G. C., Liu, D., Stamova, B., Ander, B. P., Zhan, X., Lu, A., et al. (2014). Hemorrhagic transformation after ischemic stroke in animals and humans. *Journal of Cerebral Blood Flow and Metabolism: Official Journal of the International Society of Cerebral Blood Flow and Metabolism*, *34*, 185–199.

Jin, R., Yang, G., & Li, G. (2010). Molecular insights and therapeutic targets for blood-brain barrier disruption in ischemic stroke: Critical role of matrix metalloproteinases and tissue-type plasminogen activator. *Neurobiology of Disease*, *38*, 376–385.

Jullienne, A., & Badaut, J. (2013). Molecular contributions to neurovascular unit dysfunctions after brain injuries: Lessons for target-specific drug development. *Future Neurology*, *8*, 677–689.

Kamada, H., Yu, F., Nito, C., & Chan, P. H. (2007). Influence of hyperglycemia on oxidative stress and matrix metalloproteinase-9 activation after focal cerebral ischemia/reperfusion in rats: Relation to blood-brain barrier dysfunction. *Stroke: A Journal of Cerebral Circulation*, *38*, 1044–1049.

Karolczak, K., Rozalska, S., Wieczorek, M., Labieniec-Watala, M., & Watala, C. (2012). Poly(amido)amine dendrimers generation 4.0 (PAMAM G4) reduce blood hyperglycaemia and restore impaired blood-brain barrier permeability in streptozotocin diabetes in rats. *International Journal of Pharmaceutics*, *436*, 508–518.

Kase, C. S., Furlan, A. J., Wechsler, L. R., Higashida, R. T., Rowley, H. A., Hart, R. G., et al. (2001). Cerebral hemorrhage after intra-arterial thrombolysis for ischemic stroke: The PROACT II trial. *Neurology*, *57*, 1603–1610.

Kaur, C., & Ling, E. A. (2008). Blood brain barrier in hypoxic-ischemic conditions. *Current Neurovascular Research*, *5*, 71–81.

Kaur, J., Zhao, Z., Klein, G. M., Lo, E. H., & Buchan, A. M. (2004). The neurotoxicity of tissue plasminogen activator? *Journal of Cerebral Blood Flow and Metabolism: Official Journal of the International Society of Cerebral Blood Flow and Metabolism*, *24*, 945–963.

Kelly, P. J., Morrow, J. D., Ning, M., Koroshetz, W., Lo, E. H., Terry, E., et al. (2008). Oxidative stress and matrix metalloproteinase-9 in acute ischemic stroke: The Biomarker Evaluation for Antioxidant Therapies in Stroke (BEAT-Stroke) study. *Stroke*, *39*, 100–104.

Kruyt, N. D., Biessels, G. J., Devries, J. H., & Roos, Y. B. (2010). Hyperglycemia in acute ischemic stroke: Pathophysiology and clinical management. *Nature Reviews Neurology*, *6*, 145–155.

Lakhan, S. E., Kirchgessner, A., Tepper, D., & Leonard, A. (2013). Matrix metalloproteinases and blood-brain barrier disruption in acute ischemic stroke. *Frontiers in Neurology*, *4*, 32.

Lapchak, P. A., Araujo, D. M., Song, D., Wei, J., Purdy, R., & Zivin, J. A. (2002). Effects of the spin trap agent disodium- [tert-butylimino)methyl]benzene-1,3-disulfonate N-oxide (generic NXY-059) on intracerebral hemorrhage in a rabbit Large clot embolic stroke model: Combination studies with tissue plasminogen activator. *Stroke*, *33*, 1665–1670.

Lapchak, P. A., Chapman, D. F., & Zivin, J. A. (2001). Pharmacological effects of the spin trap agents N-t-butyl-phenylnitrone (PBN) and 2,2,6, 6-tetramethylpiperidine-N-oxyl (TEMPO) in a rabbit thromboembolic stroke model: Combination studies with the thrombolytic tissue plasminogen activator. *Stroke*, *32*, 147–153.

Lee, S. R., Wang, X., Tsuji, K., & Lo, E. H. (2004a). Extracellular proteolytic pathophysiology in the neurovascular unit after stroke. *Neurological Research*, *26*, 854–861.

Lo, E. H., Broderick, J. P., & Moskowitz, M. A. (2004). tPA and proteolysis in the neurovascular unit. *Stroke*, *35*, 354–356.

Lo, E. H., Wang, X., & Cuzner, M. L. (2002a). Extracellular proteolysis in brain injury and inflammation: Role for plasminogen activators and matrix metalloproteinases. *Journal of Neuroscience Research, 69*, 1–9.

Lucke-Wold, B. P., Turner, R. C., Lucke-Wold, A. N., Rosen, C. L., & Huber, J. D. (2012). Age and the metabolic syndrome as risk factors for ischemic stroke: Improving preclinical models of ischemic stroke. *The Yale Journal of Biology and Medicine, 85*, 523–539.

MacDougall, N. J., & Muir, K. W. (2011). Hyperglycaemia and infarct size in animal models of middle cerebral artery occlusion: Systematic review and meta-analysis. *Journal of Cerebral Blood Flow and Metabolism: Official Journal of the International Society of Cerebral Blood Flow and Metabolism, 31*, 807–818.

Manna, P., & Sil, P. C. (2012). Impaired redox signaling and mitochondrial uncoupling contributes vascular inflammation and cardiac dysfunction in type 1 diabetes: Protective role of arjunolic acid. *Biochimie, 94*, 786–797.

Miller, D. J., Simpson, J. R., & Silver, B. (2011). Safety of thrombolysis in acute ischemic stroke: A review of complications, risk factors, and newer technologies. *The Neurohospitalist, 1*, 138–147.

Montaner, J., Molina, C. A., Monasterio, J., Abilleira, S., Arenillas, J. F., Ribo, M., et al. (2003). Matrix metalloproteinase-9 pretreatment level predicts intracranial hemorrhagic complications after thrombolysis in human stroke. *Circulation, 107*, 598–603.

Najjar, S., Pearlman, D. M., Devinsky, O., Najjar, A., & Zagzag, D. (2013). Neurovascular unit dysfunction with blood-brain barrier hyperpermeability contributes to major depressive disorder: A review of clinical and experimental evidence. *Journal of Neuroinflammation, 10*, 142.

Nassar, T., Akkawi, S., Shina, A., Haj-Yehia, A., Bdeir, K., Tarshis, M., et al. (2004). In vitro and in vivo effects of tPA and PAI-1 on blood vessel tone. *Blood, 103*, 897–902.

Nicole, O., Docagne, F., Ali, C., Margaill, I., Carmeliet, P., MacKenzie, E. T., et al. (2001). The proteolytic activity of tissue-plasminogen activator enhances NMDA receptor-mediated signaling. *Nature Medicine, 7*, 59–64.

Ning, R., Chopp, M., Yan, T., Zacharek, A., Zhang, C., Roberts, C., et al. (2012). Tissue plasminogen activator treatment of stroke in type-1 diabetes rats. *Neuroscience, 222*, 326–332.

Okazaki, M., Zhang, H., Tsuji, M., Morio, Y., & Oguchi, K. (1997). Blood coagulability and fibrinolysis in streptozotocin-induced diabetic rats. *Journal of Atherosclerosis and Thrombosis, 4*(1), 27–33.

Peters, S. A., Huxley, R. R., & Woodward, M. (2014). Diabetes as a risk factor for stroke in women compared with men: A systematic review and meta-analysis of 64 cohorts, including 775 385 individuals and 12 539 strokes. *Lancet, 383*(9933), 1973–1980.

Plane, J. M., Shen, Y., Pleasure, D. E., & Deng, W. (2010). Prospects for minocycline neuroprotection. *Archives of Neurology, 67*, 1442–1448.

Poppe, A. Y., Majumdar, S. R., Jeerakathil, T., Ghali, W., Buchan, A. M., & Hill, M. D. (2009). Admission hyperglycemia predicts a worse outcome in stroke patients treated with intravenous thrombolysis. *Diabetes Care, 32*, 617–622.

Pun, P. B., Lu, J., & Moochhala, S. (2009). Involvement of ROS in BBB dysfunction. *Free Radical Research, 43*, 348–364.

Radisky, D. C., Levy, D. D., Littlepage, L. E., Liu, H., Nelson, C. M., Fata, J. E., et al. (2005). Rac1b and reactive oxygen species mediate MMP-3-induced EMT and genomic instability. *Nature, 436*, 123–127.

Ribo, M., Molina, C., Montaner, J., Rubiera, M., Delgado-Mederos, R., Arenillas, J. F., et al. (2005). Acute hyperglycemia state is associated with lower tPA-induced recanalization rates in stroke patients. *Stroke: A Journal of Cerebral Circulation, 36*, 1705–1709.

Rosell, A., Foerch, C., Murata, Y., & Lo, E. H. (2008). Mechanisms and markers for hemorrhagic transformation after stroke. *Acta Neurochirurgica. Supplement, 105*, 173–178.

Rosenberg, G. A. (2002). Matrix metalloproteinases in neuroinflammation. *Glia, 39*, 279–291.

Rossi, D. J., Brady, J. D., & Mohr, C. (2007). Astrocyte metabolism and signaling during brain ischemia. *Nature Neuroscience, 10*, 1377–1386.

Rosso, C., Corvol, J. C., Pires, C., Crozier, S., Attal, Y., Jacqueminet, S., et al. (2012). Intensive versus subcutaneous insulin in patients with hyperacute stroke: Results from the randomized INSULINFARCT trial. *Stroke: A Journal of Cerebral Circulation, 43*, 2343–2349.

Sandoval, K. E., & Witt, K. A. (2008). Blood-brain barrier tight junction permeability and ischemic stroke. *Neurobiology of Disease, 32*, 200–219.

Seo, J. H., Guo, S., Lok, J., Navaratna, D., Whalen, M. J., Kim, K. W., et al. (2012). Neurovascular matrix metalloproteinases and the blood-brain barrier. *Current Pharmaceutical Design, 18*, 3645–3648.

Shao, B., & Bayraktutan, U. (2013). Hyperglycaemia promotes cerebral barrier dysfunction through activation of protein kinase C-beta. *Diabetes, Obesity & Metabolism, 15*, 993–999.

Simi, A., Tsakiri, N., Wang, P., & Rothwell, N. J. (2007). Interleukin-1 and inflammatory neurodegeneration. *Biochemical Society Transactions, 35*, 1122–1126.

Srivastava, K., Shao, B., & Bayraktutan, U. (2013). PKC-beta exacerbates in vitro brain barrier damage in hyperglycemic settings via regulation of RhoA/Rho-kinase/MLC2 pathway. *Journal of Cerebral Blood Flow and Metabolism: Official Journal of the International Society of Cerebral Blood Flow and Metabolism, 33*, 1928–1936.

Sussman, E. S., & Connolly, E. S., Jr. (2013). Hemorrhagic transformation: A review of the rate of hemorrhage in the major clinical trials of acute ischemic stroke. *Frontiers in Neurology, 4*, 69.

Thomalla, G., Kohrmann, M., Rother, J., & Schellinger, P. D. (2007). Effective acute stroke treatment beyond approval limitations: Intravenous thrombolysis within an extended time window (3–6 h) and in old patients (aged 80 or older). *Fortschritte der Neurologie-Psychiatrie, 75*, 343–350.

Thomalla, G., Schwark, C., Sobesky, J., Bluhmki, E., Fiebach, J. B., Fiehler, J., et al. (2006). Outcome and symptomatic bleeding complications of intravenous thrombolysis within 6 hours in MRI-selected stroke patients: Comparison of a German multicenter study with the pooled data of ATLANTIS, ECASS, and NINDS tPA trials. *Stroke, 37*, 852–858.

Wang, X., Lee, S. R., Arai, K., Lee, S. R., Tsuji, K., Rebeck, G. W., et al. (2003). Lipoprotein receptor-mediated induction of matrix metalloproteinase by tissue plasminogen activator. *Nature Medicine, 9*, 1313–1317.

Wang, X., & Lo, E. H. (2003a). Triggers and mediators of hemorrhagic transformation in cerebral ischemia. *Molecular Neurobiology, 28*, 229–244.

Wang, X., Rosell, A., & Lo, E. H. (2008). Targeting extracellular matrix proteolysis for hemorrhagic complications of tPA stroke therapy. *CNS & Neurological Disorders Drug Targets*, 7, 235–242.

Wang, X., Tsuji, K., Lee, S. R., Ning, M., Furie, K. L., Buchan, A. M., et al. (2004a). Mechanisms of hemorrhagic transformation after tissue plasminogen activator reperfusion therapy for ischemic stroke. *Stroke: A Journal of Cerebral Circulation, 35*, 2726–2730.

Warach, S., & Latour, L. L. (2004). Evidence of reperfusion injury, exacerbated by thrombolytic therapy, in human focal brain ischemia using a novel imaging marker of early blood-brain barrier disruption. *Stroke: A Journal of Cerebral Circulation, 35*, 2659–2661.

Weintraub, M. I. (2006). Thrombolysis (tissue plasminogen activator) in stroke: A medicolegal quagmire. *Stroke: A Journal of Cerebral Circulation, 37*, 1917–1922.

Whiteley, W. N., Thompson, D., Murray, G., Cohen, G., Lindley, R. I., Wardlaw, J., et al. (2014). Targeting recombinant tissue-type plasminogen activator in acute ischemic stroke based on risk of intracranial hemorrhage or poor functional outcome: An analysis of the third international stroke trial. *Stroke: A Journal of Cerebral Circulation, 45*, 1000–1006.

Won, S. J., Tang, X. N., Suh, S. W., Yenari, M. A., & Swanson, R. A. (2011). Hyperglycemia promotes tissue plasminogen activator-induced hemorrhage by increasing superoxide production. *Annals of Neurology*, *70*, 583–590.
Yepes, M., Sandkvist, M., Moore, E. G., Bugge, T. H., Strickland, D. K., & Lawrence, D. A. (2003). Tissue-type plasminogen activator induces opening of the blood-brain barrier via the LDL receptor-related protein. *Journal of Clinical Investigation*, *112*, 1533–1540.
Yong, V. W., Wells, J., Giuliani, F., Casha, S., Power, C., & Metz, L. M. (2004). The promise of minocycline in neurology. *Lancet Neurology*, *3*, 744–751.
Zhang, R. L., Chopp, M., Zhang, Z. G., Jiang, Q., & Ewing, J. R. (1997). A rat model of focal embolic cerebral ischemia. *Brain Research*, *766*, 83–92.
Zhang, X., Polavarapu, R., She, H., Mao, Z., & Yepes, M. (2007). Tissue-type plasminogen activator and the low-density lipoprotein receptor-related protein mediate cerebral ischemia-induced nuclear factor-kappaB pathway activation. *The American Journal of Pathology*, *171*, 1281–1290.
Zhang, L., Zalewski, A., Liu, Y., Mazurek, T., Cowan, S., Martin, J. L., et al. (2003). Diabetes-induced oxidative stress and low-grade inflammation in porcine coronary arteries. *Circulation*, *108*(4), 472–478.
Zhao, F., Hua, Y., He, Y., Keep, R. F., & Xi, G. (2011). Minocycline-induced attenuation of iron overload and brain injury after experimental intracerebral hemorrhage. *Stroke: A Journal of Cerebral Circulation*, *42*, 3587–3593.
Zhu, H., Fan, X., Yu, Z., Liu, J., Murata, Y., Lu, J., et al. (2010). Annexin A2 combined with low-dose tPA improves thrombolytic therapy in a rat model of focal embolic stroke. *Journal of Cerebral Blood Flow and Metabolism: Official Journal of the International Society of Cerebral Blood Flow and Metabolism*, *30*, 1137–1146.

CHAPTER FOURTEEN

Aging, the Metabolic Syndrome, and Ischemic Stroke: Redefining the Approach for Studying the Blood–Brain Barrier in a Complex Neurological Disease

Brandon P. Lucke-Wold[*,†], Aric F. Logsdon[†,‡], Ryan C. Turner[*,†], Charles L. Rosen[*,†], Jason D. Huber[†,‡,1]

[*]Department of Neurosurgery, West Virginia University, School of Medicine, Morgantown, West Virginia, USA

[†]The Center for Neuroscience, West Virginia University, School of Medicine, Morgantown, West Virginia, USA

[‡]Department of Basic Pharmaceutical Sciences, West Virginia University, School of Pharmacy, Morgantown, West Virginia, USA

[1]Corresponding author: e-mail address: jhuber@hsc.wvu.edu

Contents

Advances in Pharmacology, Volume 71
ISSN 1054-3589
http://dx.doi.org/10.1016/bs.apha.2014.07.001

Abstract

The blood–brain barrier (BBB) has many important functions in maintaining the brain's immune-privileged status. Endothelial cells, astrocytes, and pericytes have important roles in preserving vasculature integrity. As we age, cell senescence can contribute to BBB compromise. The compromised BBB allows an influx of inflammatory cytokines to enter the brain. These cytokines lead to neuronal and glial damage. Ultimately, the functional changes within the brain can cause age-related disease. One of the most prominent age-related diseases is ischemic stroke. Stroke is the largest cause of disability and is third largest cause of mortality in the United States. The biggest risk factors for stroke, besides age, are results of the metabolic syndrome. The metabolic syndrome, if unchecked, quickly advances to outcomes that include diabetes, hypertension, cardiovascular disease, and obesity. The contribution from these comorbidities to BBB compromise is great. Some of the common molecular pathways activated include: endoplasmic reticulum stress, reactive oxygen species formation, and glutamate excitotoxicity. In this chapter, we examine how age-related changes to cells within the central nervous system interact with comorbidities. We then look at how comorbidities lead to increased risk for stroke through BBB disruption. Finally, we discuss key molecular pathways of interest with a focus on therapeutic targets that warrant further investigation.

1. INTRODUCTION

Age is the single biggest risk factor for ischemic stroke (Denti et al., 2013). Aging disrupts collagen IV and laminin in vessel walls causing a predilection for occlusion (Hawkes et al., 2013). It has also been proposed that aging diminishes the ability of neuronal support cells to respond to injury following blood–brain barrier (BBB) disruption (Sohrabji, Bake, & Lewis, 2013). In addition, aging causes increased numbers of migrating microglia, T cells, and dendritic cells to enter the brain following middle cerebral artery occlusion (Manwani et al., 2013). The combination of these factors may account for why stroke severity is higher in the elderly (Manwani et al., 2011). Furthermore, aging leads to worse outcome and increased risk of hemorrhagic transformation following intravenous thrombolysis administration (Dharmasaroja, Muengtaweepongsa, & Dharmasaroja, 2013). Recombinant tissue plasminogen activator is currently the only FDA-approved drug for treating ischemic stroke and is limited to a 4.5-h time window following stroke onset (Fonseca, Geraldes, Almeida, & Pinhoe Melo, 2011). The lack of available interventions and the strict time window for treatment may account for why ischemic stroke is the leading cause of disability in developed nations (Fisher, Loewy, Hardy, Schlosser, & Vinogradov, 2013). Stroke not only causes motor dysfunction but also exacerbates cognitive decline in the elderly and disrupts the process of respiration (Kaffashian et al., 2013; Manor, Hu, Peng, Lipsitz, & Novak, 2012). Although age has recently been accepted as a necessary component for successfully studying stroke pathophysiology and BBB disruption, the role that aging plays in conjunction with comorbid risk factors such as coronary artery disease, hypertension, type II diabetes, and obesity has yet to be determined.

In the first part of this chapter, we examine how aging affects cell types within the central nervous system (CNS), and more importantly how these changes contribute to ischemic stroke and BBB disruption. Specifically, we look at how aging alters astrocytes, microglia, endothelial cells, and neurons. In the second part of the chapter, we examine how comorbidities interact with age to cause worse ischemic stroke outcomes. Recent findings have validated that the metabolic syndrome contributes substantially to the future development of ischemic stroke in at-risk individuals (Del Brutto et al., 2013). The metabolic syndrome consists of abdominal obesity, high blood pressure, cardiovascular disease, elevated plasma glucose, and high levels of triglycerides (Kim et al., 2013). Although many exciting projects have examined how individual components of the metabolic syndrome increase risk for ischemic stroke, few groups have looked at how age fits into the overall mixture of comorbidities. We propose that age-specific changes in the pathophysiology of cardiovascular disease, hypertension, diabetes mellitus type II (DM2), and obesity contribute to glutamate excitotoxicity, mitochondrial dysfunction, oxidative stress, BBB disruption, and endoplasmic reticulum (ER) stress following acute ischemic infarct.

2. CELL AGING

The aging process is of growing concern due to the increasing number of individuals reaching advanced age in the United States. Peripheral musculoskeletal changes are well documented and naturally occur during the aging process; however, the cognitive and memory declines are poorly understood. These declines are often the result of neuronal or glial cell death. The aging process increases the risk of cell death including: apoptosis from natural cell senescence, excitotoxicity from overactive glutamate release, and the accumulation of oxidative stressors and unfolded proteins.

Characterizing the mechanistic changes seen in each cell type within the brain during aging will help with the discovery of therapeutics that combat the unique injury paradigm seen in the aged population.

Over the past decade, a paradigm shift has occurred in the study of the CNS. Neurons were once considered as the only influential cells for brain functioning while other cells were only supportive or additive. Glial cells have recently gained prominence for the unique role they play in the brain and the BBB. Three main types of glial cells include: astrocytes, microglia, and endothelial cells. Each cell type has been extensively studied in recent years for the vital roles they play in a variety of physiological and pathological conditions.

The purpose of this section is to provide insight into each cell type and how they change in structure and function as a result of aging. The changes in functionality will be appropriated with stroke and BBB disruption. In particular, we examine how age-related changes make patients more susceptible to stroke, and ultimately how the different cell types respond to ischemic stroke in aged animals (Fig. 1). We argue that the most clinically relevant approach for studying stroke is through the use of aged animals.

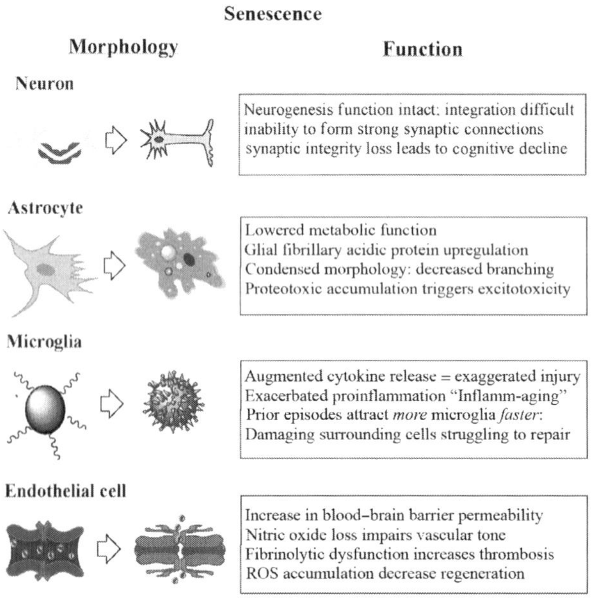
Senescence
Morphology
Function
Neuron
Neurogenesis function intact; integration difficult
inability to form strong synaptic connections
synaptic integrity loss leads to cognitive decline
Astrocyte
Lowered metabolic function
Glial fibrillary acidic protein upregulation
Condensed morphology: decreased branching
Proteotoxic accumulation triggers excitotoxicity
Microglia
Augmented cytokine release = exaggerated injury
Exacerbated proinflammation "Inflamm-aging"
Prior episodes attract more microglia faster:
Damaging surrounding cells struggling to repair
Endothelial cell
Increase in blood–brain barrier permeability
Nitric oxide loss impairs vascular tone
Fibrinolytic dysfunction increases thrombosis
ROS accumulation decrease regeneration

Figure 1 Cell-related changes with senescence.

2.1. Aging and astrocytes

The role of glia in disease has become a topic of importance in recent years (Liddell, Robinson, Dringen, & Bishop, 2010; Ramirez, Ramirez, Salazar, de Hoz, & Trivino, 2001). With a greater depth of understanding about glial cell functionality in age-related disorders such as Alzheimer's disease (AD) and Parkinson's disease (PD), the influence that age has on each glial cell type has become an emerging theme in neuroscience (Blasko et al., 2004; Ciesielska et al., 2009; Papadopoulos, Koumenis, Yuan, & Giffard, 1998). Each glial cell has an established role in the functioning of the CNS that changes as a result of the natural aging process. In this section, we discuss how age-related changes in astrocytes contribute to ischemic stroke.

The astrocyte plays important roles in neuronal maintenance (Schousboe, 2003), growth factor promotion (Le & Esquenazi, 2002), and extracellular buffering capabilities (Lian & Stringer, 2004). Other important functions include: extracellular potassium buffering (Walz, 2000), BBB maintenance (Holash, Noden, & Stewart, 1993), growth factor release (Ciccarelli et al., 1999), and neurotransmitter regulation (Westergaard, Sonnewald, & Schousboe, 1994). Recent focus has been placed on astrocyte-mediated senescence (Liddell et al., 2010; Wu, Zhang, & Yew, 2005). Much like neurons, astrocytes are subject to age-related burdens, such as oxidative stress (Brera, Serrano, & de Ceballos, 2000; Niranjan, 2013) and telomeric replication exhaustion (Bhat et al., 2012; Bitto et al., 2010). These burdens are common reference markers for a cell undergoing senescence. Astrocytes have recently been shown to contribute to cognitive deficits in aged rats (Lima et al., 2014). The cognitive decline could possibly result from age-related changes to astrocyte synaptic connections (Cotrina & Nedergaard, 2002), decreased metabolic capacities (Patel & Brewer, 2003), and altered astrocyte foot processes at the BBB (Saito et al., 2011). In aged animals, astrocytes are more condensed and distorted with decreased branch formation (Cerbai et al., 2012). The altered astrocytes in addition to BBB disruption contribute to increased neuroinflammation (Zehendner, White, Hedrich, & Luhmann, 2014).

The hallmark protein demarcating astrocyte activation is known as glial fibrilary acidic protein (GFAP) (O'Callaghan & Sriram, 2005). GFAP expression and vimentin filament production are both signs of neural injury and astrocyte activation (Fedoroff, White, Neal, Subrahmanyan, & Kalnins, 1983). The astrocyte produces these proteins in abundance when neighboring neurons are injured or are undergoing apoptosis (Cernak et al., 2010;

Suzuki, Sakata, Kato, Connor, & Morita, 2012). In the aging brain of rats, GFAP and vimentin filaments are at a higher basal level, which inhibits their mobility and functionality (Campuzano, Castillo-Ruiz, Acarin, Gonzalez, & Castellano, 2011). GFAP expression is particularly elevated in the hippocampus of aged animals (Cerbai et al., 2012). These activated astrocytes exacerbate the response to ischemia and contribute to the breakdown of the BBB.

Astrocytes are constantly releasing growth factors into the extracellular environment of the CNS, which interact with microglia and neurons. Likewise, astrocyte function is dictated by cytokines and other inflammatory components released by neurons and microglia (Dinapoli et al., 2010). This inflammatory cross talk is a primary reason for large volume strokes in aged rats (Salminen et al., 2011). Increased cytokine levels and proteotoxic aggregates overactivate astrocytes, which can lead to glutamate excitotoxicity (Morimoto, 2008). The accumulation of proteotoxic aggregates is a result of the aging process that results from the inability of the proteasome to clear aggregates within the CNS (Abd El Mohsen et al., 2005). These aggregates activate excitotoxic cascades, which ultimately lead to cell death. The maintenance of the cellular environment by astrocytes, including the BBB, is therefore compromised.

2.2. Aging and microglia

One of the major differences in microglial cell function in the aged brain is its exaggerated response to injury. In response to injury, microglia transport to the site of damage and clean up debri (Clarner et al., 2012). The process is very effective in young animals; however, in aged animals, the risk of damage to surrounding cells outweighs the potential benefit (Huizinga et al., 2012). In the aged brain, a continuous release of inflammatory cytokines disrupts the natural attempt for cell repair (McMillian, Thai, Hong, O'Callaghan, & Pennypacker, 1994). Harnessing the beneficial effect of microglia activation in response to injury without having a continuous stream of cytokine release is an ongoing focus of future research (Hefendehl et al., 2014; Hopp et al., 2014).

Microglia are essentially the immune system of the brain (Rock et al., 2004). When injury occurs in the brain, microglia change morphology and travel to the site of injury (Hayashi & Nakanishi, 2013; Ohsawa & Kohsaka, 2011). When damaged cells release chemokines, they recruit and activate nearby microglia (Bilbo, 2011). In the aged brain, neuroinflammation cascades are triggered rapidly (Njie et al., 2012). This may account for why aged animals show more deleterious signs of injury following stroke (Popa-Wagner et al., 2010). The augmented inflammatory response seen in aged animals can harm cells attempting to repair themselves. As we age, our peripheral immune system weakens as a result of a deteriorated thymus and a loss in T cells and B cells. In contrast, the immune system of the aged brain is constantly active during injury. The microglia in the aged brain participate in a positive feedback cycle. Activated microglia produce reactive oxygen species (ROS), causing cell death and an increase in glutamate levels (Trotti, Danbolt, & Volterra, 1998). The increased glutamate triggers microglia to release even more proinflammatory cytokines (Taylor, Jones, Kubota, & Pocock, 2005). This vicious cycle can easily be quelled by a young brain with full functioning astrocytes that uptake excess glutamate. Enzymes in the young brain also alleviate the dangers of ROS.

Microglia function by moving to the site of injury, releasing inflammatory cytokines to attract other macrophages, and cleaning up cellular debris (Napoli & Neumann, 2009). To measure microglia activation, a variety of antibodies can be used for immunohistochemistry and Western blot, which include: CD11β, CD45, CD68, and CD206. CD45 is expressed on all nucleated hematopoietic cells, or cells involved in CNS immunity (Penninger, Irie-Sasaki, Sasaki, & Oliveira-dos-Santos, 2001). CD11β is a marker of microglia recruitment (Perego, Fumagalli, & De Simoni, 2011), CD68 is a marker of active phagocytosis (Amanzada et al., 2013), and CD206 is expressed by activated microglia during recovery (Raes, De Baetselier, et al., 2002; Raes, Noel, et al., 2002). The other common way to measure microglia activation is to detect cytokines and other inflammatory factors known to be secreted from microglia following injury. Some of these include interleukins (IL-1β, IL-1α, 1L-6, and IL-12) as well as tumor necrosis factor alpha (TNFα) and interferon gamma (IFNγ). In the aged brain, these cytokines are commonly secreted by microglia in a variety of brain regions (Lue et al., 2001). Elevated basal levels of these cytokines are seen even without injury (Ye & Johnson, 1999). The "theory of inflamm-aging" revolves around this increase in cytokines (Bartlett et al., 2012). Inflamm-aging is due to an imbalance in homeostasis with an increase in proinflammation markers and a decrease in anti-inflammatory markers (Franceschi, 2007). Several prominent researchers are seeking to correct the imbalance and prevent the excess stimulation of the brain's immune system (Franceschi et al., 2007). Age-related disease such as stroke and AD are more common in brains that are no longer able to maintain appropriate homeostasis.

Microglia have many different phenotypic states. Each state is associated with cytokine release or the release of compounds that trigger recovery and growth. Following ischemic injury, microglia conform to the proinflammatory phenotype (Easton, 2013). This phenotype is especially common in the aged rat brain following ischemic insult (Miller & Streit, 2007). A primary reason for rapid microglia phenotype switching in the aged brain is due to preconditioning (Popa-Wagner, Carmichael, Kokaia, Kessler, & Walker, 2007). Immune reactivity following minor ischemia accelerates microglia priming in the aged brain (Badan et al., 2003). The primed microglia are geared toward rapid response during the next ischemic episode.

2.3. Aging, pericytes, and endothelial cells

Age is the biggest risk factor for stroke and cardiovascular disease. Attempts to alleviate the detrimental effects of aging have been largely unsuccessful. Aging causes changes to the endothelial cells and pericytes of the CNS. Endothelial cells cover the inner surface of vasculature and play an important role in the maintenance of the BBB. Pericytes are cells that control the contracture of endothelial cells. The integrity of the BBB is often compromised with age and has become a research topic of great interest in recent years (Takechi, Pallebage-Gamarallage, Lam, Giles, & Mamo, 2013). Damaged endothelial cells that make up the BBB of an aged brain allow drugs and proteins to enter the brain that would otherwise not have access to the immune-privileged tissue (Bartels et al., 2009).Pericytes can become compromised leading to disruption of hemostatic homeostasis. Endothelial cells also help regulate homeostasis. The endothelium is important for blood coagulation and the regulation of vascular tone. Aging affects the endothelium by impairing vascular tone through the decrease in nitric oxide and concomitant increase in endothelin (Toth et al., 2013). Aging also increases coagulation activity and decreases fibrinolytic capacity, thereby increasing the risk of coronary thrombosis (Reiner et al., 2008; Sites, 1998). ROS damage endothelial cell telomeres and decrease the number and functional progenitor cells (Heiss et al., 2005).

Aging likewise results in changes to BBB enzymes and tight junction proteins (Mooradian, Haas, & Chehade, 2003). Endothelial cells in a normal brain are rounded and robust, while endothelial cells in the aging brain are flat and figureless (Lee, Clemenson, & Gage, 2012). Pericytes likewise become shriveled with aging. This change in shape allows more proteins and drugs to pass from blood to brain. Cardiovascular repair mechanisms are impaired with aging and endothelial cells are rarely regenerated (Zhu & Joyce, 2004). Stroke often occurs in the aged population due to these faulty repair mechanisms (Sierra, Coca, & Schiffrin, 2011). The severity of stroke is increased with aging as a result of decreased endothelial and pericyte cell support (Sohrabji et al., 2013). Comorbid diseases such as diabetes and obesity affect vascular mechanisms and disrupt the endothelial cell support system as will be discussed in the second part of this chapter (Wang et al., 2009). Senescence increases the susceptibility of having a stroke and leads to worsened outcome. Attempts to protect neurons and promote recovery following stroke have failed, but new therapeutic avenues focusing on brain metabolism (Poteet et al., 2012), rather than brain vasculature, may prove to be more beneficial.

2.4. Aging and neurons

Recent focus has been placed on replacing neurons that have undergone cell death due to disease. The process of neurogenesis has long been studied in the hippocampus (Brandt & Storch, 2008). The neurogenic process is impaired as a result of the aging process (Rodriguez, Jones, & Verkhratsky, 2009). Although neurogenesis is increased in the aged hippocampus, few of these cells are ever incorporated into the functional brain (Bakirci, Kafa, Uysal, & Ayberk Kurt, 2011). The key for regenerating neurons in the aging brain is their ability to survive to full differentiation and function. Just because a neuron can be "born" from neural stem cells (NSCs) does not mean that it will be integrated into the neural network and function in a way to produce new neural connections. In the aged animal, inflammation and oxidative stress damage neuronal progenitor cells (Lee, Duan, Long, Ingram, & Mattson, 2000). The new cells generated from these progenitors struggle to incorporate into the predetermined neural networks. Future studies are needed to investigate not only how to prolong neuronal survival in the aging brain but also how to integrate cells into a potentially damaged neural network.

During development, neurons migrate to predetermined sites and develop synaptic connections over time. As the neurons age, they lose their ability to create synapses (Endres & Lessmann, 2012). Aged neurons are simply less adapted to develop complex connections. One prominent reason for the age-related decrease in functioning is telomere shortening (Ferron et al., 2009). Aging also promotes glucocorticoid production, which decreases glial cell secretion of growth factors as well as neuronal cell proliferation (Yu, Yang, Holsboer, Sousa, & Almeida, 2011). The neurons can still differentiate, but without proper proliferation recovery from neural injury and cell death is challenging. Astrocytes and microglia participate in neuronal debris clearance after neurons undergo apoptosis. Neuronal apoptosis increases in the aged brain causing astrocytes and microglia to release cytokines (Cerbai et al., 2012). The cytokines released by the microglia and astrocytes damage surrounding neurons (Buschini, Piras, Nuzzi, & Vercelli, 2011). It is still under debate whether neuronal apoptosis initially triggers the cascade or if it is the result of damaged glial cells.

3. AGE AND THE METABOLIC SYNDROME

3.1. Cardiovascular disease, aging, and ischemic stroke

Cardiovascular disease increases proportionately with age and can cause deleterious problems such as chronic kidney disease, myocardial infarction, and ischemic stroke (Hui et al., 2013). The development of cardiovascular disease is dependent on both genetics and modifiable environmental components (Yanez, Burke, Manolio, Gardin, & Polak, 2009). Interestingly, most patients diagnosed with DM2 or hypertension also have underlying atherosclerosis and cardiovascular disease (Lim et al., 2012). Aging causes an increase in DNA mutations, which is a confounding factor for cardiovascular disease (Borghini, Cervelli, Galli, & Andreassi, 2013). Aging also causes an increase in matrix metalloproteinase 2, transforming growth factor β1, and intracellular adhesion molecule-1, which leads to smooth muscle cell migration into the tunica intima (Orlandi, Bochaton-Piallat, Gabbiani, & Spagnoli, 2006). Smooth muscle cell migration in combination with dysfunctional macrophage scavenger receptors may lead to the formation of fatty foam cells (Tsimikas et al., 2012). Once fatty foam cells accumulate, a plaque will form in the vessel walls (Schwedt, 2009). The plaque results in endothelial cell senescence, and as the vessel wall ages, it becomes dangerously weakened (Costopoulos, Liew, & Bennett, 2008). A weakened vessel is more prone to rupture, which will initiate proinflammatory cascades that may eventually lead to complete vessel occlusion and BBB disruption (Lakatta, 2007) (Fig. 2).

Cardiovascular disease is associated primarily with ischemic heart disease and cerebrovascular disease (Tang et al., 2014). Cerebrovascular disease can be further broken down into two outcomes: hemorrhagic stroke or ischemic stroke (Thurston, Rewak, & Kubzansky, 2013). Eighty-six percent of all

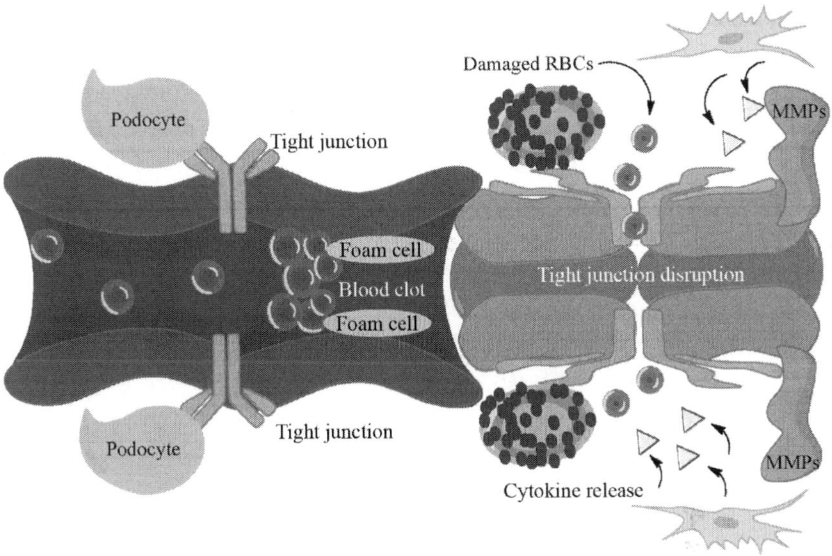

Figure 2 The metabolic syndrome significantly increases the risk for ischemic stroke and vessel occlusion. Ultimately, the BBB is compromised leading to red blood cell extravasation, matrix metalloproteinase activation, and the release of a host of inflammatory cytokines.

strokes are ischemic in nature (Shiber, Fontane, & Adewale, 2010). Not surprisingly, cardiovascular disease is reported in upwards of 67% of ischemic stroke patients (Kastorini et al., 2013). Genetic variations in chromosome 9p21 are specifically associated with ischemic stroke, whereas variations in ApoB are associated with ischemic heart disease (Ahrens et al., 2011; Calling, Ji, Sundquist, Sundquist, & Zoller, 2013). The vast majority of ischemic stroke cases, however, are mostly due to environmental factors such as smoking, sedentary lifestyle, and poor nutrition (Del Brutto et al., 2013). The American Heart Association has stated that prevention of cardiovascular disease would decrease the current number of annual ischemic strokes by 70% (Folsom et al., 2011). A key for success in treating cardiovascular disease complications in the elderly is secondary prevention. Secondary prevention involves antiplatelet therapy, anticoagulation therapy, blood pressure lowering agents, and the use of statins (Alhusban & Fagan, 2011). Currently, secondary prevention is underutilized in the elderly (Lin, Lee, Soo, & Lin, 2011). By increasing the use of secondary prevention, the incidence of ischemic strokes would drastically decrease (Castilla-Guerra, Fernandez-Moreno Mdel, & Alvarez-Suero, 2009).

3.2. Hypertension, aging, and ischemic stroke

Besides age itself, hypertension is one of the biggest risk factors for ischemic stroke (Rietbrock, Heeley, Plumb, & van Staa, 2008). The percentage of people with hypertension increases significantly with age, especially in postmenopausal women (Cohen, Curhan, & Forman, 2012). One underlying factor responsible for the increase in hypertension with age is vessel wall stiffening possibly due to increased basal activity in the renal angiotensin system (Kral et al., 2013; Vaidya & Williams, 2012). Such vessel wall stiffening can eventually lead to renal insufficiency and congestive heart failure (Joseph, Koka, & Aronow, 2008) The additional comorbidities increase the likelihood of potential vascular disturbance (Munshi et al., 2010). Risk for vascular occlusion is particularly elevated at systolic blood pressures above 180 mm Hg (Giantin et al., 2011). Inadequately treated hypertension substantially contributes to worse outcome following a vascular event (Auriel et al., 2011).

Hypertension, unlike other components of the metabolic syndrome, is not heavily dependent on genetic predisposition (Laloux, Ossemann, & Jamart, 2007). The biggest risk factors for hypertension are associated with lifestyle dynamics such as lack of physical activity, excessive alcohol consumption, and smoking (Howard et al., 2010). These factors are also directly associated with risk for ischemic stroke, and may help account for why hypertension is reported in 82% of patients with ischemic stroke (Giantin et al., 2011). Outcome severity following a stroke can be best predicted by the initial systolic blood pressure reading at admission (Soares, Abecasis, & Ferro, 2011). Hypertension ultimately results in larger infarct volumes and worse clinical outcome (Lee et al., 2014). By treating hypertension, the risk for stroke is decreased by 43% (Hisham & Bayraktutan, 2013). Hypertension can also be acutely treated following stroke but care should be made to not drop the heightened blood pressure too quickly (Feldstein, 2013). The goal is to improve neurological functional scores quickly after infarct because better acute scores correlate with improved long-term survival (Yeo et al., 2013).

3.3. Diabetes mellitus type II, aging, and ischemic stroke

DM2 decreases longevity and contributes too less successful aging (Hodge, Flicker, O'Dea, English, & Giles, 2013). A primary reason for this less successful aging is the development of peripheral neuropathy (Nguyen, Pham, Chemla, Valensi, & Cosson, 2013). Furthermore, DM2 contributes to cognitive decline by the formation of advanced glycosylated end products and ROS (Roriz-Filho et al., 2009). The molecular events cause changes in synaptic plasticity that lead to memory deficits (Artola, 2008). The accelerated brain aging has been described as diabetic encephalopathy (Biessels, van der Heide, Kamal, Bleys, & Gispen, 2002). As part of this syndrome, angiogenin is released resulting in increased risk for stroke and BBB disruption (Ning et al., 2014).

DM2 has increased over fourfold in the elderly population over the last half century (Graham et al., 2009). After age 65, the risk for ischemic stroke within 5 years for a DM2 patient is significantly elevated (Malaguarnera, Vacante, Frazzetto, & Motta, 2012). The hazard ratio for ischemic stroke is 1.83 for DM2 patients compared to a nondiabetic cohort (Murakami et al., 2012). DM2 causes worse motor outcomes and increased loss of vision following ischemic stroke, which contributes to long-term disability (Golden, Hill-Briggs, Williams, Stolka, & Mayer, 2005). In addition, DM2 negates the beneficial effects of acute recombinant tissue plasminogen factor treatment (Ning et al., 2012). Prevention and successful management of DM2 is the best solution for improving healthy aging and decreasing stroke risk (Liu et al., 2013). Pioglitazone treatment has been shown to both prevent stroke in DM2 patients and to reduce the severity of poststroke outcome (Yoshii et al., 2014).

3.4. Obesity, aging, and stroke

The prevalence of obesity has doubled in the past 30 years (Cavuoto & Nussbaum, 2014). The adjusted odds ratio for disability with a diagnosis of obesity is 1.81 (Dixon-Ibarra & Horner-Johnson, 2014). Unfortunately, this increase in disability contributes to a decreased quality of life with aging (Warkentin et al., 2014). One of the reasons for this decreased quality of life is due to the adverse role of saturated fats in the brain with time (Haast & Kiliaan, 2014). Saturated fats contribute to the formation of ROS that act on endothelial cells (Shiroto et al., 2014). The damaged endothelial cells can bind platelets and form clots (McEwen, 2014). It has been proposed that endothelial cells in obese individuals are genetically more susceptible to ROS-induced damage (Glogowska-Ligus, Dabek, Zych-Twardowska, & Tkacz, 2013). As a partially heritable disease, interventions can be implicated early in people at-risk for obesity (Samantha Sevilla & Hubal, 2014). Environmental factors such as physical inactivity, poor nutrition, drinking sugary carbonated beverages, and alcohol consumption also contribute to the epidemic of obesity (Holden et al., 2014; Martin-Calvo et al., 2014). Obesity is associated with a low level of adiponectin in the circulation leading to worsened health outcomes (Kishida, Funahashi, & Shimomura, 2014). The most adverse events such as stroke, myocardial infarction, and cardiac arrest are highest in people with both hypertension and obesity (Seimon et al., 2014). It is important to consider the entire metabolic profile because not all overweight individuals have comorbidities (van Vliet-Ostaptchouk et al., 2014).

Obese individuals with low socioeconomic status are most at risk for stroke (Piccolo, Yang, Bliwise, Yaggi, & Araujo, 2013). Vasomotor reactivity is decreased with increased body mass index predisposing to vessel occlusion (Rodriguez-Flores, Garcia-Garcia, Cano-Nigenda, & Cantu-Brito, 2014). Visceral fat, in particular, causes an increase in cerebral small vessel disease (Yamashiro et al., 2014). The most reliable measurements for visceral fat are waist circumference and waist-to-hip ratio (St Pie et al., 2014). In order to prevent serious long-term outcomes, aggressive approaches are often necessary to manage obesity. Bariatric surgery decreases the relative risk for stroke by 34% (Droste & Keipes, 2013). Roux-en-Y gastric bypass is most effective in decreasing obesity related comorbidities, but has a higher risk for complications than the commonly used sleeve gastrectomy (Li et al., 2014). Bariatric surgery has an overall success rate of 80% for long-term weight loss (Gibson, Le Page, & Taylor, 2013). Treatment must be given early since advanced age is associated with poor outcome (Pontiroli, Alberto, Paganelli, Saibene, & Busetto, 2013). Other commonly used treatments include medications, improved diet, and increased physical activity (Wissing & Pipeleers, 2013).

3.5. Comorbidities and the BBB

The BBB is highly dependent on vascular stabilization and integrity. Comorbidities compromise small vessels by making them leaky and at risk for plaque development. In particular, atherosclerosis can cause tight junction proteins to decrease (Zhou et al., 2014). ZO-1, claudin-5, and occludin are essential for BBB maintenance, but synthesis and integration of these proteins are severely disrupted by comorbidities. Endothelial cells undergo the blunt of chronic disease and monolayer permeability drastically increases over time (Krouwer, Hekking, Langelaar-Makkinje, Regan-Klapisz, & Post, 2012). It is the infiltration of peripheral macrophages and toxins that can have long-lasting detrimental effects on the brain (Kim, Kim, Kim,

Kang, & Kang, 2012). Managing comorbidities is therefore essential to maintaining brain health over time.

4. LINKING METABOLIC SYNDROME AND AGING

While age is the greatest risk factor for ischemic stroke (Sacco et al., 1997), hypertension, dyslipidemia, diabetes, and more specifically, the metabolic syndrome represent perhaps the greatest modifiable risk factor. Elimination of metabolic syndrome is predicted to reduce overall stroke rates by 19% and up to 35% in certain ethnic subpopulations (Boden-Albala et al., 2008). In middle-aged men, the metabolic syndrome is responsible for a 2.16 times higher risk for ischemic stroke specifically, further indicating the significant contribution the metabolic syndrome makes to ischemic stroke risk across gender and age categories (Kurl et al., 2006). As such, there is an increasing need not only understanding how both age and the metabolic syndrome contribute to ischemic stroke pathophysiology independently, but also in combination as age and metabolic syndrome are closely related in prevalence (Lucke-Wold, Turner, Lucke-Wold, Rosen, & Huber, 2012). In fact, a study by Hildrum and colleagues showed that metabolic syndrome incidence increased from 11.0% to 47.2% in men at ages 20–29 and 80–89 years old, respectively (Hildrum, Mykletun, Hole, Midthjell, & Dahl, 2007). Similar findings were observed in women with the incidence increasing from 9.2% to 64.4% in corresponding age groups (Hildrum et al., 2007). While a clear link between age and metabolic syndrome exists, particularly in relation to ischemic stroke risk, it remains unclear how precisely each contributes to not only ischemic stroke risk but also disease pathophysiology and outcome. In sections 4.1 through 4.6, after a brief discussion of available models combining metabolic syndrome and aging, we explore some of the most common and promising mechanisms of ischemic injury and how these mechanisms may be altered by aging and/or metabolic syndrome.

4.1. Cerebrovascular disease

Hypertension can cause vessel damage and expose the underlying collagen meshwork. Collagen attracts platelets to the site of injury, but comorbidities can contribute to insufficient vessel repair. During sleep, blood pressure falls, and the small vessels are at increased risk for embolic or thrombic events (Morley, 2014). Occlusion of a diseased vessel quickly contributes to ischemic infarct. As tissue dies, the remaining vasculature becomes leaky and tight junctions begin to break down. Without administration of neuroprotective agents, permanent vessel damage can result. Managing comorbidities will decrease the likelihood of adverse events and limit the damage that may result from cerebrovascular disease.

4.2. Utilizing animal models to study metabolic syndrome and aging

Addressing both aging processes and metabolic syndrome within one experimental animal model, particularly with regard to ischemic stroke, remains largely uninvestigated. While the reasons for the lack of investigation, despite the significant clinical relevance, are not entirely clear, one likely reason is the cost. Acquiring and maintaining an aging colony frequently results in a cost exceeding $200 per animal, making the study of aging expensive in isolation and in many cases, prohibitive. The cost would likely be driven up further through inclusion of the metabolic syndrome both directly, via unique animal strains or special diets, and indirectly with regard to ischemic stroke due to the heightened mortality rate in the combined metabolic syndrome and aged animals. In fact, aged animals alone exhibit worsened outcome following ischemia and a higher mortality rate, in comparison to healthy young-adult animals, necessitating increased animal numbers for experimental paradigms and consequently, an elevated cost (Dinapoli, Rosen, Nagamine, & Crocco, 2006; Rosen, Dinapoli, Nagamine, & Crocco, 2005). Regardless, methods to overcome the potential cost limitations precluding the investigation of aging and metabolic syndrome in combination with ischemic stroke need to be investigated. One potential alternative may be the use of animal strains shown to develop metabolic syndrome as a consequence of normal aging. Aged Wistar rats have been shown to develop some signs of the metabolic syndrome, namely adiposity, dyslipidemia, and elevated serum glucose, despite being maintained on what was described to be a standard rodent diet (Ghezzi et al., 2012). Whether these animals developed hypertension, an important component of the metabolic syndrome, is unclear.

4.3. Glutamate excitotoxicity

The onset of ischemia, a consequence of blood flow cessation due to thrombotic or embolic disruption, is associated with a rapid decline in oxygen and glucose delivery to the brain. The nearly immediate shortage of the main sources of energy production, glucose and oxygen, results in the decoupling of oxidative phosphorylation and a consequent decline of ATP production. This decrease is reported within only 2 min of ischemic onset (Stankowski & Gupta, 2011). Diminished ATP availability within the cell leads to a disruption in ionic pump function, perhaps the most well studied being the Na-K ATPase. Failure of the Na-K ATPase to maintain homeostatic ionic gradients results in elevated cytosolic Na^+ and a decrease in cytosolic K^+, producing rapid depolarization of the neuronal membrane. Depolarization results in a swift influx of Ca^{2+} and subsequent release of excitotoxic amino acids such as glutamate into the synaptic cleft. Here, the glutamate binds NMDA and AMPA receptors on the postsynaptic membrane, leading to depolarization of the postsynaptic neuron and propagating waves of depolarization (Lo, Dalkara, & Moskowitz, 2003). In fact, these propagating waves of depolarization, termed periinfarct depolarizations, have been shown to persist for at least 6–8 h. Therefore, the initial 3 h after ischemic onset may predict final infarct volume (Hossmann, 2006).

The influx of calcium results in activation of a host of enzymes, either directly or indirectly, including phospholipases, proteases, and endonucleases (Hossmann, 2009; Kristian & Siesjo, 1998). Membranes, proteins, and genetic material essential for cell survival and/or function may be degraded following ischemia. Besides being involved in enzyme activation, the heightened level of intracellular calcium combined with improper functioning of the mitochondrial uniporter and $2Na^+$-Ca^{2+} exchanger, results in elevated mitochondrial calcium levels (Kristian & Siesjo, 1998). Elevated mitochondrial calcium levels can produce opening of the mitochondrial permeability transition pore found on the inner mitochondrial membrane leading to osmotic swelling, subsequent rupture of the mitochondrial outer membrane, and release of cytochrome *C*, a key player in initiation of apoptotic cascades (Turner, Dodson, Rosen, & Huber, 2013). Finally, the influx of calcium and mitochondrial disruption can lead to generation of ROS via unspecified mechanisms (Turner et al., 2013).

How these processes are altered by aging and how these changes may contribute to ischemic pathophysiology remain under investigation and may play a role in future therapeutic development. It is generally accepted that molecular and cellular changes occur with aging that impair normal functioning of various ionic ATPases and other transporters for glutamate and glucose, leading to both oxidative and metabolic stressors (Mattson & Magnus, 2006). Hof and colleagues showed that while aging neurons have lower levels of GluR2 than in young individuals, aging was associated with a higher ratio of NMDAR1 to GluR2, potentially rendering the aged neuron more prone to glutamate-mediated excitotoxicity (Hof et al., 2002). Similarly, disruptions and/or impairments in cellular energetics predispose the aged neuron to excitotoxic events. In other neurodegenerative diseases, such as AD, PD, and Huntington's disease, disease-specific changes in Aβ, dopamine, mutant huntingtin, and mutant Cu/Zn-superoxide dismutase (SOD) have been shown to increase neuronal susceptibility to excitotoxicity. Subsequently, excitotoxicity has been identified as a potential key mechanism in rodent models of these neurodegenerative conditions (Cleveland & Rothstein, 2001; Cookson, 2005; Mattson, 2004; Mattson & Magnus, 2006; Moore, West, Dawson, & Dawson, 2005; Sieradzan & Mann, 2001). While the effect of the metabolic syndrome on glutamate excitotoxicity following ischemic stroke has not been investigated to the best of our knowledge, components of the metabolic syndrome, such as diabetes, have been studied in animal models. Di Luca and colleagues showed that while transcript levels of NR1 and NR2A subunits of the NMDA receptor remained unchanged, immunoreactivity of the NR2B subunit was reduced by 40% with a diabetic duration of 3 months in comparison to age-matched control rats (Di Luca et al., 1999). Insulin only partially restored this deficit and notably, long-term potentiation (LTP), an electrophysiological correlate of learning and memory, is diminished in diabetic animals. Aging, in combination with diabetes, was associated with a more severe impairment in LTP than either condition alone, indicating that diabetes may lead to an "accelerated" brain aging (Biessels et al., 2002). While the direct relationship between these findings and glutamate excitotoxicity following ischemic stroke is unclear, what is apparent is that both aging and components of the metabolic syndrome, namely diabetes, alter neurotransmission through actions on the NMDA receptor. These changes may predispose to increased susceptibility to excitotoxicity following ischemic stroke.

4.4. Oxidative stress

In addition to glutamate-mediated excitotoxicity and associated enzymatic activation due to the influx of calcium, oxidative stress represents another prominent component of ischemic injury. Oxidative stress is induced largely via mitochondrial dysfunction and impairment of normal cellular respiration, resulting in the production of free radicals. Release of free radicals leads to peroxidation of plasma membranes and intracellular organelle membranes, ultimately causing release of biologically active free fatty acids, like arachidonic acid. Similarly, ROS production leads to the induction of ER stress and fragmentation of DNA, events that may directly and indirectly influence cellular survival.

How oxidative stress is altered by the presence of the metabolic syndrome and the aging process remains under investigation but it is clear that oxidative stress plays a role in the increased risk for ischemic stroke, and worsened outcome following ischemic stroke, associated with both conditions. Diabetes, one component of the metabolic syndrome, has been described as a prooxidant state, consistent with an increase in LDL oxidation, the presence of increased monocyte superoxide, elevated nitrotyrosine, and urinary F2-isoprostanes (Devaraj, Goyal, & Jialal, 2008). The more encompassing metabolic syndrome appears to exhibit many of these prooxidant markers as well with various studies reporting findings ranging from increased lipid peroxidation products to elevation of carbonylated proteins to an increase in enzymes responsible for generating ROS such as catalase and nicotinamide adenine dinucleotide phosphate (NADPH)-oxidases (NOXs) (Bedard & Krause, 2007; Cardona et al., 2008; Devaraj et al., 2008; Fortuno et al., 2006; Gomes, Casella-Filho, Chagas, & Tanus-Santos, 2008). Levels of antioxidant molecules on the other hand, such as glutathione (GSH), are decreased in metabolic syndrome (Devaraj et al., 2008).

Aging is also associated with increased levels of oxidant markers, leading to the theory of "inflam-aging." It is theorized that heightened inflammation and oxidative stress, and a decreased capacity for handling these processes, leads to the negative consequences associated with aging, such as increased risk for stroke as well as cardiovascular and neurodegenerative disease. The cause of the increased oxidative stress associated with aging is not entirely clear, but evidence indicates not only excessive free radical production but also diminished capacity for handling the increased radical production. Specifically, aging is associated with an increase in mitochondrial O_2^- and H_2O_2 production concomitant with diminished enzymatic activities of gamma-glutamylcysteine synthetase (γ-GCS), glutathione reductase, glutathione peroxidase, gamma-glutamyl transpeptidase, glutathione-S-transferase, catalase, SOD, and glutathione (GSH) (Sandhu & Kaur, 2002). While the mechanisms leading to reduced radical scavenging remain under investigation, reduced gene expression of γ-GCS has been observed in aged rats by Liu and colleagues, likely contributing to diminished synthesis and scavenging capability (Liu & Choi, 2000). The decline in γ-GCS was accompanied by a decrease in total GSH content as well (Liu & Choi, 2000), an important finding due to the association between GSH decline in the mitochondria and diminished levels of ATP (Sandhu & Kaur, 2002). Loss of ATP in the mitochondria may predispose neural cells to cellular damage, particularly in times of cellular stress, such as stroke and other neurodegenerative disease (Floyd & Hensley, 2002).

Aging is not only associated with alterations in the synthesis and scavenging of radicals but also the cellular response to these events. One of the most well-studied responses is the effect of oxidative stress on heat-shock protein (Hsp) induction and/or expression. Hsp70 is attenuated during the aging process, a finding associated with reduced survival, whereas elevated levels of Hsp70 have been associated with survival of cellular stress (Finkel & Holbrook, 2000; Richardson & Holbrook, 1996). In contrast, the basal expression of other Hsp's may be increased with aging and may help counter the elevated oxidative load imposed by the aging process. Other pathways are also altered in aging, such as extracellular signal-regulated kinase (ERK) signaling. ERK signaling is attenuated with aging and much like Hsp70, this effect appears deleterious as ERK activation generally exerts a prosurvival (or antiapoptotic) signal during periods of cellular stress (Finkel & Holbrook, 2000; Guyton et al., 1998; Guyton, Liu, Gorospe, Xu, & Holbrook, 1996).

Interestingly, the combination of aging and the metabolic syndrome, or at least components of the metabolic syndrome, may lead to synergistic effects with regard to the physiological response to injurious mechanisms. Specifically, aging has been shown to worsen obesity-induced systemic inflammation and BBB disruption, leading to an increase in the circulation of proinflammatory cytokines, microglial activation, and elevated levels of oxidative stress (Tucsek et al., 2013). Aging was also associated with increased oxidative stress and inflammation, exemplified by increased macrophage infiltration, in periaortic adipose tissue (Bailey-Downs et al., 2013). These findings would appear to support the notion that systemic inflammation induced by the presence of the metabolic syndrome may be worsened by the aging process, predisposing individuals to an elevated ischemic stroke risk and likely worsened outcome following ischemia.

4.5. ER stress

Perhaps, one of the most exciting in terms of therapeutic development, but least studied and understood areas at the forefront of the interface among age, metabolic syndrome, and neural injury, is ER stress. ER stress, triggered by the accumulation of newly synthesized unfolded or misfolded proteins, has been linked to not only various disease states ranging from diabetes to AD

(Ozcan & Tabas, 2012) but also the aging process in general, often times providing a potential link between aging and the development of degenerative disease (Brown & Naidoo, 2012). How precisely ER stress is triggered and how it contributes to the risk for ischemic stroke and/or modulates outcome from ischemic stroke presently remains unclear and under further investigation.

ER stress and the subsequent unfolded protein response comprise three distinct, but often overlapping, pathways termed the PERK, IRE1α, and ATF6 pathways. These pathways ultimately influence progression to cell survival or apoptosis and in doing so, modulate a number of inflammatory and stress signaling pathways that include NF-κB-IκB kinase (IKK), JNK-AP1, among others, including those that regulate oxidative stress (Hotamisligil, 2010) (Fig. 3). Whether ER stress is the precipitating factor leading to the development of disease or simply acts to propagate the disease remains unclear in many cases, but numerous reports from preclinical and clinical studies alike implicate ER stress in disease pathophysiology.

Studies of atherosclerosis, a common component of the metabolic syndrome due to the association of the metabolic syndrome with hyperlipidemia, have shown a clear association between atherosclerotic lesions and markers of ER stress in humans, particularly in regions of endothelium exhibiting concentrated levels of oxidized phospholipids (Ozcan & Tabas, 2012). Perhaps, most notably with regard to contribution to ischemic stroke risk is the fact that chronic ER stress has been linked to macrophage apoptosis in atherosclerosis (Ozcan & Tabas, 2012), a finding consistent with

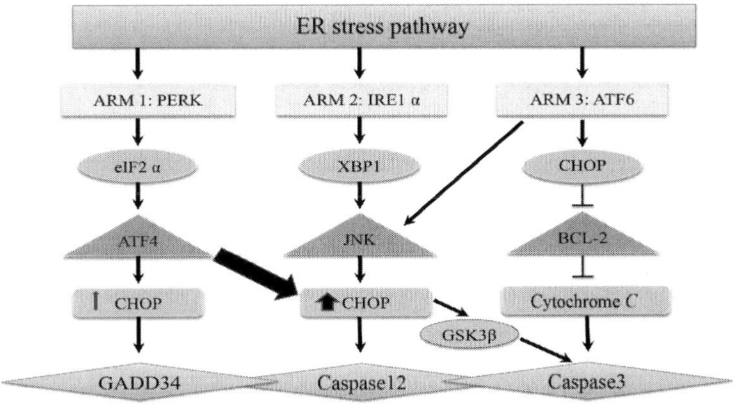

Figure 3 Three arms of the ER stress pathway. Arm 1 is neuroprotective while arms 2 and 3 trigger apoptosis.

elevated risk for plaque necrosis and embolization. Myoishi et al. and Erbay et al. have also provided evidence that expression of markers of ER stress are associated with not only plaque vulnerability in human coronary artery lesions but also that a deficiency in fatty acid-binding protein-4, a protein required for induction of ER stress in the presence of lipids, reduces atherosclerotic lesion size (Ozcan & Tabas, 2012). In addition to ER stress being required for lesion expansion, evidence indicates that ER stress is required for maximum inflammatory gene expression in atherosclerotic lesions, a characteristic that has been modulated successfully *in vitro* using modulators of ER stress (Gargalovic et al., 2006). Consequently, the suggestion has been made that ER stress plays a crucial role in mediating cardiovascular inflammation and subsequent dysfunction of the endothelium in atherosclerosis (Gargalovic et al., 2006).

ER stress involvement is not limited to atherosclerosis either. In fact, studies show that animals genetically predisposed to obesity as well as those with obesity promoted through diet exhibit increased ER stress in both adipose and liver tissue. These findings are consistent with human studies in which markers of ER stress and downstream signaling components (Grp78, XBP1s, phospho-eIF2α, and phospho-JNK) are elevated in insulin-resistant nondiabetic humans. Notably, these changes are reduced following surgically induced weight loss (Ozcan & Tabas, 2012).

Another condition closely related to the metabolic syndrome, type II diabetes, has also been linked to alterations in ER stress. Specifically, both genetic modifications leading to obesity as well as diet-induced obesity, key risk factors for the development of diabetes have been shown to correlate with increased ER stress in liver and adipose tissue. Looking at insulin resistance in particular, activation of JNK, a downstream component of ER stress, has been shown to phosphorylate insulin receptor substrate-1 (IRS1) on Ser307. This phosphorylation causes reduced tyrosine phosphorylation and activation of IRS1. This direct implication between ER stress and insulin resistance is consistent with findings in insulin-resistant humans in which numerous ER stress parameters (Grp78, XBP1s, phospho-eIF2α, and phospho-JNK) are elevated in liver and adipose tissue. Finally, work in animal models of type II diabetes has implicated ER stress mechanistically in glycemic control, as CHOP ablation resulted in improved control and an expanded beta cell population. In contrast, XBP1 is believed to be protective as selective deletion of XBP1 in beta cells triggers hyperglycemia and beta cell loss. Therefore, much like other aspects of ER stress, it appears that ER stress can serve both protective and detrimental roles, likely a product of the duration of physiological stress (Ozcan & Tabas, 2012). Looking at the metabolic syndrome in its entirety, short-term induction of ER stress over 3 days using thapsigargin infusion in the brain resulted in glucose intolerance, insulin resistance (systemic and hepatic), and an increase in blood pressure. Interestingly, inhibition of ER stress in the brain using tauroursodeoxycholic acid (TUDCA) partially diminished metabolic and blood pressure changes (Purkayastha et al., 2011).

ER stress is also altered during the aging process, much like it is in the metabolic syndrome and/or facets of the metabolic syndrome. This is particularly true in many of the diseases associated with accumulation of insoluble fibrils or plaques that occur at a higher rate in the aged population such as AD, PD, and type II diabetes. How these fibrils and plaques develop remains under continual investigation but recent evidence has implicated a decline in protein folding and chaperoning systems with age (Brown & Naidoo, 2012; Ozcan & Tabas, 2012). Prior studies have identified a particular decline in BiP (Naidoo, 2009), PDI, calnexin, and GRP94 with aging. Similarly, PERK mRNA is reduced in aged rats and the function of PKR, an eIF2α kinase, is impaired as well. Furthermore, GADD34, a downstream regulator of eIF2α phosphorylation state, is increased in aged mice. Perhaps most importantly with regard to the overall function of the ER stress pathway in aging, CHOP expression is increased with age and can be further induced, in conjunction with caspase-12, in stressed aged rats but not young (Brown & Naidoo, 2012). These findings indicate the potential interaction between age and metabolic syndrome with regard to neural injury in that the added physiological stress imposed by the two conditions in conjunction may lead to not only increased risk for ischemic stroke but also worsened outcome, a concept illustrated previously in a study of age and traumatic brain injury (Sandhir & Berman, 2010). In fact, studies have shown a clear link between ER stress and autophagy defects in a model of overnutrition-induced neuroinflammation. These same studies even indicate a potential therapeutic approach in which central inhibition of ER stress attenuates pathological effects of overnutrition through inhibition of NF-κB, furthering the concept of a connection between stress and inflammation related to disease (Cai, 2013).

4.6. Inflammation

Understanding and subsequently modulating inflammation for therapeutic development for ischemic stroke remains an area of continued investigation.

Inflammation has long been recognized as being altered in both aging and the metabolic syndrome with the details of each individually beyond the scope of this review. More importantly, recent studies have illustrated a clear link between aging and metabolic syndrome with regard to inflammation and in particular, aspects of inflammation that may modulate both risk and outcomes related to ischemic stroke. Tucsek and colleagues, comparing mice fed high-fat diets to induce obesity at 7 months and 24 months of age, showed that aging was responsible for a dramatic increase in both systemic inflammation and BBB disruption, based on circulating levels of inflammatory cytokines and extravasated immunoglobulin, respectively (Tucsek et al., 2013). Additional changes were observed within the brain in conjunction with BBB disruption and these included activation of microglia, elevated levels of oxidative stress, and release of inflammatory cytokines (Tucsek et al., 2013). Notably, the changes associated with aging in the brain appear to be systemically induced as treatment of cultured primary microglia with sera from young animals demonstrating increased activation and oxidative stress (Tucsek et al., 2013). Therefore, it appears that systemic inflammation, a documented product of obesity, results in CNS changes (Tucsek et al., 2013). Furthermore, studies have shown that exposing arteries from young, healthy control rodents to inflammatory components released from perivascular fat tissue of aged rodents result in significant oxidative and inflammatory changes, replicating what is most often seen in aging (Bailey-Downs et al., 2013). Importantly, modulation of inflammation induced by the metabolic syndrome has been shown to be protective with regard to the development of age-associated neurodegenerative disease (Cai, Yan, & Wang, 2013). This concept was shown to be accurate by Cai and colleagues via the administration of minocycline, a tetracycline derivative and known anti-inflammatory agent, to rodents suffering from a diabetic-like metabolic disorder. Minocycline was shown to reduce the development of β-amyloid and tauopathy in this model, indicating the relevance and potential for metabolic syndrome-induced inflammation in the development of neurodegenerative and other forms of neurological disease (Cai et al., 2013).

5. CONCLUSION

In summary, the BBB is compromised with aging. Astrocytes and pericytes maintain barrier homeostasis, but with age, barrier support is compromised and may contribute to increased permeability. Microglia are more active with age and contribute to heightened levels of inflammation within the aged brain that compromise tight junctions. Oxidative stress from damaged glial cells can harm endothelial cells. Endothelial cells help maintain BBB integrity, but with n drugs and exogenous toxins enter and harm the brain. These toxins cause neurons to die in an aging brain and although NSCs seek to replenish the cells, the problem of integration continues to be a challenge. Ultimately, the aging process has a profound effect on glial cell activation, BBB permeability, neurogenesis, and apoptosis. Better animal models, age-specific treatment approaches, and increased understanding about aging will contribute to improved care over the coming decades.

Aging also contributes to poor outcomes seen with the metabolic syndrome. We examined cardiovascular disease, hypertension, DM2, and obesity. The growing concern across the nation is the rapidly increasing prevalence of these comorbidities. In order to prevent serious long-term outcomes such as ischemic stroke and myocardial infarction, it is necessary to implement lifestyle, medical, and community changes. Research into how the BBB is altered by these comorbidities is essential as we move forward. Better models are necessary to improve our understanding of the aged neurovascular unit. Consideration of injury cascades such as glutamate excitotoxity, oxidative stress, and ER stress is crucial in the enhancement of better pharmaceutical agents as we progress forward.

CONFLICT OF INTEREST

No authors contributing to this manuscript have a conflict of interest or financial disclosure.

REFERENCES

Abd El Mohsen, M. M., Iravani, M. M., Spencer, J. P., Rose, S., Fahim, A. T., Motawi, T. M., et al. (2005). Age-associated changes in protein oxidation and proteasome activities in rat brain: Modulation by antioxidants. *Biochemical and Biophysical Research Communications*, *336*(2), 386–391. http://dx.doi.org/10.1016/j.bbrc.2005.07.201.

Ahrens, L., Shoeib, M., Harner, T., Lane, D. A., Guo, R., & Reiner, E. J. (2011). Comparison of annular diffusion denuder and high volume air samplers for measuring per- and polyfluoroalkyl substances in the atmosphere. *Analytical Chemistry*, *83*(24), 9622–9628. http://dx.doi.org/10.1021/ac202414w.

Alhusban, A., & Fagan, S. C. (2011). Secondary prevention of stroke in the elderly: A review of the evidence. *The American Journal of Geriatric Pharmacotherapy*, *9*(3), 143–152. http://dx.doi.org/10.1016/j.amjopharm.2011.04.002.

Amanzada, A., Malik, I. A., Blaschke, M., Khan, S., Rahman, H., Ramadori, G., et al. (2013). Identification of CD68(+) neutrophil granulocytes in in vitro model of acute inflammation and inflammatory bowel disease. *International Journal of Clinical and Experimental Pathology*, *6*(4), 561–570.

Artola, A. (2008). Diabetes-, stress- and ageing-related changes in synaptic plasticity in hippocampus and neocortex—The same metaplastic process? *European Journal of Pharmacology, 585*(1), 153–162. http://dx.doi.org/10.1016/j.ejphar.2007.11.084.

Auriel, E., Gur, A. Y., Uralev, O., Brill, S., Shopin, L., Karni, A., et al. (2011). Characteristics of first ever ischemic stroke in the very elderly: Profile of vascular risk factors and clinical outcome. *Clinical Neurology and Neurosurgery, 113*(8), 654–657. http://dx.doi.org/10.1016/j.clineuro.2011.05.011.

Badan, I., Buchhold, B., Hamm, A., Gratz, M., Walker, L. C., Platt, D., et al. (2003). Accelerated glial reactivity to stroke in aged rats correlates with reduced functional recovery. *Journal of Cerebral Blood Flow and Metabolism, 23*(7), 845–854. http://dx.doi.org/10.1097/01.WCB.0000071883.63724.A7.

Bailey-Downs, L. C., Tucsek, Z., Toth, P., Sosnowska, D., Gautam, T., Sonntag, W. E., et al. (2013). Aging exacerbates obesity-induced oxidative stress and inflammation in perivascular adipose tissue in mice: A paracrine mechanism contributing to vascular redox dysregulation and inflammation. *The Journals of Gerontology. Series A, Biological Sciences and Medical Sciences, 68*(7), 780–792. http://dx.doi.org/10.1093/gerona/gls238. Epub 2012 Dec 3.

Bakirci, S., Kafa, I. M., Uysal, M., & Ayberk Kurt, M. (2011). Increased adult neurogenesis in the subventricular zone in a rat model of sepsis. *Neuroscience Letters, 497*(1), 27–31. http://dx.doi.org/10.1016/j.neulet.2011.04.014.

Bartels, A. L., Kortekaas, R., Bart, J., Willemsen, A. T., de Klerk, O. L., de Vries, J. J., et al. (2009). Blood-brain barrier P-glycoprotein function decreases in specific brain regions with aging: A possible role in progressive neurodegeneration. *Neurobiology of Aging, 30*(11), 1818–1824. http://dx.doi.org/10.1016/j.neurobiolaging.2008.02.002.

Bartlett, D. B., Firth, C. M., Phillips, A. C., Moss, P., Baylis, D., Syddall, H., et al. (2012). The age-related increase in low-grade systemic inflammation (inflamm-aging) is not driven by cytomegalovirus infection. *Aging Cell, 11*(5), 912–915. http://dx.doi.org/10.1111/j.1474-9726.2012.00849.x.

Bedard, K., & Krause, K. H. (2007). The NOX family of ROS-generating NADPH oxidases: Physiology and pathophysiology. *Physiological Reviews, 87*(1), 245–313. http://dx.doi.org/10.1152/physrev.00044.2005, 87/1/245 [pii].

Bhat, R., Crowe, E. P., Bitto, A., Moh, M., Katsetos, C. D., Garcia, F. U., et al. (2012). Astrocyte senescence as a component of Alzheimer's disease. *PLoS One, 7*(9), e45069. http://dx.doi.org/10.1371/journal.pone.0045069.

Biessels, G. J., van der Heide, L. P., Kamal, A., Bleys, R. L., & Gispen, W. H. (2002). Ageing and diabetes: Implications for brain function. *European Journal of Pharmacology, 441*(1–2), 1–14.

Bilbo, S. D. (2011). How cytokines leave their mark: The role of the placenta in developmental programming of brain and behavior. *Brain, Behavior, and Immunity, 25*(4), 602–603. http://dx.doi.org/10.1016/j.bbi.2011.01.018.

Bitto, A., Sell, C., Crowe, E., Lorenzini, A., Malaguti, M., Hrelia, S., et al. (2010). Stress-induced senescence in human and rodent astrocytes. *Experimental Cell Research, 316*(17), 2961–2968. http://dx.doi.org/10.1016/j.yexcr.2010.06.021.

Blasko, I., Stampfer-Kountchev, M., Robatscher, P., Veerhuis, R., Eikelenboom, P., & Grubeck-Loebenstein, B. (2004). How chronic inflammation can affect the brain and support the development of Alzheimer's disease in old age: The role of microglia and astrocytes. *Aging Cell, 3*(4), 169–176. http://dx.doi.org/10.1111/j.1474-9728.2004.00101.x.

Boden-Albala, B., Sacco, R. L., Lee, H. S., Grahame-Clarke, C., Rundek, T., Elkind, M. V., et al. (2008). Metabolic syndrome and ischemic stroke risk: Northern Manhattan study. *Stroke, 39*(1), 30–35. http://dx.doi.org/10.1161/STROKEAHA.107.496588, STROKEAHA.107.496588 [pii].

Borghini, A., Cervelli, T., Galli, A., & Andreassi, M. G. (2013). DNA modifications in atherosclerosis: From the past to the future. *Atherosclerosis*, *230*(2), 202–209. http://dx.doi.org/10.1016/j.atherosclerosis.2013.07.038.

Brandt, M. D., & Storch, A. (2008). Neurogenesis in the adult brain: From bench to bedside? *Fortschritte der Neurologie-Psychiatrie*, *76*(9), 517–529. http://dx.doi.org/10.1055/s-2008-1038218.

Brera, B., Serrano, A., & de Ceballos, M. L. (2000). Beta-amyloid peptides are cytotoxic to astrocytes in culture: A role for oxidative stress. *Neurobiology of Disease*, 7(4), 395–405. http://dx.doi.org/10.1006/nbdi.2000.0313.

Brown, M. K., & Naidoo, N. (2012). The endoplasmic reticulum stress response in aging and age-related diseases. *Frontiers in Physiology*, *3*, 263. http://dx.doi.org/10.3389/fphys.2012.00263.

Buschini, E., Piras, A., Nuzzi, R., & Vercelli, A. (2011). Age related macular degeneration and drusen: Neuroinflammation in the retina. *Progress in Neurobiology*, *95*(1), 14–25. http://dx.doi.org/10.1016/j.pneurobio.2011.05.011.

Cai, D. (2013). Neuroinflammation and neurodegeneration in overnutrition-induced diseases. *Trends in Endocrinology and Metabolism*, *24*(1), 40–47. http://dx.doi.org/10.1016/j.tem.2012.11.003, S1043-2760(12)00203-2 [pii].

Cai, Z., Yan, Y., & Wang, Y. (2013). Minocycline alleviates beta-amyloid protein and tau pathology via restraining neuroinflammation induced by diabetic metabolic disorder. *Clinical Interventions in Aging*, *8*, 1089–1095. http://dx.doi.org/10.2147/CIA.S46536, cia-8-1089 [pii].

Calling, S., Ji, J., Sundquist, J., Sundquist, K., & Zoller, B. (2013). Shared and non-shared familial susceptibility of coronary heart disease, ischemic stroke, peripheral artery disease and aortic disease. *International Journal of Cardiology*, *168*(3), 2844–2850. http://dx.doi.org/10.1016/j.ijcard.2013.03.149.

Campuzano, O., Castillo-Ruiz, M. M., Acarin, L., Gonzalez, B., & Castellano, B. (2011). Decreased myeloperoxidase expressing cells in the aged rat brain after excitotoxic damage. *Experimental Gerontology*, *46*(9), 723–730. http://dx.doi.org/10.1016/j.exger.2011.05.003.

Cardona, F., Tunez, I., Tasset, I., Montilla, P., Collantes, E., & Tinahones, F. J. (2008). Fat overload aggravates oxidative stress in patients with the metabolic syndrome. *European Journal of Clinical Investigation*, *38*(7), 510–515. http://dx.doi.org/10.1111/j.1365-2362.2008.01959.x, ECI1959 [pii].

Castilla-Guerra, L., Fernandez-Moreno Mdel, C., & Alvarez-Suero, J. (2009). Secondary stroke prevention in the elderly: New evidence in hypertension and hyperlipidemia. *European Journal of Internal Medicine*, *20*(6), 586–590. http://dx.doi.org/10.1016/j.ejim.2009.06.005.

Cavuoto, L. A., & Nussbaum, M. A. (2014). The influences of obesity and age on functional performance during intermittent upper extremity tasks. *Journal of Occupational and Environmental Hygiene*. http://dx.doi.org/10.1080/15459624.2014.887848.

Cerbai, F., Lana, D., Nosi, D., Petkova-Kirova, P., Zecchi, S., Brothers, H. M., et al. (2012). The neuron-astrocyte-microglia triad in normal brain ageing and in a model of neuroinflammation in the rat hippocampus. *PLoS One*, 7(9), e45250. http://dx.doi.org/10.1371/journal.pone.0045250.

Cernak, I., Chang, T., Ahmed, F. A., Cruz, M. I., Vink, R., Stoica, B., et al. (2010). Pathophysiological response to experimental diffuse brain trauma differs as a function of developmental age. *Developmental Neuroscience*, *32*(5–6), 442–453. http://dx.doi.org/10.1159/000320085.

Ciccarelli, R., Di Iorio, P., Bruno, V., Battaglia, G., D'Alimonte, I., D'Onofrio, M., et al. (1999). Activation of A(1) adenosine or mGlu3 metabotropic glutamate receptors enhances the release of nerve growth factor and S-100beta protein from cultured astrocytes. *Glia, 27*(3), 275–281.

Ciesielska, A., Joniec, I., Kurkowska-Jastrzebska, I., Cudna, A., Przybylkowski, A., Czlonkowska, A., et al. (2009). The impact of age and gender on the striatal astrocytes activation in murine model of Parkinson's disease. *Inflammation Research, 58*(11), 747–753. http://dx.doi.org/10.1007/s00011-009-0026-6.

Clarner, T., Diederichs, F., Berger, K., Denecke, B., Gan, L., van der Valk, P., et al. (2012). Myelin debris regulates inflammatory responses in an experimental demyelination animal model and multiple sclerosis lesions. *Glia, 60*(10), 1468–1480. http://dx.doi.org/10.1002/glia.22367.

Cleveland, D. W., & Rothstein, J. D. (2001). From Charcot to Lou Gehrig: Deciphering selective motor neuron death in ALS. *Nature Reviews. Neuroscience, 2*(11), 806–819. http://dx.doi.org/10.1038/35097565, 35097565 [pii].

Cohen, L., Curhan, G. C., & Forman, J. P. (2012). Influence of age on the association between lifestyle factors and risk of hypertension. *Journal of the American Society of Hypertension, 6*(4), 284–290. http://dx.doi.org/10.1016/j.jash.2012.06.002.

Cookson, M. R. (2005). The biochemistry of Parkinson's disease. *Annual Review of Biochemistry, 74,* 29–52. http://dx.doi.org/10.1146/annurev.biochem.74.082803.133400.

Costopoulos, C., Liew, T. V., & Bennett, M. (2008). Ageing and atherosclerosis: Mechanisms and therapeutic options. *Biochemical Pharmacology, 75*(6), 1251–1261. http://dx.doi.org/10.1016/j.bcp.2007.10.006.

Cotrina, M. L., & Nedergaard, M. (2002). Astrocytes in the aging brain. *Journal of Neuroscience Research, 67*(1), 1–10.

Del Brutto, O. H., Montalvan, M., Tettamanti, D., Penaherrera, E., Santibanez, R., Pow-Chon-Long, F., et al. (2013). The "know your numbers" program in Atahualpa–a pilot study aimed to reduce cardiovascular diseases and stroke burden in rural communities of developing countries. *International Journal of Cardiology, 168*(3), 3123–3124. http://dx.doi.org/10.1016/j.ijcard.2013.04.049.

Del Brutto, O. H., Zambrano, M., Penaherrera, E., Montalvan, M., Pow-Chon-Long, F., & Tettamanti, D. (2013). Prevalence of the metabolic syndrome and its correlation with the cardiovascular health status in stroke- and ischemic heart disease-free Ecuadorian natives/mestizos aged >/=40 years living in Atahualpa: A population-based study. *Diabetes & Metabolic Syndrome*, 7(4), 218–222. http://dx.doi.org/10.1016/j.dsx.2013.10.006.

Denti, L., Artoni, A., Scoditti, U., Caminiti, C., Giambanco, F., Casella, M., et al. (2013). Impact of gender-age interaction on the outcome of ischemic stroke in an Italian cohort of patients treated according to a standardized clinical pathway. *European Journal of Internal Medicine, 24*(8), 807–812. http://dx.doi.org/10.1016/j.ejim.2013.07.015.

Devaraj, S., Goyal, R., & Jialal, I. (2008). Inflammation, oxidative stress, and the metabolic syndrome. *US Endocrinology, 4*(2), 32–37.

Dharmasaroja, P. A., Muengtaweepongsa, S., & Dharmasaroja, P. (2013). Intravenous thrombolysis in Thai patients with acute ischemic stroke: Role of aging. *Journal of Stroke and Cerebrovascular Diseases, 22*(3), 227–231. http://dx.doi.org/10.1016/j.jstrokecerebrovasdis.2011.08.001.

Di Luca, M., Ruts, L., Gardoni, F., Cattabeni, F., Biessels, G. J., & Gispen, W. H. (1999). NMDA receptor subunits are modified transcriptionally and post-translationally in the brain of streptozotocin-diabetic rats. *Diabetologia, 42*(6), 693–701. http://dx.doi.org/10.1007/s001250051217.

Dinapoli, V. A., Benkovic, S. A., Li, X., Kelly, K. A., Miller, D. B., Rosen, C. L., et al. (2010). Age exaggerates proinflammatory cytokine signaling and truncates signal transducers and activators of transcription 3 signaling following ischemic stroke in the rat. *Neuroscience, 170*(2), 633–644. http://dx.doi.org/10.1016/j.neuroscience.2010.07.011.

Dinapoli, V. A., Rosen, C. L., Nagamine, T., & Crocco, T. (2006). Selective MCA occlusion: A precise embolic stroke model. *Journal of Neuroscience Methods*, *154*(1–2), 233–238. http://dx.doi.org/10.1016/j.jneumeth.2005.12.026, S0165-0270(06)00007-0 [pii].

Dixon-Ibarra, A., & Horner-Johnson, W. (2014). Disability status as an antecedent to chronic conditions: National health interview survey, 2006–2012. *Preventing Chronic Disease*, *11*, E15. http://dx.doi.org/10.5888/pcd11.130251.

Droste, D. W., & Keipes, M. (2013). The reduction of stroke risk, risk of myocardial infarction and death by healthy diet and physical activity. *Bulletin de la Société des Sciences Médicales du Grand-Duché de Luxembourg*, *2*, 51–62.

Easton, A. S. (2013). Neutrophils and stroke—Can neutrophils mitigate disease in the central nervous system? *International Immunopharmacology*, *17*(4), 1218–1225. http://dx.doi.org/10.1016/j.intimp.2013.06.015.

Endres, T., & Lessmann, V. (2012). Age-dependent deficits in fear learning in heterozygous BDNF knock-out mice. *Learning & Memory*, *19*(12), 561–570. http://dx.doi.org/10.1101/lm.028068.112.

Fedoroff, S., White, R., Neal, J., Subrahmanyan, L., & Kalnins, V. I. (1983). Astrocyte cell lineage. II. Mouse fibrous astrocytes and reactive astrocytes in cultures have vimentin- and GFP-containing intermediate filaments. *Brain Research*, *283*(2–3), 303–315.

Feldstein, C. A. (2013). Early treatment of hypertension in acute ischemic and intracerebral hemorrhagic stroke: Progress achieved, challenges, and perspectives. *Journal of the American Society of Hypertension*. http://dx.doi.org/10.1016/j.jash.2013.09.004.

Ferron, S. R., Marques-Torrejon, M. A., Mira, H., Flores, I., Taylor, K., Blasco, M. A., et al. (2009). Telomere shortening in neural stem cells disrupts neuronal differentiation and neuritogenesis. *The Journal of Neuroscience*, *29*(46), 14394–14407. http://dx.doi.org/10.1523/JNEUROSCI.3836-09.2009.

Finkel, T., & Holbrook, N. J. (2000). Oxidants, oxidative stress and the biology of ageing. *Nature*, *408*(6809), 239–247. http://dx.doi.org/10.1038/35041687.

Fisher, M., Loewy, R., Hardy, K., Schlosser, D., & Vinogradov, S. (2013). Cognitive interventions targeting brain plasticity in the prodromal and early phases of schizophrenia. *Annual Review of Clinical Psychology*, *9*, 435–463. http://dx.doi.org/10.1146/annurev-clinpsy-032511-143134.

Floyd, R. A., & Hensley, K. (2002). Oxidative stress in brain aging. Implications for therapeutics of neurodegenerative diseases. *Neurobiology of Aging*, *23*(5), 795–807, S0197458002000192 [pii].

Folsom, A. R., Yatsuya, H., Nettleton, J. A., Lutsey, P. L., Cushman, M., Rosamond, W. D., et al. (2011). Community prevalence of ideal cardiovascular health, by the American Heart Association definition, and relationship with cardiovascular disease incidence. *Journal of the American College of Cardiology*, *57*(16), 1690–1696. http://dx.doi.org/10.1016/j.jacc.2010.11.041.

Fonseca, A. C., Geraldes, R., Almeida, V., & Pinhoe Melo, T. (2011). Treatment with rtPA of stroke associated with intravenous immunoglobulins perfusion. *Journal of Neurological Science*, *308*(1–2), 180–181. http://dx.doi.org/10.1016/j.jns.2011.05.037.

Fortuno, A., San Jose, G., Moreno, M. U., Beloqui, O., Diez, J., & Zalba, G. (2006). Phagocytic NADPH oxidase overactivity underlies oxidative stress in metabolic syndrome. *Diabetes*, *55*(1), 209–215, 55/1/209 [pii].

Franceschi, C. (2007). Inflamm-aging as a major characteristic of old people: Can it be prevented or cured? *Nutrition Reviews*, *65*(12 Pt. 2), S173–S176.

Franceschi, C., Capri, M., Monti, D., Giunta, S., Olivieri, F., Sevini, F., et al. (2007). Inflamm-aging and anti-inflammaging: A systemic perspective on aging and longevity emerged from studies in humans. *Mechanisms of Ageing and Development*, *128*(1), 92–105. http://dx.doi.org/10.1016/j.mad.2006.11.016.

Gargalovic, P. S., Gharavi, N. M., Clark, M. J., Pagnon, J., Yang, W. P., He, A., et al. (2006). The unfolded protein response is an important regulator of inflammatory genes in endothelial cells. *Arteriosclerosis, Thrombosis, and Vascular Biology*, *26*(11), 2490–2496. http://dx.doi.org/10.1161/01.ATV.0000242903.41158.a1, 01.ATV.0000242903.41158.a1 [pii].

Ghezzi, A. C., Cambri, L. T., Botezelli, J. D., Ribeiro, C., Dalia, R. A., & de Mello, M. A. (2012). Metabolic syndrome markers in wistar rats of different ages. *Diabetology & Metabolic Syndrome*, *4*(1), 16. http://dx.doi.org/10.1186/1758-5996-4-16.

Giantin, V., Semplicini, A., Franchin, A., Simonato, M., Baccaglini, K., Attanasio, F., et al. (2011). Outcome after acute ischemic stroke (AIS) in older patients: Effects of age, neurological deficit severity and blood pressure (BP) variations. *Archives of Gerontology and Geriatrics*, *52*(3), e185–e191. http://dx.doi.org/10.1016/j.archger.2010.11.002.

Gibson, S. C., Le Page, P. A., & Taylor, C. J. (2013). Laparoscopic sleeve gastrectomy: Review of 500 cases in single surgeon Australian practice. *ANZ Journal of Surgery*. http://dx.doi.org/10.1111/ans.12483.

Glogowska-Ligus, J., Dabek, J., Zych-Twardowska, E., & Tkacz, M. (2013). Expression analysis of intercellular adhesion molecule-2 (ICAM-2) in the context of classical cardiovascular risk factors in acute coronary syndrome patients. *Archives of Medical Science*, *9*(6), 1035–1039. http://dx.doi.org/10.5114/aoms.2012.28808.

Golden, S. H., Hill-Briggs, F., Williams, K., Stolka, K., & Mayer, R. S. (2005). Management of diabetes during acute stroke and inpatient stroke rehabilitation. *Archives of Physical Medicine and Rehabilitation*, *86*(12), 2377–2384. http://dx.doi.org/10.1016/j.apmr.2005.07.306.

Gomes, V. A., Casella-Filho, A., Chagas, A. C., & Tanus-Santos, J. E. (2008). Enhanced concentrations of relevant markers of nitric oxide formation after exercise training in patients with metabolic syndrome. *Nitric Oxide*, *19*(4), 345–350. http://dx.doi.org/10.1016/j.niox.2008.08.005, S1089-8603(08)00365-0 [pii].

Graham, J. E., Ripsin, C. M., Deutsch, A., Kuo, Y. F., Markello, S., Granger, C. V., et al. (2009). Relationship between diabetes codes that affect medicare reimbursement (tier comorbidities) and outcomes in stroke rehabilitation. *Archives of Physical Medicine and Rehabilitation*, *90*(7), 1110–1116. http://dx.doi.org/10.1016/j.apmr.2009.01.014.

Guyton, K. Z., Gorospe, M., Wang, X., Mock, Y. D., Kokkonen, G. C., Liu, Y., et al. (1998). Age-related changes in activation of mitogen-activated protein kinase cascades by oxidative stress. *The Journal of Investigative Dermatology*, *3*(1), 23–27.

Guyton, K. Z., Liu, Y., Gorospe, M., Xu, Q., & Holbrook, N. J. (1996). Activation of mitogen-activated protein kinase by H2O2. Role in cell survival following oxidant injury. *The Journal of Biological Chemistry*, *271*(8), 4138–4142.

Haast, R. A., & Kiliaan, A. J. (2014). Impact of fatty acids on brain circulation, structure and function. *Prostaglandins, Leukotrienes, and Essential Fatty Acids*. http://dx.doi.org/10.1016/j.plefa.2014.01.002.

Hawkes, C. A., Michalski, D., Anders, R., Nissel, S., Grosche, J., Bechmann, I., et al. (2013). Stroke-induced opposite and age-dependent changes of vessel-associated markers in co-morbid transgenic mice with Alzheimer-like alterations. *Experimental Neurology*, *250*, 270–281. http://dx.doi.org/10.1016/j.expneurol.2013.09.020.

Hayashi, Y., & Nakanishi, H. (2013). Microglia and synaptic reorganization: Focus on the movement and functions of microglial processes. *Nihon Yakurigaku Zasshi*, *142*(5), 231–235.

Hefendehl, J. K., Neher, J. J., Suhs, R. B., Kohsaka, S., Skodras, A., & Jucker, M. (2014). Homeostatic and injury-induced microglia behavior in the aging brain. *Aging Cell*, *13*(1), 60–69. http://dx.doi.org/10.1111/acel.12149.

Heiss, C., Keymel, S., Niesler, U., Ziemann, J., Kelm, M., & Kalka, C. (2005). Impaired progenitor cell activity in age-related endothelial dysfunction. *Journal of the American College of Cardiology*, *45*(9), 1441–1448. http://dx.doi.org/10.1016/j.jacc.2004.12.074.

Hildrum, B., Mykletun, A., Hole, T., Midthjell, K., & Dahl, A. A. (2007). Age-specific prevalence of the metabolic syndrome defined by the international diabetes federation and the national cholesterol education program: The Norwegian HUNT 2 study. *BMC Public Health*, 7, 220. http://dx.doi.org/10.1186/1471-2458-7-220, 1471-2458-7-220 [pii].

Hisham, N. F., & Bayraktutan, U. (2013). Epidemiology, pathophysiology, and treatment of hypertension in ischaemic stroke patients. *Journal of Stroke and Cerebrovascular Diseases*, *22*(7), e4–e14. http://dx.doi.org/10.1016/j.jstrokecerebrovasdis.2012.05.001.

Hodge, A. M., Flicker, L., O'Dea, K., English, D. R., & Giles, G. G. (2013). Diabetes and ageing in the Melbourne collaborative cohort study (MCCS). *Diabetes Research and Clinical Practice*, *100*(3), 398–403. http://dx.doi.org/10.1016/j.diabres.2013.03.024.

Hof, P. R., Duan, H., Page, T. L., Einstein, M., Wicinski, B., He, Y., et al. (2002). Age-related changes in GluR2 and NMDAR1 glutamate receptor subunit protein immunoreactivity in corticocortically projecting neurons in macaque and patas monkeys. *Brain Research*, *928*(1–2), 175–186, S0006899301033455 [pii].

Holash, J. A., Noden, D. M., & Stewart, P. A. (1993). Re-evaluating the role of astrocytes in blood-brain barrier induction. *Developmental Dynamics*, *197*(1), 14–25. http://dx.doi.org/10.1002/aja.1001970103.

Holden, C. A., Collins, V. R., Handelsman, D. J., Jolley, D., Pitts, M., & Men in Australia Telephone Survey Working, Group. (2014). Healthy aging in a cross-sectional study of Australian men: What has sex got to do with it? *The Aging Male*. http://dx.doi.org/10.3109/13685538.2013.843167.

Hopp, S. C., Royer, S., Brothers, H. M., Kaercher, R. M., D'Angelo, H., Bardou, I., et al. (2014). Age-associated alterations in the time-dependent profile of pro- and anti-inflammatory proteins within the hippocampus in response to acute exposure to interleukin-1beta. *Journal of Neuroimmunology*, *267*(1–2), 86–91. http://dx.doi.org/10.1016/j.jneuroim.2013.12.010.

Hossmann, K. A. (2006). Pathophysiology and therapy of experimental stroke. *Cellular and Molecular Neurobiology*, *26*(7–8), 1057–1083. http://dx.doi.org/10.1007/s10571-006-9008-1.

Hossmann, K. A. (2009). Pathophysiological basis of translational stroke research. *Folia Neuropathologica*, *47*(3), 213–227, 13176 [pii].

Hotamisligil, G. S. (2010). Endoplasmic reticulum stress and the inflammatory basis of metabolic disease. *Cell*, *140*(6), 900–917. http://dx.doi.org/10.1016/j.cell.2010.02.034, S0092-8674(10)00187-X [pii].

Howard, V. J., Woolson, R. F., Egan, B. M., Nicholas, J. S., Adams, R. J., Howard, G., et al. (2010). Prevalence of hypertension by duration and age at exposure to the stroke belt. *Journal of the American Society of Hypertension*, *4*(1), 32–41. http://dx.doi.org/10.1016/j.jash.2010.02.001.

Hui, X., Matsushita, K., Sang, Y., Ballew, S. H., Fulop, T., & Coresh, J. (2013). CKD and cardiovascular disease in the atherosclerosis risk in communities (ARIC) study: Interactions with age, sex, and race. *American Journal of Kidney Diseases*, *62*(4), 691–702. http://dx.doi.org/10.1053/j.ajkd.2013.04.010.

Huizinga, R., van der Star, B. J., Kipp, M., Jong, R., Gerritsen, W., Clarner, T., et al. (2012). Phagocytosis of neuronal debris by microglia is associated with neuronal damage in multiple sclerosis. *Glia*, *60*(3), 422–431. http://dx.doi.org/10.1002/glia.22276.

Joseph, J., Koka, M., & Aronow, W. S. (2008). Prevalence of moderate and severe renal insufficiency in older persons with hypertension, diabetes mellitus, coronary artery disease, peripheral arterial disease, ischemic stroke, or congestive heart failure in an academic nursing home. *Journal of the American Medical Directors Association*, *9*(4), 257–259. http://dx.doi.org/10.1016/j.jamda.2008.01.002.

Kaffashian, S., Dugravot, A., Brunner, E. J., Sabia, S., Ankri, J., Kivimaki, M., et al. (2013). Midlife stroke risk and cognitive decline: A 10-year follow-up of the Whitehall II cohort study. *Alzheimers Dement*, *9*(5), 572–579. http://dx.doi.org/10.1016/j.jalz.2012.07.001.

Kastorini, C. M., Georgousopoulou, E., Vemmos, K. N., Nikolaou, V., Kantas, D., Milionis, H. J., et al. (2013). Comparative analysis of cardiovascular disease risk factors influencing nonfatal acute coronary syndrome and ischemic stroke. *The American Journal of Cardiology*, *112*(3), 349–354. http://dx.doi.org/10.1016/j.amjcard.2013.03.039.

Kim, O. J., Hong, S. H., Jeon, Y. J., Oh, S. H., Kim, H. S., Park, Y. S., et al. (2013). Gene-environment interactions between methylenetetrahydrofolate reductase (MTHFR) 677C>T and metabolic syndrome for the prevalence of ischemic stroke in Koreans. *Neuroscience Letters*, *533*, 11–16. http://dx.doi.org/10.1016/j.neulet.2012.11.031.

Kim, M. S., Kim, D. S., Kim, H. S., Kang, S. W., & Kang, Y. H. (2012). Inhibitory effects of luteolin on transendothelial migration of monocytes and formation of lipid-laden macrophages. *Nutrition*, *28*(10), 1044–1054. http://dx.doi.org/10.1016/j.nut.2011.12.003.

Kishida, K., Funahashi, T., & Shimomura, I. (2014). Adiponectin as a routine clinical biomarker. *Best Practice & Research. Clinical Endocrinology & Metabolism*, *28*(1), 119–130. http://dx.doi.org/10.1016/j.beem.2013.08.006.

Kral, M., Sanak, D., Veverka, T., Hutyra, M., Vindis, D., Kuncarova, A., et al. (2013). Troponin T in acute ischemic stroke. *The American Journal of Cardiology*, *112*(1), 117–121. http://dx.doi.org/10.1016/j.amjcard.2013.02.067.

Kristian, T., & Siesjo, B. K. (1998). Calcium in ischemic cell death. *Stroke*, *29*(3), 705–718.

Krouwer, V. J., Hekking, L. H., Langelaar-Makkinje, M., Regan-Klapisz, E., & Post, J. A. (2012). Endothelial cell senescence is associated with disrupted cell-cell junctions and increased monolayer permeability. *Vascular Cell*, *4*(1), 12. http://dx.doi.org/10.1186/2045-824X-4-12.

Kurl, S., Laukkanen, J. A., Niskanen, L., Laaksonen, D., Sivenius, J., Nyyssonen, K., et al. (2006). Metabolic syndrome and the risk of stroke in middle-aged men. *Stroke*, *37*(3), 806–811. http://dx.doi.org/10.1161/01.STR.0000204354.06965.44, 01.STR.0000204354.06965.44 [pii].

Lakatta, E. G. (2007). Central arterial aging and the epidemic of systolic hypertension and atherosclerosis. *Journal of the American Society of Hypertension*, *1*(5), 302–340. http://dx.doi.org/10.1016/j.jash.2007.05.001.

Laloux, P., Ossemann, M., & Jamart, J. (2007). Family history of hypertension is not an independent genetic factor predisposing to ischemic stroke subtypes. *Clinical Neurology and Neurosurgery*, *109*(3), 247–249. http://dx.doi.org/10.1016/j.clineuro.2006.09.005.

Le, R., & Esquenazi, S. (2002). Astrocytes mediate cerebral cortical neuronal axon and dendrite growth, in part, by release of fibroblast growth factor. *Neurological Research*, *24*(1), 81–92. http://dx.doi.org/10.1179/016164102101199459.

Lee, S. W., Clemenson, G. D., & Gage, F. H. (2012). New neurons in an aged brain. *Behavioural Brain Research*, *227*(2), 497–507. http://dx.doi.org/10.1016/j.bbr.2011.10.009.

Lee, J., Duan, W., Long, J. M., Ingram, D. K., & Mattson, M. P. (2000). Dietary restriction increases the number of newly generated neural cells, and induces BDNF expression, in the dentate gyrus of rats. *Journal of Molecular Neuroscience*, *15*(2), 99–108. http://dx.doi.org/10.1385/JMN:15:2:99.

Lee, J. T., Liu, H. L., Yang, J. T., Yang, S. T., Lin, J. R., & Lee, T. H. (2014). Longitudinal MR imaging study in the prediction of ischemic susceptibility after cerebral hypoperfusion in rats: Influence of aging and hypertension. *Neuroscience*, *257*, 31–40. http://dx.doi.org/10.1016/j.neuroscience.2013.10.066.

Li, J. F., Lai, D. D., Lin, Z. H., Jiang, T. Y., Zhang, A. M., & Dai, J. F. (2014). Comparison of the long-term results of roux-en-Y gastric bypass and sleeve gastrectomy for morbid obesity: A systematic review and meta-analysis of randomized and nonrandomized trials.

Surgical Laparoscopy, Endoscopy & Percutaneous Techniques, *24*(1), 1–11. http://dx.doi.org/10.1097/SLE.0000000000000041.

Lian, X. Y., & Stringer, J. L. (2004). Astrocytes contribute to regulation of extracellular calcium and potassium in the rat cerebral cortex during spreading depression. *Brain Research*, *1012*(1–2), 177–184. http://dx.doi.org/10.1016/j.brainres.2004.04.011.

Liddell, J. R., Robinson, S. R., Dringen, R., & Bishop, G. M. (2010). Astrocytes retain their antioxidant capacity into advanced old age. *Glia*, *58*(12), 1500–1509. http://dx.doi.org/10.1002/glia.21024.

Lim, S., Choi, H. J., Shin, H., Khang, A. R., Kang, S. M., Yoon, J. W., et al. (2012). Subclinical atherosclerosis in a community-based elderly cohort: The Korean longitudinal study on health and aging. *International Journal of Cardiology*, *155*(1), 126–133. http://dx.doi.org/10.1016/j.ijcard.2011.05.054.

Lima, A., Sardinha, V. M., Oliveira, A. F., Reis, M., Mota, C., Silva, M. A., et al. (2014). Astrocyte pathology in the prefrontal cortex impairs the cognitive function of rats. *Molecular Psychiatry*, *1*. http://dx.doi.org/10.1038/mp.2013.182.

Lin, T. Y., Lee, W. C., Soo, K. M., & Lin, H. L. (2011). Predictors of intracranial hemorrhage in patients taking anticoagulant and antiplatelet medication. *Journal of Trauma*, *70*(3), 764. http://dx.doi.org/10.1097/TA.0b013e318206cb18.

Liu, R., & Choi, J. (2000). Age-associated decline in gamma-glutamylcysteine synthetase gene expression in rats. *Free Radical Biology & Medicine*, *28*(4), 566–574.

Liu, K. P., Wong, D., Chung, A. C., Kwok, N., Lam, M. K., Yuen, C. M., et al. (2013). Effectiveness of a workplace training programme in improving social, communication and emotional skills for adults with autism and intellectual disability in Hong Kong—a pilot study. *Occupational Therapy International*, *20*(4), 198–204. http://dx.doi.org/10.1002/oti.1356.

Lo, E. H., Dalkara, T., & Moskowitz, M. A. (2003). Mechanisms, challenges and opportunities in stroke. *Nature Reviews. Neuroscience*, *4*(5), 399–415. http://dx.doi.org/10.1038/nrn1106, nrn1106 [pii].

Lucke-Wold, B. P., Turner, R. C., Lucke-Wold, A. N., Rosen, C. L., & Huber, J. D. (2012). Age and the metabolic syndrome as risk factors for ischemic stroke: Improving preclinical models of ischemic stroke. *The Yale Journal of Biology and Medicine*, *85*(4), 523–539.

Lue, L. F., Rydel, R., Brigham, E. F., Yang, L. B., Hampel, H., Murphy, G. M., Jr., et al. (2001). Inflammatory repertoire of Alzheimer's disease and nondemented elderly microglia in vitro. *Glia*, *35*(1), 72–79.

Malaguarnera, M., Vacante, M., Frazzetto, P. M., & Motta, M. (2012). The role of diabetes and aging in the determinism of hypertension and the related cerebrovascular complications. *Archives of Gerontology and Geriatrics*, *55*(2), 221–225. http://dx.doi.org/10.1016/j.archger.2011.08.008.

Manor, B. D., Hu, K., Peng, C. K., Lipsitz, L. A., & Novak, V. (2012). Posturo-respiratory synchronization: Effects of aging and stroke. *Gait & Posture*, *36*(2), 254–259. http://dx.doi.org/10.1016/j.gaitpost.2012.03.002.

Manwani, B., Liu, F., Scranton, V., Hammond, M. D., Sansing, L. H., & McCullough, L. D. (2013). Differential effects of aging and sex on stroke induced inflammation across the lifespan. *Experimental Neurology*, *249*, 120–131. http://dx.doi.org/10.1016/j.expneurol.2013.08.011.

Manwani, B., Liu, F., Xu, Y., Persky, R., Li, J., & McCullough, L. D. (2011). Functional recovery in aging mice after experimental stroke. *Brain, Behavior, and Immunity*, *25*(8), 1689–1700. http://dx.doi.org/10.1016/j.bbi.2011.06.015.

Martin-Calvo, N., Martinez-Gonzalez, M. A., Bes-Rastrollo, M., Gea, A., Ochoa, M. C., Marti, A., et al. (2014). Sugar-sweetened carbonated beverage consumption and

childhood/adolescent obesity: A case-control study. *Public Health Nutrition, 1–9*. http://dx.doi.org/10.1017/S136898001300356X.
Mattson, M. P. (2004). Pathways towards and away from Alzheimer's disease. *Nature, 430*(7000), 631–639. http://dx.doi.org/10.1038/nature02621, nature02621 [pii].
Mattson, M. P., & Magnus, T. (2006). Ageing and neuronal vulnerability. *Nature Reviews Neuroscience*, 7(4), 278–294. http://dx.doi.org/10.1038/nrn1886, nrn1886 [pii].
McEwen, B. J. (2014). The influence of diet and nutrients on platelet function. *Seminars in Thrombosis and Hemostasis*. http://dx.doi.org/10.1055/s-0034-1365839.
McMillian, M. K., Thai, L., Hong, J. S., O'Callaghan, J. P., & Pennypacker, K. R. (1994). Brain injury in a dish: A model for reactive gliosis. *Trends in Neurosciences, 17*(4), 138–142.
Miller, K. R., & Streit, W. J. (2007). The effects of aging, injury and disease on microglial function: A case for cellular senescence. *Neuron Glia Biology, 3*(3), 245–253. http://dx.doi.org/10.1017/S1740925X08000136.
Mooradian, A. D., Haas, M. J., & Chehade, J. M. (2003). Age-related changes in rat cerebral occludin and zonula occludens-1 (ZO-1). *Mechanisms of Ageing and Development, 124*(2), 143–146.
Moore, D. J., West, A. B., Dawson, V. L., & Dawson, T. M. (2005). Molecular pathophysiology of Parkinson's disease. *Annual Review of Neuroscience, 28*, 57–87. http://dx.doi.org/10.1146/annurev.neuro.28.061604.135718.
Morimoto, R. I. (2008). Proteotoxic stress and inducible chaperone networks in neurodegenerative disease and aging. *Genes & Development, 22*(11), 1427–1438. http://dx.doi.org/10.1101/gad.1657108.
Morley, J. E. (2014). Treatment of hypertension in older persons: What is the evidence? *Drugs & Aging, 31*(5), 331–337. http://dx.doi.org/10.1007/s40266-014-0171-7.
Munshi, A., Sharma, V., Kaul, S., Rajeshwar, K., Babu, M. S., Shafi, G., et al. (2010). Association of the -344C/T aldosterone synthase (CYP11B2) gene variant with hypertension and stroke. *Journal of the Neurological Sciences, 296*(1–2), 34–38. http://dx.doi.org/10.1016/j.jns.2010.06.013.
Murakami, Y., Huxley, R. R., Lam, T. H., Tsukinoki, R., Fang, X., Kim, H. C., et al. (2012). Diabetes, body mass index and the excess risk of coronary heart disease, ischemic and hemorrhagic stroke in the Asia pacific cohort studies collaboration. *Preventive Medicine, 54*(1), 38–41. http://dx.doi.org/10.1016/j.ypmed.2011.10.010.
Naidoo, N. (2009). ER and aging-protein folding and the ER stress response. *Ageing Research Reviews, 8*(3), 150–159. http://dx.doi.org/10.1016/j.arr.2009.03.001, S1568-1637(09)00017-8 [pii].
Napoli, I., & Neumann, H. (2009). Microglial clearance function in health and disease. *Neuroscience, 158*(3), 1030–1038. http://dx.doi.org/10.1016/j.neuroscience.2008.06.046.
Nguyen, M. T., Pham, I., Chemla, D., Valensi, P., & Cosson, E. (2013). Decreased stroke volume-brachial pulse pressure ratio in patients with type 2 diabetes over 50 years: The role of peripheral neuropathy. *Nutrition, Metabolism, and Cardiovascular Diseases, 23*(11), 1093–1100. http://dx.doi.org/10.1016/j.numecd.2013.01.008.
Ning, R., Chopp, M., Yan, T., Zacharek, A., Zhang, C., Roberts, C., et al. (2012). Tissue plasminogen activator treatment of stroke in type-1 diabetes rats. *Neuroscience, 222*, 326–332. http://dx.doi.org/10.1016/j.neuroscience.2012.07.018.
Ning, R., Chopp, M., Zacharek, A., Yan, T., Zhang, C., Roberts, C., et al. (2014). Neamine induces neuroprotection after acute ischemic stroke in type one diabetic rats. *Neuroscience, 257*, 76–85. http://dx.doi.org/10.1016/j.neuroscience.2013.10.071.
Niranjan, R. (2013). The role of inflammatory and oxidative stress mechanisms in the pathogenesis of Parkinson's disease: Focus on astrocytes. *Molecular Neurobiology*. http://dx.doi.org/10.1007/s12035-013-8483-x.
Njie, E. G., Boelen, E., Stassen, F. R., Steinbusch, H. W., Borchelt, D. R., & Streit, W. J. (2012). Ex vivo cultures of microglia from young and aged rodent brain reveal

age-related changes in microglial function. *Neurobiology of Aging*, *33*(1), 195.e1–195.e12. http://dx.doi.org/10.1016/j.neurobiolaging.2010.05.008.

O'Callaghan, J. P., & Sriram, K. (2005). Glial fibrillary acidic protein and related glial proteins as biomarkers of neurotoxicity. *Expert Opinion on Drug Safety*, *4*(3), 433–442. http://dx.doi.org/10.1517/14740338.4.3.433.

Ohsawa, K., & Kohsaka, S. (2011). Dynamic motility of microglia: Purinergic modulation of microglial movement in the normal and pathological brain. *Glia*, *59*(12), 1793–1799. http://dx.doi.org/10.1002/glia.21238.

Orlandi, A., Bochaton-Piallat, M. L., Gabbiani, G., & Spagnoli, L. G. (2006). Aging, smooth muscle cells and vascular pathobiology: Implications for atherosclerosis. *Atherosclerosis*, *188*(2), 221–230. http://dx.doi.org/10.1016/j.atherosclerosis.2006.01.018.

Ozcan, L., & Tabas, I. (2012). Role of endoplasmic reticulum stress in metabolic disease and other disorders. *Annual Review of Medicine*, *63*, 317–328. http://dx.doi.org/10.1146/annurev-med-043010-144749.

Papadopoulos, M. C., Koumenis, I. L., Yuan, T. Y., & Giffard, R. G. (1998). Increasing vulnerability of astrocytes to oxidative injury with age despite constant antioxidant defenses. *Neuroscience*, *82*(3), 915–925.

Patel, J. R., & Brewer, G. J. (2003). Age-related changes in neuronal glucose uptake in response to glutamate and beta-amyloid. *Journal of Neuroscience Research*, *72*(4), 527–536. http://dx.doi.org/10.1002/jnr.10602.

Penninger, J. M., Irie-Sasaki, J., Sasaki, T., & Oliveira-dos-Santos, A. J. (2001). CD45: New jobs for an old acquaintance. *Nature Immunology*, *2*(5), 389–396. http://dx.doi.org/10.1038/87687.

Perego, C., Fumagalli, S., & De Simoni, M. G. (2011). Temporal pattern of expression and colocalization of microglia/macrophage phenotype markers following brain ischemic injury in mice. *Journal of Neuroinflammation*, *8*, 174. http://dx.doi.org/10.1186/1742-2094-8-174.

Piccolo, R. S., Yang, M., Bliwise, D. L., Yaggi, H. K., & Araujo, A. B. (2013). Racial and socioeconomic disparities in sleep and chronic disease: Results of a longitudinal investigation. *Ethnicity & Disease*, *23*(4), 499–507.

Pontiroli, A. E., Alberto, M., Paganelli, M., Saibene, A., & Busetto, L. (2013). Metabolic syndrome, hypertension, and diabetes mellitus after gastric banding: The role of aging and of duration of obesity. *Surgery for Obesity and Related Diseases*, *9*(6), 894–900. http://dx.doi.org/10.1016/j.soard.2013.04.001.

Popa-Wagner, A., Carmichael, S. T., Kokaia, Z., Kessler, C., & Walker, L. C. (2007). The response of the aged brain to stroke: too much, too soon? *Current Neurovascular Research*, *4*(3), 216–227.

Popa-Wagner, A., Pirici, D., Petcu, E. B., Mogoanta, L., Buga, A. M., Rosen, C. L., et al. (2010). Pathophysiology of the vascular wall and its relevance for cerebrovascular disorders in aged rodents. *Current Neurovascular Research*, 7(3), 251–267.

Poteet, E., Winters, A., Yan, L. J., Shufelt, K., Green, K. N., Simpkins, J. W., et al. (2012). Neuroprotective actions of methylene blue and its derivatives. *PLoS One*, 7(10), e48279. http://dx.doi.org/10.1371/journal.pone.0048279.

Purkayastha, S., Zhang, H., Zhang, G., Ahmed, Z., Wang, Y., & Cai, D. (2011). Neural dysregulation of peripheral insulin action and blood pressure by brain endoplasmic reticulum stress. *Proceedings of the National Academy of Sciences of the United States of America*, *108*(7), 2939–2944. http://dx.doi.org/10.1073/pnas.1006875108, 1006875108 [pii].

Raes, G., De Baetselier, P., Noel, W., Beschin, A., Brombacher, F., & Hassanzadeh Gh, G. (2002). Differential expression of FIZZ1 and Ym1 in alternatively versus classically activated macrophages. *Journal of Leukocyte Biology*, *71*(4), 597–602.

Raes, G., Noel, W., Beschin, A., Brys, L., de Baetselier, P., & Hassanzadeh, G. H. (2002). FIZZ1 and Ym as tools to discriminate between differentially activated macrophages. *Developmental Immunology*, *9*(3), 151–159.

Ramirez, J. M., Ramirez, A. I., Salazar, J. J., de Hoz, R., & Trivino, A. (2001). Changes of astrocytes in retinal ageing and age-related macular degeneration. *Experimental Eye Research*, *73*(5), 601–615. http://dx.doi.org/10.1006/exer.2001.1061.

Reiner, A. P., Carty, C. L., Jenny, N. S., Nievergelt, C., Cushman, M., Stearns-Kurosawa, D. J., et al. (2008). PROC, PROCR and PROS1 polymorphisms, plasma anticoagulant phenotypes, and risk of cardiovascular disease and mortality in older adults: The Cardiovascular Health Study. *Journal of Thrombosis and Haemostasis*, *6*(10), 1625–1632. http://dx.doi.org/10.1111/j.1538-7836.2008.03118.x.

Richardson, A., & Holbrook, N. J. (1996). *Aging and the cellular response to stress: Reduction in the heat shock response* (1st ed.). New York, NY: Wiley-Liss.

Rietbrock, S., Heeley, E., Plumb, J., & van Staa, T. (2008). Chronic atrial fibrillation: Incidence, prevalence, and prediction of stroke using the congestive heart failure, hypertension, age >75, diabetes mellitus, and prior stroke or transient ischemic attack (CHADS2) risk stratification scheme. *American Heart Journal*, *156*(1), 57–64. http://dx.doi.org/10.1016/j.ahj.2008.03.010.

Rock, R. B., Gekker, G., Hu, S., Sheng, W. S., Cheeran, M., Lokensgard, J. R., et al. (2004). Role of microglia in central nervous system infections. *Clinical Microbiology Reviews*, *17*(4), 942–964. http://dx.doi.org/10.1128/CMR.17.4.942-964.2004 (table of contents).

Rodriguez, J. J., Jones, V. C., & Verkhratsky, A. (2009). Impaired cell proliferation in the subventricular zone in an Alzheimer's disease model. *Neuroreport*, *20*(10), 907–912. http://dx.doi.org/10.1097/WNR.0b013e32832be77d.

Rodriguez-Flores, M., Garcia-Garcia, E., Cano-Nigenda, C. V., & Cantu-Brito, C. (2014). Relationship of obesity and insulin resistance with the cerebrovascular reactivity: A case control study. *Cardiovascular Diabetology*, *13*(1), 2. http://dx.doi.org/10.1186/1475-2840-13-2.

Roriz-Filho, J. S., Sa-Roriz, T. M., Rosset, I., Camozzato, A. L., Santos, A. C., Chaves, M. L., et al. (2009). (Pre)diabetes, brain aging, and cognition. *Biochimica et Biophysica Acta*, *1792*(5), 432–443. http://dx.doi.org/10.1016/j.bbadis.2008.12.003.

Rosen, C. L., Dinapoli, V. A., Nagamine, T., & Crocco, T. (2005). Influence of age on stroke outcome following transient focal ischemia. *Journal of Neurosurgery*, *103*(4), 687–694. http://dx.doi.org/10.3171/jns.2005.103.4.0687.

Sacco, R. L., Benjamin, E. J., Broderick, J. P., Dyken, M., Easton, J. D., Feinberg, W. M., et al. (1997). American Heart Association Prevention Conference IV. Prevention and rehabilitation of stroke. Risk factors. *Stroke*, *28*(7), 1507–1517.

Saito, T., Shibasaki, K., Kurachi, M., Puentes, S., Mikuni, M., & Ishizaki, Y. (2011). Cerebral capillary endothelial cells are covered by the VEGF-expressing foot processes of astrocytes. *Neuroscience Letters*, *497*(2), 116–121. http://dx.doi.org/10.1016/j.neulet.2011.04.043.

Salminen, A., Ojala, J., Kaarniranta, K., Haapasalo, A., Hiltunen, M., & Soininen, H. (2011). Astrocytes in the aging brain express characteristics of senescence-associated secretory phenotype. *European Journal of Neuroscience*, *34*(1), 3–11. http://dx.doi.org/10.1111/j.1460-9568.2011.07738.x.

Samantha Sevilla, M., & Hubal, M. J. (2014). Genetic modifiers of obesity and bariatric surgery outcomes. *Seminars in Pediatric Surgery*, *23*(1), 43–48. http://dx.doi.org/10.1053/j.sempedsurg.2013.10.017.

Sandhir, R., & Berman, N. E. (2010). Age-dependent response of CCAAT/enhancer binding proteins following traumatic brain injury in mice. *Neurochemistry International*, *56*(1), 188–193. http://dx.doi.org/10.1016/j.neuint.2009.10.002, S0197-0186(09)00282-4 [pii].

Sandhu, S. K., & Kaur, G. (2002). Alterations in oxidative stress scavenger system in aging rat brain and lymphocytes. *Biogerontology*, *3*(3), 161–173.

Schousboe, A. (2003). Role of astrocytes in the maintenance and modulation of glutamatergic and GABAergic neurotransmission. *Neurochemical Research*, *28*(2), 347–352.

Schwedt, T. J. (2009). The migraine association with cardiac anomalies, cardiovascular disease, and stroke. *Neurologic Clinics*, *27*(2), 513–523. http://dx.doi.org/10.1016/j.ncl.2008.11.006.

Seimon, R. V., Espinoza, D., Ivers, L., Gebski, V., Finer, N., Legler, U. F., et al. (2014). Changes in body weight and blood pressure: Paradoxical outcome events in overweight and obese subjects with cardiovascular disease. *International Journal of Obesity*. http://dx.doi.org/10.1038/ijo.2014.2.

Shiber, J. R., Fontane, E., & Adewale, A. (2010). Stroke registry: Hemorrhagic vs ischemic strokes. *American Journal of Emergency Medicine*, *28*(3), 331–333. http://dx.doi.org/10.1016/j.ajem.2008.10.026.

Shiroto, T., Romero, N., Sugiyama, T., Sartoretto, J. L., Kalwa, H., Yan, Z., et al. (2014). Caveolin-1 is a critical determinant of autophagy, metabolic switching, and oxidative stress in vascular endothelium. *PLoS One*, *9*(2), e87871. http://dx.doi.org/10.1371/journal.pone.0087871.

Sieradzan, K. A., & Mann, D. M. (2001). The selective vulnerability of nerve cells in Huntington's disease. *Neuropathology and Applied Neurobiology*, *27*(1), 1–21, nan299 [pii].

Sierra, C., Coca, A., & Schiffrin, E. L. (2011). Vascular mechanisms in the pathogenesis of stroke. *Current Hypertension Reports*, *13*(3), 200–207. http://dx.doi.org/10.1007/s11906-011-0195-x.

Sites, C. K. (1998). Hormone replacement therapy: Cardiovascular benefits for aging women. *Coronary Artery Disease*, *9*(12), 789–793.

Soares, I., Abecasis, P., & Ferro, J. M. (2011). Outcome of first-ever acute ischemic stroke in the elderly. *Archives of Gerontology and Geriatrics*, *53*(2), e81–e87. http://dx.doi.org/10.1016/j.archger.2010.06.019.

Sohrabji, F., Bake, S., & Lewis, D. K. (2013). Age-related changes in brain support cells: Implications for stroke severity. *Neurochemistry International*, *63*(4), 291–301. http://dx.doi.org/10.1016/j.neuint.2013.06.013.

St Pie, M., St Pie, A., Wlaze, R. N., Paradowski, M., Banach, M., & Rysz, J. (2014). Obesity indices and inflammatory markers in obese non-diabetic normo- and hypertensive patients: A comparative pilot study. *Lipids in Health and Disease*, *13*(1), 29. http://dx.doi.org/10.1186/1476-511X-13-29.

Stankowski, J. N., & Gupta, R. (2011). Therapeutic targets for neuroprotection in acute ischemic stroke: Lost in translation? *Antioxidants & Redox Signaling*, *14*(10), 1841–1851. http://dx.doi.org/10.1089/ars.2010.3292.

Suzuki, T., Sakata, H., Kato, C., Connor, J. A., & Morita, M. (2012). Astrocyte activation and wound healing in intact-skull mouse after focal brain injury. *European Journal of Neuroscience*, *36*(12), 3653–3664. http://dx.doi.org/10.1111/j.1460-9568.2012.08280.x.

Takechi, R., Pallebage-Gamarallage, M. M., Lam, V., Giles, C., & Mamo, J. C. (2013). Aging-related changes in blood-brain barrier integrity and the effect of dietary fat. *Neuro-Degenerative Diseases*, *12*(3), 125–135. http://dx.doi.org/10.1159/000343211.

Tang, Z., Zhou, T., Luo, Y., Xie, C., Huo, D., Tao, L., et al. (2014). Risk factors for cerebrovascular disease mortality among the elderly in Beijing: A competing risk analysis. *PLoS One*, *9*(2), e87884. http://dx.doi.org/10.1371/journal.pone.0087884.

Taylor, D. L., Jones, F., Kubota, E. S., & Pocock, J. M. (2005). Stimulation of microglial metabotropic glutamate receptor mGlu2 triggers tumor necrosis factor alpha-induced neurotoxicity in concert with microglial-derived Fas ligand. *The Journal of Neuroscience*, *25*(11), 2952–2964. http://dx.doi.org/10.1523/JNEUROSCI.4456-04.2005.

Thurston, R. C., Rewak, M., & Kubzansky, L. D. (2013). An anxious heart: Anxiety and the onset of cardiovascular diseases. *Progress in Cardiovascular Diseases*, *55*(6), 524–537. http://dx.doi.org/10.1016/j.pcad.2013.03.007.

Toth, P., Tucsek, Z., Sosnowska, D., Gautam, T., Mitschelen, M., Tarantini, S., et al. (2013). Age-related autoregulatory dysfunction and cerebromicrovascular injury in mice with angiotensin II-induced hypertension. *Journal of Cerebral Blood Flow and Metabolism, 33*(11), 1732–1742. http://dx.doi.org/10.1038/jcbfm.2013.143.

Trotti, D., Danbolt, N. C., & Volterra, A. (1998). Glutamate transporters are oxidant-vulnerable: A molecular link between oxidative and excitotoxic neurodegeneration? *Trends in Pharmacological Sciences, 19*(8), 328–334.

Tsimikas, S., Willeit, P., Willeit, J., Santer, P., Mayr, M., Xu, Q., et al. (2012). Oxidation-specific biomarkers, prospective 15-year cardiovascular and stroke outcomes, and net reclassification of cardiovascular events. *Journal of the American College of Cardiology, 60*(21), 2218–2229. http://dx.doi.org/10.1016/j.jacc.2012.08.979.

Tucsek, Z., Toth, P., Sosnowska, D., Gautam, T., Mitschelen, M., Koller, A., et al. (2013). Obesity in aging exacerbates blood-brain barrier disruption, neuroinflammation, and oxidative stress in the mouse hippocampus: Effects on expression of genes involved in beta-amyloid generation and Alzheimer's disease. *The Journals of Gerontology. Series A, Biological Sciences and Medical Sciences.* http://dx.doi.org/10.1093/gerona/glt177, glt177 [pii].

Turner, R. C., Dodson, S. C., Rosen, C. L., & Huber, J. D. (2013). The science of cerebral ischemia and the quest for neuroprotection: Navigating past failure to future success. *Journal of Neurosurgery, 118*(5), 1072–1085. http://dx.doi.org/10.3171/2012.11.JNS12408.

Vaidya, A., & Williams, J. S. (2012). The relationship between vitamin D and the renin-angiotensin system in the pathophysiology of hypertension, kidney disease, and diabetes. *Metabolism, 61*(4), 450–458. http://dx.doi.org/10.1016/j.metabol.2011.09.007.

van Vliet-Ostaptchouk, J. V., Nuotio, M. L., Slagter, S. N., Doiron, D., Fischer, K., Foco, L., et al. (2014). The prevalence of metabolic syndrome and metabolically healthy obesity in Europe: A collaborative analysis of ten large cohort studies. *BMC Endocrine Disorders, 14*(1), 9. http://dx.doi.org/10.1186/1472-6823-14-9.

Walz, W. (2000). Role of astrocytes in the clearance of excess extracellular potassium. *Neurochemistry International, 36*(4–5), 291–300.

Wang, C. Y., Kim, H. H., Hiroi, Y., Sawada, N., Salomone, S., Benjamin, L. E., et al. (2009). Obesity increases vascular senescence and susceptibility to ischemic injury through chronic activation of Akt and mTOR. *Science Signaling, 2*(62), 11. http://dx.doi.org/10.1126/scisignal.2000143.

Warkentin, L. M., Majumdar, S. R., Johnson, J. A., Agborsangaya, C. B., Rueda-Clausen, C., Sharma, A. M., et al. (2014). Predictors of health-related quality of life in 500 severely obese patients: An assessment using three validated instruments. *Obesity (Silver Spring).* http://dx.doi.org/10.1002/oby.20694.

Westergaard, N., Sonnewald, U., & Schousboe, A. (1994). Release of alpha-ketoglutarate, malate and succinate from cultured astrocytes: Possible role in amino acid neurotransmitter homeostasis. *Neuroscience Letters, 176*(1), 105–109.

Wissing, K. M., & Pipeleers, L. (2013). Obesity, metabolic syndrome and diabetes mellitus after renal transplantation: Prevention and treatment. *Transplantation Reviews (Orlando, Fla).* http://dx.doi.org/10.1016/j.trre.2013.12.004.

Wu, Y., Zhang, A. Q., & Yew, D. T. (2005). Age related changes of various markers of astrocytes in senescence-accelerated mice hippocampus. *Neurochemistry International, 46*(7), 565–574. http://dx.doi.org/10.1016/j.neuint.2005.01.002.

Yamashiro, K., Tanaka, R., Tanaka, Y., Miyamoto, N., Shimada, Y., Ueno, Y., et al. (2014). Visceral fat accumulation is associated with cerebral small vessel disease. *European Journal of Neurology.* http://dx.doi.org/10.1111/ene.12374.

Yanez, N. D., Burke, G. L., Manolio, T., Gardin, J. M., & Polak, J. (2009). Sibling history of myocardial infarction or stroke and risk of cardiovascular disease in the elderly: The cardiovascular health study. *Annals of Epidemiology*, *19*(12), 858–866. http://dx.doi.org/10.1016/j.annepidem.2009.07.095, CHS Collaborative Research Group.

Ye, S. M., & Johnson, R. W. (1999). Increased interleukin-6 expression by microglia from brain of aged mice. *Journal of Neuroimmunology*, *93*(1–2), 139–148.

Yeo, L. L., Paliwal, P., Teoh, H. L., Seet, R. C., Chan, B. P., Wakerley, B., et al. (2013). Early and continuous neurologic improvements after intravenous thrombolysis are strong predictors of favorable long-term outcomes in acute ischemic stroke. *Journal of Stroke and Cerebrovascular Diseases*, *22*(8), e590–e596. http://dx.doi.org/10.1016/j.jstrokecerebrovasdis.2013.07.024.

Yoshii, H., Onuma, T., Yamazaki, T., Watada, H., Matsuhisa, M., Matsumoto, M., et al. (2014). Effects of pioglitazone on macrovascular events in patients with type 2 diabetes mellitus at high risk of stroke: The PROFIT-J study. *Journal of Atherosclerosis and Thrombosis*, *21*, 563–573.

Yu, S., Yang, S., Holsboer, F., Sousa, N., & Almeida, O. F. (2011). Glucocorticoid regulation of astrocytic fate and function. *PLoS One*, *6*(7), e22419. http://dx.doi.org/10.1371/journal.pone.0022419.

Zehendner, C. M., White, R., Hedrich, J., & Luhmann, H. J. (2014). A neurovascular blood-brain barrier in vitro model. *Methods in Molecular Biology*, *1135*, 403–413. http://dx.doi.org/10.1007/978-1-4939-0320-7_33.

Zhou, T., He, Q., Tong, Y., Zhan, R., Xu, F., Fan, D., et al. (2014). Phospholipid transfer protein (PLTP) deficiency impaired blood-brain barrier integrity by increasing cerebrovascular oxidative stress. *Biochemical and Biophysical Research Communications*, *445*(2), 352–356. http://dx.doi.org/10.1016/j.bbrc.2014.01.194.

Zhu, C., & Joyce, N. C. (2004). Proliferative response of corneal endothelial cells from young and older donors. *Investigative Ophthalmology & Visual Science*, *45*(6), 1743–1751.

CHAPTER FIFTEEN

Drug Abuse and the Neurovascular Unit

Richard D. Egleton*,[1], Thomas Abbruscato†,[1]
*Department of Pharmacology, Physiology and Toxicology, Joan C. Edwards School of Medicine, Marshall University, Huntington, West Virginia, USA
†Department of Pharmaceutical Sciences, School of Pharmacy, Texas Tech University Health Sciences Center, Amarillo, Texas, USA
[1]Corresponding author: e-mail address: egleton@marshall.edu; thomas.abbruscato@ttuhsc.edu

Contents

Abstract

Drug abuse continues to create a major international epidemic affecting society. A great majority of past drug abuse research has focused mostly on the mechanisms of addiction and the specific effects of substance use disorders on brain circuits and pathways that modulate reward, motivation, craving, and decision making. Few studies have focused on the neurobiology of acute and chronic substance abuse as it relates to the neurovascular unit (brain endothelial cell, neuron, astrocyte, microglia, and pericyte).

Advances in Pharmacology, Volume 71
ISSN 1054-3589
http://dx.doi.org/10.1016/bs.apha.2014.06.019

Increasing research indicates that all cellular components of the neurovascular unit play a pivotal role in both the process of addiction and how drug abuse affects the brain response to diseases. This review will focus on the specific effects of opioids, amphetamines, alcohol, and nicotine on the neurovascular unit and its role in addiction and adaption to brain diseases. Elucidation of the role of the neurovascular unit on the neurobiology associated with drug addiction will help to facilitate the development of better therapeutic approaches for drug-dependent individuals.

1. INTRODUCTION

Drug abuse has become a major international epidemic, with an estimated 6% of the World population (aged 15–64) using illicit drugs in 2011 resulting in a mortality rate of around 4.6 per 100,000 population globally (United Nations World Drug Report, 2013). Within the United States, this number is even higher with an estimated 8.9% of the population (12 and older) having used illicit drugs in 2010 (CDC), with a resultant death rate of almost 14 per 100,000. This is further complicated by the fact that an estimated 4.8% of adults in the United States are heavy drinkers and 18% use tobacco products (Centers for Disease Control and Prevention, 2013). Studies on the effects of substances of abuse have largely focused on their mechanisms of addiction and overdose and effects on either the respiratory or cardiovascular system. The few studies that have looked at the various cellular components of the neurovascular unit (NVU) do however indicate that the NVU can be significantly altered in the addiction process and could play a role in the risk for substance-induced neurological disorders.

2. MOLECULAR TARGETS OF COMMON SUBSTANCES OF ABUSE

There are a large number of substances that are abused within modern society. The drug of choice is generally based on several factors that include the agent (availability, cost, purity/potency, and route of administration), the host (age, genetics, metabolism, and psychiatric symptoms), and the environment (rural vs. urban, socioeconomic status, employment, and education). In this review, we will focus on some of the more commonly abused substances, including opioids, amphetamines, alcohol, and nicotine.

2.1. Opioids

Opioids are one of the major drugs abused and are responsible for the majority of drug-related poisoning deaths in the United States (Calcaterra, Glanz, & Binswanger, 2013). Endogenous opioids have been proposed to play an important role in regulating a range of processes including ion homeostasis during environmental stress, cell proliferation, inflammation, pain response, and addiction (Feng et al., 2012). Opioids, such as morphine and oxycodone, are used predominantly for the alleviation of pain, however, the role of opioid receptors in the regulation of dopamine within the nucleus accumbens make them highly addictive drugs. The majority of opioid actions are via four g-protein-coupled receptors the μ, δ, κ, and nociceptin receptors (Al-Hasani & Bruchas, 2011). Acutely following activation, opioid receptors induce inhibition of adenylyl cyclase and voltage-gated (P/Q and N-type) Ca^{2+} channels, in conjunction with an activation of inwardly rectifying K^{+} (Kir) channels. This results in presynaptic inhibition and postsynaptic hyperpolarization (Al-Hasani & Bruchas, 2011). Opioid receptor activation also leads to the activation of a number of signaling cascades which can have a significant effect on cellular function. This includes activation of various transcription factors including CREB, c-Fos, STAT-1, and JUN, thus cells that express opioid receptors can be significantly regulated during addiction. Recent studies indicate that some (McLaughlin & Zagon, 2012) opioids may also work via other nontraditional opioid receptors including the opioid growth factor receptor (OGFR) and potentially toll-like receptors (TLRs) (Hutchinson et al., 2010). Additionally, activation of other receptor systems, such as the peripheral sigma 1 receptor, may result in potentiation of opioid analgesia without significant increases in the unwanted opioid side effect of constipation (Sanchez-Fernandez et al., 2014).

2.2. Amphetamines

Amphetamine use continues to be a worldwide problem and widespread use continues to increase (United Nations, 2013). Amphetamines act via increasing the synaptic levels of monoamine neurotransmitters dopamine, norepinephrine, and serotonin (Panenka et al., 2013). This is accomplished by the systematic redistribution of neurotransmitters from vesicular storage, the reverse transport of transmitters into the synapse, inhibition of reuptake, and finally inhibition of monoamine oxidase (Panenka et al., 2013). This combination of neurotransmitter redistribution and enzymatic inhibition can lead to significant changes in neurotransmission both centrally and peripherally and have a profound effect on the cardiovasculature via activation of the sympathetic nervous system and the hypothalamic-pituitary-axis (Panenka et al., 2013). Users of methamphetamine experience a sense of euphoria, increased stimulation, productivity, hypersexuality, and decreased anxiety after acute intake, which lasts for several hours (Homer et al., 2008). Long-term use ultimately results in amphetamine dependence, memory problems, and overall cognitive dysfunction (Rendell, Mazur, & Henry, 2009).

2.3. Alcohol

Alcohol is probably the most used substance of abuse in the western world. A recent report based on a representative survey indicates that in the United States approximately 11% of 24 to 35-year-olds abuse alcohol (Haberstick et al., 2014). The acute effect of alcohol is via multiple mechanisms ranging from altering membrane dynamics to being an allosteric modulator of ligand-gated ion channels including $GABA_A$, nACh, and $5HT_3$ (Doyon, Thomas, Ostroumov, Dong, & Dani, 2013). K^+ channels have also been linked to alcohol's activity including an inward rectifying channel, Ca^{2+}-activated K^+ channels, and voltage-gated K^+ channels (Harris, 1999). At recreational doses of alcohol, the predominant targets are nACh and $GABA_A$ receptors, though other transport systems can be activated at nonfatal doses of ethanol (Harris, 1999). The metabolites of alcohol, acetylaldehyde and acetate, are toxic and can regulate cellular functions via multiple mechanisms including protein adduct formation, neurotransmitter adducts (including dopamine), mitochondrial dysfunction, and the production of reactive oxygen species (Manzo-Avalos & Saavedra-Molina, 2010). Chronically, these changes can result in organ dysfunction especially the liver leading to steatosis and eventually cirrhosis, which can have a significant impact on neurological function.

2.4. Tobacco (nicotine)

Cigarette smoke travels to the lungs on tar droplets (particulate matter) when inhaled. Nicotine is quickly absorbed in the lungs and on average 1 mg of nicotine is absorbed from one cigarette (Hukkanen, Jacob, & Benowitz, 2005). Upon absorption, nicotine follows the pulmonary venous circulation arriving to the left ventricle of the heart and continues along the arterial circulation ultimately reaching the brain within 10–20 s after each puff

(Hukkanen et al., 2005). Although many components of tobacco smoke are toxic, nicotine is the primary chemical component responsible for addiction and smoking behavior (Benowitz, 2008). Nicotine acts on nicotinic acetylcholine receptors (nAChRs) which are found throughout the body and the brain. nAChR are ligand-gated ion channels that are pentameric proteins of either homomeric or heteromeric subunits (Egleton, Brown, & Dasgupta, 2009). Activation of nAChRs ultimately causes brain release of dopamine and other neurotransmitter systems that facilitate addiction (Benowitz, 2008). Cytochrome P450 2A6 is primarily responsible for the oxidation of nicotine to cotinine in the liver (Hukkanen et al., 2005). The half-life of nicotine in the plasma averages ~2 h and cotinine ranges from 13 to 19 h. Cotinine is oftentimes utilized as a diagnostic test for the use of tobacco and/or nicotine products. Interestingly, considerable individual variability exists with regard to the ability to metabolize nicotine primarily by CYP2A6 and this can be determined by genetic, racial, and sex differences. Ultimately, slow metabolism appears to be correlated with a lower level of nicotine dependence (Malaiyandi, Sellers, & Tyndale, 2005).

Recent studies also indicate that nicotine can have a profound effect on angiogenesis via regulating VEGF and MMPs (Dom et al., 2011).

3. THE NEUROVASCULAR UNIT

In the last 20 years, it has become apparent that the blood brain barrier (BBB) is not the static barrier that it was once considered, with major regulatory input from both pericytes and astrocytes. Further in the last decade, the vital role of cells not previously considered to play a major role in barrier function including neurons and microglia has become an area of considerable research. This in combination with the apparent role of the BBB in neurological disorder progression has resulted in the concept of the NVU. The NVU concept takes into account the dynamic role of neurons, microglia, basement membrane, plasma, and cellular components of the blood in maintaining BBB phenotype and thus brain homeostasis (see Fig. 1). This leads to a complex cellular and paracrine interaction within the NVU that regulates barrier function and dysfunction (Hawkins & Davis, 2005). It is also likely, that the NVU will be different in each brain region as the neuronal input varies dependent on brain location. For example, several studies have investigated the innervation of blood vessels in the brain by serotonergic nerve fibers and have found a number of regional differences. In the frontal cortex, 10% of all serotonergic nerve terminals are associated with

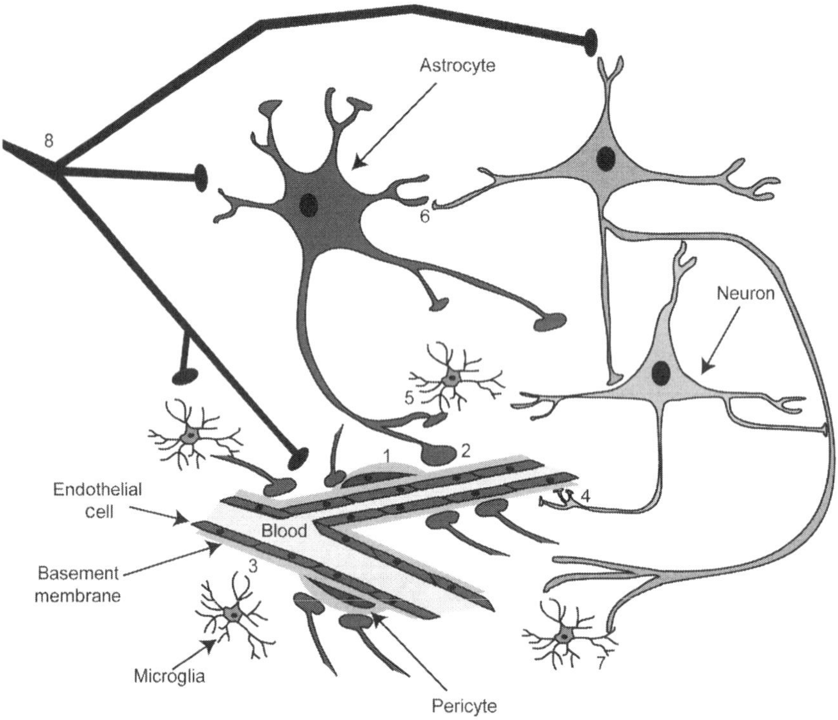

Figure 1 The cells and interactions of the neurovascular unit (NVU). The NVU composes of a complex interaction between the cells of the brain and the cells and components of the blood. The endothelial cells carry out the major barrier functions of the NVU and are regulated via interactions with the basement membrane, astrocytes, pericytes, microglia, and neurons. Further each of the other cellular components of the NVU can also interact and thus coordinate their regulation of barrier function. The interaction of the cells of the NVU can have a regional variation (see text for details) dependent on different receptor and neurotransmitter expression levels on the cellular components. The major interactions that can regulate localized NVU function include endothelial pericyte (1), endothelial astrocyte (2), endothelial microglia (3), endothelial-local neuron (4), astrocyte microglia (5), astrocyte-local neuron (6), microglia-local neuron (7). There is also considerable evidence for regulation of the NVU on a more global scale by several brain regions that have efferent connections throughout the brain (8). This includes the locus coeruleus and the raphe nuclei. The role of the above interactions (1–8) on regulating NVU function during substance abuse is outlined in the text.

microvessels compared to only 4% in the hippocampus. Furthermore, the serotonergic terminals are considerably closer to microvessels in the cortex compared to hippocampus (Cohen, Bonvento, Lacombe, & Hamel, 1996) thus the response to serotonin activation in these regions may vary and alter the BBB response accordingly. It is thus important to consider what the local environment for the NVU is when considering response to endogenous and exogenous stimuli, such as acute or chronic exposure to substances of abuse. With drugs of abuse, this concept is particularly vital as these substances target multiple cells and organs and thus can regulate barrier functions both directly and indirectly.

Not only is the local neurovascular niche important when you consider regulation of the NVU, but it is also essential to consider the effects of global and distant regulation of the NVU. Within the brain there are several key regions that project fibers to anatomically distant brain regions. Perhaps the most important when we consider potential NVU changes in drug abuse would be the locus coeruleus (LC). The LC has norepinephrine efferent fibers that link to most brain regions and has been related to the stress response to withdrawal associated with most drugs of abuse. In the cortex, norepinephrine synaptic boutons are found in close association with astrocytes and also with microvessels at sites of glial end-feet discontinuations (Paspalas & Papadopoulos, 1998). There have been several studies that indicate a role for the LC in direct regulation of endothelial function at the NVU. Acute electrical stimulation of the LC also induces increased mannitol (Pavlasek, Haburcak, Haburcakova, Orlicky, & Mikulajova, 1998) and sodium fluorescein (Sarmento, Borges, & Lima, 1994) permeability at the BBB. Chemical lesions of NE fibers in the LC-induced astrogliosis and loss of BBB tight junctions (Kalinin et al., 2006), indicating an important role for the LC in regulating the BBB.

4. TRANSPORT OF DRUGS OF ABUSE INTO THE BRAIN

Transport of drugs into the brain can occur via multiple pathways, including diffusion and carrier-mediated transport. Efflux transporters can also play a significant role in limiting drug delivery to the brain.

4.1. Opioids

Morphine has a relatively low uptake into the brain when given peripherally, early studies comparing *in situ* brain uptake with LogP values indicated that morphine entry into the brain was below what would be expected for its lipophilicity (Cornford, Braun, Oldendorf, & Hill, 1982), indicating that there was an acting efflux mechanism limiting morphine's uptake. Subsequent studies indicate that the ABC transporter MDR1 plays an important role in limiting brain uptake of morphine (Dagenais, Graff, & Pollack, 2004).

Several studies have shown that modulation of endothelial MDR1 alters the distribution of morphine to the brain. This can either during pathophysiological situations or via drug–drug interactions. Inflammatory pain results in a change in barrier function at the BBB, including increasing MDR1 expression and function resulting in reduced morphine brain uptake (Seelbach, Brooks, Egleton, & Davis, 2007) as does increased levels of brain VEGF (Hawkins, Sykes, & Miller, 2010). In contrast, the immunosuppressive agent cyclosporine A is also a MDR1 inhibitor which promotes morphine entry to the brain (Hawkins et al., 2010). Heroin, the diacetyl analog of morphine, in contrast has an uptake which is more than would be expected by lipophilicity-based diffusion (Cornford et al., 1982). Early studies that characterized the BBB penetration of morphine in comparison to heroin after carotid injection speculated that the rapid penetration of the BBB by heroin is a large contributor to the addictive properties of this drug (Oldendorf, Hyman, Braun, & Oldendorf, 1972). There also appears to be a higher uptake in neonatal animals compared to adult (Cornford et al., 1982). This suggests that maternal use of opioids may provide substantial neonatal exposure.

4.2. Amphetamines

Amphetamine uptake into the brain is via diffusion (Mosnaim, Callaghan, Hudzik, & Wolf, 2013). Its uptake distribution is relatively uniform throughout the brain (Mosnaim et al., 2013). Methamphetamine, the methylated analog, has a higher uptake into the brain than amphetamine based on its lipophilicity with approximately 10% of a dose delivered to the brain (Volkow et al., 2010).

4.3. Alcohol

Ethanol is lipophilic and its uptake correlates well with its lipophilicity, indicating that its transport is via diffusion (Cornford et al., 1982).

4.4. Nicotine

Nicotine uptake into the brain occurs via a saturable mechanism indicating the presence of a transporter-mediated uptake, at normal smoking levels of nicotine approximately 79% of transport was via a storable mechanism (Cisternino et al., 2013). Several studies have tried to identify the specific transporter, and though the specific transporter has not been identified, it is sensitive to pyrilamine (Tega, Akanuma, Kubo, Terasaki, & Hosoya,

2013), diphenhydramine (Cisternino et al., 2013), and coupled to H^+ ions (Cisternino et al., 2013). This putative transporter based on its kinetics is probably a low-affinity high-capacity transporter (Cisternino et al., 2013). Even with this putative transport mechanism for nicotine, a large portion of nicotine and the principle metabolite, cotinine, do enter into the brain by passive diffusion (Lockman et al., 2005). Interestingly, comparison of the brain influx data measured for the both nicotine and cotinine suggests that cotinine enters the brain at amounts approximately 40% of that compared to nicotine. These *in vivo* brain influx measurements were not affected by prior nicotine exposure for 28 days, suggesting that chronic nicotine exposed animals retain a restrictive BBB (Lockman et al., 2005).

5. REGULATION OF THE NVU BY DRUGS OF ABUSE

5.1. Opioids

There is evidence for opioid receptors expression by all of the cellular components of the NVU. Only a few studies have specifically shown expression of opioid receptors on brain endothelial cells including μ-opioid (OPRM1) (Wilbert-Lampen, Trapp, Barth, Plasse, & Leistner, 2007) and the nociception receptor (OPRL1) (Granata et al., 2003). There are however many functional studies that show brain endothelial cells are reactive to a host of opioids. Morphine treatment of endothelial cells leads to a range of functional changes; initially morphine leads to a rapid increase in intracellular Ca^{2+}, characteristic of opioid receptor activation (Mahajan, et al., 2008b). This is followed by changes in barrier function including reduced electrical resistance (Mahajan, et al., 2008b), coupled with reduced occludin and ZO-1 and increased JAM-2 (Mahajan, et al., 2008b; Wen, Lu, Yao, & Buch, 2011). These changes were in part due to opioid activation of ERK1/2- and JNK MAPK-activated pathways (Wen et al., 2011), and could be blocked by the nonspecific opioid receptor antagonist naltrexone (Wen et al., 2011). There is also evidence that morphine can regulate growth factor expression in brain endothelial cells, which may play a role in the reported change in function. During development, endogenous opioids play an important role in vascular development. Dynorphin and κ-opioid tone have been shown to be important factors in development of the vasculature and κ receptors are expressed in endothelial progenitor cells (Yamamizu et al., 2011), activation of κ receptors significantly reduces differentiation and vessel growth, so it is likely that morphine a mixed μ/κ agonist may also regulate vessel growth or repair.

Morphine treatment induces a significant increase in platelet-derived growth factor, which induces the reported changes in permeability and tight junction proteins (Wen et al., 2011). Morphine also significantly regulates the endothelial endothelin system by increasing levels of ET-1 and also one of its receptors ET-A (Van Woerkom et al., 2004). Interestingly naloxone, an opioid antagonist, downregulates ET-1 and ET-A and increases ET-B in the absence of morphine (Van Woerkom et al., 2004), indicating that in endothelial cells there is a basal activity of opioid receptor signaling. The endothelin system has been linked with morphine tolerance (Puppala, Matwyshyn, Bhalla, & Gulati, 2004) and this provides a novel mechanism that regulates brain entry of opioids. ET-1 application has been reported to lead to an initial reduction of MDR1 activity in brain microvessels followed by an increase in both the protein levels and activity resulting in increased efflux of MDR1 substrates (Bauer, Hartz, & Miller, 2007). Morphine does induce MDR1 expression in brain endothelial cells (Mahajan, et al., 2008b), possibly by the paracrine effect of endothelial-produced ET-1. Inflammation also seems to be an important regulator of this action as TNF-α shows a similar effect to ET-1 on MDR1 response (Bauer et al., 2007), in other studies acute morphine has been shown to potentiate the response of lipopolysaccharide (LPS) to brain endothelial permeability (Liu, Anday, House, & Chang, 2004). In contrast, peripheral morphine has been shown to inhibit LPS-induced endothelial responses indicating that opioids can regulate TLR activity; perhaps this differential response is due to differential receptor levels and types. LPS is not the only pathogen protein that regulates opioid activity. There have been several studies that show that HIV-1 proteins can interact with opioids to regulate endothelial cell function. Coadministration of morphine and HIV-1 TAT has an additive effect on barrier disruption *in vitro* (Mahajan, et al., 2008b).

Astrocytes express μ, κ, and δ-opioid receptors (Sargeant, Miller, & Day, 2008) as well as the OGFR (Campbell, Zagon, & McLaughlin, 2013) and opioid signaling has been clearly linked to astrocyte proliferation (Sargeant et al., 2008). Further there is good evidence for differential expression of opioid receptors on astrocytes based on both cell cycle and developmental stages (Stiene-Martin et al., 2001). Astrocytes become more sensitive to morphine inhibition of proliferation as they develop (Stiene-Martin et al., 2001). It is also important to understand that there is also a regional differential expression of opioid receptors based on mRNA profiles (Ruzicka et al., 1995). δ and κ receptors are expressed at a much higher level than μ in astrocytes isolated from all brain regions (Ruzicka et al., 1995). The highest levels of total opioid mRNA were found in cortex astrocytes, which also have the area of highest μ expression (Ruzicka et al., 1995). This may play a vital role in how astrocytes interact with endothelial cells during opioid exposure, potentially promoting a regional response. Opioids induce a number of responses in astrocytes. In spinal cord astrocytes, studies have shown that morphine can promote the production of sphingolipids, including sphingosine-1-phosphate (S1P) (Muscoli et al., 2010). S1P is a known regulator of brain endothelial cell function via the S1P receptor activation which reduces the activity of MDR1 (Cannon, Peart, Hawkins, Campos, & Miller, 2012). Chronic morphine, also promotes the expression of astrocytic tissue plasminogen activator (tPA) in astrocytes (Berta, Liu, Xu, & Ji, 2013). Endothelial tight junction disruption via tPA has been reported and has been linked to breakdown of occludin (Reijerkerk et al., 2008). Opioids can also regulate the release of cytokines from astrocytes including CCL5 (Avdoshina, Biggio, Palchik, Campbell, & Mocchetti, 2010) and the activity of cytokines on astrocytes including TNF-α (Akhter, Nix, Abdul, Singh, & Husain, 2013). In a study comparing morphine, fentanyl, and β-funaltrexamine on their ability to regulate TNF-induced CXCL10 release form astrocytes, it was shown that β-funaltrexamine a potent μ-antagonist and a κ agonist was considerably more effective than both morphine and fentanyl at reducing release (Davis, Buck, Saffarian, & Stevens, 2007). Perhaps, pointing again to the importance of κ-receptors in astrocytes, in contrast both morphine and fentanyl are potent μ agonists. Chemokines such as CCl5, TNF-α, and CXCl10 are important regulators of endothelial activation and immune cell diapedesis into the CNS (Biernacki, Prat, Blain, & Antel, 2004; Ubogu, Callahan, Tucky, & Ransohoff, 2006). TNF-α induces the release of MMP-2 from optic nerve astrocytes, which can be blocked via the δ-opioid agonist SNC-121 (Akhter et al., 2013). During opioid dependence and withdrawal, increased levels of MMP-9 in astrocytes of the dorsal horn have also been reported (Liu et al., 2010). MMPs have been linked to the progression of barrier disruption during stroke (Lenglet, Montecucco, & Mach, 2013) and are a vital components of barrier remodeling and angiogenesis, thus any change in there activity can have a significant effect on NVU function. Interestingly, several studies have used opioids as a treatment option for animal models of stroke. In one such study, biphalin a mixed μ/δ opioid agonist reduces stroke volume in the rat middle cerebral artery occlusion model by almost 60%, though this is linked to the $Na^+/K^+/2Cl^-$ cotransporter (Yang, Shah, Wang, Karamyan, & Abbruscato, 2011), it is possible that regulation of astrocytic MMP release may also be involved. Studies looking at more specific agonists showed similar responses when μ, δ, or κ-receptors where targeted (Yang, Wang, Shah, Karamyan, & Abbruscato, 2011), although the neuroprotective efficacy was greater using the mixed opioid receptor agonist, biphalin. Future studies are warranted to investigate the potential neuroprotective target of the opioid receptor system in the ischemic brain. It will be important to elucidate the both regional and cellular expression of opioid receptor types at the ischemic, NVU so that these therapeutic targets could potentially be activated for both neuroprotection and/or neurorestoration.

Pericytes are in close proximity to the endothelial cells and have been shown to be of importance for both development and maintenance of barrier function. There have been no studies that focus on opioid interaction with pericytes, however, there is likely to be at the very least an indirect regulation of barrier function due to the role of pericytes in brain inflammation and the interaction of opioids with the immune system (Hurtado-Alvarado, Cabanas-Morales, & Gomez-Gonzalez, 2014).

Microglia are the primary immune cell of the brain and are pharmacologically responsive to μ, δ, and κ-agonists. Morphine has been shown to both increase microglia migration (Horvath & DeLeo, 2009) and activation (Horvath, Romero-Sandoval, & De Leo, 2010) via a μ-receptor-mediated regulation of purinergic receptors (Horvath & DeLeo, 2009; Horvath et al., 2010). Morphine-induced activation leads to an enhanced immune response following LPS activation (Merighi et al., 2013). Autopsy studies also show a significant brain inflammation in heroin overdose patients (Neri et al., 2013). This opioid-induced increase in inflammation is believed to be due to microglia activation and an epigenetic programming of microglia response (Schwarz, Hutchinson, & Bilbo, 2011). Microglia activation and the associated release of MMPs and cytokines are a key factor in barrier dysfunction. Opioids are also known to regulate TLR function. Morphine regulation of TLR function in HIV models increases bacterial load in the brain via a combination of reduced clearance and increased bacterial load (Dutta et al., 2012). The increased levels of bacterial load are likely due to enhanced entry because of microglia proinflammatory responses promoting increased BBB opening (Dutta et al., 2012). Inhibition of microglia activation via drugs such as minocycline can prevent BBB dysfunction (Yenari, Xu, Tang, Qiao, & Giffard, 2006). Rat opioid-withdrawal models have shown that there is a proinflammatory stress response mediated by microglia that promotes neuronal damage (Campbell, Avdoshina, Rozzi, & Mocchetti,

2013). This coincides with the reported changes in BBB permeability due to withdrawal (Sharma, Sjoquist, & Ali, 2010) that can be ameliorated via antioxidant treatment (Sharma et al., 2010). This suggests that the proinflammatory microglia response following withdrawal from chronic opioids regulates barrier function, potentially via inflammation-induced increases in ROS.

Opioids can have a profound effect on neuronal function and development and are involved in regulating numerous functions including pain response, feeding and satiety, learning and memory, stress responses, and addiction (Bodnar, 2012). During opioid abuse, many of these function abnormally and can lead to significant changes in behavior. Further, during drug abuse there is a cycle of drug stimulation and acute withdrawal which can also have profound effects. The role of neuronal regulation of the BBB during opioid abuse has not been studied in much depth; however, several studies point to an important role of changes in neuronal signaling and barrier alterations. The LC expresses the three primary opioid receptors and their endogenous activation has been linked to stress responses (Benarroch, 2012). During withdrawal to opioids, there is an acute increase in norepinephrine release in areas innervated by LC following withdrawal, including the cortex (Devoto, Flore, Pira, Diana, & Gessa, 2002). Morphine withdrawal as stated above also leads to increased permeability of the BBB to Evans blue albumin and lanthanum (Sharma & Ali, 2006); the areas reported all have high LC innervation. It is thus likely that opioid-induced stimulation either during acute opioid use or during withdrawal may promote BBB changes via LC norepinephrine projections.

5.2. Amphetamines

Changes in catecholamine signaling are the hallmark of amphetamines. During amphetamine abuse, there is a dose-dependent increase in the levels off all catecholamines in the synapse as outlined above. Functionally in brain endothelial cells, activation of α-adrenergic receptors induces an increase in monolayer permeability, while β-adrenergic stimulation decreases permeability (Borges, Shi, Azevedo, & Audus, 1994). Subsequent studies both molecular and functional showed that microvessels have a variety of both α and β-adrenergic receptors. Brain endothelium also has functional dopamine receptors from the D1 and D2 families, with a differential expression dependent on vessel size, especially for the D1 subtype (large = small vessel > capillary) (Bacic, Uematsu, McCarron, & Spatz, 1991). Further, some of the molecular targets for amphetamines are present at the endothelial cells including both the serotonin- and norepinephrine-reuptake transporters, though not dopamine reuptake (Wakayama, Ohtsuki, Takanaga, Hosoya, & Terasaki, 2002). Thus, it is likely that amphetamines such as methamphetamine may have a significant effect on endothelial function at the BBB. Methamphetamine treatment leads to an induction of HSP72 in endothelial cells of the brain that was maintained for more than 24 h (Goto et al., 1993), indicating that methamphetamine stresses the endothelial cells. Further studies indicated that methamphetamine induces activation of redox-sensitive transcription factors AP-1 and NFκB in endothelial cells, resulting in increased expression of proinflammatory genes (Lee, Hennig, Yao, & Toborek, 2001). Methamphetamine endothelial oxidative stress induced a reduction in monolayer TEER, which could be ameliorated with antioxidant therapy (Zhang, Banerjee, Banks, & Ercal, 2009). The reduction in TEER is dose dependent and is a result of both reorganization and loss of tight junction proteins (Mahajan, et al., 2008a; Park, Kim, Lim, Wylegala, & Toborek, 2013; Ramirez et al., 2009). Interestingly, much like observed with opioids, there is a synergistic effect on tight junction loss with coincubation with HIV proteins (Mahajan, et al., 2008a). So how does methamphetamine induce oxidative stress in endothelial cells? Cerebral microvessel expresses a number of the enzymes responsible for monoamine synthesis and degradation, including tyrosine hydroxylase, dopa-decarboxylase, and monoamine oxidase (Hardebo, Emson, Falck, Owman, & Rosengren, 1980). Peripheral endothelial cells are capable of synthesizing and releasing catecholamines (Sorriento et al., 2012); thus, it is likely that brain endothelial cells can also do this. Metamphetamine-induced oxidative stress has been proposed to be in part via a buildup of extracellular dopamine that leads to an increase in dopamine quinone production and reactive oxygen species (Perfeito, Cunha-Oliveira, & Rego, 2013). This results in lipid peroxidation, mitochondrial dysfunction, and iNOS induction, all of which have been reported during brain endothelial treatment with methamphetamine (Lee et al., 2001; Martins et al., 2013; Ramirez et al., 2009; Zhang et al., 2009).

Astrocytes express adrenergic, dopaminergic, and serotonergic receptors (Hertz, Schousboe, Hertz, & Schousboe, 1984) and also the various targets for methamphetamine (Inazu, Takeda, & Matsumiya, 2003; Malynn, Campos-Torres, Moynagh, & Haase, 2013; Oliva, Fernandez, & Martin, 2013). Methamphetamine treatment of cultured astrocytes induces astrocyte activation and a differential oxidative stress depending on which brain regions astrocytes are isolated from (Lau, Senok, & Stadlin, 2000). Reactive astrocytes (Abbruscato, Lopez, Mark, Hawkins, & Davis, 2002), as noted with opioids, can produce a range of cytokines and factors that can regulate endothelial function. In astrocytes, dopamine has been reported to induce oxidative stress in astrocytes (Vaarmann, Gandhi, & Abramov, 2010), so it is likely that the mechanism is related to increased dopamine releases in the cultures.

Chronic methamphetamine leads to reactive microgliosis in human abusers (Sekine et al., 2008), indicating that it induces a long-lasting brain inflammation. This activation has been linked to methamphetamine increasing levels of dopamine and subsequently dopamine quinone increases. In microglia, dopamine quinones induce a significant change in gene expression especially in inflammatory genes (Kuhn, Francescutti-Verbeem, & Thomas, 2006). Chronic activation of microglia and the associated neuroinflammation is a common component of neurological disorders (Cunningham, 2013). As noted above in Section 5.1, many of the factors released by reactive microglia can regulate both basement membranes and endothelial function. Thus, this chronic inflammation may have a profound effect on endothelial function.

The primary effect of methamphetamine is the increase of catecholamines in the synapse of neurons. This can thus have a profound effect on synaptic transmission and neuronal function. The increase in neurotransmitters can as described for the other cell types induce reactive oxygen species and dopamine quinone production resulting in significant oxidative damage and neuronal death. Though much of this is via dopamine metabolism induced ROS, other mechanisms are also involved as significant oxidative stress is seen in both dopamine-rich and dopamine-poor brain regions (Horner, Gilbert, & Cline, 2011). Changes in synaptic neurotransmitters will not only supply the dopamine of quinone formation that can induce oxidative stress in neurons, it can also drive the oxidative damage of the other cells of the NVU, and it can also stimulate various receptor systems. The various components of the NVU express an array of catecholamine receptors that can regulate their function. One such system could be the LC norepinephrine system outlined in Section 5.1.

5.3. Alcohol

Chronic ethanol consumption can lead to considerable endothelial disruption. Chronic consumption leads to significant morphological changes including enlarged nuclei, increased mitochondria, and vesicles (Karwacka, 1980). There is also evidence of perivascular edema perhaps indicating tight junction disruption (Karwacka, 1980). *In vitro* treatment of endothelia cells with either ethanol or its metabolites, confirm the tight junction involvement. Ethanol induces a reorganization of tight junctions and a loss of both occludin and claudin-5 (Haorah et al., 2005), leading to a decrease in transmembrane electrical resistance. The ethanol-induced tight junction changes have been linked to endothelial metabolism of ethanol leading to reactive oxygen species production and subsequent activation of myosin-light chain kinase (Haorah et al., 2005). This change in myosin-light chain kinase is proposed to be via an IP3-mediated Ca^{2+} release (Haorah, Knipe, Gorantla, Zheng, & Persidsky, 2007). Ethanol can also regulate the activity of a number of ligand-gated ion channels GABA and nACh. At recreational doses where ethanol plasma levels are below 10 mM, $GABA_A$ and α7-nACh receptors are the primary targets. At more chronic and elevated doses, a whole host of channels may be affected (Crews, Morrow, Criswell, & Breese, 1996; Harris, 1999). To date, little is known about the regulation of these channels in brain endothelial cells, though several of them are known to be expressed at the BBB including the nACh α7 (Abbruscato et al., 2002; Hawkins, Egleton, & Davis, 2005), GABA (Gragera, Muniz, & Martinez-Rodriguez, 1993), and NMDA (Neuhaus et al., 2012); thus, it is likely that this may contribute to alcohol regulation of brain endothelial cells.

During chronic ethanol consumption, astrocytic end feet display a swollen morphology indicative of a response to brain edema (Karwacka, 1980). In astrocytes, ethanol exposure can regulate the expression and function of genes that promote the inflammatory response. Ethanol exposure leads to an activation of TLR4 in astrocytes that can promote neuroinflammation (Blanco, Valles, Pascual, & Guerri, 2005; Floreani et al., 2010). This response is regulated via ethanol metabolites (Floreani et al., 2010). Ethanol treatment leads to a rapid activation of NFκB- and AP-1-mediated activation of genes such as *NOS2* and *PTGS2* (Blanco et al., 2005). This indicates that ethanol, much like the other abusive agents discussed, can regulate astrocyte immune response, and thus alter the communication between astrocytes and endothelial cells. The role of ligand-gated and other ion channels in astrocytic response to ethanol has been less well characterized, however, as astrocytes express many of these proteins there is likely to be an effect. There is evidence for ethanol-regulated signaling via muscarinic receptor signaling in astrocytes. Muscarinic receptor activation in astrocytes induces proliferation; this response is inhibited via ethanol, potentially via an

NFκB-mediated pathway (Guizzetti et al., 2003). Electrophysiological studies show that ethanol regulates Ca^{2+}-insensitive K^{+} channels and also has a prolonged effect on astrocytic gap junctions (Adermark & Lovinger, 2006). Astrocytes can form gap junctions with endothelial cells, so does ethanol also effect this interaction? These gap junctions have been linked to NVU dysfunction during disease (Orellana et al., 2011), and thus could play a role in alcohol-induced NVU dysfunction.

Microglia have been implicated as a key regulator in CNS damage induced by ethanol and inhibition of microglia activation is protective against acute ethanol effects (Wu et al., 2011). Acutely ethanol induces a TLR4-mediated MYD88-independent microglia response (Fernandez-Lizarbe, Pascual, & Guerri, 2009). This leads to microglia activation and a release of TNF-α, IL-1β, and NO (Fernandez-Lizarbe et al., 2009), though the reported response was not as robust as classic TLR4 activators, conditioned media from ethanol-treated microglia can induce neuronal apoptosis(Fernandez-Lizarbe et al., 2009) and are thus likely able to regulate endothelial function as well.

Neuronal response to ethanol and thus its effect on the NVU is likely to be regional based on the relative expression of the receptors and channels that ethanol regulates and the relative doses of ethanol ingested. There have been reports of regional variations of GABA (Criswell, Ming, Kelm, & Breese, 2008) and NMDA (Randoll, Wilson, Weaver, Spuhler-Phillips, & Leslie, 1996) signaling induced by ethanol. Further, adolescent drinking in rats has been associated with altered neurotransmitter levels in adult animals. This can include a reduction of cholinergic-related gene expression (Coleman, He, Lee, Styner, & Crews, 2011), particularly in the basal forebrain. Chronic ethanol consumption in rats also leads to a reduction in LC neuron content (Lu et al., 1997) and can thus potentially have a profound effect on LC control of NVU function.

5.4. Nicotine

Nicotine, the major component of tobacco smoke can have a considerable effect both *in vitro* and *in vivo* on brain endothelial function. Brain endothelial cells express several nicotinic receptor subunits including the α3, α5 α7, β2, and β3 subunits (Abbruscato et al., 2002). Nicotine and/or cotinine (nicotine major metabolite) increased paracellular permeability of brain endothelial monolayers and also attenuated the expression of the tight junction protein Z0-1 (Abbruscato et al., 2002). Oxidative stress has been reported to promote the effects of nicotine on tight junction modulation (Hutamekalin et al., 2008). In animal models, a similar response is seen in permeability changes coupled to altered tight junction function (Hawkins et al., 2004). Both the *in vitro*- and *in vivo*-induced permeability changes could be prevented by treatment with specific α7 antagonists (Abbruscato et al., 2002; Hawkins et al., 2004, 2005). In hypoxia studies, nicotine promoted the observed tight junction changes (Abbruscato et al., 2002), indicating that this could play a role in smoking's promotion of stroke. Further, nicotine promoted bacterial entry in cellular models of bacterial meningitis (Chen et al., 2002) via a nicotinic receptor-mediated cytoskeletal rearrangement. Nicotinic receptors have also been implicated in regulating BBB ion transport in response to noxious insults such as stroke. During hypoxic models of stroke, there is an increase in the activity the BBB $Na^+/K^+/2Cl^-$ cotransporter (NKCC), presumably as a protective measure to reduce edema formation (Abbruscato, Lopez, Roder, & Paulson, 2004). Nicotine has been shown to inhibit the hypoxia-induced increased NKCC activity (Abbruscato et al., 2004) via a PKC-mediated phosphorylation pathway (Yang, Roder, Bhat, Thekkumkara, & Abbruscato, 2006). This regulation of NKCC during hypoxia was also seen when endothelial cells were treated with nicotine-containing smoke extract, but not with nicotine-free smoke extract (Paulson et al., 2006). *In vivo* studies treating rats with the smoke extracts indicate that similar changes in NKCC and its activity occur *in vivo* (Paulson et al., 2006). In animal models of focal stroke, such as the middle cerebral artery occlusion, nicotine exposure increased the infarct sizes and edema compared to control animals (Paulson et al., 2010). These results suggest that nAChRs modulate cellular functions outside synaptic transmission and could play a significant role in the nicotinic effects on the BBB during brain ischemia. Further studies have also shown that nicotine produces increases in both cytotoxic and vasogenic brain edema using both a hippocampal slice OGD model and an *in vivo* focal ischemia model to simulate brain ischemia (Paulson et al., 2010). Nicotine also regulates the expression of Notch-4 in brain endothelial cells (Manda, Mittapalli, Geldenhuys, & Lockman, 2010). Notch-4 has been linked to maintaining BBB phenotype, thus the reduced levels of Notch-4 induced by nicotine treatment are evidence for a reduced stability of the barrier (Manda et al., 2010). In a closely related system, the blood retinal barrier, nicotine exposure leads to an α7-mediated increase in angiogenesis (Dom et al., 2011). This is via an increase in the activity of MMP2 and MMP9 (Dom et al., 2011) and a promotion of early growth response gene-1 (Brown et al.,

2012). Interestingly, several studies have now also linked nicotinic stimulation of the α7 nicotine receptor with increased invasion of *Escherichia coli* in meningitis via a caveolin-1 raft recruitment (Chi, Wang, Zheng, Jong, & Huang, 2011).

Astrocytes express α3, α4, α5, α6, α7, β2, and β4 subunits (Gahring et al., 2004; Ono, Toyono, & Inenaga, 2008), though there is variation within brain region, specific region in astrocyte subpopulations and strain of mouse (Gahring et al., 2004; Ono et al., 2008), and also smoking status in humans. In chronic smokers, there is a downregulation of astrocytic α7 (Teaktong, Graham, Johnson, Court, & Perry, 2004). Astrocytic response to nicotine is also dependent on the local environment. Cortical astrocytes grown in monoculture are considerably less responsive to nicotine than those grown in co-culture with endothelial cells (Delbro, Westerlund, Bjorklund, & Hansson, 2009). Nicotine has been linked as a protective agent against both Parkinson's and Alzheimer's disease. This is potentially due to nicotine inhibition of astrocyte activation via an α7-mediated mechanism (Liu et al., 2012). In contrast, in already activated astrocytes, there is a reduced Ca^{2+} response to nicotine stimulation (Delbro et al., 2009).

Nicotine also regulates microglia activation. Preincubation of microglia with nicotine leads to a dose-dependent decrease in LPS-stimulated activation (Shytle et al., 2004) via an α7-mediated mechanism. Activation of α7 modulates the cell activation via PLC/IP3-mediated pathway and promotes a proneuroprotection response (Suzuki et al., 2006). Not only does α7 activation inhibit proinflammatory response but it also promotes the production of prostaglandin E2 (De Simone, Ajmone-Cat, Carnevale, & Minghetti, 2005), a suppressor of acute inflammatory mediators such as cytokines (Kalinski, 2012); perhaps, explaining why nicotine promotes HIV-1 levels in infected microglia (Rock et al., 2008).

The cholinergic system has connections throughout the brain, thus nicotine can have profound effect on neuronal activity and consequently neuronal regulation of the NVU. The LC again may be an important player in BBB regulation due to nicotine. The LC has two distinct populations of neurons that express nAChR (Lena et al., 1999). One group of neurons (type A) expresses predominantly α3 and β4 with a minor expression of α5 and β2, while the other group (type B) expresses α6, β2, and β3 (Lena et al., 1999). This expression difference leads to different electrophysiological properties (Lena et al., 1999). Based on morphological characteristics, the type A neurons have projections throughout the brain, while the type B largely connects with the hippocampus and cortex (Lena et al., 1999).

It is possible that this difference in nAChR distribution is responsible for the differential LC-activation response seen with low- and high-dose nicotine studies (Engberg & Hajos, 1994). Activation of the LC by nicotine induces an increased release of norepinephrine and also an induction of LC tyrosine hydroxylase, a key enzyme in norepinephrine synthesis (Matta, Valentine, & Sharp, 1997; Sun, Chen, Xu, Sterling, & Tank, 2004). Thus nicotine's ability to regulate the LC norepinephrine output may also play a role in regulating NVU function.

6. CONCLUSION

Substance abuse has long been characterized by activation of brain-reward circuitry located in the cortico-striatal-limbic brain regions and it is known that chronic use causes significant biochemical and structural abnormalities in addicted individuals. It has also been known for years that the BBB provides a central "gatekeeper" function regulating access into the brain of most drugs from the blood. This restrictive permeability prevents the greater majority of drugs ~98% from gaining CNS access. Although some lipid-soluble molecules, such as heroin, methamphetamine, alcohol, and nicotine, can gain brain entry, mostly by lipid-mediated diffusion, it is apparent that the rapid onset of action and BBB permeability of these drugs has a significant impact on the addiction liability of these agents. The known brain structural alterations of these molecules can have long-term effects on how the NVU functions both during normal brain physiology and pathogenic states related to neurodegenerative conditions, such as acute and chronic pain, stroke, Alzheimer's and Parkinson's disease, and HIV and bacterial infection. Future research will need to understand the cellular pathology of continued use of opioids, amphetamine, alcohol, and nicotine, specifically at the NVU, and not solely the effects of drugs of abuse on neuronal circuits. It is apparent that acute and chronic effects of illicit drug use reaches beyond these neuronal circuits and encompasses most all components of the NVU; brain endothelial cells, astrocytes, pericytes, and microglia. Receptor systems that are targeted by common drugs of abuse can also regulate important adaptive cellular process in the brain microenvironment, including proliferation, angiogenesis, and inflammation. Some biologic targets of drugs of abuse, nAChRs and opioid receptors, expressed in cells that comprise the NVU, might even provide useful therapeutic targets for a number of potential brain disorders. Future research will need to incorporate a neurovascular approach to understand the mechanisms of addiction and the long-term effects of activating these pathways on brain disease.

CONFLICT OF INTEREST

The authors have no conflicts.

REFERENCES

Abbruscato, T. J., Lopez, S. P., Mark, K. S., Hawkins, B. T., & Davis, T. P. (2002). Nicotine and cotinine modulate cerebral microvascular permeability and protein expression of ZO-1 through nicotinic acetylcholine receptors expressed on brain endothelial cells. *Journal of Pharmaceutical Sciences*, *91*(12), 2525–2538. http://dx.doi.org/10.1002/jps.10256.

Abbruscato, T. J., Lopez, S. P., Roder, K., & Paulson, J. R. (2004). Regulation of blood-brain barrier Na, K,2Cl-cotransporter through phosphorylation during in vitro stroke conditions and nicotine exposure. *Journal of Pharmacology and Experimental Therapeutics*, *310*(2), 459–468. http://dx.doi.org/10.1124/jpet.104.066274.

Adermark, L., & Lovinger, D. M. (2006). Ethanol effects on electrophysiological properties of astrocytes in striatal brain slices. *Neuropharmacology*, *51*(7–8), 1099–1108. http://dx.doi.org/10.1016/j.neuropharm.2006.05.035.

Akhter, N., Nix, M., Abdul, Y., Singh, S., & Husain, S. (2013). Delta-opioid receptors attenuate TNF-alpha-induced MMP-2 secretion from human ONH astrocytes. *Investigative Ophthalmology & Visual Science*, *54*(10), 6605–6611. http://dx.doi.org/10.1167/iovs.13-12196.

Al-Hasani, R., & Bruchas, M. R. (2011). Molecular mechanisms of opioid receptor-dependent signaling and behavior. *Anesthesiology*, *115*(6), 1363–1381. http://dx.doi.org/10.1097/ALN.0b013e318238bba6.

Avdoshina, V., Biggio, F., Palchik, G., Campbell, L. A., & Mocchetti, I. (2010). Morphine induces the release of CCL5 from astrocytes: Potential neuroprotective mechanism against the HIV protein gp120. *Glia*, *58*(13), 1630–1639. http://dx.doi.org/10.1002/glia.21035.

Bacic, F., Uematsu, S., McCarron, R. M., & Spatz, M. (1991). Dopaminergic receptors linked to adenylate cyclase in human cerebromicrovascular endothelium. *Journal of Neurochemistry*, *57*(5), 1774–1780.

Bauer, B., Hartz, A. M., & Miller, D. S. (2007). Tumor necrosis factor alpha and endothelin-1 increase P-glycoprotein expression and transport activity at the blood-brain barrier. *Molecular Pharmacology*, *71*(3), 667–675. http://dx.doi.org/10.1124/mol.106.029512.

Benarroch, E. E. (2012). Endogenous opioid systems: Current concepts and clinical correlations. *Neurology*, *79*(8), 807–814. http://dx.doi.org/10.1212/WNL.0b013e3182662098.

Benowitz, N. L. (2008). Neurobiology of nicotine addiction: Implications for smoking cessation treatment. *American Journal of Medicine*, *121*(4 Suppl 1), S3–S10. http://dx.doi.org/10.1016/j.amjmed.2008.01.015.

Berta, T., Liu, Y. C., Xu, Z. Z., & Ji, R. R. (2013). Tissue plasminogen activator contributes to morphine tolerance and induces mechanical allodynia via astrocytic IL-1beta and ERK signaling in the spinal cord of mice. *Neuroscience*, *247*, 376–385. http://dx.doi.org/10.1016/j.neuroscience.2013.05.018.

Biernacki, K., Prat, A., Blain, M., & Antel, J. P. (2004). Regulation of cellular and molecular trafficking across human brain endothelial cells by Th1- and Th2-polarized lymphocytes. *Journal of Neuropathology and Experimental Neurology*, *63*(3), 223–232.

Blanco, A. M., Valles, S. L., Pascual, M., & Guerri, C. (2005). Involvement of TLR4/type I IL-1 receptor signaling in the induction of inflammatory mediators and cell death induced by ethanol in cultured astrocytes. *Journal of Immunology, 175*(10), 6893–6899.

Bodnar, R. J. (2012). Endogenous opiates and behavior: 2011. *Peptides, 38*(2), 463–522. http://dx.doi.org/10.1016/j.peptides.2012.09.027.

Borges, N., Shi, F., Azevedo, I., & Audus, K. L. (1994). Changes in brain microvessel endothelial cell monolayer permeability induced by adrenergic drugs. *European Journal of Pharmacology, 269*(2), 243–248.

Brown, K. C., Lau, J. K., Dom, A. M., Witte, T. R., Luo, H., Crabtree, C. M., et al. (2012). MG624, an alpha7-nAChR antagonist, inhibits angiogenesis via the Egr-1/FGF2 pathway. *Angiogenesis, 15*(1), 99–114. http://dx.doi.org/10.1007/s10456-011-9246-9.

Calcaterra, S., Glanz, J., & Binswanger, I. A. (2013). National trends in pharmaceutical opioid related overdose deaths compared to other substance related overdose deaths: 1999–2009. *Drug and Alcohol Dependence, 131*(3), 263–270. http://dx.doi.org/10.1016/j.drugalcdep.2012.11.018.

Campbell, L. A., Avdoshina, V., Rozzi, S., & Mocchetti, I. (2013). CCL5 and cytokine expression in the rat brain: Differential modulation by chronic morphine and morphine withdrawal. *Brain, Behavior, and Immunity, 34*, 130–140. http://dx.doi.org/10.1016/j.bbi.2013.08.006.

Campbell, A. M., Zagon, I. S., & McLaughlin, P. J. (2013). Astrocyte proliferation is regulated by the OGF-OGFr axis in vitro and in experimental autoimmune encephalomyelitis. *Brain Research Bulletin, 90*, 43–51. http://dx.doi.org/10.1016/j.brainresbull.2012.09.001.

Cannon, R. E., Peart, J. C., Hawkins, B. T., Campos, C. R., & Miller, D. S. (2012). Targeting blood-brain barrier sphingolipid signaling reduces basal P-glycoprotein activity and improves drug delivery to the brain. *Proceedings of the National Academy of Sciences of the United States of America, 109*(39), 15930–15935. http://dx.doi.org/10.1073/pnas.1203534109.

Chen, Y. H., Chen, S. H., Jong, A., Zhou, Z. Y., Li, W., Suzuki, K., et al. (2002). Enhanced Escherichia coli invasion of human brain microvascular endothelial cells is associated with alternations in cytoskeleton induced by nicotine. *Cellular Microbiology, 4*(8), 503–514.

Chi, F., Wang, L., Zheng, X., Jong, A., & Huang, S. H. (2011). Recruitment of alpha7 nicotinic acetylcholine receptor to caveolin-1-enriched lipid rafts is required for nicotine-enhanced Escherichia coli K1 entry into brain endothelial cells. *Future Microbiology, 6*(8), 953–966. http://dx.doi.org/10.2217/FMB.11.65.

Cisternino, S., Chapy, H., Andre, P., Smirnova, M., Debray, M., & Scherrmann, J. M. (2013). Coexistence of passive and proton antiporter-mediated processes in nicotine transport at the mouse blood-brain barrier. *The AAPS Journal, 15*(2), 299–307. http://dx.doi.org/10.1208/s12248-012-9434-6.

Cohen, Z., Bonvento, G., Lacombe, P., & Hamel, E. (1996). Serotonin in the regulation of brain microcirculation. *Progress in Neurobiology, 50*(4), 335–362.

Coleman, L. G., Jr., He, J., Lee, J., Styner, M., & Crews, F. T. (2011). Adolescent binge drinking alters adult brain neurotransmitter gene expression, behavior, brain regional volumes, and neurochemistry in mice. *Alcoholism: Clinical and Experimental Research, 35*(4), 671–688. http://dx.doi.org/10.1111/j.1530-0277.2010.01385.x.

Cornford, E. M., Braun, L. D., Oldendorf, W. H., & Hill, M. A. (1982). Comparison of lipid-mediated blood-brain-barrier penetrability in neonates and adults. *American Journal of Physiology, 243*(3), C161–C168.

Crews, F. T., Morrow, A. L., Criswell, H., & Breese, G. (1996). Effects of ethanol on ion channels. *International Review of Neurobiology, 39*, 283–367.

Criswell, H. E., Ming, Z., Kelm, M. K., & Breese, G. R. (2008). Brain regional differences in the effect of ethanol on GABA release from presynaptic terminals. *Journal of Pharmacology and Experimental Therapeutics, 326*(2), 596–603. http://dx.doi.org/10.1124/jpet.107.135418.

Cunningham, C. (2013). Microglia and neurodegeneration: The role of systemic inflammation. *Glia, 61*(1), 71–90. http://dx.doi.org/10.1002/glia.22350.

Dagenais, C., Graff, C. L., & Pollack, G. M. (2004). Variable modulation of opioid brain uptake by P-glycoprotein in mice. *Biochemical Pharmacology, 67*(2), 269–276.

Davis, R. L., Buck, D. J., Saffarian, N., & Stevens, C. W. (2007). The opioid antagonist, beta-funaltrexamine, inhibits chemokine expression in human astroglial cells. *Journal of Neuroimmunology, 186*(1–2), 141–149. http://dx.doi.org/10.1016/j.jneuroim.2007.03.021.

De Simone, R., Ajmone-Cat, M. A., Carnevale, D., & Minghetti, L. (2005). Activation of alpha7 nicotinic acetylcholine receptor by nicotine selectively up-regulates cyclooxygenase-2 and prostaglandin E2 in rat microglial cultures. *Journal of Neuroinflammation, 2*(1), 4. http://dx.doi.org/10.1186/1742-2094-2-4.

Delbro, D., Westerlund, A., Bjorklund, U., & Hansson, E. (2009). In inflammatory reactive astrocytes co-cultured with brain endothelial cells nicotine-evoked Ca(2+) transients are attenuated due to interleukin-1beta release and rearrangement of actin filaments. *Neuroscience, 159*(2), 770–779. http://dx.doi.org/10.1016/j.neuroscience.2009.01.005.

Devoto, P., Flore, G., Pira, L., Diana, M., & Gessa, G. L. (2002). Co-release of noradrenaline and dopamine in the prefrontal cortex after acute morphine and during morphine withdrawal. *Psychopharmacology, 160*(2), 220–224. http://dx.doi.org/10.1007/s00213-001-0985-y.

Dom, A. M., Buckley, A. W., Brown, K. C., Egleton, R. D., Marcelo, A. J., Proper, N. A., et al. (2011). The alpha7-nicotinic acetylcholine receptor and MMP-2/-9 pathway mediate the proangiogenic effect of nicotine in human retinal endothelial cells. *Investigative Ophthalmology & Visual Science, 52*(7), 4428–4438. http://dx.doi.org/10.1167/iovs.10-5461.

Doyon, W. M., Thomas, A. M., Ostroumov, A., Dong, Y., & Dani, J. A. (2013). Potential substrates for nicotine and alcohol interactions: A focus on the mesocorticolimbic dopamine system. *Biochemical Pharmacology, 86*(8), 1181–1193. http://dx.doi.org/10.1016/j.bcp.2013.07.007.

Dutta, R., Krishnan, A., Meng, J., Das, S., Ma, J., Banerjee, S., et al. (2012). Morphine modulation of toll-like receptors in microglial cells potentiates neuropathogenesis in a HIV-1 model of coinfection with pneumococcal pneumoniae. *Journal of Neuroscience, 32*(29), 9917–9930. http://dx.doi.org/10.1523/JNEUROSCI.0870-12.2012.

Egleton, R. D., Brown, K. C., & Dasgupta, P. (2009). Angiogenic activity of nicotinic acetylcholine receptors: Implications in tobacco-related vascular diseases. *Pharmacology and Therapeutics, 121*(2), 205–223. http://dx.doi.org/10.1016/j.pharmthera.2008.10.007.

Engberg, G., & Hajos, M. (1994). Nicotine-induced activation of locus coeruleus neurons—An analysis of peripheral versus central induction. *Naunyn-Schmiedeberg's Archives of Pharmacology, 349*(5), 443–446.

Feng, Y., He, X., Yang, Y., Chao, D., Lazarus, L. H., & Xia, Y. (2012). Current research on opioid receptor function. *Current Drug Targets, 13*(2), 230–246.

Fernandez-Lizarbe, S., Pascual, M., & Guerri, C. (2009). Critical role of TLR4 response in the activation of microglia induced by ethanol. *Journal of Immunology, 183*(7), 4733–4744. http://dx.doi.org/10.4049/jimmunol.0803590.

Floreani, N. A., Rump, T. J., Abdul Muneer, P. M., Alikunju, S., Morsey, B. M., Brodie, M. R., et al. (2010). Alcohol-induced interactive phosphorylation of Src and toll-like receptor regulates the secretion of inflammatory mediators by human astrocytes.

Journal of Neuroimmune Pharmacology, *5*(4), 533–545. http://dx.doi.org/10.1007/s11481-010-9213-z.
Gahring, L. C., Persiyanov, K., Dunn, D., Weiss, R., Meyer, E. L., & Rogers, S. W. (2004). Mouse strain-specific nicotinic acetylcholine receptor expression by inhibitory interneurons and astrocytes in the dorsal hippocampus. *Journal of Comparative Neurology*, *468*(3), 334–346. http://dx.doi.org/10.1002/cne.10943.
Goto, S., Korematsu, K., Oyama, T., Yamada, K., Hamada, J., Inoue, N., et al. (1993). Neuronal induction of 72-kDa heat shock protein following methamphetamine-induced hyperthermia in the mouse hippocampus. *Brain Research*, *626*(1–2), 351–356.
Gragera, R. R., Muniz, E., & Martinez-Rodriguez, R. (1993). Electron microscopic immunolocalization of GABA and glutamic acid decarboxylase (GAD) in cerebellar capillaries and their microenvironment. *Cellular and Molecular Biology (Noisy-le-Grand, France)*, *39*(8), 809–817.
Granata, F., Potenza, R. L., Fiori, A., Strom, R., Caronti, B., Molinari, P., et al. (2003). Expression of OP4 (ORL1, NOP1) receptors in vascular endothelium. *European Journal of Pharmacology*, *482*(1–3), 17–23.
Guizzetti, M., Bordi, F., Dieguez-Acuna, F. J., Vitalone, A., Madia, F., Woods, J. S., et al. (2003). Nuclear factor kappaB activation by muscarinic receptors in astroglial cells: Effect of ethanol. *Neuroscience*, *120*(4), 941–950.
Haberstick, B. C., Young, S. E., Zeiger, J. S., Lessem, J. M., Hewitt, J. K., & Hopfer, C. J. (2014). Prevalence and correlates of alcohol and cannabis use disorders in the United States: Results from the national longitudinal study of adolescent health. *Drug and Alcohol Dependence*, *136*, 158–161. http://dx.doi.org/10.1016/j.drugalcdep.2013.11.022.
Haorah, J., Heilman, D., Knipe, B., Chrastil, J., Leibhart, J., Ghorpade, A., et al. (2005). Ethanol-induced activation of myosin light chain kinase leads to dysfunction of tight junctions and blood-brain barrier compromise. *Alcoholism: Clinical and Experimental Research*, *29*(6), 999–1009.
Haorah, J., Knipe, B., Gorantla, S., Zheng, J., & Persidsky, Y. (2007). Alcohol-induced blood-brain barrier dysfunction is mediated via inositol 1,4,5-triphosphate receptor (IP3R)-gated intracellular calcium release. *Journal of Neurochemistry*, *100*(2), 324–336. http://dx.doi.org/10.1111/j.1471-4159.2006.04245.x.
Hardebo, J. E., Emson, P. C., Falck, B., Owman, C., & Rosengren, E. (1980). Enzymes related to monoamine transmitter metabolism in brain microvessels. *Journal of Neurochemistry*, *35*(6), 1388–1393.
Harris, R. A. (1999). Ethanol actions on multiple ion channels: Which are important? *Alcoholism: Clinical and Experimental Research*, *23*(10), 1563–1570.
Hawkins, B. T., Abbruscato, T. J., Egleton, R. D., Brown, R. C., Huber, J. D., Campos, C. R., et al. (2004). Nicotine increases in vivo blood-brain barrier permeability and alters cerebral microvascular tight junction protein distribution. *Brain Research*, *1027*(1–2), 48–58. http://dx.doi.org/10.1016/j.brainres.2004.08.043.
Hawkins, B. T., & Davis, T. P. (2005). The blood-brain barrier/neurovascular unit in health and disease. *Pharmacological Reviews*, *57*(2), 173–185. http://dx.doi.org/10.1124/pr.57.2.4.
Hawkins, B. T., Egleton, R. D., & Davis, T. P. (2005). Modulation of cerebral microvascular permeability by endothelial nicotinic acetylcholine receptors. *American Journal of Physiology Heart and Circulatory Physiology*, *289*(1), H212–H219. http://dx.doi.org/10.1152/ajpheart.01210.2004.
Hawkins, B. T., Sykes, D. B., & Miller, D. S. (2010). Rapid, reversible modulation of blood-brain barrier P-glycoprotein transport activity by vascular endothelial growth factor. *Journal of Neuroscience*, *30*(4), 1417–1425. http://dx.doi.org/10.1523/JNEUROSCI.5103-09.2010.

Hertz, L., Schousboe, I., Hertz, L., & Schousboe, A. (1984). Receptor expression in primary cultures of neurons or astrocytes. *Progress in Neuropsychopharmacology and Biological Psychiatry*, *8*(4–6), 521–527.

Homer, B. D., Solomon, T. M., Moeller, R. W., Mascia, A., DeRaleau, L., & Halkitis, P. N. (2008). Methamphetamine abuse and impairment of social functioning: A review of the underlying neurophysiological causes and behavioral implications. *Psychological Bulletin*, *134*(2), 301–310. http://dx.doi.org/10.1037/0033-2909.134.2.301.

Horner, K. A., Gilbert, Y. E., & Cline, S. D. (2011). Widespread increases in malondialdehyde immunoreactivity in dopamine-rich and dopamine-poor regions of rat brain following multiple, high doses of methamphetamine. *Frontiers in Systems Neuroscience*, *5*, 27. http://dx.doi.org/10.3389/fnsys.2011.00027.

Horvath, R. J., & DeLeo, J. A. (2009). Morphine enhances microglial migration through modulation of P2X4 receptor signaling. *Journal of Neuroscience*, *29*(4), 998–1005. http://dx.doi.org/10.1523/JNEUROSCI.4595-08.2009.

Horvath, R. J., Romero-Sandoval, E. A., & De Leo, J. A. (2010). Inhibition of microglial P2X4 receptors attenuates morphine tolerance, Iba1, GFAP and mu opioid receptor protein expression while enhancing perivascular microglial ED2. *Pain*, *150*(3), 401–413. http://dx.doi.org/10.1016/j.pain.2010.02.042.

Hukkanen, J., Jacob, P., 3rd., & Benowitz, N. L. (2005). Metabolism and disposition kinetics of nicotine. *Pharmacological Reviews*, *57*(1), 79–115. http://dx.doi.org/10.1124/pr.57.1.3.

Hurtado-Alvarado, G., Cabanas-Morales, A. M., & Gomez-Gonzalez, B. (2014). Pericytes: Brain-immune interface modulators. *Frontiers in Integrative Neuroscience*, 7, 80. http://dx.doi.org/10.3389/fnint.2013.00080.

Hutamekalin, P., Farkas, A. E., Orbok, A., Wilhelm, I., Nagyoszi, P., Veszelka, S., et al. (2008). Effect of nicotine and polyaromtic hydrocarbons on cerebral endothelial cells. *Cell Biology International*, *32*(2), 198–209. http://dx.doi.org/10.1016/j.cellbi.2007.08.026.

Hutchinson, M. R., Zhang, Y., Shridhar, M., Evans, J. H., Buchanan, M. M., Zhao, T. X., et al. (2010). Evidence that opioids may have toll-like receptor 4 and MD-2 effects. *Brain, Behavior, and Immunity*, *24*(1), 83–95. http://dx.doi.org/10.1016/j.bbi.2009.08.004.

Inazu, M., Takeda, H., & Matsumiya, T. (2003). Functional expression of the norepinephrine transporter in cultured rat astrocytes. *Journal of Neurochemistry*, *84*(1), 136–144.

Kalinin, S., Feinstein, D. L., Xu, H. L., Huesa, G., Pelligrino, D. A., & Galea, E. (2006). Degeneration of noradrenergic fibres from the locus coeruleus causes tight-junction disorganisation in the rat brain. *European Journal of Neuroscience*, *24*(12), 3393–3400. http://dx.doi.org/10.1111/j.1460-9568.2006.05223.x.

Kalinski, P. (2012). Regulation of immune responses by prostaglandin E2. *Journal of Immunology*, *188*(1), 21–28. http://dx.doi.org/10.4049/jimmunol.1101029.

Karwacka, H. (1980). Ultrastructural and biochemical studies of the brain and other organs in rats after chronic ethanol administration. I. Electronmicroscopic investigations of the morphologic elements of the blood-brain barrier in the rat after ethanol intoxication. *Experimental Pathology (Jena)*, *18*(2), 118–126.

Kuhn, D. M., Francescutti-Verbeem, D. M., & Thomas, D. M. (2006). Dopamine quinones activate microglia and induce a neurotoxic gene expression profile: Relationship to methamphetamine-induced nerve ending damage. *Annals of the New York Academy of Sciences*, *1074*, 31–41. http://dx.doi.org/10.1196/annals.1369.003.

Lau, J. W., Senok, S., & Stadlin, A. (2000). Methamphetamine-induced oxidative stress in cultured mouse astrocytes. *Annals of the New York Academy of Sciences*, *914*, 146–156.

Lee, Y. W., Hennig, B., Yao, J., & Toborek, M. (2001). Methamphetamine induces AP-1 and NF-kappaB binding and transactivation in human brain endothelial cells. *Journal of Neuroscience Research, 66*(4), 583–591.

Lena, C., de Kerchove D'Exaerde, A., Cordero-Erausquin, M., Le Novere, N., del Mar Arroyo-Jimenez, M., & Changeux, J. P. (1999). Diversity and distribution of nicotinic acetylcholine receptors in the locus ceruleus neurons. *Proceedings of the National Academy of Sciences of the United States of America, 96*(21), 12126–12131.

Lenglet, S., Montecucco, F., & Mach, F. (2013). Role of matrix metalloproteinases in animal models of ischemic stroke. *Current Vascular Pharmacology*. Epub ahead of print.

Liu, H. C., Anday, J. K., House, S. D., & Chang, S. L. (2004). Dual effects of morphine on permeability and apoptosis of vascular endothelial cells: Morphine potentiates lipopolysaccharide-induced permeability and apoptosis of vascular endothelial cells. *Journal of Neuroimmunology, 146*(1–2), 13–21.

Liu, W. T., Han, Y., Liu, Y. P., Song, A. A., Barnes, B., & Song, X. J. (2010). Spinal matrix metalloproteinase-9 contributes to physical dependence on morphine in mice. *Journal of Neuroscience, 30*(22), 7613–7623. http://dx.doi.org/10.1523/JNEUROSCI.1358-10.2010.

Liu, Y., Hu, J., Wu, J., Zhu, C., Hui, Y., Han, Y., et al. (2012). Alpha7 nicotinic acetylcholine receptor-mediated neuroprotection against dopaminergic neuron loss in an MPTP mouse model via inhibition of astrocyte activation. *Journal of Neuroinflammation, 9*, 98. http://dx.doi.org/10.1186/1742-2094-9-98.

Lockman, P. R., McAfee, G., Geldenhuys, W. J., Van der Schyf, C. J., Abbruscato, T. J., & Allen, D. D. (2005). Brain uptake kinetics of nicotine and cotinine after chronic nicotine exposure. *Journal of Pharmacology and Experimental Therapeutics, 314*(2), 636–642. http://dx.doi.org/10.1124/jpet.105.085381.

Lu, W., Jaatinen, P., Rintala, J., Sarviharju, M., Kiianmaa, K., & Hervonen, A. (1997). Effects of lifelong ethanol consumption on rat locus coeruleus. *Alcohol and Alcoholism, 32*(4), 463–470.

Mahajan, S. D., Aalinkeel, R., Sykes, D. E., Reynolds, J. L., Bindukumar, B., Adal, A., et al. (2008a). Methamphetamine alters blood brain barrier permeability via the modulation of tight junction expression: Implication for HIV-1 neuropathogenesis in the context of drug abuse. *Brain Research, 1203*, 133–148. http://dx.doi.org/10.1016/j.brainres.2008.01.093.

Mahajan, S. D., Aalinkeel, R., Sykes, D. E., Reynolds, J. L., Bindukumar, B., Fernandez, S. F., et al. (2008b). Tight junction regulation by morphine and HIV-1 tat modulates blood-brain barrier permeability. *Journal of Clinical Immunology, 28*(5), 528–541. http://dx.doi.org/10.1007/s10875-008-9208-1.

Malaiyandi, V., Sellers, E. M., & Tyndale, R. F. (2005). Implications of CYP2A6 genetic variation for smoking behaviors and nicotine dependence. *Clinical Pharmacology and Therapeutics*, 77(3), 145–158. http://dx.doi.org/10.1016/j.clpt.2004.10.011.

Malynn, S., Campos-Torres, A., Moynagh, P., & Haase, J. (2013). The pro-inflammatory cytokine TNF-alpha regulates the activity and expression of the serotonin transporter (SERT) in astrocytes. *Neurochemical Research, 38*(4), 694–704. http://dx.doi.org/10.1007/s11064-012-0967-y.

Manda, V. K., Mittapalli, R. K., Geldenhuys, W. J., & Lockman, P. R. (2010). Chronic exposure to nicotine and saquinavir decreases endothelial Notch-4 expression and disrupts blood-brain barrier integrity. *Journal of Neurochemistry, 115*(2), 515–525. http://dx.doi.org/10.1111/j.1471-4159.2010.06948.x.

Manzo-Avalos, S., & Saavedra-Molina, A. (2010). Cellular and mitochondrial effects of alcohol consumption. *International Journal of Environmental Research and Public Health*, 7(12), 4281–4304. http://dx.doi.org/10.3390/ijerph7124281.

Martins, T., Burgoyne, T., Kenny, B. A., Hudson, N., Futter, C. E., Ambrosio, A. F., et al. (2013). Methamphetamine-induced nitric oxide promotes vesicular transport in blood-brain barrier endothelial cells. *Neuropharmacology*, *65*, 74–82. http://dx.doi.org/10.1016/j.neuropharm.2012.08.021.

Matta, S. G., Valentine, J. D., & Sharp, B. M. (1997). Nicotine activates NPY and catecholaminergic neurons in brainstem regions involved in ACTH secretion. *Brain Research*, *759*(2), 259–269.

McLaughlin, P. J., & Zagon, I. S. (2012). The opioid growth factor-opioid growth factor receptor axis: Homeostatic regulator of cell proliferation and its implications for health and disease. *Biochemical Pharmacology*, *84*(6), 746–755. http://dx.doi.org/10.1016/j.bcp.2012.05.018.

Merighi, S., Gessi, S., Varani, K., Fazzi, D., Stefanelli, A., & Borea, P. A. (2013). Morphine mediates a proinflammatory phenotype via mu-opioid receptor-PKCvarepsilon-Akt-ERK1/2 signaling pathway in activated microglial cells. *Biochemical Pharmacology*, *86*(4), 487–496. http://dx.doi.org/10.1016/j.bcp.2013.05.027.

Mosnaim, A. D., Callaghan, O. H., Hudzik, T., & Wolf, M. E. (2013). Rat brain-uptake index for phenylethylamine and various monomethylated derivatives. *Neurochemical Research*, *38*(4), 842–846. http://dx.doi.org/10.1007/s11064-013-0988-1.

Muscoli, C., Doyle, T., Dagostino, C., Bryant, L., Chen, Z., Watkins, L. R., et al. (2010). Counter-regulation of opioid analgesia by glial-derived bioactive sphingolipids. *Journal of Neuroscience*, *30*(46), 15400–15408. http://dx.doi.org/10.1523/JNEUROSCI.2391-10.2010.

Neri, M., Panata, L., Bacci, M., Fiore, C., Riezzo, I., Turillazzi, E., et al. (2013). Cytokines, chaperones and neuroinflammatory responses in heroin-related death: What can we learn from different patterns of cellular expression? *International Journal of Molecular Sciences*, *14*(10), 19831–19845. http://dx.doi.org/10.3390/ijms141019831.

Neuhaus, W., Burek, M., Djuzenova, C. S., Thal, S. C., Koepsell, H., Roewer, N., et al. (2012). Addition of NMDA-receptor antagonist MK801 during oxygen/glucose deprivation moderately attenuates the upregulation of glucose uptake after subsequent reoxygenation in brain endothelial cells. *Neuroscience Letters*, *506*(1), 44–49. http://dx.doi.org/10.1016/j.neulet.2011.10.045.

Oldendorf, W. H., Hyman, S., Braun, L., & Oldendorf, S. Z. (1972). Blood-brain barrier: Penetration of morphine, codeine, heroin, and methadone after carotid injection. *Science*, *178*(4064), 984–986.

Oliva, I., Fernandez, M., & Martin, E. D. (2013). Dopamine release regulation by astrocytes during cerebral ischemia. *Neurobiology of Disease*, *58*, 231–241. http://dx.doi.org/10.1016/j.nbd.2013.06.007.

Ono, K., Toyono, T., & Inenaga, K. (2008). Nicotinic receptor subtypes in rat subfornical organ neurons and glial cells. *Neuroscience*, *154*(3), 994–1001. http://dx.doi.org/10.1016/j.neuroscience.2008.04.028.

Orellana, J. A., Figueroa, X. F., Sanchez, H. A., Contreras-Duarte, S., Velarde, V., & Saez, J. C. (2011). Hemichannels in the neurovascular unit and white matter under normal and inflamed conditions. *CNS & Neurological Disorders Drug Targets*, *10*(3), 404–414.

Panenka, W. J., Procyshyn, R. M., Lecomte, T., MacEwan, G. W., Flynn, S. W., Honer, W. G., et al. (2013). Methamphetamine use: A comprehensive review of molecular, preclinical and clinical findings. *Drug and Alcohol Dependence*, *129*(3), 167–179. http://dx.doi.org/10.1016/j.drugalcdep.2012.11.016.

Park, M., Kim, H. J., Lim, B., Wylegala, A., & Toborek, M. (2013). Methamphetamine-induced occludin endocytosis is mediated by the Arp2/3 complex-regulated actin rearrangement. *Journal of Biological Chemistry*, *288*(46), 33324–33334. http://dx.doi.org/10.1074/jbc.M113.483487.

Paspalas, C. D., & Papadopoulos, G. C. (1998). Ultrastructural evidence for combined action of noradrenaline and vasoactive intestinal polypeptide upon neurons, astrocytes, and blood vessels of the rat cerebral cortex. *Brain Research Bulletin*, *45*(3), 247–259.

Paulson, J. R., Roder, K. E., McAfee, G., Allen, D. D., Van der Schyf, C. J., & Abbruscato, T. J. (2006). Tobacco smoke chemicals attenuate brain-to-blood potassium transport mediated by the Na, K,2Cl-cotransporter during hypoxia-reoxygenation. *Journal of Pharmacology and Experimental Therapeutics*, *316*(1), 248–254. http://dx.doi.org/10.1124/jpet.105.090738.

Paulson, J. R., Yang, T., Selvaraj, P. K., Mdzinarishvili, A., Van der Schyf, C. J., Klein, J., et al. (2010). Nicotine exacerbates brain edema during in vitro and in vivo focal ischemic conditions. *Journal of Pharmacology and Experimental Therapeutics*, *332*(2), 371–379. http://dx.doi.org/10.1124/jpet.109.157776.

Pavlasek, J., Haburcak, M., Haburcakova, C., Orlicky, J., & Mikulajova, M. (1998). Mannitol derivate used as a marker for voltammetrically monitored transport across the blood-brain barrier under condition of locus coeruleus stimulation. *General Physiology and Biophysics*, *17*(4), 309–322.

Perfeito, R., Cunha-Oliveira, T., & Rego, A. C. (2013). Reprint of: Revisiting oxidative stress and mitochondrial dysfunction in the pathogenesis of Parkinson disease-resemblance to the effect of amphetamine drugs of abuse. *Free Radical Biology and Medicine*, *62*, 186–201. http://dx.doi.org/10.1016/j.freeradbiomed.2013.05.042.

Puppala, B. L., Matwyshyn, G., Bhalla, S., & Gulati, A. (2004). Role of endothelin in neonatal morphine tolerance. *Journal of Cardiovascular Pharmacology*, *44*(Suppl. 1), S383–S385.

Ramirez, S. H., Potula, R., Fan, S., Eidem, T., Papugani, A., Reichenbach, N., et al. (2009). Methamphetamine disrupts blood-brain barrier function by induction of oxidative stress in brain endothelial cells. *Journal of Cerebral Blood Flow and Metabolism*, *29*(12), 1933–1945. http://dx.doi.org/10.1038/jcbfm.2009.112.

Randoll, L. A., Wilson, W. R., Weaver, M. S., Spuhler-Phillips, K., & Leslie, S. W. (1996). N-methyl-D-aspartate-stimulated increases in intracellular calcium exhibit brain regional differences in sensitivity to inhibition by ethanol. *Alcoholism: Clinical and Experimental Research*, *20*(2), 197–200.

Reijerkerk, A., Kooij, G., van der Pol, S. M., Leyen, T., van Het Hof, B., Couraud, P. O., et al. (2008). Tissue-type plasminogen activator is a regulator of monocyte diapedesis through the brain endothelial barrier. *Journal of Immunology*, *181*(5), 3567–3574.

Rendell, P. G., Mazur, M., & Henry, J. D. (2009). Prospective memory impairment in former users of methamphetamine. *Psychopharmacology*, *203*(3), 609–616. http://dx.doi.org/10.1007/s00213-008-1408-0.

Rock, R. B., Gekker, G., Aravalli, R. N., Hu, S., Sheng, W. S., & Peterson, P. K. (2008). Potentiation of HIV-1 expression in microglial cells by nicotine: Involvement of transforming growth factor-beta 1. *Journal of Neuroimmune Pharmacology*, *3*(3), 143–149. http://dx.doi.org/10.1007/s11481-007-9098-7.

Ruzicka, B. B., Fox, C. A., Thompson, R. C., Meng, F., Watson, S. J., & Akil, H. (1995). Primary astroglial cultures derived from several rat brain regions differentially express mu, delta and kappa opioid receptor mRNA. *Brain Research Molecular Brain Research*, *34*(2), 209–220.

Sanchez-Fernandez, C., Montilla-Garcia, A., Gonzalez-Cano, R., Nieto, F. R., Romero, L., Artacho-Cordon, A., et al. (2014). Modulation of peripheral mu-opioid analgesia by sigma1 receptors. *Journal of Pharmacology and Experimental Therapeutics*, *348*(1), 32–45. http://dx.doi.org/10.1124/jpet.113.208272.

Sargeant, T. J., Miller, J. H., & Day, D. J. (2008). Opioidergic regulation of astroglial/neuronal proliferation: Where are we now? *Journal of Neurochemistry*, *107*(4), 883–897. http://dx.doi.org/10.1111/j.1471-4159.2008.05671.x.

Sarmento, A., Borges, N., & Lima, D. (1994). Influence of electrical stimulation of locus coeruleus on the rat blood-brain barrier permeability to sodium fluorescein. *Acta Neurochirurgica (Wien)*, *127*(3–4), 215–219.

Schwarz, J. M., Hutchinson, M. R., & Bilbo, S. D. (2011). Early-life experience decreases drug-induced reinstatement of morphine CPP in adulthood via microglial-specific epigenetic programming of anti-inflammatory IL-10 expression. *Journal of Neuroscience, 31*(49), 17835–17847. http://dx.doi.org/10.1523/JNEUROSCI.3297-11.2011.

Seelbach, M. J., Brooks, T. A., Egleton, R. D., & Davis, T. P. (2007). Peripheral inflammatory hyperalgesia modulates morphine delivery to the brain: A role for P-glycoprotein. *Journal of Neurochemistry, 102*(5), 1677–1690. http://dx.doi.org/10.1111/j.1471-4159.2007.04644.x.

Sekine, Y., Ouchi, Y., Sugihara, G., Takei, N., Yoshikawa, E., Nakamura, K., et al. (2008). Methamphetamine causes microglial activation in the brains of human abusers. *Journal of Neuroscience, 28*(22), 5756–5761. http://dx.doi.org/10.1523/JNEUROSCI.1179-08.2008.

Sharma, H. S., & Ali, S. F. (2006). Alterations in blood-brain barrier function by morphine and methamphetamine. *Annals of the New York Academy of Sciences, 1074*, 198–224. http://dx.doi.org/10.1196/annals.1369.020.

Sharma, H. S., Sjoquist, P. O., & Ali, S. F. (2010). Alterations in blood-brain barrier function and brain pathology by morphine in the rat. Neuroprotective effects of antioxidant H-290/51. *Acta Neurochirurgica Supplementum, 106*, 61–66. http://dx.doi.org/10.1007/978-3-211-98811-4_10.

Shytle, R. D., Mori, T., Townsend, K., Vendrame, M., Sun, N., Zeng, J., et al. (2004). Cholinergic modulation of microglial activation by alpha 7 nicotinic receptors. *Journal of Neurochemistry, 89*(2), 337–343. http://dx.doi.org/10.1046/j.1471-4159.2004.02347.x.

Sorriento, D., Santulli, G., Del Giudice, C., Anastasio, A., Trimarco, B., & Iaccarino, G. (2012). Endothelial cells are able to synthesize and release catecholamines both in vitro and in vivo. *Hypertension, 60*(1), 129–136. http://dx.doi.org/10.1161/HYPERTENSIONAHA.111.189605.

Stiene-Martin, A., Knapp, P. E., Martin, K., Gurwell, J. A., Ryan, S., Thornton, S. R., et al. (2001). Opioid system diversity in developing neurons, astroglia, and oligodendroglia in the subventricular zone and striatum: Impact on gliogenesis in vivo. *Glia, 36*(1), 78–88.

Sun, B., Chen, X., Xu, L., Sterling, C., & Tank, A. W. (2004). Chronic nicotine treatment leads to induction of tyrosine hydroxylase in locus ceruleus neurons: The role of transcriptional activation. *Molecular Pharmacology, 66*(4), 1011–1021. http://dx.doi.org/10.1124/mol.104.001974.

Suzuki, T., Hide, I., Matsubara, A., Hama, C., Harada, K., Miyano, K., et al. (2006). Microglial alpha7 nicotinic acetylcholine receptors drive a phospholipase C/IP3 pathway and modulate the cell activation toward a neuroprotective role. *Journal of Neuroscience Research, 83*(8), 1461–1470. http://dx.doi.org/10.1002/jnr.20850.

Teaktong, T., Graham, A. J., Johnson, M., Court, J. A., & Perry, E. K. (2004). Selective changes in nicotinic acetylcholine receptor subtypes related to tobacco smoking: an immunohistochemical study. *Neuropathology and Applied Neurobiology, 30*(3), 243–254. http://dx.doi.org/10.1046/j.0305-1846.2003.00528.x.

Tega, Y., Akanuma, S., Kubo, Y., Terasaki, T., & Hosoya, K. (2013). Blood-to-brain influx transport of nicotine at the rat blood-brain barrier: Involvement of a pyrilamine-sensitive organic cation transport process. *Neurochemistry International, 62*(2), 173–181. http://dx.doi.org/10.1016/j.neuint.2012.11.014.

Ubogu, E. E., Callahan, M. K., Tucky, B. H., & Ransohoff, R. M. (2006). Determinants of CCL5-driven mononuclear cell migration across the blood-brain barrier Implications for therapeutically modulating neuroinflammation. *Journal of Neuroimmunology, 179*(1–2), 132–144. http://dx.doi.org/10.1016/j.jneuroim.2006.06.004.

UNODC, World Drug Report 2013 (United Nations publication, Sales No. E.13.XI.6).

U.S. Department of Health and Human Services, Centers for Disease Control and Prevention, National Center for Health Statistics. (2013). *Health, United States, 2012: With special feature on emergency care.* MD: Hyattsville.

Vaarmann, A., Gandhi, S., & Abramov, A. Y. (2010). Dopamine induces Ca2 + signaling in astrocytes through reactive oxygen species generated by monoamine oxidase. *Journal of Biological Chemistry, 285*(32), 25018–25023. http://dx.doi.org/10.1074/jbc.M110.111450.
Van Woerkom, R., Beharry, K. D., Modanlou, H. D., Parker, J., Rajan, V., Akmal, Y., et al. (2004). Influence of morphine and naloxone on endothelin and its receptors in newborn piglet brain vascular endothelial cells: Clinical implications in neonatal care. *Pediatric Research, 55*(1), 147–151. http://dx.doi.org/10.1203/01.PDR.0000100756.32861.60.
Volkow, N. D., Fowler, J. S., Wang, G. J., Shumay, E., Telang, F., Thanos, P. K., et al. (2010). Distribution and pharmacokinetics of methamphetamine in the human body: Clinical implications. *PLoS One, 5*(12), e15269. http://dx.doi.org/10.1371/journal.pone.0015269.
Wakayama, K., Ohtsuki, S., Takanaga, H., Hosoya, K., & Terasaki, T. (2002). Localization of norepinephrine and serotonin transporter in mouse brain capillary endothelial cells. *Neuroscience Research, 44*(2), 173–180.
Wen, H., Lu, Y., Yao, H., & Buch, S. (2011). Morphine induces expression of platelet-derived growth factor in human brain microvascular endothelial cells: Implication for vascular permeability. *PLoS One, 6*(6), e21707. http://dx.doi.org/10.1371/journal.pone.0021707.
Wilbert-Lampen, U., Trapp, A., Barth, S., Plasse, A., & Leistner, D. (2007). Effects of beta-endorphin on endothelial/monocytic endothelin-1 and nitric oxide release mediated by mu1-opioid receptors: A potential link between stress and endothelial dysfunction? *Endothelium, 14*(2), 65–71. http://dx.doi.org/10.1080/10623320701346585.
Wu, Y., Lousberg, E. L., Moldenhauer, L. M., Hayball, J. D., Robertson, S. A., Coller, J. K., et al. (2011). Attenuation of microglial and IL-1 signaling protects mice from acute alcohol-induced sedation and/or motor impairment. *Brain, Behavior, and Immunity, 25*(Suppl. 1), S155–S164. http://dx.doi.org/10.1016/j.bbi.2011.01.012.
Yamamizu, K., Furuta, S., Katayama, S., Narita, M., Kuzumaki, N., Imai, S., et al. (2011). The kappa opioid system regulates endothelial cell differentiation and pathfinding in vascular development. *Blood, 118*(3), 775–785. http://dx.doi.org/10.1182/blood-2010-09-306001.
Yang, T., Roder, K. E., Bhat, G. J., Thekkumkara, T. J., & Abbruscato, T. J. (2006). Protein kinase C family members as a target for regulation of blood-brain barrier Na, K,2Cl-cotransporter during in vitro stroke conditions and nicotine exposure. *Pharmaceutical Research, 23*(2), 291–302. http://dx.doi.org/10.1007/s11095-005-9143-2.
Yang, L., Shah, K., Wang, H., Karamyan, V. T., & Abbruscato, T. J. (2011). Characterization of neuroprotective effects of biphalin, an opioid receptor agonist, in a model of focal brain ischemia. *Journal of Pharmacology and Experimental Therapeutics, 339*(2), 499–508. http://dx.doi.org/10.1124/jpet.111.184127.
Yang, L., Wang, H., Shah, K., Karamyan, V. T., & Abbruscato, T. J. (2011). Opioid receptor agonists reduce brain edema in stroke. *Brain Research, 1383*, 307–316. http://dx.doi.org/10.1016/j.brainres.2011.01.083.
Yenari, M. A., Xu, L., Tang, X. N., Qiao, Y., & Giffard, R. G. (2006). Microglia potentiate damage to blood-brain barrier constituents: Improvement by minocycline in vivo and in vitro. *Stroke, 37*(4), 1087–1093. http://dx.doi.org/10.1161/01.STR.0000206281.77178.ac.
Zhang, X., Banerjee, A., Banks, W. A., & Ercal, N. (2009). N-Acetylcysteine amide protects against methamphetamine-induced oxidative stress and neurotoxicity in immortalized human brain endothelial cells. *Brain Research, 1275*, 87–95. http://dx.doi.org/10.1016/j.brainres.2009.04.008.

INDEX

Note: Page numbers followed by "*f*" indicate figures and "*t*" indicate tables.

A

B

D

J

L

M

P

R

T

CPI Antony Rowe
Eastbourne, UK
November 12, 2014